ANXIETY DISORDERS

ANXIETY DISORD ERS

...spectives on ...eatment

MD, PhD

...dical Institute
...ioral Sciences
...cine

...ne, MD

...nd Affective Neuroscience

...lth

...Rothbaum, PhD, ABPP

...avioral Sciences
...ecovery Program
...sychopharmacology
...dicine

UNIVERSITY PRESS

OXFORD
UNIVERSITY PRESS

Oxford University Press is a department of the University of
Oxford. It furthers the University's objective of excellence in research,
scholarship, and education by publishing worldwide.

Oxford   New York
Auckland   Cape Town   Dar es Salaam   Hong Kong   Karachi
Kuala Lumpur   Madrid   Melbourne   Mexico City   Nairobi
New Delhi   Shanghai   Taipei   Toronto

With offices in
Argentina   Austria   Brazil   Chile   Czech Republic   France   Greece
Guatemala   Hungary   Italy   Japan   Poland   Portugal   Singapore
South Korea   Switzerland   Thailand   Turkey   Ukraine   Vietnam

Oxford is a registered trademark of Oxford University Press
in the UK and certain other countries.

Published in the United States of America by
Oxford University Press
198 Madison Avenue, New York, NY 10016

Library of Congress Cataloging-in-Publication Data
Cataloging-in-Publication data is on file at the Library of Congress
978–0–19–939512–5

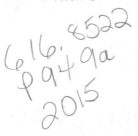
9 8 7 6 5 4 3 2 1
Printed in the United States of America
on acid-free paper

CONTENTS

FOREWORD: ANXIETY DISORDERS, BIG SCIENCE, AND BIG DATA: THE NEXT GENERATION OF SCIENCE AND PRACTICE

For some thirty-five years, the Anxiety and Depression Association of America (ADAA) provided inspiration to patients with anxiety disorders, the clinicians treating them, and clinical scientists committed to improving the knowledge base in this academic field. An interdisciplinary organization from its origins, the ADAA today brings together leaders from psychology, psychiatry, social work, epidemiology, and the neurosciences who are dedicated to mitigating the impact of anxiety and mood disorders on society. The interdisciplinary nature of this group, with its focus on these prevalent disorders, makes it unique among all professional organizations. The initiative represented in this volume is edited by members of our Board of Directors: Kerry J. Ressler of Emory University, Daniel S. Pine of the National Institute Mental Health, Barbara O. Rothbaum, and Alies Muskin, the Executive Director of the ADAA. Written by key clinical and scientific members of our professional community, the chapters in this text highlight recent new knowledge with important directions for the future. Critically, the volume crosses all levels of scientific analysis from the genetic to the molecular to the physiological substrates and on to treatment outcome research and to the newest level of analysis, termed implementation science.

Contributors were selected to participate in the completion of this volume based upon their clinical and research contributions to the field of anxiety disorders over many decades. Each is a recognized leader in the field, whether on the basis of their clinical expertise, research achievements, or their ability to educate new generations through teaching, writing, or supervision. All are outstanding members of the professional community, and all hail from a wide range of disciplines. The astute synthesis of information that is apparent in the chapters, coupled with the clear exposition of principles and concepts, suggests that the care by the Editors in selecting these particular contributors was well worth the effort. This text will have a lasting impact on the field of anxiety disorders if not even more broadly to the greater mental health field itself.

Why is now the time for an edited collection of work on the anxiety disorders? The answer is simply that scientific knowledge in these conditions has exploded in the past two decades, so much so that it is far beyond any single scholar to summarize and synthesize the literature in either clinical practice or clinical science. The era of a sole author writing across the many disorders of anxiety and across all levels of analysis is long gone. The scientific literature is too vast and the clinical knowledge is too broad for any single individual to master all of the details necessary to write a compelling tome on this topic.

This was true more than a decade ago when psychologist David Barlow (2002) edited rather than rewrote his tome on anxiety disorders when it was time for a second edition. The Editors, here, selected groups of contributors who are experts in the specific topic of importance in the field of anxiety disorders. We benefit from their contributions in terms of clinical updates, research reviews, and the forward thinking of outstanding professionals in the field.

Era of Big Science and Big Data. We are entering the period in health and clinical science when many of the easiest problems are solved but answers to the more complex chronic problems, as represented by psychiatric conditions, remain a formidable challenge. The mapping of the human genome, the development of mass spectroscopy, and the availability of increasingly powerful neuroimaging capacity give us opportunities to view molecular processes and neural circuitry in ways unimaginable a decade or more ago. Yet with these newer measurement capabilities come additional scientific and conceptual challenges for those engaged in the scientific process. The vast increases in computational power represent opportunities for the field to advance knowledge across multiple levels of scientific analyses. Even a decade ago, few places in the world could actually begin to manage the huge data bases drawn from different measurement tools in order to answer increasingly precise questions of mechanism and process. Today we possess this type of computational power. As a result, clinicians and scientists can pose very different types of questions and can expect answers in real time.

The questions in front of us are those reminiscent of the early aims of behavior therapy as stated by psychologist Gordon Paul, who famously articulated the objective of behavioral assessment as "finding . . . what treatment for which patient with what problem will work optimally under which conditions" (Paul, 1966). With the advent of big science and big data one can visualize a future where more precise treatments and more precise treatment targets are possible in the interest of maximizing patient outcomes. For example, might a blood test examining genetic expression, proteomics, amino acids, metabolomics, and psychophysiological parameters be matched with structural and functional neuroimaging to map out the optimal treatment for someone with obsessive compulsive disorder? Will the optimal treatment for an individual with posttraumatic stress disorder be exposure therapy or cognitive processing therapy, the former treatment demonstrably focused upon eliciting anxiety in order to promote recovery, while the latter treatment purports to challenge cognitive distortions when teaching alternative perspectives that are more rational? Perhaps the era of big data with its remarkable capabilities will permit real-time analyses of these complex factors and provide answers to these big clinical and scientific questions.

The era of big science in mental health is already upon us. Statistical modeling permits the projection of treatment effects, allowing us to determine the needed sample sizes for clinical trials. With increasing precision in measurement across domains (i.e., behavioral, cognitive, and physiological) comes the need for larger samples, which highlights the need for multisite clinical trials where patients and therapists are available to deliver care in order to answer desired scientific questions. More emphasis is now placed on head-to-head comparative effectiveness trials, where two or more active interventions are examined rather than comparing an active treatment to an attention placebo or a delayed treatment group. This approach demands large samples in virtually all cases, requiring data sharing across geographic regions within a single study. Efforts to ensure double-blind (and sometimes even triple-blind) studies require different teams at each site to conduct the evaluations and the treatments. When pharmacotherapy is involved, these designs require research pharmacies equipped with contemporary methods to ensure adequate dosing and distribution of the medication utilized. Studies involving both psychotherapy and psychopharmacology represent even higher levels of scientific precision and analysis owing to the need for including an examination of treatment fidelity, therapy compliance, adherence to medication, and proper assessment throughout the trial and its follow-up period. The approach needed to address all components of scientific trials of this size and scope constitutes big science. This is already the status of psychological and psychiatric science today.

Data analyses are also becoming necessarily more complex. With expanded computing capacity different questions are now possible. Which treatments are most successful for which phenotypes? Do psychological or pharmacological treatments change behavior, cognition, physiology? Are these changes visible using functional magnetic resonance imaging? Is it possible to change structural patterns with pharmacotherapy? Similarly, is it possible for psychotherapy to change the structure and function of the brain? With sufficient statistical power and adequate computational power, these questions and others become not only possible, they become the next generation of important scientific questions in the field of anxiety disorders.

Big science and big data are also permitting us to examine anxiety and its disorders in ways that have been possible only recently. Prior decades saw advances in the study of human emotions predominantly from a single perspective. Emphases often depended upon the theoretical model from which the scholar operated. Emotion could be studied as a set of expressive behaviors, as a cognitive process of perception and appraisal, or from a neurobiological perspective. Today, it is possible and indeed important to draw information in an integrative way from all three of these models of emotion when studying anxiety and its disorders. As behavioral, cognitive, and neurobiological measures become more complex, the need for large samples and big data processing become key to answering integrative questions. As this book suggests, there is no turning back from big science and big data. Chapter after chapter underscores the need for addressing the big scientific questions of our time with suitable models and methods in order to provide the best understanding of anxiety disorders and to ultimately deliver optimal treatments to patients across the world. The vision of a clinician in one corner of the world using biological and psychological analyses to devise the best approach to ameliorating one or another of the anxiety disorders is aspirational at this time, yet it is also inspirational. We can and must proceed down this road to understand the limits of our scientific methods and to improve the health of the populations for which we are responsible.

Preliminary Glimpses of the Future. Several recent studies offer a glimpse into what the future might hold in the era of big science and big data. Walkup, et al. (2008) in the *New England Journal of Medicine* reported on a multisite randomized control trial of sertraline (a selective serotonin reuptake inhibitor; SSRI), a cognitive behavioral treatment approach for childhood anxiety, and their combination. They studied nearly 500 children and adolescents with anxiety disorders. This innovative study found that combination therapy was substantially better than either of the monotherapies alone in mitigating anxiety and improving outcomes across measurement domains. Understanding that the combination of these therapies was strikingly better than either alone (and better than a placebo!) is a critically important advance for the entire field. Participating in this clinical trial were expert psychopharmacologists and expert cognitive behavior therapists, so the comparative therapy trial stands as a paragon of methodological rigor. As important a study as that of Walkup, et al. is, however, future studies will combine phenotypic, genotypic, and neuroimaging data and require substantially greater numbers of participants in order to determine which treatment is better for which participants with which anxiety disorders.

In a 2013 study published in *Molecular Psychiatry,* the Major Depressive Disorder Working Group of the Psychiatric Genome Wide Association Study (GWAS) Consortium conducted a mega-analysis for major depressive disorder (MDD) with the hope that increasing power would increase the likelihood of identifying genetic loci underpinning the disorder. Using nearly 20,000 total cases and non-cases in the test sample and over 50,000 in the cross-validation sample, these investigators were unable to stably identify robust and replicable findings for depression in these samples. Their interpretation of this inability to identify specific genetic loci associated with MDD centered on the complex trait that is depression and the need for even larger samples to find stable genetic factors related to MDD. Is this the case, or do we need more precise measures of the products of the genome in order to delve into the contributions of genes to the onset and severity of MDD?

Another example of future directions comes from the Cross-Disorder Group of the Psychiatric Genomics Consortium (2013) published in the *Lancet.* Again employing GWAS, this group examined genetic variants underlying genetic effects shared among the five disorders assigned to their study group: autism spectrum disorder, attention deficit-hyperactivity disorder, bipolar disorder, MDD, and schizophrenia. Examining a total of some 60,000 cases and controls, the investigators identified single nucleotide polymorphisms (SNPs) that were associated with the range of psychiatric conditions studied. Specificity of the SNPs to a single psychiatric condition, despite suggestions from prior studies, was unstable in this large sample of cases and controls. The findings suggested common genetic factors associated with these divergent psychiatric conditions. Is this the case for other psychiatric disorders? Are descriptions of psychopathology as heralded by the third edition of the *Diagnostic and Statistics Manual,* (American Psychiatric Association, 1980) outmoded? Might studying other traits such as neuroticism, internality, externality, and other personality variables be a more fruitful direction?

The National Institute of Mental Health (NIMH) is providing an alternative way to classify psychiatric conditions that may help us study and understand these disorders apart from the classification scheme offered by the DSM or International Classification of Diseases. The Research Domain Criteria (RDoC) is a new way to classify conditions for purposes of scientific study. Expressly developed to assist in the identification of the etiology of the many disabling psychiatric disorders, RDoC proposes a matrix that is dimensional in nature and is likely to be more relevant for studying genetic, neural and behavioral features of disorders. It is fundamentally an integrative schema that will ultimately include cognitive processes, social processes, arousal and regulatory systems, and positive and negative valence systems in the study of psychopathology. Ultimately, it will require big science and big data approaches to identify signal to noise in understanding the many levels of analyses responsible for human psychological suffering. As the genetic studies above suggest, the complexity of the tasks ahead of us are great and the challenges to innovate are many. Successes and failures in an era like this will be equally informative as the questions before us are foundational.

Many of the chapters contained in this volume are testing the limits of our scientific knowledge to date. Conceptual models of psychopathology abound and, importantly, most are becoming integrative across levels of scientific analysis. This is essential as we move from single domain analysis of the emotions. Behavioral, cognitive, and neurobiological domains need to be included as we move into the next era of scientific exploration of anxiety disorders and mental health more broadly.

Culture and Psychopathology. Will we find that the same genetic variants, cognitive, behavioral, and physiological substrates underlie the various forms of psychopathology in Western, highly developed countries and in the developing, understudied world? Will the same underlying factors be responsible for the differential prevalence rates noted in anxiety disorders between women and men in the West? Or are there culturally specific contributants to the development and maintenance of anxiety disorders across national boundaries? It is appealing to think that there are commonalities across all of these conditions, as the task for intervening becomes more systematic if this is the case. Yet cultural beliefs and historical understanding of these conditions vary considerably and it's widely accepted that emotional disorders are expressed very differently across cultures. Will the treatment of a panic attack in the city of Boston be approached in the same way as *ataque de nervios* in someone from the Dominican Republic or elsewhere in the Caribbean? No matter the similarities in the phenotypic behavior observed, incorporating cultural meaning will probably need to be a component of any successful treatment.

Devon Hinton, a psychiatrist and anthropologist at the Massachusetts General Hospital, studied the mental health problems of refugees from the Killing Fields of Cambodia extensively. Predominantly interested in the development of PTSD secondary to the mass murdering by the Khmer Rouge, Hinton and colleagues noticed a panic disorder-like syndrome that was termed "sore neck" as it presented with orthostatic dizziness, panic symptoms, and sore neck (Hinton, Ba, Peou, & Um, 2000). The Khmer view their bodies as possessing vessels of blood and wind. Wind overload represented a systemic dysregulation and mediated the catastrophic cognitions that accompanied "sore neck." The imbalance of blood and wind determines what symptoms, physiological and psychological, one experiences. These cultural idioms are fundamental to the Cambodian population so affected, and many other culturally specific idioms exist across the world. Taking these into account in devising interventions appears to be critically important to the ultimate engagement of the patients in treatment. Treatment engagement and the therapeutic alliance may well depend upon the extent to which clinicians accept and respect the cultural legacies and beliefs of the index society. In short, culture matters and incorporating aspects of culture into the scientific study of emotion (i.e., anxiety, etc.) is essential for progress in understanding etiology and in successful treatment.

Future Near-Term Directions. There are many questions that remain to be solved pertaining to the nature and treatment of anxiety disorders. Decades will be required for answering the most complicated questions. In the near term, we are left with addressing the needs of patients with anxiety disorders with the tools that we have. The psychological needs of the returning war veterans are paramount in the minds of clinicians, researchers, and the American public. We cannot wait for decades for the scientific method to provide answers to the problems with which these men and women present. Dissemination of existing assessment approaches and therapeutic tools to clinicians across the country is a priority. Moreover, the use of newer forms of delivery is essential to provide the best possible treatment for these returning war veterans. VetChange (Brief, et al., 2013) is one such initiative that uses the Internet from the National Center for PTSD to treat veterans with risky alcohol use and PTSD symptomatology. The reach of this Internet treatment to hundreds of participants in a randomized clinical trial was remarkable: we recruited some 600 veterans in six weeks' time into the trial. Importantly, these war veterans came for this treatment, they stayed in high numbers to complete the modules, and their alcohol symptoms and PTSD symptoms improved dramatically. Does the near-term future include the use of computerized interventions either alone or in combination with face-to-face health care? It surely will. The faithful delivery of cognitive behavioral treatments is every bit as important as accurate dosing and trials of pharmacotherapy. The technologies available today will improve and enhance treatment outcomes in the very near term. As our knowledge base across levels of scientific analysis improves, these cognitive behavioral interventions will remain important as one component of the next generation of treatments. The time is now to develop these and to disseminate them widely. Adaptations across culture, language, gender, race, and ethnicity are needed. We already have the tools to accomplish this important work.

We live in an age and era of great anxiety. While it is sobering to understand what lies ahead of us, it is encouraging to see all that has already been achieved. This book, from international leaders in the study of anxiety and its disorders, represents the state of the art today in 2014. One short decade from now, I can say with a degree of certainty, our intellectual understanding of anxiety disorders and their treatment will be greatly advanced. The authors of these chapters lay out the map for all to follow.

Terence M. Keane, PhD
VA National Center for Posttraumatic Stress Disorder,
VA Boston Healthcare System, Boston University School of Medicine

REFERENCES

American Psychiatric Association (1980). *Diagnostic and statistical manual of mental disorders, 3rd edition*. Washington, DC: American Psychiatric Association Press .

Barlow, D. H. (2002). *Anxiety and its disorders*. New York: Guilford Press.

Brief, D. J., Rubin, A., Keane, T. M., Enggasser, J., Roy, M., Helmuth, E., Hermos, J., et al. (2013). Web intervention for OEF-OIF veterans with problem drinking and PTSD symptoms. *J Consult and Clin Psychol, 81,* 890–900.

Cross Disorder Work Group of Psychiatric Genetics Consortium (2013). Identification of risk loci with shared effects on five major psychiatric disorders: A genome wide analysis. *Lancet, 381* (9875), 1371–1379.

Hinton, D., Ba, P., Peou, S., & Um, K. (2000). Panic disorder among Cambodian refugees attending a psychiatric clinic. *Gen Hosp Psychiatry, 22,* 437–444.

Major Depressive Disorder Working Group of the Psychiatric GWAS Consortium (2013). A mega-analysis of genome-wide association studies for major depressive disorder. *Mol Genet, 18,* 497–511.

Paul, G. (1966). *Insight v. desensitization in psychotherapy: An experiment in anxiety reduction*. Stanford, CA: Stanford University Press.

Walkup, J. T., Albano, A. M., Piacentini, J., et al., & Kendall, P. C. (2008) Cognitive behavioral therapy, sertraline, or a combination in childhood anxiety. *New Engl J Med, 359,* 2753–2766.

CONTRIBUTORS

James L. Abelson, MD, PhD
Department of Psychiatry
University of Michigan
    Medical School
Ann Arbor, Michigan, USA

Susanne E. Ahmari, MD, PhD
Department of Psychiatry
University of Pittsburgh
Pittsburgh, Pennsylvania, USA

Erik Andersson, PhD
Department of Clinical
    Neuroscience
Division of Psychiatry
    and Psychology
Karolinska Institutet
Stockholm, Sweden

Gordon J. G. Asmundson, PhD
Department of Psychology
University of Regina
Regina, Saskatchewan, Canada

Sudie E. Back, PhD
Department of Psychiatry and
    Behavioral Sciences
Medical University of
    South Carolina
Charleston, South Carolina, USA
Ralph H. Johnson Veterans Affairs
    Medical Center
Charleston, South Carolina, USA

Jafar Bakhshaie, MD
Department of Psychology
University of Houston
Houston, Texas, USA

Kathleen T. Brady, MD, PhD
Department of Psychiatry and
    Behavioral Sciences
Medical University of South Carolina
Charleston, South Carolina, USA
Ralph H. Johnson Veterans Affairs
    Medical Center
Charleston, South Carolina, USA

Charles Brandt, MA
Department of Psychology
University of Houston
Houston, Texas, USA

Bridget L. Callaghan, PhD
Department of Psychology
Columbia University
New York, New York, USA

Amanda W. Calkins, PhD
Department of Psychiatry
Massachusetts General Hospital
Harvard Medical School
Boston, MA

Allison A. Campbell, BA
Department of Psychiatry
Massachusetts General Hospital
Harvard Medical School
Boston, MA

Karen Lynn Cassiday, PhD
The Anxiety Treatment Center of
    Greater Chicago
Clinical Assistant Professor
Department of Psychology
Rosalind Franklin University of
    Medicine and Science
Chicago, Illinois, USA

Felecia E. Cerrato, MPH
Department of Psychology
Psychiatric and Neurodevelopmental
   Genetics Unit
Center for Human Genetic Research
Massachusetts General Hospital
Boston, Massachusetts, USA

Andrew A. Cooper, PhD
Department of Psychological
   Sciences
Case Western Reserve University
Cleveland, Ohio, USA

Kara K. Cover, BA
Department of Psychiatry
Harvard Medical School
Massachusetts General Hospital
Boston, Massachusetts, USA

Michelle G. Craske, PhD
Department of Psychology
University of California,
   Los Angeles
Los Angeles, California, USA

Christina A. D'Ambrosio, BS
Department of Psychology
University of Regina
Regina, Saskatchewan, Canada

Daniel G. Dillon, PhD
Department of Psychiatry
Harvard Medical School and
   McLean Hospital
Belmont, Massachusetts, USA

Darin D. Dougherty, MD
Department of Psychiatry
Massachusetts General Hospital
Harvard Medical School
Boston, Massachusetts, USA

Sheila M. Dowd, PhD
Department of Psychiatry
Rush University Medical Center
Chicago, Illinois, USA

Boadie W. Dunlop, MD
Department of Psychiatry and
   Behavioral Sciences
Emory University
Atlanta, Georgia, USA

Amit Etkin, MD, PhD
Department of Psychiatry and
   Behavioral Sciences
Stanford University
Palo Alto, California, USA
Sierra-Pacific Mental Illness Research,
   Education, and Clinical
   Center (MIRECC)
Veterans Affairs Palo Alto Health
   Care System
Palo Alto, California, USA

Norah C. Feeny, PhD
Department of Psychological
   Sciences
Case Western Reserve University
Cleveland, Ohio, USA

Edna B. Foa, PhD
Department of Psychiatry
School of Medicine
University of Pennsylvania
Philadelphia, Pennsylvania, USA

Cara H. Fuchs, PhD, MPH
Department of Psychiatry and
   Human Behavior
Alpert Medical School of
   Brown University
Providence, Rhode Island, USA

Emmanuel Garcia, MA
Department of Psychology
The Graduate Center, City University
   of New York
New York, New York, USA
Department of Psychology
Hunter College, City University
   of New York
New York, NY, USA

Anett Gyurak, PhD
Department of Psychiatry and
   Behavioral Sciences
Department of Psychology
Stanford University
Palo Alto, California, USA
Sierra-Pacific Mental Illness Research,
   Education, and Clinical Center
   (MIRECC)
Veterans Affairs Palo Alto Health
   Care System
Palo Alto, California, USA

Asala Halaj, MA
Department of Psychiatry
New York State Psychiatric Institute
New York, New York, USA

Lisa R. Hale, PhD
Kansas City Center for Anxiety
   Treatment, P.A. (KCCAT)
Overland Park, Kansas, USA
Department of Psychology
University of Missouri-Kansas City
Kansas City, Missouri, USA

Erik Hedman, PhD
Department of Clinical Neuroscience
Division of Psychology
Division of Psychology, Osher Center
   for Integrative Medicine
Karolinska Institutet
Stockholm, Sweden

John M. Hettema, MD, PhD
Department of Psychiatry
Virginia Institute for Psychiatric and
   Behavioral Genetics
Virginia Commonwealth University
Richmond, Virginia, USA

Stefan G. Hofmann, PhD
Department of Psychological and
   Brain Sciences
Boston University
Boston, Massachusetts, USA

Arash Javanbakht, MD
Department of Psychiatry
University of Michigan Medical School
Ann Arbor, Michigan, USA

Elizabeth C. Kaiser, MA
Department of Psychiatry
Rush University Medical Center
Chicago, Illinois, USA

Terence M. Keane, PhD
National Center for Posttraumatic
   Stress Disorder
VA Boston Healthcare System & Boston
   University School of Medicine
Rush University Medical Center
Chicago, Illinois, USA

Ryan J. Kimmel, MD
Department of Psychiatry and
   Behavioral Sciences
University of Washington
Seattle, Washington, USA

Kathryn D. Kriegshauser, PhD
Kansas City Center for Anxiety Treatment,
   P.A. (KCCAT)
Overland Park, Kansas, USA

Israel Liberzon, MD
VA Ann Arbor Healthcare System
Departments of Psychiatry and Psychology
University of Michigan Medical School
Ann Arbor, Michigan, USA

R. Bruce Lydiard, PhD, MD
Department of Psychiatry and
   Behavioral Sciences
Medical University of South Carolina
Charleston, South Carolina, USA

Luminita Luca, MD, PhD
Department of Psychiatry and
   Behavioral Sciences
Miller School of Medicine
   University of Miami
Miami, Florida, USA

Jenna L. McCauley, PhD
Department of Psychiatry and
    Behavioral Sciences
Medical University of
    South Carolina
Charleston, South Carolina, USA

Douglas S. Mennin, PhD
Department of Psychology
Hunter College, City University of
    New York
New York, New York, USA
Department of Psychology
The Graduate Center, City University
    of New York
New York, New York, USA

Mohammed R. Milad, PhD
Department of Psychiatry
Harvard Medical School
Massachusetts General Hospital
Boston, Massachusetts, USA

Charles B. Nemeroff, MD, PhD
Department of Psychiatry and
    Behavioral Sciences
Miller School of Medicine
University of Miami
Miami, Florida, USA

Matthew K. Nock, PhD
Department of Psychology
Harvard University
Cambridge, Massachusetts, USA

Holly A. Parkerson, PhD
Department of Psychology
University of Regina
Regina, Saskatchewan, Canada

K. Luan Phan, MD
Departments of Psychiatry,
    Psychology and Anatomy
    and Cell Biology
University of Illinois at Chicago
Chicago, Illinois, USA
Mental Health Service Line
Jesse Brown VA Medical Center
Chicago, Illinois, USA

Daniel S. Pine, MD
Section on Development and
    Affective Neuroscience
Intramural Research Program
National Institute of Mental
    Health (NIMH)
Bethesda, Maryland, USA

Diego A. Pizzagalli, PhD
Department of Psychiatry
Harvard Medical School and
    McLean Hospital
Belmont, Massachusetts, USA

Mark H. Pollack, MD
Department of Psychiatry
Rush University Medical Center
Chicago, Illinois, USA

Scott L. Rauch, MD
Department of Psychiatry
Harvard Medical School and
    McLean Hospital
Belmont, Massachusetts, USA

Sheila A. M. Rauch, PhD
VA Ann Arbor Healthcare System
Department of Psychiatry
University of Michigan
    Medical School
Ann Arbor, Michigan, USA

Megan E. Renna, BA
Department of Psychology
The Graduate Center, City University
    of New York
New York, New York, USA

Kerry J. Ressler, MD, PhD
Department of Psychiatry and
    Behavioral Sciences
Emory University
Atlanta, Georgia, USA

Jessica D. Ribeiro, PhD
Department of Psychology
Harvard University
Cambridge, Massachusetts, USA

Rick Richardson, PhD
School of Psychology
The University of New South Wales
Sydney, Australia

Andrew H. Rogers, BA
Department of Psychiatry
Massachusetts General Hospital
Harvard Medical School
Boston, MA

Isabelle M. Rosso, PhD
Department of Psychiatry
Harvard Medical School and
    McLean Hospital
Belmont, Massachusetts, USA

Barbara O. Rothbaum, PhD, ABPP
Department of Psychiatry and
    Behavioral Sciences
Emory University
Atlanta, Georgia, USA

Blake L. Rosenbaum, BS
Department of Psychiatry
Harvard Medical School
Massachusetts General Hospital
Boston, Massachusetts, USA

Peter P. Roy-Byrne, MD
Department of Psychiatry and
    Behavioral Sciences
University of Washington
    School of Medicine
Seattle, Washington, USA
Psychiatric Medicine Associates
Seattle, Washington, USA

Christian Rück, PhD
Department of Clinical Neuroscience
Division of Psychiatry
Karolinska Institutet
Stockholm, Sweden

Gerard Sanacora, MD, PhD
Department of Psychiatry
Yale Depression Research Program
Yale University
New Haven, Connecticut, USA

Franklin Schneier, MD
Department of Psychiatry
New York State Psychiatric Institute
Columbia University Medical Center
New York, New York, USA

Naomi M. Simon, MD, MSc
Department of Psychiatry
Massachusetts General Hospital
Harvard Medical School
Boston, MA

H. Blair Simpson, MD, PhD
Department of Psychiatry
Columbia University
New York State Psychiatric Institute
New York, New York, USA

Jordan W. Smoller, MD, ScD
Department of Psychiatry
Psychiatric and Neurodevelopmental
    Genetics Unit
Center for Human Genetic Research
Massachusetts General Hospital
Boston, Massachusetts, USA
Stanley Center for Psychiatric Research
Broad Institute
Boston, Massachusetts, USA

Huijin Song, PhD
Department of Psychiatry
Massachusetts General Hospital
Harvard Medical School
Boston, Massachusetts, USA

Lindsay K. Staples-Bradley, MA
Department of Psychology
University of California, Los Angeles
Los Angeles, CA

Dan J. Stein, MD, PhD
Department of Psychiatry
University of Cape Town
Cape Town, South Africa

Michael Treanor, PhD
Department of Psychology
University of California, Los Angeles
Los Angeles, CA

Sarah L. Weatherall, BA
Department of Psychiatry
Psychiatric and Neurodevelopmental
    Genetics Unit
Center for Human
    Genetic Research
Massachusetts General Hospital
Boston, Massachusetts, USA

Risa B. Weisberg, PhD
VA Boston Healthcare System
Boston, MA, USA
Department of Psychiatry and
    Human Behavior
Department of Family Medicine
Alpert Medical School of
    Brown University
Providence, Rhode Island, USA

Wendol Williams, MD
Department of Psychiatry
Yale Depression Research Program
Yale University
New Haven, Connecticut, USA

Alyson K. Zalta, PhD
Departments of Psychiatry and
    Behavioral Science
Rush University Medical Center
Chicago, Illinois, USA

Michael J. Zvolensky, PhD
Department of Psychology
University of Houston
Houston, Texas, USA
Department of Behavioral Science
The University of Texas MD Anderson
    Cancer Center

OVERVIEW OF ANXIETY AND RELATED ILLNESSES

ANXIETY AND RELATED DISORDERS IN DSM-5

DAN J. STEIN

INTRODUCTION

Since the introduction of operational diagnostic criteria in the third edition of the *Diagnostic and Statistical Manual of Mental Disorders* (DSM), this classification system has not only drawn closely on research findings but has also played a key role in influencing clinical practice and research studies. DSM-III, published in 1980, was significantly influenced by new developments in the psychopharmacology of these conditions (Klein, 1987) and played a key role in formalizing the idea that the anxiety disorders comprised a distinct and important set of conditions. DSM-IV, published 14 years later in 1994, drew on a substantial body of research that had explored DSM-III diagnostic criteria, as well as the psychobiology and treatment of the anxiety disorders, and further refined the criteria for these conditions. DSM-5, published after a 19-year gap in 2013, provided a timely opportunity to review a continuously accumulating set of studies on anxiety and related disorders and helped set new standards for future diagnosis and research. This chapter reviews key decisions taken by DSM-5 (American Psychiatric Association, 2013) and the relevant evidence base used to support them.

THE DSM-5 METASTRUCTURE

A first key issue facing DSM-5 was the so-called "metastructure": the way in which the manual divides disorders into distinct clusters. The DSM-5 chairs encouraged workgroups to think creatively about their task, attend to recent neuroscientific research, and consider dimensional and developmental approaches to diagnosis (Regier et al., 2009). Along these lines, a DSM-5 preparatory research conference focused on the notion of stress-induced and fear circuitry disorders as a new grouping (Andrews et al., 2009). Another DSM-5 preparatory research conference focused on the considerable overlap of depression and generalized anxiety disorder (D. Goldberg et al., 2010), and indeed an early proposal was for DSM-5 to include an emotional cluster of disorders, encompassing both depression and generalized anxiety disorder, on the basis that these conditions are characterized by negative affect and high comorbidity, as well as by overlapping risk factors (Goldberg et al., 2009).

The DSM-5 workgroup on anxiety, obsessive-compulsive spectrum, posttraumatic stress, and dissociative disorders undertook a number of reviews addressing the metastructure (Craske et al., 2009; Friedman et al., 2011b; Phillips et al., 2010a; Stein et al., 2010c). A first conclusion was that anxiety disorders are characterized by increased sensitivity to threat as reflected in self-reported fear and anxiety, as well as by heightened biobehavioral responses to threatening stimuli, and that although dimensional approaches are clearly important, it remains premature to divide these conditions into fear disorders and anxious misery disorders (Craske et al., 2009). On the basis that DSM-5 would have only a limited number of chapters, an early proposal was that the anxiety disorders be relabelled "anxiety and obsessive-compulsive disorders" to reflect important distinctions between these groups of conditions (Stein et al., 2010c). However, when it became apparent that DSM-5 would allow for more than 10 chapters, the workgroup proposed separating anxiety disorders into anxiety disorders, obsessive-compulsive and related disorders (OCRDs), and trauma- and stressor-related disorders (Table 1.1), arguing that this would maximize the diagnostic validity and clinical utility of the manual. At the same time, the workgroup advocated that the three sets of disorders be placed next to one another in the manual in order to highlight their close relationship (Stein et al., 2011).

Given the constraints of a linear classification system, any particular solution to the metastructure question arguably has both pros and cons (Stein, 2008a). There are a

TABLE 1.1 Anxiety, Obsessive-Compulsive and Related Disorders, and Trauma- and Stressor-Disorders in DSM-5

ANXIETY DISORDERS	OBSESSIVE-COMPULSIVE AND RELATED DISORDERS (OCRD)	TRAUMA- AND STRESSOR-RELATED DISORDERS
Separation anxiety disorder	Obsessive-compulsive disorder	Reactive attachment disorder
Selective mutism	Body dysmorphic disorder	Disinhibited social engagement disorder
Specific phobia	Hoarding disorder	Posttraumatic stress disorder
Social anxiety disorder (social phobia)	Trichotillomania (hair-pulling disorder)	Acute stress disorder
Panic disorder	Excoriation (skin-picking) disorder	Adjustment disorders
Agoraphobia	—	—
Generalized anxiety disorder	—	—
Substance/medication-induced anxiety disorder	Substance/medication-induced OCRD	—
Anxiety disorder due to another medical condition	OCRD due to another medical disorder	—
Other specified anxiety disorder	Other specified OCRD	Other specified trauma- and stressor-related disorder
Unspecified anxiety disorder	Unspecified OCRD	Unspecified trauma- and stressor-related disorder

number of apparent advantages of the DSM-5 approach. First, there are significant differences in the underlying neurocircuitry of many of the anxiety disorders (e.g., panic disorder, social anxiety disorder) and of obsessive-compulsive disorder (Stein et al., 2010c). Second, having a section on OCRDs provides a mechanism for recognizing a range of underdiagnosed and undertreated disorders that have significant comorbidities, as well as commonalities in underlying psychobiology and in treatment approach (Phillips et al., 2010b). Third, having a section on trauma and stressor-related disorders reflects a growing recognition of trauma as a precipitant, thus making the classification more etiological in nature and helping provide clinicians with tools for recognizing and approaching a range of overlooked conditions, including the adjustment disorders (Friedman et al., 2011b).

At the same time, there are also potential disadvantages. First, obsessive-compulsive disorder (OCD) and posttraumatic stress disorder (PTSD) have similar symptom structures to other anxiety disorders in that they are characterized by fear and avoidance symptoms; therefore, each of these disorders responds to analogous cognitive-behavior interventions that address these symptom structures (Storch et al., 2008; Zoellner et al., 2011). Second, there are significant differences in underlying psychobiology and treatment approaches across the OCRDs (Storch et al., 2008). Third, although it is true that PTSD begins in the aftermath of trauma, a broad range of different disorders are associated with increased likelihood of onset after trauma, and there is relatively little support for an independent stressor meta-construct (Zoellner et al., 2011). There may also be unintended consequences of such a division; for example, the Anxiety Disorders Association of America has been a useful forum for those interested in the anxiety disorders to share their ongoing work; will OCD and PTSD researchers decrease their attendance at such meetings, and will fewer productive cross-disorder collaborations ensue—or will a new construct of "anxiety and related disorders" prove fruitful?

Adding to the complexity of decision making about the metastructure is the point that, at times, different considerations can be in conflict. DSM-5 review papers considered various diagnostic validators, each of which may provide contradictory information. Thus, neurocircuitry findings may suggest one way of grouping disorders (for example, that obsessive-compulsive disorder and tic disorders fall into separate groupings), while family history data may suggest another (for example, that obsessive-compulsive disorder and tic disorders fall into the same grouping). Considerations of diagnostic validity (for example, several OCRDs respond selectively to serotonin reuptake inhibitors) may conflict with considerations of clinical utility (for example, both anxiety disorders and OCD respond to similar cognitive-behavioral techniques). Furthermore, considerations of clinical utility may be influenced by context; in a well-resourced setting, a specialized clinician may benefit from a classification system with finely drawn distinctions between different conditions, but in a poorly resourced setting, a primary care clinician may well prefer a nosology that employs broad brushstrokes. DSM as well as ICD are unable to carve nature at her joints, but rather must aim for an optimal solution at any particular time point, balancing arguments for "splitting" versus those for "lumping."

ANXIETY DISORDERS

One notable aspect of the new DSM-5 chapter on anxiety disorders is the use of a similarly structured set of diagnostic criteria for many of these conditions

(Table 1.2). A first criterion often emphasizes that there is "marked fear or anxiety" about one or another situation, consistent with a literature differentiating the phenomenology and psychobiology of these two constructs (Dias et al., 2013). Subsequent criteria may emphasize that these situations almost always provoke fear or anxiety and that these situations are avoided or endured with intense fear or anxiety, consistent with a literature emphasizing that fear/anxiety and avoidance have a different neurocircuitry and that both deserve treatment (Craske et al., 2009). A contextual criterion may note that the fear is out of proportion to the actual threat posed by the situation and to the sociocultural context—a useful criterion given that DSM-IV symptoms sometimes ignored context and culture (Lewis-Fernandez et al., 2010; Wakefield and First, 2012). There is also no longer the requirement in specific phobia and social anxiety that individuals over the age of 18 recognize their anxiety as excessive or unreasonable, consistent with a growing recognition that insight in anxiety and related disorders can be impaired or absent (Leckman et al., 2010; Phillips et al., 2014).

A duration criterion in many of the anxiety disorders notes that the fear, anxiety, or avoidance is persistent, typically lasting 6 months or more. Although it has been argued that there is benefit to allowing for the shorter duration of some anxiety disorders (Kessler et al., 2005), the 6-month criterion arguably helps differentiate these conditions

TABLE 1.2 Comparison of Diagnostic Criteria Across the Anxiety Disorders

	FOCUS OF FEAR	MINIMAL DURATION	CLINICAL CRITERION	MEDICAL EXCLUSION CRITERION	PSYCHIATRIC EXCLUSION CRITERION
Separation Anxiety Disorder	Separation from those to whom the individual is attached	4 weeks in children/adolescents, 6 months in adults	√		√
Selective Mutism		1 month	√		√
Specific Phobia	Specific object or situation	6 months	√		√
Social Anxiety Disorder (Social Phobia)	Social situations with possible scrutiny	6 months	√	√	√
Panic Disorder				√	√
Agoraphobia	2 or more of 5 agoraphobic situations	6 months	√	√	√
Generalized Anxiety Disorder	Number of events or activities	6 months	√	√	√

from adjustment or other more transient disorders. A clinical criterion typically emphasizes that the fear, anxiety, or avoidance causes clinically significant distress or impairment. While the DSM-5 taskforce considered the potential value of divorcing diagnosis (based purely on symptoms) and disability (based on impairment), in the case of the symptoms of anxiety disorders, which fall on a spectrum with normal phenomena, this is sometimes difficult to do, and the clinical criterion arguably helps avoid false positives (Kessler et al., 2003; Zimmerman et al., 2004). A medical exclusion criterion may note that the fear, anxiety, or avoidance is not attributable to the physiological effects of a substance or another medical condition. Finally, a psychiatric exclusion criterion may note that the fear, anxiety, or avoidance is not better explained by the symptoms of another mental disorder.

This similarly structured set of diagnostic criteria across the anxiety disorders is clinically useful insofar as it provides the clinician a framework for assessing key aspects of the symptoms of these conditions. Although DSM has been criticized for its checklist approach to diagnosis, the advantage of such a checklist arguably lies in providing the clinician with careful reminders about the importance of including key defining symptoms and excluding crucially important medical and psychiatric conditions, thus ensuring that relevant differential diagnoses are rigorously considered. The evaluation of fear, anxiety, and avoidance symptoms also provides the clinician a useful framework for initiating a comprehensive assessment (including evaluating the severity of symptoms) and treatment plan. The diagnostic criteria provide a foundation for screening and diagnostic questionnaires, as well as for the dimensional assessment of symptom severity across the anxiety disorders, and indeed the brief self-rated scales developed by the DSM-5 workgroup for these conditions are consistent in content and structure (LeBeau et al., 2012).

The DSM-5 section on anxiety disorders has a number of other features that also differentiate it from DSM-IV. First, separation anxiety disorder and selective mutism are now included as anxiety disorders. This is consistent with a growing body of research on the importance of these conditions and their links to other anxiety conditions (Bogels et al., 2010; 2013). Second, there is a delinking of panic disorder and agoraphobia, and it is emphasized that the presence of panic attacks can be a specifier applicable to all DSM-5 disorders. This change is again evidence based, reflecting a growing awareness of the diagnostic validity of agoraphobia as an independent diagnosis, and of the clinical utility of assessing panic symptoms in a range of psychiatric disorders (Craske et al., 2010). Third, there are a number of changes to anxiety disorder specifiers; for example, the "generalized" specifier for social anxiety disorder has been deleted and replaced with a "performance only" specifier. There is a growing awareness that social anxiety symptoms fall on a spectrum of severity, and there is no specific cut-point that differentiates generalized from nongeneralized social anxiety disorder (Stein et al., 2010d).

OBSESSIVE-COMPULSIVE AND RELATED DISORDERS

The chapter on OCRDs is new to DSM-5, and it reflects a growing evidence base pointing to the diagnostic validity and clinical utility of classifying this set of conditions in the same diagnostic grouping (Phillips et al., 2010b). The OCRDs arguably fall into two main categories: those characterized by obsessions or preoccupations (and often also by compulsive behaviors or mental acts) and those characterized by body-focused repetitive behaviors. The former category includes OCD, body dysmorphic disorder (BDD), and hoarding disorder, while the latter category includes trichotillomania (hair-pulling disorder) and excoriation (skin-picking) disorder. Hoarding disorder and excoriation disorder are also new to DSM-5, reflecting growing research on the clinical importance of these conditions (Grant et al., 2012; Mataix-Cols et al., 2010). The addition of this chapter also required the creation of the new disorders of substance/medication-induced OCRD and OCRD due to another medical disorder in order to be consistent with the structure of other DSM-5 chapters.

The argument regarding diagnostic validity of the chapter on OCRDs (OCRDs) emphasizes that there is significant overlap in the phenomenology and psychobiology of these conditions (Phillips et al., 2010b) (Table 1.3). Certainly, as already noted, OCD appears to be mediated by a different neurocircuitry from that of the anxiety disorders, and there are elements in common between the neurocircuitry and neurochemistry of OCD and a number of the OCRDs, including involvement of cortico-striatal-thalamic-cortical (CSTC) circuitry and selective response to serotonin reuptake inhibitors (SRIs). Furthermore, as emphasized in a secondary analysis commissioned by the workgroup, the OCRDs also share higher than expected comorbidity and familiality (Bienvenu et al., 2012). At the same time, it should be acknowledged that the psychobiology of many OCRDs is very poorly understood and that the hypothesis that all OCRDs selectively respond to SRIs has not entirely withstood empirical testing. On the whole, however, the subworkgroup argued that it made more sense, from the perspective of diagnostic validity, to have these disorders in one category rather than to keep OCD, BDD, and trichotillomania in separate chapters.

One potential weakness of the DSM-5 on OCRDs is the exclusion of Tourette's disorder and of hypochondriasis. Tourette's disorder is in some ways the central exemplar of an OCRD; there are phenomenological similarities between compulsions and complex tics, many patients with Tourette's have comorbid OCD and many patients with OCD have

TABLE 1.3 Comparison of Diagnostic Criteria Across the OCRDs

	OBSESSION/ PREOCCUPATION	COMPULSION/ REPETITIVE ACT	CLINICAL CRITERION	MEDICAL EXCLUSION CRITERION	PSYCHIATRIC EXCLUSION CRITERION
Obsessive-compulsive disorder	Recurrent persistent thoughts, urges or images	Repetitive behaviors or mental acts	√	√	√
Body dysmorphic disorder	Perceived defects or flaws in physical appearance	Behaviors or mental acts in response to such concerns	√		√
Hoarding disorder	Need to save items	Accumulation of possessions	√	√	√
Trichotillomania (hair-pulling disorder)		Hair-pulling	√	√	√
Excoriation (skin-picking) disorder		Skin-picking	√	√	√

comorbid tics, there are clear genetic relationships between the two conditions, and there are some overlaps across the disorders in approach to treatment (Walkup et al., 2010). At the same time, there are certainly arguments for having tic disorders in the DSM-5 chapter on neurodevelopmental disorders; it is a group of disorders with early onset, there is comorbidity between tic disorders and other neurodevelopmental disorders such as attention deficit–hyperactivity disorder, there are important differences in the genetics of Tourette's and OCD, and there are key differences in the treatment approach to the two conditions (Walkup et al., 2010). Although the decision was taken to not include Tourette's in the chapter on OCRDs, OCD does have a new tic-related specifier, reflecting knowledge of the importance of this relationship.

Hypochondriasis was classified in the DSM-IV chapter on somatoform disorders. However, unlike other somatoform disorders, the disorder is not characterized by predominant somatic symptoms. Instead individuals with hypochondriasis present with preoccupations about having or developing a medical disorder, as well as repetitive behaviors (e.g., checking medical textbooks) or mental acts (e.g., scanning of the body). At the same time, there is overlap between hypochondriasis and the anxiety disorders, insofar as many patients with panic disorder have somatic concerns, and patients with hypochondriasis may have panic symptoms. Although psychobiological data on hypochondriasis are scant, some work points to an overlap in neurocircuitry between hypochondriasis, OCD, and panic disorder. While treatment research is also at a relatively early stage, there is some suggestion that overlapping approaches are efficacious in hypochondriasis and OCD (Stein, 2012). In DSM-5, however, the construct of hypochondriasis was changed to "illness anxiety disorder," and this disorder is classified in the chapter on somatic symptom and related disorders.

The argument regarding clinical utility of the OCRDs emphasizes that the significant overlap in phenomenology and psychobiology across these disorders leads to important similarities in the clinical approach to diagnosis and treatment, so that having a single OCRD grouping may improve recognition of and intervention for these underdiagnosed and undertreated conditions. Thus, for example, when screening for OCRDs or when assessing a patient with any OCRD, it may be useful to ask about repetitive intrusive phenomena (e.g., obsessions in OCD, sensory phenomena in skin-picking), as well as about repetitive behaviors or mental acts (e.g., checking for danger in OCD, mirror checking in BDD). It is also clinically important to ask patients with any one OCRD about comorbidity with, and family history of, other OCRDs. The DSM-5 insight specifiers for OCD, BDD, and hoarding disorder are comparable, again reflecting overlaps in clinical assessment across these conditions. Similarly, the DSM-5 workgroup developed brief self-rated symptom severity scales for the OCRDs that are consistent in content and structure (LeBeau et al., 2013).

At the same time, clinicians do need to be aware of key differences in assessment and treatment approach across the OCRDs. Although those disorders characterized by body-focused repetitive behaviors, such as trichotillomania and excoriation disorder, may be precipitated by specific stimuli, they are not characterized by obsessions (Stein et al., 2010b). Furthermore, they may require quite different cognitive-behavioral interventions (i.e., they respond to habit-reversal techniques) and psychopharmacological treatments (i.e., they do not appear to respond as well as OCD to SRIs, and they may respond to treatment with n-acetyl-cysteine). Although patients with OCRDs may be characterized by no insight, this is far more common in some conditions (e.g., BDD) than in others (e.g., OCD) (Phillips et al., 2014). While such differences are clearly important, it may be noted that clinical distinctions across different disorders are apparent in each

DSM-5 chapter; there are key differences in the assessment and treatment approach, for example, across the psychotic, mood, and eating disorders.

TRAUMA- AND STRESSOR-RELATED DISORDERS

The new DSM-5 chapter on trauma- and stressor-related disorders includes a range of conditions in which exposure to a traumatic or stressful event is a diagnostic criterion. These conditions include reactive attachment disorder, disinhibited social engagement disorder, posttraumatic stress disorder (PTSD), acute stress disorder, and adjustment disorders (Table 1.4). The chapter starts by noting that psychological distress following exposure to a traumatic or stressful event is quite variable, and that while some individuals exhibit fear and anxiety symptoms, others have a phenotype characterized by anhedonic and dysphoric symptoms, externalizing angry or aggressive symptoms, or dissociative symptoms. It is also important to note that many individuals suffer from a combination of these different symptoms (Friedman et al., 2011b).

Social neglect, or the absence of adequate caregiving during childhood, is arguably the trauma/stressor with the most disruptive and persistent consequences. The literature describing the phenomenology and psychobiology of animal maternal separation and of human social neglect constitutes one of the foundational elements of the translational approach to anxiety and related disorders. Social neglect is a diagnostic criterion in both reactive attachment disorder and disinhibited social engagement disorder. Reactive

TABLE 1.4 Comparison of Diagnostic Criteria Across the Trauma- and Stressor-Related Disorders

	TRAUMA/ STRESSOR	MINIMAL DURATION	CLINICAL CRITERION	MEDICAL EXCLUSION CRITERION	PSYCHIATRIC EXCLUSION CRITERION
Reactive attachment disorder	Extremes of insufficient care				√
Disinhibited social engagement disorder	Extremes of insufficient care				
Posttraumatic stress disorder	Actual or threatened death, serious injury, or sexual violence	1 month	√	√	
Acute stress disorder	Actual or threatened death, serious injury, or sexual violence	3 days	√	√	√
Adjustment disorders	Identifiable stressor		√		√

attachment disorder can, however, be characterized as an internalizing disorder with depressive symptoms and withdrawn behavior, while disinhibited social engagement disorder can be characterized as an externalizing disorder with disinhibition (American Psychiatric Association, 2013).

A number of key nosological issues regarding the trauma- and stressor-related disorders have been debated in the literature (Friedman et al., 2011a). A first, foundational issue is whether PTSD and adjustments disorders should be considered as normal responses to abnormal events or as abnormal responses to quite common events (Yehuda and McFarlane, 1995). Although it is certainly important to recognize the evolutionary value of the stress response, epidemiological data have confirmed the ubiquity of traumatic and stressful events. Furthermore, psychobiological data have confirmed that PTSD is characterized by significant alterations, which respond to intervention. Thus, the DSM-5 view that PTSD and a range of related conditions should be recognized as disorders now seems indisputable.

Second, there is the question of whether it is best to conceptualize PTSD as a narrow disorder (characterized by intrusive, avoidant, and hyperarousal phenomena) in order to delineate it from other responses to trauma, or whether it is best to expand the criteria to include a range of different symptoms given the heterogeneity of posttraumatic stress responses. Spitzer and colleagues have argued for a narrow approach (Rosen et al., 2008), and this has been supported in an ICD-11 proposal (Maercker et al., 2013). However, members of the DSM-5 workgroup argued for a broader version, which includes a fourth cluster of symptoms characterized by negative alterations in cognitions and mood (Friedman et al., 2011a). In a comparison of DSM-IV, DSM-5, ICD-10, and ICD-11 criteria from around the world, it was found that each diagnostic criteria set identified somewhat different individuals, but that each of these subsets of individuals had a clinically relevant condition (Stein et al., 2014). For now, then, the evidence would seem to support the value of somewhat broader approaches, whether in clinical practice or in research.

Third, and partly related, there is the question of whether some form of complex PTSD should be recognized by the nosology (Friedman et al., 2011a; Maercker et al., 2013). Individuals with complex PTSD have been exposed to severe and long-lasting trauma (e.g., childhood sexual abuse) and may suffer a wide range of symptoms, including impulsivity, affective lability, dissociation, and somatization. DSM-5 PTSD is characterized by an expansion of diagnostic criteria to include additional symptoms such as aggression, as well as by a new specifier for dissociative symptoms, arguably helping to bridge the gap between a narrower concept of PTSD and a broader construct of PTSD (as entailed by the notion of complex PTSD). This is consistent with a growing understanding of the psychobiology of dissociative PTSD, as well as a growing appreciation of its clinical associations (Stein et al., 2013).

CONTROVERSY AND CRITICISM

The DSM-5 process has involved a range of controversies, and a number of criticisms have been put forward from within and without the field. It is worth reviewing briefly a number of the more common of these controversies and criticisms.

First, there is a group of concerns including the idea that DSM-5 is mired in conflicts of interest with the pharmaceutical industry, that decisions are made on the basis of "political" considerations rather than scientific evidence, and that such decisions take place behind closed doors rather than in the open (Cosgrove and Krimsky, 2012). Versions of these concerns emphasize that the DSM-5 is an American process rather than an international one, that it ignores the inputs and concerns of clinicians other than psychiatrists, and that key stakeholders such as consumers are ignored. Each of these criticisms fails to pass muster when the evidence is examined. DSM-5 workgroup members were carefully vetted for conflicts of interest, proposed diagnostic criteria were posted on the Internet for feedback, and a range of clinicians and international colleagues participated in the process (Kupfer et al., 2008). This is not to say that medical and psychiatric diagnoses do not involve values; rather it is to indicate that such values can be rigorously considered and debated (Stein, 2008b).

A particularly interesting debate concerns the role of consumer advocates in nosology. Some have argued that it is crucial to include consumers in decision-making about psychiatric diagnoses, while others have countered that this is politically correct nonsense (Sadler and Fulford, 2004; Spitzer, 2004). However, there is growing consensus among nosologists, clinicians, and researchers that psychiatric diagnosis and treatment is dependent on first-person accounts, that understanding and appreciating individual voices and experiences is key, and that it is useful to include people with psychiatric disorders as collaborators in clinical and research processes (Stein and Phillips, 2013). In the case of the DSM-5 workgroup, feedback from patients and patient advocates played a useful role in influencing some of the recommendations. For example, many individuals who suffered from excoriation disorder posted messages on the American Psychiatric Association website; this input usefully supported the view that the available scientific data were sufficient to add this disorder to DSM-5 (Stein and Phillips, 2013).

Second, there is a related group of concerns that DSM-5 involves a medicalization of problems of living, with an expanding number of diagnoses with each edition, ultimately benefitting clinicians and the pharmaceutical industry and deflecting more appropriate interventions from reaching sufferers, at the expense of society as a whole. One version of these criticisms is that the United States is exporting its particular brand of disease-mongering to the rest of the world. This set of concerns raises the key conceptual question of "What is a psychiatric disorder?" (Stein et al., 2010a). In addressing this question, it is important to concede that symptoms of anxiety and related disorders are highly prevalent in the community, that there is a fuzzy border between normality and pathology, and that the clinical criterion (which emphasizes distress and impairment) must still be relied on. It is also crucial to emphasize the evolutionary roots and adaptive nature of anxiety (Nesse and Stein, 2012). At the same time, the boundaries of mental disorder are not necessarily arbitrary, nor are they set at too low a threshold (Kessler et al., 2003). Indeed, throughout the world, anxiety and related disorders remain underdiagnosed and undertreated.

DSM-5 work on anxiety and related disorders paid particular attention to cultural issues (Lewis-Fernandez et al., 2010). This is exemplified in the criteria for social anxiety disorder, as well as in the description of panic attacks. Thus, in social anxiety disorder, DSM-IV wording has been changed to note in DSM-5 that the individual fears that he or she will act or show anxiety symptoms in a way that will be negatively evaluated, that will be humiliating or embarrassing, or that will lead to rejection or offend others. This wording combines the DSM-IV emphasis on humiliating or embarrassing symptoms with the Eastern construct of *taijin kyofusho*, or anthrophobia, where social anxieties center around a concern with the offense of others (Stein, 2009). In the description of panic attacks, the list of symptoms has been expanded to be consistent with the variability in panic symptoms that has been reported around the world (Lewis-Fernandez et al., 2010).

Third, there is a debate about the extent to which DSM-5 could or should have been an iterative process or a paradigm shift. First (2010) points out that despite the scientific advances that have occurred since the descriptive approach was first introduced in DSM-III, the field lacks a sufficiently deep understanding of mental disorders to justify abandoning this approach in favor of a more etiologically based alternative. Furthermore, he points out that despite the increased reference to dimensional constructs in DSM-5, this is neither paradigm shifting, given that simpler versions of such dimensions are already a component of DSM-IV, nor likely to be used by busy clinicians without evidence that they improve clinical outcomes. Ultimately DSM-5 required a high threshold of evidence for making changes to the nosology; for example, proposed changes to the diagnostic criteria for generalized anxiety disorder (Andrews et al., 2010) were rejected.

In the sections on anxiety and related disorders, there were, however, a number of important incremental changes. Perhaps the largest change was one that did not involve changes to the diagnostic criteria, but rather the splitting of anxiety and related disorders into three separate chapters. Furthermore, despite DSM-5 having set very high thresholds for the introduction of new disorders, on the strength of the scientific evidence, several new disorders were in fact included in these sections. The inclusion of a "no insight/delusional" specifier in the chapter on OCRDs effectively moves some individuals who would be conceptualized as having a psychotic disorder in DSM-IV into the section on OCRDs in DSM-5, a fairly substantial shift in conceptualization. Thus, although there was perhaps no dramatic paradigm shift, and some disorders such as generalized anxiety disorder remained unchanged, on the whole DSM-5 has brought some substantive and important changes to the field of anxiety and related disorders.

Fourth, and partly related, there is a debate about the extent to which DSM-5 can and will promote translational neuroscience (Hyman, 2007). It has long been argued that for a truly biological psychiatry to progress, clinician-researchers need to look beyond diagnostic categories, aiming rather to delineate the psychobiology of symptom dimensions that cut across various disorders (Van Praag et al., 1990). Certainly, there are few data to suggest that disorders such as schizophrenia are homogenous entities, or that they will map closely to specific genetic variants. The Research Domain Criteria (RDoC) framework has been proposed as a key translational neuroscience approach to bio-behavioral dimensional assessment (Rauch, Chapter 9, this volume). It seems clear that for work on the optimal classification, evaluation, and treatment of anxiety and related disorders to progress, the field will need to understand the cognitive-affective neuroscience of these conditions and of relevant endophenotypes in much greater detail.

That said, it is relevant to note that the importance of focusing on biologically based symptom dimensions has been stated for many years now. Indeed, since DSM-IV, there has been significant progress in understanding constructs such as behavioral inhibition, fear conditioning, and cognitive flexibility, which are relevant to a range of anxiety and related disorders. However, the neurobiology of such constructs has proven complex, and although laboratory-based measures have been key in advancing research they have not always proven to have as much clinical utility as might have been hoped. While dimensional assessment approaches are key in research (Brown and Barlow, 2009; Shear et al., 2007), categorical diagnoses remain central to clinical practice. Furthermore, in DSM-5, the formulation of such categories and their diagnostic criteria has relied heavily on the basic and clinical neuroscience literature. For the foreseeable future, we will arguably need to rely on DSM-5, RDoC, and a range of other conceptual approaches in order to continue to drive forward a translational approach to those suffering from anxiety symptoms and related disorders (Stein, 2014).

ACKNOWLEDGMENTS

Dan J. Stein is supported by the Medical Research Council of South Africa. In the past three years, Dr. Stein has received research grants and/or consultancy honoraria from AMBRF, Biocodex, Cipla, Lundbeck, National Responsible Gambling Foundation, Novartis, Servier, and Sun.

REFERENCES

American Psychiatric Association (2013). *Diagnostic and statistical manual of mental disorders, fifth edition.* Arlington, VA: American Psychiatric Association.

Andrews, G., Charney, D. S., Sirovatka, P. J., and Regier, D. A. (Eds.). (2009). *Stress-induced and fear circuitry disorders: Refining the research agenda for DSM-V.* Arlington, VA: American Psychiatric Association.

Andrews, G., Hobbs, M. J., Borkovec, T. D., Beesdo, K., Craske, M. G., Heimberg, R. G.,... Stanley, M. A. (2010). Generalized worry disorder: A review of DSM-IV generalized anxiety disorder and options for DSM-V. *Depress Anxiety, 27* (2), 134–147.

Bienvenu, O. J., Samuels, J. F., Wuyek, L. A., Liang, K. Y., Wang, Y., Grados, M. A.,... Nestadt, G. (2012). Is obsessive-compulsive disorder an anxiety disorder, and what, if any, are spectrum conditions? A family study perspective. *Psychol Med, 42* (1), 1–13.

Bogels, S. M., Knappe, S., and Clark, L. A. (2013). Adult separation anxiety disorder in DSM-5. *Clin Psychol Rev, 33* (5), 663–674.

Bogels, S. M., Alden, L., Beidel, D. C., Clark, L. A., Pine, D. S., Stein, M. B., and Voncken, M. (2010). Social anxiety disorder: questions and answers for the DSM-V. *Depress Anxiety, 27* (2), 168–189.

Brown, T. A., and Barlow, D. H. (2009). A proposal for a dimensional classification system based on the shared features of the DSM-IV anxiety and mood disorders: Implications for assessment and treatment. *Psychol Assess, 21* (3), 256–271.

Cosgrove, L., and Krimsky, S. (2012). A comparison of DSM-IV and DSM-5 panel members' financial associations with industry: A pernicious problem persists. *PLoS Med, 9* (3), e1001190.

Craske, M. G., Kircanski, K., Epstein, A., Wittchen, H. U., Pine, D. S., Lewis-Fernandez, R., ... Dissociative Disorder Work Group (2010). Panic disorder: A review of DSM-IV panic disorder and proposals for DSM-V. *Depress Anxiety, 27* (2), 93–112.

Craske, M. G., Rauch, S. L., Ursano, R., Prenoveau, J., Pine, D. S., and Zinbarg, R. E. (2009). What is an anxiety disorder? *Depress Anxiety, 26* (12), 1066–1085.

Dias, B. G., Banerjee, S. B., Goodman, J. V., and Ressler, K. J. (2013). Towards new approaches to disorders of fear and anxiety. *Curr Opin Neurobiol, 23* (3), 346–352.

First, M. B. (2010). Paradigm shifts and the development of the diagnostic and statistical manual of mental disorders: past experiences and future aspirations. *Can J Psychiatry, 55* (11), 692–700.

Friedman, M. J., Resick, P. A., Bryant, R. A., and Brewin, C. R. (2011a). Considering PTSD for DSM-5. *Depress Anxiety, 28* (9), 750–769.

Friedman, M. J., Resick, P. A., Bryant, R. A., Strain, J., Horowitz, M., and Spiegel, D. (2011b). Classification of trauma and stressor-related disorders in DSM-5. *Depress Anxiety, 28* (9), 737–749.

Goldberg, D., Kendler, K. S., Sirovatka, P. J., and Regier, D. A. (2010). *Diagnostic issues in depression and generalized anxiety disorder: Refining the research agenda for DSM-V.* Arlington, VA: American Psychiatric Publishing.

Goldberg, D. P., Krueger, R. F., Andrews, G., and Hobbs, M. J. (2009). Emotional disorders: Cluster 4 of the proposed meta-structure for DSM-V and ICD-11. *Psychol Med, 39* (12), 2043–2059.

Grant, J. E., Odlaug, B. L., Chamberlain, S. R., Keuthen, N. J., Lochner, C., and Stein, D. J. (2012). Skin picking disorder. *Am J Psychiatry, 169* (11), 1143–1149.

Hyman, S. E. (2007). Can neuroscience be integrated into the DSM-V? *Nat Rev Neurosci, 8* (9), 725–732.

Kessler, R. C., Brandenburg, N., Lane, M., Roy-Byrne, P., Stang, P. D., Stein, D. J., and Wittchen, H. U. (2005). Rethinking the duration requirement for generalized anxiety disorder: Evidence from the National Comorbidity Survey Replication. *Psychol Med, 35* (7), 1073–1082.

Kessler, R. C., Merikangas, K. R., Berglund, P., Eaton, W. W., Koretz, D. S., and Walters, E. E. (2003). Mild disorders should not be eliminated from the DSM-V. *Arch Gen Psychiatry, 60* (11), 1117–1122.

Klein, D. F. (1987). Anxiety reconceptualized. Gleaning from pharmacological dissection—early experience with imipramine and anxiety. *Mod Probl Pharmacopsychiatry, 22*, 1–35.

Kupfer, D. J., Regier, D. A., and Kuhl, E. A. (2008). On the road to DSM-V and ICD-11. *Eur Arch Psychiatry Clin Neurosci, 258*, Suppl 5, 2–6.

LeBeau, R. T., Glenn, D. E., Hanover, L. N., Beesdo-Baum, K., Wittchen, H. U., and Craske, M. G. (2012). A dimensional approach to measuring anxiety for DSM-5. *Int J Methods Psychiatr Res, 21* (4), 258–272.

LeBeau, R. T., Mischel, E. R., Simpson, H. B., Mataix-Cols, D., Phillips, K. A., Stein, D. J., and Craske, M. G. (2013). Preliminary assessment of obsessive-compulsive spectrum scales for DSM-5. *J Obsess Compul Rel Dis, 2*, 114–118.

Leckman, J. F., Denys, D., Simpson, H. B., Mataix-Cols, D., Hollander, E.,... Stein, D. J. (2010). Obsessive-compulsive disorder: A review of the diagnostic criteria and possible subtypes and dimensional specifiers for DSM-V. *Depress Anxiety, 27* (6), 507–527.

Lewis-Fernandez, R., Hinton, D. E., Laria, A. J., Patterson, E. H., Hofmann, S. G., Craske, M. G.,... Liao, B. (2010). Culture and the anxiety disorders: Recommendations for DSM-V. *Depress Anxiety, 27* (2), 212–229.

Maercker, A., Brewin, C. R., Bryant, R. A., Cloitre, M., van Ommeren, M., Jones, L. M.,... Reed, G. M. (2013). Diagnosis and classification of disorders specifically associated with stress: Proposals for ICD-11. *World Psychiatry, 12* (3), 198–206.

Mataix-Cols, D., Frost, R. O., Pertusa, A., Clark, L. A., Saxena, S., Leckman, J. F.,... Wilhelm, S. (2010). Hoarding disorder: A new diagnosis for DSM-V? *Depress Anxiety, 27* (6), 556–572.

Nesse, R. M., and Stein, D. J. (2012). Towards a genuinely medical model for psychiatric nosology. *BMC Med, 10*, 5.

Phillips, K. A., Friedman, M. J., Stein, D. J., and Craske, M. (2010a). Special DSM-V issues on anxiety, obsessive-compulsive spectrum, posttraumatic, and dissociative disorders." *Depress Anxiety, 27* (2), 91–92.

Phillips, K. A., Hart, A. S., Simpson, H. B., and Stein, D. J. (2014). Delusional versus nondelusional body dysmorphic disorder: Recommendations for DSM-5. *CNS Spectr, 19* (1), 10–20.

Phillips, K. A., Stein, D. J., Rauch, S. L., Hollander, E., Fallon, B. A., Barsky, A.,... Leckman, J. (2010b). Should an obsessive-compulsive spectrum grouping of disorders be included in DSM-V? *Depress Anxiety, 27* (6), 528–555.

Regier, D. A., Narrow, W. E., Kuhl, E. A., and Kupfer, D. J. (2009). "The conceptual development of DSM-V. *Am J Psychiatry, 166* (6), 645–650.

Rosen, G. M., Spitzer, R. L., and McHugh, P. R. (2008). Problems with the post-traumatic stress disorder diagnosis and its future in DSM V. *Br J Psychiatry, 192* (1), 3–4.

Sadler, J. Z., and Fulford, B. (2004). Should patients and their families contribute to the DSM-V process? *Psychiatr Serv, 55* (2), 133–138.

Shear, M. K., Bjelland, I., Beesdo, K., Gloster, A. T., and Wittchen, H. U. (2007). Supplementary dimensional assessment in anxiety disorders. *Int J Methods Psychiatr Res, 16* Suppl 1, S52–S64.

Spitzer, R. L. (2004). Good idea or politically correct nonsense? *Psychiatr Serv, 55* (2), 113.

Stein, D. J. (2008a). Is disorder X in category or spectrum Y? General considerations and application to the relationship between obsessive-compulsive disorder and anxiety disorders. *Depress Anxiety, 25* (4), 330–335.

———(2008b). *Philosophy of psychopharmacology.* Cambridge: Cambridge University Press.

———(2009). Social anxiety disorder in the West and in the East. *Ann Clin Psychiatry, 21* (2), 109–117.

———(2012). Hypochondriasis in ICD-11. *World Psychiatry, 11* (S1), 99–103.

——— (2014). An integrative approach to psychiatric diagnosis and research. *World Psychiatry, 13* (1), 51–53.

Stein, D. J., and Phillips, K. A. (2013). Patient advocacy and DSM-5. *BMC Med, 11,* 133.

Stein, D. J., Craske, M. G., Friedman, M. J., and Phillips, K. A. (2011). Meta-structure issues for the DSM-5: How do anxiety disorders, obsessive-compulsive and related disorders, post-traumatic disorders, and dissociative disorders fit together? *Curr Psychiatry Rep, 13* (4), 248–250.

Stein, D. J., Fineberg, N. A., Bienvenu, O. J., Denys, D., Lochner, C., Nestadt, G.,. . . Phillips, K. A. (2010c). Should OCD be classified as an anxiety disorder in DSM-V? *Depress Anxiety, 27* (6), 495–506.

Stein, D. J., Grant, J. E., Franklin, M. E., Keuthen, N., Lochner, C., Singer, H. S., and Woods, D. W. (2010b). Trichotillomania (hair pulling disorder), skin picking disorder, and stereotypic movement disorder: Toward DSM-V. *Depress Anxiety, 27* (6), 611–626.

Stein, D. J., Koenen, K. C., Friedman, M. J., Hill, E., McLaughlin, K. A., Petukhova, M.,. . . Kessler, R. C. (2013). Dissociation in posttraumatic stress disorder: Evidence from the world mental health surveys. *Biol Psychiatry, 73* (4), 302–312.

Stein, D. J., McLaughlin, K. A., Koenen, K. C., Atwoli, L., Friedman, M. J., Hill, E. D.,. . . Kessler, R. C. (2014). DSM-5 and ICD-11 definitions of posttraumatic stress disorder: Investigating 'narrow' and 'broad' approaches. *Depress Anxiety, 31* (6), 494–505.

Stein, D. J., Phillips, K. A., Bolton, D., Fulford, K. W., Sadler, J. Z., and Kendler, K. S. (2010a). What is a mental/psychiatric disorder? From DSM-IV to DSM-V. *Psychol Med, 40* (11), 1759–1765.

Stein, D. J., Ruscio, A. M., Lee, S., Petukhova, M., Alonso, J., Andrade, L. H.,. . . Kessler, R. C. (2010d). Subtyping social anxiety disorder in developed and developing countries. *Depress Anxiety, 27* (4), 390–403.

Storch, E. A., Abramowitz, J., and Goodman, W. K. (2008). Where does obsessive-compulsive disorder belong in DSM-V? *Depress Anxiety, 25* (4), 336–347.

Van Praag, H. M., Asnis, G. M., Kahn, R. S., Brown, S. L., Korn, M., Friedman, J. M., and Wetzler, S. (1990). Nosological tunnel vision in biological psychiatry. A plea for a functional psychopathology. *Ann NY Acad Sci, 600,* 501–510.

Wakefield, J. C., and First, M. B. (2012). Placing symptoms in context: The role of contextual criteria in reducing false positives in Diagnostic and Statistical Manual of Mental Disorders diagnoses. *Compr Psychiatry, 53* (2), 130–139.

Walkup, J. T., Ferrao, Y., Leckman, J. F., Stein, D. J., and Singer, H. (2010). Tic disorders: Some key issues for DSM-V. *Depress Anxiety, 27* (6), 600–610.

Yehuda, R., and McFarlane, A. C. (1995). Conflict between current knowledge about posttraumatic stress disorder and its original conceptual basis. *Am J Psychiatry, 152* (12), 1705–1713.

Zimmerman, M., Chelminski, I., and Young, D. (2004). On the threshold of disorder: A study of the impact of the DSM-IV clinical significance criterion on diagnosing depressive and anxiety disorders in clinical practice. *J Clin Psychiatry, 65* (10), 1400–1405.

Zoellner, L. A., Rothbaum, B. O., and Feeny, N. C. (2011). PTSD not an anxiety disorder? DSM committee proposal turns back the hands of time. *Depress Anxiety, 28* (10), 853–856.

2

TRANSLATIONAL PERSPECTIVES ON ANXIETY DISORDERS AND THE RESEARCH DOMAIN CRITERIA CONSTRUCT OF POTENTIAL THREAT

ISABELLE M. ROSSO, DANIEL G. DILLON,
DIEGO A. PIZZAGALLI, AND SCOTT L. RAUCH

INTRODUCTION

Anxiety disorders are the most prevalent mental illnesses in the United States and a common presenting complaint in both primary and secondary medical care settings. Disorders that have anxiety as a central aspect of phenomenology are generalized anxiety disorder (GAD), obsessive compulsive disorder (OCD), panic disorder, posttraumatic stress disorder (PTSD), specific phobia, and social anxiety disorder (SAD). Most of these conditions appear during childhood and subsequently persist for years or even decades, usually following a chronic or recurring course in which full symptomatic remission is the exception rather than the rule. Over time, anxiety symptoms and disorders take their toll in the form of persistent distress, impaired social and occupational function, accumulation of comorbid conditions, and increased suicide risk (Garner, Mohler, Stein, Mueggler, and Baldwin, 2009).

Treatment for anxiety disorders is challenging because existing interventions are neither consistently beneficial nor particularly precise. Although first-line pharmacological and psychological therapies are highly efficacious for some individuals, many are left with significant residual symptoms or cannot tolerate the side effects. For instance, the most effective psychotherapy for anxiety-related disorders is cognitive-behavior therapy (CBT); however, 40% to 50% of patients do not benefit from this treatment (Walkup et al., 2008). Moreover, anti-anxiety agents are not targeted medications for particular anxiety disorders but instead are used across a number of anxiety, mood, and other psychiatric disorders. At present, clinicians have no way to reliably predict which patients will respond to which treatments, and they must therefore go through a trial-and-error process of treatment selection that often results in suboptimal treatment and high dropout rates. To date, there are no objective diagnostic tests or pathognomonic markers that can be used to diagnose any of the anxiety disorders or predict treatment response.

This state of affairs is particularly vexing given the explosion of neuroscience and genetics research that is relevant to conceptualizing the pathophysiology of psychiatric illness. Our understanding of brain circuits and their relationship with genetic and environmental factors has increased over recent decades, and we now have a grasp on the mechanisms that support behavior and cognition. We know that genes influence risk for mental illnesses, including anxiety-related disorders, and that many current psychiatric categories share genetic underpinnings (Smoller, 2013). Similarly, stress and environmental influences such as adverse life events increase the probability of multiple psychiatric disorders and interact with genetic factors to alter neural mechanisms involved in cognition and emotional processing (Gregory, Lau, and Eley, 2008).

Of relevance to anxiety disorders, there are well-replicated basic science findings on the neural circuitry that mediates functions such as aversive conditioning, context representation, physiological arousal, emotional modulation of memory, threat detection, and cognitive regulation of emotional experience (Casey, Oliveri, and Insel, 2014; Craig, 2009; Milad and Quirk, 2012; Nitschke et al., 2009; Ochsner and Gross, 2005). In parallel, the clinical literature has produced strong evidence that some aspects of anxiety disorders reflect disruptions in the neural mechanisms that underlie these processes. For example, anxiety disorders with prominent fear-related symptoms, perhaps most convincingly PTSD, involve a disruption of normative brain mechanisms that mediate fear conditioning and extinction (Rauch, Shin, & Phelps, 2006). Altogether, there is now a wealth of neuroscience data indicating that many aspects of the pathophysiology of anxiety disorders are better represented as quantitative deviations from normal cognitive-affective brain mechanisms than as qualitatively distinct patterns of brain and behavior.

The current psychiatric nosology does not reflect these advances in scientific knowledge, and its diagnostic categories have limited neurobiological validity. This should come as no surprise, because the *Diagnostic and Statistical Manual of Mental Disorders* (DSM), now in its fifth edition (American Psychiatric Association, 2013), was designed to categorize disorders based on symptoms rather than pathophysiology. In the absence of sufficient knowledge of underlying mechanisms or objective diagnostic tests, the manual created a coherent set of symptom-based categories that provided a common language for clinicians and researchers, as well as standard criteria that yielded reliable psychiatric diagnoses. Since its inception, the DSM has performed its intended functions reasonably effectively, and it remains the standard from which to diagnose and treat mental illness. At the same time, because symptom-based DSM categories do not principally reflect underlying biology, these categories have limited potential for advancing research into biological mechanisms of brain health and disease.

Indeed, none of the mechanisms enumerated above "map onto" a specific DSM diagnosis. Rather, any particular mechanism, such as deficient extinction of conditioned fear or enhanced threat appraisal bias, is implicated in not one but multiple DSM entities, thus yielding pathophysiological overlap and clinical comorbidity *across* disorders. Furthermore, each DSM category captures dysfunction in multiple mechanisms, thus yielding pathophysiological and clinical heterogeneity *within* disorders. These problems have been the subject of considerable discussion and scholarship. Prominent thought leaders, including the two most recent National Institutes of Mental Health (NIMH) directors, have characterized the DSM nosology as an impediment to progress in translational psychiatric research (Hyman, 2010; Insel et al., 2010). In short, in order to take advantage of breakthroughs in neuroscience and genetics, researchers must continue to move away from diagnoses based on symptoms and toward an understanding of psychiatric illness as emerging from deviations in the functioning of brain systems.

The Research Domain Criteria (RDoC) model embraces this perspective. Unveiled by the NIMH in 2010 (Insel et al., 2010), RDoC represents a paradigm shift by considering psychopathology from a translational point of view. Instead of symptom-based categories, RDoC offers a matrix of fundamental dimensions of behavior (rows) that were selected based on empirical evidence of both their construct validity *as well as* their correspondence with brain circuitry (Table 2.1; Cuthbert, 2014). These rows represent broad domains of function: Positive Valence Systems, Negative Valence Systems, Cognitive Systems, Systems for Social Processes, and Arousal/Regulatory Systems. The columns of the matrix list levels of analysis that can be applied to the investigation of each domain: genes, molecules, cells, circuits, physiology, behavior, and self-report. This matrix has already inspired several theoretical and empirical publications (e.g., Dillon et al., 2014; Simpson, 2012).

Importantly, the dimensional RDoC model represents mental disorders as continuous with each other and with adaptive behavioral functioning. This contrasts with the DSM approach of defining mental disorders as discrete entities, separate from each other and discontinuous from mental health. This dimensional approach reflects scientific evidence that (many) symptoms of mental illness represent quantitative variations in traits and occurrences that are normally distributed in the population (Hyman, 2010). Accordingly, psychopathology—at the group and individual level—can be characterized across levels of analysis as varying degrees of dysfunction (or deviation) in one or more of the RDoC's domains of function. Prominent alterations in Negative Valence Systems (e.g., threat processing) are well established as central to anxiety, but it is also clear that a complete clinical picture may need to incorporate dysfunctions in Positive Valence (e.g., anhedonia in PTSD), Arousal and Regulatory Systems (e.g., hyperarousal in panic disorder), Cognitive Systems (e.g., cognitive control in OCD), and Social Processes (e.g., theory of mind in SAD). In the short-term, the RDoC research framework will enable collection of data on mental (dys)function and identification of treatment targets within a neuroscientifically valid framework. In the long term, the RDoC and its descendants should support an approach that can characterize treatment-seeking individuals along each dimension, thus facilitating interventions tailored to the particular combination of behavioral and neurobiological mechanisms dysfunctional in the individual.

THE RESEARCH DOMAIN CRITERIA APPROACH TO PATHOLOGICAL ANXIETY

To illustrate how the RDoC initiative stands to reshape our approach to pathological anxiety, we focus the rest of this chapter on the RDoC domain of "potential threat," which is nested within Negative Valence Systems. "Potential threat" is a construct that relates to a key element of the phenomenology of anxiety—namely, apprehension about danger that is suspected, but remains uncertain, ambiguous, or delayed (Woody & Szechtman, 2011). We selectively review basic, translational, and clinical literatures germane to threat detection and explore how the behavioral patterns and neurocircuitry

TABLE 2.1 The RDoC Matrix

DOMAINS/CONSTRUCTS	UNITS OF ANALYSIS							
	GENES	MOLECULES	CELLS	CIRCUITS	PHYSIOLOGY	BEHAVIOR	SELF-REPORTS	PARADIGMS
NEGATIVE VALENCE SYSTEMS								
Active Threat ("fear")								
Potential threat ("anxiety")								
Sustained threat								
Loss								
Frustrative nonreward								
POSITIVE VALENCE SYSTEMS								
Approach motivation								
Initial responsiveness to reward								
Sustained responsiveness to reward								
Reward learning								
Habit								
COGNITIVE SYSTEMS								
Attention								
Perception								
Working memory								
Declarative memory								
Language behavior								
Cognitive (effortful) control								
SYSTEMS FOR SOCIAL PROCESSES								
Affiliation/attachment								
Social communication								
Perception/understanding of self								
Perception/understanding of others								
AROUSAL/MODULATORY SYSTEMS								
Arousal								
Biological rhythms								
Sleep-wake								

Source: Cuthbert (2014).

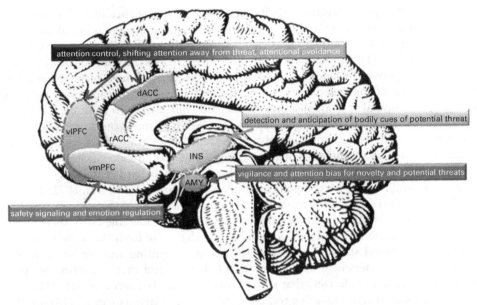

FIGURE 2.1 A schematic depiction of key brain areas involved in potential threat detection and regulation. *Note:* AMY: amygdala; INS: insula; dACC: dorsal anterior cingulate cortex; rACC: rostral anterior cingulate cortex; vlPFC: ventrolateral prefrontal cortex; vmPFC: ventromedial prefrontal cortex.

associated with this construct contribute to a dimensional, transdiagnostic approach to pathological anxiety.

Potential Threat and Its Relevance to Anxiety

Anxiety is a future-oriented affective state in which the individual prepares to cope with an uncertain but possible negative event, often in the absence of a triggering stimulus. As such, the state captured by the construct of "potential threat" can be differentiated from the fear response elicited by actual and imminent danger, which is represented separately in the RDoC matrix as the dimension of "active threat." The validity of this dichotomy is supported by factor analytic studies that show fear and anxiety as separate, though related, constructs and by animal and human neuroimaging evidence of partially disso-ciable neural systems for signaling manifest versus potential threat (Craske et al., 2009). Next we examine the potential threat construct at the behavioral and neural circuit levels of analysis and discuss therapeutic translations (Figure 2.1, see also Dillon et al., 2014).

Potential Threat as a Translational Construct: Risk Assessment Across Mammalian Species

In the wild, danger is ever present and lapses in vigilance can be deadly; thus organisms must have systems to detect threats. Anxiety is experienced when a threat is suspected, but the full-fledged fear response typically emerges only when an imminent threat is detected (Eilam, Izhar, and Mort, 2011; Woody and Szechtman, 2011). Consequently, survival depends on the organism possessing a motivational system that emphasizes threat assessment and that is biased toward perceiving threats, even at the expense of a high false alarm rate (Eilam et al., 2011).

Suspicion of a potential threat elicits an orchestrated sequence of "risk assessment" behaviors in all mammalian species. Specifically, animals immediately orient toward the threat and engage in sustained vigilance and risk analysis (Blanchard, Griebel, Pobbe, and Blanchard, 2011). The outcome of this assessment shapes the selection of an adaptive behavioral response. If a potential threat is still suspected, the most adaptive behavioral response is one of continued risk analysis and engagement of precautionary behaviors that keep the animal at a safe distance (Blanchard et al., 2011). In contrast, if a threat's existence is confirmed, a defensive response is elicited to move the animal away from the danger (flight, freeze) or to directly attack (fight). Importantly, if a potential threat is determined to be absent or innocuous, disengagement of threat assessment behaviors and a return to nondefensiveness is the adaptive route (Blanchard et al., 2011).

Anxiety and fear are homologous in animals and humans (Darwin, 1872; Eilam et al., 2011). With respect to potential threat, humans engage risk assessment processes similar to those of other mammals, and there is also considerable cross-species overlap in the precautionary and defensive behaviors that arise from threat detection. An ambiguous or novel stimulus will draw attentional orienting and vigilant scanning, followed by risk assessment and exploratory behavior, and then activation of appropriate precautionary behaviors that will ultimately generate a sense of safety (Eilam et al., 2011). Interestingly, adaptive responses to potential threats can be characterized as early as the second year of life, and they have been described as a temperamental phenotype called behavioral inhibition or anxious temperament (Fox and Kalin, 2014; Kagan, Reznick, and Snidman, 1987). Behavioral inhibition manifests as timid and cautious behavior upon exposure to novel stimuli that are neutral and ambiguous. Children with extreme behavioral inhibition, meaning that they react to novelty with excessive shyness and avoidance, are at heightened risk of later developing an anxiety disorder, particularly social anxiety.

Anxiety-related disorders are marked by increased vigilance to potential threats. Pathological anxiety is characterized by faster attentional engagement to threat cues, impaired disengagement from threat, biased appraisal of neutral stimuli as threatening, and attentional avoidance of threat stimuli (Bar-Haim, Lamy, Pergamin, Bakermans-Kranenburg, and Van Ijzendoorn, 2007; Cisler and Koster, 2010; Craske et al., 2009). Moreover, an attentional threat bias seems to be a common feature across adult anxiety disorders, although the content of the bias varies between disorders (e.g., bodily symptoms in panic disorder, trauma-related cues in PTSD, angry faces in SAD). A meta-analysis of studies that used attention-capture paradigms (e.g., emotional Stroop, dot-probe task) concluded that clinically and subclinically anxious children and adults show a reliable threat-related attention bias (Bar-Haim et al., 2007), a bias that is exaggerated in comparison to a normative threat detection system that already leans toward false alarms. Interestingly, some research suggests that this threat sensitivity may manifest as an early attention-orienting response toward threat, followed by a shifting of attention away from threat (Mueller et al., 2009). In addition, the nature of the attentional bias appears to vary across development, as clinically anxious children exhibit a greater attentional bias *away* from threat, in contrast to the bias toward threat that is observed in anxious adults (Monk et al., 2006; Pine et al., 2005).

These empirical findings converge with longstanding cognitive models of anxiety disorder-related behaviors as arising from biased threat assessment and exaggerated precautionary or defensive behaviors (e.g., Beck & Clark, 1997). For instance, excessive worry in GAD, hypervigilance in PTSD, and obsessions in OCD reflect excessive engagement of risk assessment systems and/or failure to disengage these behaviors, together with a sustained (but illusory) sense of threat (Blanchard et al., 2011; Eilam et al., 2011). Similarly, the rituals and compulsions seen in OC spectrum disorders may represent a failure to cease precautionary behaviors due to an absence of feedback or "sense of knowing" that the necessary precautions have been completed (Woody & Szechtman, 2011).

In summary, there is evidence that anxiety-related disorders as operationalized in the DSM all involve aberrant detection and orienting toward potential threat, and/or failure to disengage threat assessment mechanisms appropriately, perhaps depending upon the context or the type of threat (e.g., threat of injury, contamination, social status loss, or homeostatic disruption). In this case, neurobiological mechanisms of threat detection and precautionary action could serve as pathophysiologically relevant dimensions and intermediate phenotypes in a new research framework (and ultimately nosology).

Brain Circuitry of Potential Threat

The amygdala–ventrolateral prefrontal cortex (vlPFC) circuit plays a critical role in mediating vigilance for threat. Long implicated in threat appraisal during fear conditioning, the amygdala is now more broadly conceptualized as playing a role in stimulus-driven (bottom-up) attentional capture of emotionally evocative stimuli, including (but not restricted to) cues of potential threat (LeDoux, 1996). Also relevant is the amygdala's involvement in the evaluation of uncertainty and ambiguity (Whalen et al., 1998). For instance, intolerance of uncertainty is associated with significantly higher amygdala activity in both healthy subjects and patients with pathological anxiety (Krain et al., 2008). Similarly, adults who had displayed extreme behavioral inhibition at 2 years old show a stronger bilateral amygdala response to novel faces than their uninhibited counterparts (Schwartz, Wright, Shin, Kagan, & Rauch, 2003). Amygdala hyperactivity is seen across a number of DSM anxiety-related disorders (e.g., Etkin et al., 2004; Rauch, Shin, and Wright, 2003; Stein, Simmons, Feinstein, and Paulus, 2007), suggesting that it may relate to shared phenotype(s) such as attentional threat biases. In functional magnetic resonance imaging (fMRI) paradigms designed to measure such biases, subjects with anxiety disorders show increased amygdala activation that is positively correlated with both anxiety levels and attentional threat bias (Monk et al., 2006, 2008). Clinically anxious patients also show higher activation of the amygdala than healthy subjects while anticipating potentially aversive stimuli (Nitschke et al., 2009). In addition, compared to nonanxious individuals, highly anxious adults generate a stronger amygdala response to fearful, angry, and *happy* faces, consistent with the concept that they detect threats where none exist (Stein et al., 2007). Overall, there is a strong foundation for considering amygdala function as related to an individual's automatic detection and vigilance to potential threats.

The vlPFC is thought to facilitate emotional regulation by controlling top-down attentional control during threat processing, which modulates amygdala engagement (Britton, Lissek, Grillon, Norcross, and Pine, 2011; Monk et al., 2006, 2008). Indeed, there is substantial animal and human neuroimaging work showing that the vlPFC regulates amygdala activity during threat processing (Monk et al., 2008). In fMRI studies, activity and connectivity of the vlPFC and amygdala are negatively correlated during threat processing (Monk et al., 2008). In response to cues of potential threat, anxious adolescents show less negative coupling of vlPFC and amygdala activity, as well as greater activity of the vlPFC than nonanxious control subjects (Britton et al., 2011; Monk et al., 2006, 2008). Moreover, aberrant response of the vlPFC to threat cues is correlated with behavioral threat bias scores in anxious subjects (Fani et al., 2012; Monk et al., 2008). These and other studies suggest that vlPFC modulation of amygdala activity is disrupted in clinical anxiety and represents underlying mechanism(s) of observable attentional threat biases in anxious individuals. Increased recruitment of lateral prefrontal cortex and functionally related areas, such as anterior cingulate cortex, have been posited as mechanisms of particular relevance to difficulties with regulation of attentional control, including difficulty disengaging attention from threat and attentional avoidance of threatening stimuli (Cisler & Koster, 2010; Fani et al., 2012). Altogether this suggests that individual differences in lateral frontal function are relevant to understanding human variation in anxiety-related disruption of attentional biases to threat, including the ability to volitionally direct attention toward or away from threatening stimuli.

There is substantial evidence that medial aspects of the frontal cortex also play a role in top-down regulation of responses to potential threats. Medial frontal areas, including the subgenual and rostral anterior cingulate, are involved in dampening emotional responses that are driven by the amygdala (Rauch et al., 2006). Anxiety-prone individuals show reduced activation of these areas in response to ambiguous affective stimuli (Simmons, Matthews, Paulus, and Stein, 2008), as do individuals with PTSD (Etkin & Wager, 2007; Shin, Rauch, and Pitman, 2006). Moreover, activation of the ventromedial prefrontal cortex is negatively correlated with amygdala activation to emotional stimuli in PTSD (Shin et al., 2006), suggesting reduced capacity to maintain effective top-down regulation of limbic reactivity (Rauch et al., 2006). In healthy subjects viewing predictable and unpredictable negative and neutral pictures, medial frontal/anterior cingulate response is stronger when anxiety is lowest (neutral/predictable condition) and weaker when anxiety is highest (negative/unpredictable condition) (Somerville et al., 2013). Overall, the literature supports a role for the medial prefrontal cortex in safety signaling, accomplished by dampening the threat signaling generated by the amygdala.

The neuroimaging literature has also implicated the insula, particularly its anterior extent, as a neural substrate of anticipation of potential threats (Carlson, Greenberg, Rubin, and Mujica-Parodi, 2011). This is consistent with a literature showing that the anterior insula mediates individuals' conscious appraisal and prediction of their interoceptive and affective feeling states, including aversive bodily sensations and anxiety (Craig, 2002). Paulus and Stein (2006) have summarized evidence that individuals who are prone to anxiety show a biased appraisal of internal bodily sensations as dangerous, leading to erroneous predictions of future aversive bodily states, which ultimately manifests as anxiety. These errors in appraising the interoceptive state are posited to be due to increased sensitivity to physical sensations of anxiety, a trait known as anxiety sensitivity (Stein et al., 2007). Functional MRI studies have shown that higher anxiety sensitivity is associated with increased activation of the bilateral insula in both healthy and anxiety-disordered subjects (Killgore et al., 2011; Simmons et al., 2008). Insula activation is also observed when anticipating aversive and neutral auditory stimuli, altogether suggesting that the insula is critical in processing many aspects of potential threat, including ambiguity, uncertainty, and anticipation. Moreover, there is evidence that anterior insula volume and thickness are significantly correlated with anxiety sensitivity in both healthy subjects and clinically anxious patients (Rosso et al., 2010). Thus, variability in insula function and structure appears to be sensitive to individual differences in a proclivity to monitor the internal environment for potential "threats," such as bodily sensations of anxiety.

In summary, we have highlighted some of the brain regions and circuits that have emerged from functional imaging research on the neural basis of potential threat detection. There is evidence that limbic and subcortical structures, including the amygdala and insular cortex, mediate automatic vigilance and detection of threatening cues and that their heightened activity in anxiety-related disorders underlies excessive or facilitated detection of threat. Similarly, several frontal cortical regions have been implicated in attentional control and emotion regulatory mechanisms, and dysfunction of these areas is related to difficulty determining that a stimulus is safe and decreased ability to adaptively direct attention toward and away from threat.

TARGETING POTENTIAL THREAT IN THERAPY: NEUROBIOLOGICALLY INFORMED TREATMENT SELECTION

There is burgeoning evidence that manipulating attentional threat biases modulates anxiety levels. Research has shown that teaching clinically anxious individuals to attend preferentially to non-threat cues can ameliorate their attentional threat biases and reduce their anxiety. These findings are fueling excitement about attention-bias-modification treatment (ABMT), a computer-based attention training program, as a promising treatment for individuals with clinical anxiety (for reviews of attention bias models and ABMT, see (Cisler & Koster, 2010; Hakamata et al., 2010). One aspect that is particularly relevant to translational approaches such as RDoC is that ABMT was developed based on the behavioral and neuroscience literatures on threat detection, and that it targets neural mechanisms of threat-related attentional biases.

Based on neurocognitive models of attention control (Cisler and Koster, 2010), the therapeutic effects of ABMT and similar interventions could be mediated by alterations of either subcortical threat signaling or prefrontal cortical regulation. Among two studies that examined how ABMT modifies neural systems of threat detection, both found evidence that training affected top-down attentional processes mediated by higher-order cortical areas including the lateral prefrontal cortex (Browning, Holmes, Murphy, Goodwin, and Harmer, 2010; Eldar et al., 2012). In a parallel literature, mindfulness-based interventions, which also focus on redirecting attention, have been shown capable of modulating the activation and connectivity of brain regions implicated in bottom-up threat reactivity and regulation, including the amygdala, insula, anterior cingulate cortex, and medial and lateral prefrontal cortices (reviewed in Chiesa, Serretti, and Jakobsen, 2013). Thus, while many early studies have aimed to test whether attention training affects threat biases via bottom-up *versus* top-down mechanisms, there seems to be a strong case building for both possibilities.

CONCLUSIONS

Unlike many fields of medicine, psychiatry has not yet reached the goal of providing precision or personalized treatment based on knowledge of pathophysiology (Insel et al., 2010). However, we do have considerable understanding of the mechanisms that underlie many behavioral, cognitive, and affective functions known to be centrally implicated in psychopathology. Consequently, the NIMH's RDoC research matrix has emerged from both need and readiness to provide a biologically meaningful way to organize symptoms of mental illness, specifically on the basis of dimensional measures of behavior and brain circuitry, that represent a full range of normal to abnormal functioning. This is a broad departure from the symptom-based categorical DSM approach. Currently RDoC is positioned not as a diagnostic system, but as a research framework for facilitating the translation of basic and clinical neuroscience findings to clinical diagnosis and treatment. Ultimately, this approach is expected to lead to an improved nosology and the development of personalized treatments.

We have presented in this chapter an overview of how clinical anxiety symptoms can be related to attentional threat biases and to dysfunction of the neurocircuitry that supports threat detection and regulation mechanisms. These mechanisms include automatic processes that facilitate detection of potential threats, as well as volitional processes that allow strategic attentional allocation toward and away from threat in order to modulate emotional response. Although the attentional bias literature is still an evolving one, it provides a useful heuristic for understanding how RDoC stands to reshape our approach to anxiety in a manner that supports translation from mechanism to treatment. That is, identifying individuals based on a behavioral measure such as attentional threat bias, as opposed to self-reported symptoms, should produce a more homogeneous group in terms of underlying brain mechanism(s) and therefore represent a more useful target for treatment selection. Similarly, development of novel treatments can also target specific mechanisms, which would be relevant to specific symptoms rather than particular DSM disorders. Importantly, designing RDoC studies presents many challenges and requires sweeping changes in research design. The NIMH provides examples of RDoC studies on its website to aid researchers with this transition (including the task of ascertaining subject samples differently than the traditional recruitment based on categorical diagnosis). As the research field transitions progressively toward RDoC formulations that can incorporate knowledge of brain-behavior relationships, there is reason for optimism that a new generation of neurobiologically inspired treatments of mental illness will emerge.

DISCLOSURE STATEMENT

Over the past three years, Dr. Pizzagalli has received honoraria/consulting fees from Advanced Neuro Technology North America, AstraZeneca, Pfizer, and Servier for activities unrelated to this project. Drs. Rosso, Dillon, and Rauch have no conflicts of interest to report.

ACKNOWLEDGMENTS

Dr. Rosso was partially supported by NIMH R01 MH096987 as well as a Brain and Immuno-Imaging grant from the Dana Foundation. Dr. Dillon was partially supported by NIMH grant R00 MH094438. Dr. Pizzagalli was partially supported by NIMH grants R01 MH101521 and R01 MH068376, as well as a Clinical Neuroscience Research Grant from the Dana Foundation. Dr. Rauch was partially supported by DOD grant W81XWH-12-1-0109.

REFERENCES

American Psychiatric Association (2013). *Diagnostic and statistical manual of mental disorders, fifth edition*. Arlington, VA: American Psychiatric Publishing.

Bar-Haim, Y., Lamy, D., Pergamin, L., Bakermans-Kranenburg, M. J., and Van Ijzendoorn, M. H. (2007). Threat-related attentional bias in anxious and nonanxious individuals: A meta-analytic study. *Psychol Bull, 133* (1), 1. Retrieved from http://people.socsci.tau.ac.il/mu/anxietytrauma/files/2013/08/Bar-Haim-et-al-2007-Psychological-Bulletin.pdf

Beck, A. T., and Clark, D. A. (1997). An information processing model of anxiety: Automatic and strategic processes. *Behav Res Ther, 35*(1), 48–58. Retrieved from http://www.sciencedirect.com/science/article/pii/S0005796796000691

Blanchard, D. C., Griebel, G., Pobbe, R., and Blanchard, R. J. (2011). Risk assessment as an evolved threat detection and analysis process. *Neurosci Biobehav Rev, 35* (4), 991–998. doi:10.1016/j.neubiorev.2010.10.016

Britton, J. C., Lissek, S., Grillon, C., Norcross, M. A., and Pine, D. S. (2011). Development of anxiety: The role of threat appraisal and fear learning. *Depress Anxiety, 28* (1), 5–17. doi:10.1002/da.20733

Browning, M., Holmes, E. A., Murphy, S. E., Goodwin, G. M., and Harmer, C. J. (2010). Lateral prefrontal cortex mediates the cognitive modification of attentional bias. *Biol Psychiatry, 67* (10), 919–925. doi:10.1016/j.biopsych.2009.10.031

Carlson, J. M., Greenberg, T., Rubin, D., and Mujica-Parodi, L. R. (2011). Feeling anxious: anticipatory amygdalo-insular response predicts the feeling of anxious anticipation. *Soc Cogn Affect Neurosci, 6*(1), 74–81.

Casey, B. J., Oliveri, M. E., and Insel, T. (2014). A Neurodevelopmental perspective on the research domain criteria (RDoC) framework. *Biol Psychiatry, 76* (5), 350–353. doi:10.1016/j.biopsych.2014.01.006

Chiesa, A., Serretti, A., and Jakobsen, J. C. (2013). Mindfulness: Top-down or bottom-up emotion regulation strategy? *Clin Psychol Rev, 33* (1), 82–96. doi:10.1016/j.cpr.2012.10.006

Cisler, J. M., and Koster, E. H. (2010). Mechanisms of attentional biases towards threat in anxiety disorders: An integrative review. *Clin Psychol Rev, 30* (2), 203–216. doi:10.1016/j.cpr.2009.11.003

Craig, A. D. (2002). How do you feel? Interoception: The sense of the physiological condition of the body. *Nat Rev Neurosci, 3* (8), 655–666. doi:10.1038/nrn894

Craig, A. D. (2009). How do you feel—now? The anterior insula and human awareness. *Nat Rev Neurosci, 10* (1), 59–70. doi:10.1038/nrn2555

Craske, M. G., Rauch, S. L., Ursano, R., Prenoveau, J., Pine, D. S., and Zinbarg, R. E. (2009). What is an anxiety disorder? *Depress Anxiety, 26* (12), 1066–1085. doi:10.1002/da.20633

Cuthbert, B. N. (2014). The RDoC framework: Facilitating transition from ICD/DSM to dimensional approaches that integrate neuroscience and psychopathology. *World Psychiatry, 13,* 28–35. doi:10.1002/wps.20087

Darwin, C. (1998/1872). *The expression of emotions in man and animals.* New York: Oxford University Press.

Dillon, D. G., Rosso, I. M., Pechtel, P., Killgore, W. D., Rauch, S. L., and Pizzagalli, D. A. (2014). Peril and pleasure: An RDoC-inspired examination of threat responses and reward processing in anxiety and depression. *Depress Anxiety, 31* (3), 233–249. doi:10.1002/da.22202

Eilam, D., Izhar, R., and Mort, J. (2011). Threat detection: Behavioral practices in animals and humans. *Neurosci Biobehav Rev, 35* (4), 999–1006. doi:10.1016/j.neubiorev.2010.08.002

Eldar, S., Apter, A., Lotan, D., Edgar, K. P., Naim, R., Fox, N. A., . . . Bar-Haim, Y. (2012). Attention bias modification treatment for pediatric anxiety disorders: A randomized controlled trial. *American Journal of Psychiatry, 169,* 213–220. doi:10.1176/appi.ajp.2011.11060886

Etkin, A., Klemenhagen, K. C., Dudman, J. T., Rogan, M. T., Hen, R., Kandel, E. R., and Hirsch, J. (2004). Individual differences in trait anxiety predict the response of the basolateral amygdala to unconsciously processed fearful faces. *Neuron, 44* (6), 1043–1055. doi:10.1016/j.neuron.2004.12.006

Etkin, A., and Wager, T. D. (2007). Functional neuroimaging of anxiety: A meta-analysis of emotional processing in PTSD, social anxiety disorder, and specific phobia. *Am J Psychiatry, 164* (10), 1476–1488. doi:10.1176/appi.ajp.2007.07030504

Fani, N., Jovanovic, T., Ely, T. D., Bradley, B., Gutman, D., Tone, E. B., and Ressler, K. J. (2012). Neural correlates of attention bias to threat in post-traumatic stress disorder. *Biol Psychol, 90* (2), 134–142. doi:10.1016/j.biopsycho.2012.03.001

Fox, A. S., & Kalin, N. H. (2014). A translational neuroscience approach to understanding the development of social anxiety disorder and its pathophysiology. *Am J Psychiatry.* doi: 10.1176/appi.ajp.2014.14040449. [Epub ahead of print]

Garner, M., Mohler, H., Stein, D. J., Mueggler, T., and Baldwin, D. S. (2009). Research in anxiety disorders: From the bench to the bedside. *Eur Neuropsychopharmacol, 19* (6), 381–390. doi:10.1016/j.euroneuro.2009.01.011

Gregory, A. M., Lau, J. Y., and Eley, T. C. (2008). Finding gene-environment interactions for generalised anxiety disorder. *Eur Arch Psychiatry Clin Neurosci, 258* (2), 69–75. doi:10.1007/s00406-007-0785-4

Hakamata, Y., Lissek, S., Bar-Haim, Y., Britton, J. C., Fox, N. A., Leibenluft, E., . . . Pine, D. S. (2010). Attention bias modification treatment: A meta-analysis toward the establishment of novel treatment for anxiety. *Biol Psychiatry, 68* (11), 982–990. doi:10.1016/j.biopsych.2010.07.021

Hyman, S. E. (2010). The diagnosis of mental disorders: The problem of reification. *Annu Rev Clin Psychol, 6*, 155–179. doi:10.1146/annurev.clinpsy.3.022806.091532

Insel, T., Cuthbert, B., Garvey, M., Heinssen, R., Pine, D. S., Quinn, K., . . . Wang, P. (2010). Research domain criteria (RDoC): Toward a new classification framework for research on mental disorders. *Am J Psychiatry, 167* (7), 748–751. doi:10.1176/appi.ajp.2010.09091379

Kagan, J., Reznick, J. S., and Snidman, N. (1987). The physiology and psychology of behavioral inhibition in children. *Child Dev, 58*, 1459–1473. doi:10.2307/1130685

Killgore, W. D., Britton, J. C., Price, L. M., Gold, A. L., Deckersbach, T., and Rauch, S. L. (2011). Neural correlates of anxiety sensitivity during masked presentation of affective faces. *Depress Anxiety, 28* (3), 243–249. doi:10.1002/da.20788

Krain, A. L., Gotimer, K., Hefton, S., Ernst, M., Castellanos, F. X., Pine, D. S., and Milham, M. P. (2008). A functional magnetic resonance imaging investigation of uncertainty in adolescents with anxiety disorders. *Biol Psychiatry, 63* (6), 563–568. doi:10.1016/j.biopsych.2007.06.011

LeDoux, J. E. (1996). *The emotional brain: the mysterious underpinnings of emotional life.* New York: Simon and Schuster.

Milad, M. R., & Quirk, G. J. (2012). Fear extinction as a model for translational neuroscience: Ten years of progress. *Annu Rev Psychol, 63*, 129–151. doi:10.1146/annurev.psych.121208.131631

Monk, C. S., Nelson, E. E., McClure, E. B., Mogg, K., Bradley, B. P., Leibenluft, E., . . . Pine, D. S. (2006). Ventrolateral prefrontal cortex activation and attentional bias in response to angry faces in adolescents with generalized anxiety disorder. *Am J Psychiatry, 163* (6), 1091–1097. doi:10.1176/appi.ajp.163.6.1091

Monk, C. S., Telzer, E. H., Mogg, K., Bradley, B. P., Mai, X., Louro, H. M., . . . Pine, D. S. (2008). Amygdala and ventrolateral prefrontal cortex activation to masked angry faces in children and adolescents with generalized anxiety disorder. *Arch Gen Psychiatry, 65* (5), 568–576. doi:10.1001/archpsyc.65.5.568

Mueller, E. M., Hofmann, S. G., Santesso, D. L., Meuret, A. E., Bitran, S., and Pizzagalli, D. A. (2009). Electrophysiological evidence of attentional biases in social anxiety disorder. *Psychological Medicine, 39*, 1141–1152. doi:10.1017/S0033291708004820

Nitschke, J. B., Sarinopoulos, I., Oathes, D. J., Johnstone, T., Whalen, P. J., Davidson, R. J., and Kalin, N. H. (2009). Anticipatory activation in the amygdala and anterior cingulate in generalized anxiety disorder and prediction of treatment response. *Am J Psychiatry, 166* (3), 302–310. doi:10.1176/appi.ajp.2008.07101682

Ochsner, K. N., and Gross, J. J. (2005). The cognitive control of emotion. *Trends Cogn Sci, 9* (5), 242–249. doi:10.1016/j.tics.2005.03.010

Paulus, M. P., and Stein, M. B. (2006). An insular view of anxiety. *Biol Psychiatry, 60* (4), 383–387. doi:10.1016/j.biopsych.2006.03.04210.1016/j.biopsych.2006.03.042

Pine, D. S., Mogg, K., Bradley, B. P., Montgomery, L., Monk, C. S., McClure, E., . . . Kaufman, J. (2005). Attention bias to threat in maltreated children: Implications for vulnerability to stress-related psychopathology. *Am J Psychiatry, 162* (2), 291–296. doi:10.1176/appi.ajp.162.2.291

Rauch, S. L., Shin, L. M., and Phelps, E. A. (2006). Neurocircuitry models of posttraumatic stress disorder and extinction: human neuroimaging research—past, present, and future. *Biol Psychiatry, 60* (4), 376–382. doi:10.1016/j.biopsych.2006.06.004

Rauch, S. L., Shin, L. M., and Wright, C. I. (2003). Neuroimaging studies of amygdala function in anxiety disorders. *Ann N Y Acad Sci, 985*, 389–410. Retrieved from http://www.ncbi.nlm.nih.gov/entrez/query.fcgi?cmd=Retrieve&db=PubMed&dopt=Citation&list_uids=12724173

Rosso, I. M., Makris, N., Britton, J. C., Price, L. M., Gold, A. L., Zai, D., ... Rauch, S. L. (2010). Anxiety sensitivity correlates with two indices of right anterior insula structure in specific animal phobia. *Depress Anxiety, 27* (12), 1104–1110. doi:10.1002/da.20765

Schwartz, C. E., Wright, C. I., Shin, L. M., Kagan, J., and Rauch, S. L. (2003). Inhibited and uninhibited infants "grown up": Adult amygdalar response to novelty. *Science, 300,* 1952–1953. doi:10.1126/science.1083703

Shin, L. M., Rauch, S. L., and Pitman, R. K. (2006). Amygdala, medial prefrontal cortex, and hippocampal function in PTSD. *Ann N Y Acad Sci, 1071,* 67–79. doi:10.1196/annals.1364.007

Simmons, A., Matthews, S. C., Paulus, M. P., and Stein, M. B. (2008). Intolerance of uncertainty correlates with insula activation during affective ambiguity. *Neurosci Lett, 430* (2), 92–97. doi:10.1016/j.neulet.2007.10.030 10.1016/j.neulet.2007.10.030

Simpson, H. B. (2012). The RDoC project: A new paradigm for investigating the pathophysiology of anxiety. *Depress Anxiety, 29* (4), 251–252. doi:10.1002/da.21935

Smoller, J. W. (2013). Disorders and borders: Psychiatric genetics and nosology. *American Journal of Medical Genetics, Part B: Neuropsychiatric Genetics, 162,* 559–578. doi:10.1002/ajmg.b.32174

Somerville, L. H., Wagner, D. D., Wig, G. S., Moran, J. M., Whalen, P. J., and Kelley, W. M. (2013). Interactions between transient and sustained neural signals support the generation and regulation of anxious emotion. *Cereb Cortex, 23* (1), 49–60. doi:10.1093/cercor/bhr373

Stein, M. B., Simmons, A. N., Feinstein, J. S., and Paulus, M. P. (2007). Increased amygdala and insula activation during emotion processing in anxiety-prone subjects. *Am J Psychiatry, 164* (2), 318–327. doi:10.1176/appi.ajp.164.2.318 10.1176/appi.ajp.164.2.318

Walkup, J. T., Albano, A. M., Piacentini, J., Birmaher, B., Compton, S. N., Sherrill, J. T., ... Kendall, P. C. (2008). Cognitive behavioral therapy, sertraline, or a combination in childhood anxiety. *The New England Journal of Medicine, 359,* 2753–2766. doi:10.1056/NEJMoa0804633

Whalen, P. J., Rauch, S. L., Etcoff, N. L., McInerney, S. C., Lee, M. B., and Jenike, M. A. (1998). Masked presentations of emotional facial expressions modulate amygdala activity without explicit knowledge. *J Neurosci, 18* (1), 411–418. Retrieved from http://www.ncbi.nlm.nih.gov/entrez/query.fcgi?cmd=Retrieve&db=PubMed&dopt=Citation&list_uids=9412517

Woody, E. Z., and Szechtman, H. (2011). Adaptation to potential threat: The evolution, neurobiology, and psychopathology of the security motivation system. *Neurosci Biobehav Rev, 35*(4), 1019–1033. doi:10.1016/j.neubiorev.2010.08.003

NEUROBIOLOGY AND NEURAL CIRCUITRY OF ANXIETY DISORDERS

3

NEUROBIOLOGY AND NEUROIMAGING OF FEAR AND ANXIETY CIRCUITRY

K. LUAN PHAN

INTRODUCTION

Anxiety can be conceived as a broad set of responses (subjective self-report, peripheral reactions, and unpleasant sensation) that reflect reactions to a sense of threat—external or internal. This sense can be temporally sustained/free-floating or acute/phasic. Responses involving anxiety and/or fear are often adaptive, but when they are out of context, exaggerated, inappropriately timed, and/or irrational, they can cause dysfunction. A comprehensive understanding of the continuum of anxiety and fear, from adaptive to maladaptive forms, incorporates both expression and regulation of these negative emotions. Moreover, it should also incorporate the current thinking about nosology, the *Diagnostic and Statistical Manual of Mental Disorders* (DSM-5), and the National Institute of Mental Health's Research Domain Criteria (RDoC) initiative (see Section 1). Anxiety disorders include specific phobia (SP), panic disorder (PD), social anxiety disorder (SAD), generalized anxiety disorder (GAD), posttraumatic stress disorder (PTSD), and obsessive compulsive disorder (OCD).

This chapter reviews data from neuroimaging, neuroendocrinology, and neuropsychopharmacology. By using positron emission tomography (PET), magnetic resonance imaging (MRI, functional and structural) and magnetic resonance spectroscopy (MRS), scientists can map multiple aspects of the brain and leverage knowledge in basic neuroscience (Box 3.1). Historically, psychiatric neuroscience has pursued disorder-specific approaches, which reveal complexity and heterogeneity of findings. While some anxiety disorders have been investigated at greater depth than others, there is both consistency and convergence in the available research.

Imaging studies have used behavioral paradigms to probe threat perception (e.g., angry/fearful faces), fear acquisition (e.g., pairing aversive stimuli and neutral stimuli to produce a conditioned response), and aversive-affect processing (e.g., emotional pictures, imagery). More recently, paradigms examine the regulation of these processes. Sufficient data have accrued to support quantitative meta-analyses that relate anxiety to individual differences in several key regions—amygdala, insula (INS), hippocampus (HPC), ventral striatum (VS), bed nucleus stria terminalis (BNST), anterior cingulate cortex (ACC), ventral and dorsal medial prefrontal cortex (VMPFC and DMPFC, respectively), dorsolateral prefrontal cortex (DLPFC), and ventro-lateral prefrontal cortex (VLPFC) (Figure 3.1) (see reviews/meta-analyses in healthy controls: Phan et al., 2002; Kober et al., 2008; Sabatinelli et al., 2011; Diekhof et al., 2011; Etkin et al., 2011; Calder, Lawrence, and Young, 2001; Costafreda et al., 2008; Sergerie et al., 2008; Etkin 2007; and across anxiety disorders: Etkin and Wager, 2007; Etkin, 2010; Shin and Liberzon, 2010; Engel et al., 2009). Complementary neuroimaging approaches support models of dynamic interactions among brain regions. These models suggest that fear-generating and fear-processing brain structures (amygdala, INS, VS, BNST, ACC) integrate sensory, affective, and motivational signals; they are regulated by higher cognitive centers of the brain (VMPFC, DMPFC, DLPFC, VLPFC) to support appraisal, planning, decision making, cognitive, and attentional control. In particular, the amygdala has been consistently implicated in the perception of danger cues and the generation of fear/anxiety, while the INS and BNST have been posited to instantiate the integration of interoceptive states and the anticipation of aversive states (e.g., pending danger, unpredictable

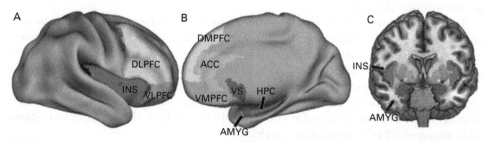

FIGURE 3.1 Key brain regions involved in fear, anxiety, and negative affect and their regulation: (A) lateral view; (B) medial view; (C) coronal view. Amygdala (amygdala), insula (INS), hippocampus (HPC), ventral striatum (VS), anterior cingulate cortex (ACC), ventral medial prefrontal cortex (VMPFC), dorsal medial prefrontal cortex and (DMPFC), dorsolateral prefrontal cortex (DLPFC), ventro-lateral prefrontal cortex (VLPFC).

threat). Although precisely how these interconnected regions produce anxiety and fear remains poorly understood, a growing number of data implicate neurotransmitters, such as γ-amino-butyric-acid (GABA), glutamate (Glu), serotonin (5-hydroxytryptamine, 5-HT), norepinephrine (NE), and dopamine (DA), as well as neuropeptides such as cholecystokinin (CCK), neuropeptide Y (NPY), arginine vasopressin (AVP), oxytocin (OXT), and cortico-tropin-releasing factor (CRF); and neurohormones/neurosteroids such as adrenocorticotropic hormone (ACTH), cortisol (CORT), and allopregnano-lone/pregnanolone (ALLO) (see reviews/meta-analyses: Bakermans-Kranenburg and van IJzendoorn, 2013; Cortese and Phan, 2005; Durant et al., 2010; Griebel and Holmes, 2013; Kim and Gorman, 2005; Kormos and Gaszner, 2013; Martin et al., 2010; Pego et al., 2010; Pitman et al., 2012; Risbrough and Stein, 2006; Elnazer and Baldwin, 2014; Neumann and Landgraf, 2012).

Recent developments emphasize the neural systems level, which leverages the multi-layered, interconnected nature of these findings. As reflected in this chapter, this empha-sis allows scientists to aggregate the anxiety disorders based on shared features while highlighting the distinctions.

NEUROCIRCUITRY OF FEAR AND EMOTION

Contemporary brain-based models of fear, anxiety, and other negative emotional states consider a fronto-limbic circuit involving prefrontal (DLPFC, VLPFC, DMPFC, VMPFC including orbitofrontal cortex [OFC]), limbic (amygdala, HPC, VS, ACC), and paralimbic areas such as INS and BNST. This chapter reviews aspects of these models relevant to fear, anxiety, and their regulation (Phan et al., 2002; Sabatinelli et al., 2011; Diekhof et al., 2011; Etkin et al., 2011; Calder and Lawrence, 2001; Costafreda et al., 20008; Sergerie et al., 2008; Etkin 2007).

Key among the subcortical structures is the amygdala, a phylogenetically old "alarm" sys-tem implicated in the detection and perception of stimuli relevant to an organism's goals, including the acquisition of learned fear (Calder and Lawrence, 2001; Davis and Whalen, 2001; Pessoa and Adolphs, 2010). Because some studies have shown that the amygdala is especially sensitive to threat-related information, the amygdala has been characterized as functioning to protect the organism from danger. However, other data temper these views. First, damage to the amygdala does not necessarily change the subjective experience of fear. Second, the amygdala appears to play a prominent role in positive emotions. Third, other "emotional" stimuli engage the amygdala, including neutral and surprised faces, suggest-ing involvement in vigilance or the decoding of ambiguity. That said, these caveats do not exclude the link of amygdala and fear, given that danger and threats evoking fear and anxi-ety just happen to be the most salient, motivational signals requiring immediate attention and disambiguation. Within the medial temporal lobe, the HPC communicates with the amygdala to support consolidation of declarative information and other aspects of memory. Similarly, the INS communicates somatic sensations elicited by emotional stimuli that are linked to homeostasis (Craig, 2002). The INS has been associated with visceral states and interoceptive awareness and, more broadly, the experience of negative emotion. Increasing evidence has implicated the insula as particularly important for "internally generated" emo-tions, such as aversive anticipation, somatic sensations, and anxiety sensitivity (Paulus and Stein, 2006).

The prefrontal cortex (PFC) is located anterior to the brain's motor areas; it is involved in higher-level cognitive tasks and interacts with limbic cortices through rich anatomical connections (Fuster et al., 2013). The medial prefrontal cortex (MPFC) is commonly activated during emotional tasks and is associated with the cognitive aspects of emotion processing. Specifically, the MPFC may integrate affective estimations of the stimulus generated by the amygdala and VS with valuations from other regions of the brain, including medial temporal regions (e.g., HPC); the VLPFC may allocate attention to salient stimuli. The DLPFC relays goal-related information and regulates emotion as appropriate. By contextualizing the affective valuation of a stimulus in terms of prior experience and current behavioral goals, the MPFC contributes to adaptive behavior. Specifically, the dorsal MPFC (DMPFC) has been associated with self-awareness and perspective taking, whereas the ventral MPFC (VMPFC) is associated with personal and social decision making, regulation of emotional behavior including fear extinction, and its recall (Beer et al., 2006; Milad and Quirk, 2012). More broadly, the VMPFC may provide "somatic markers" that enable individuals to learn from environmental experience (Bechara and Damasio, 2000; Damasio, 1996). The ACC, part of the "frontal" limbic system, is believed to be involved in monitoring and evaluating the outcomes of actions—including error detection—and responds to effortful tasks, including effortful emotion regulation (Bush et al., 2000). Although previously thought be functionally divided along caudal-dorsal "cognitive" and rostral-ventral "affective" lines, new evidence suggests that emotion, even fear expression, engages the caudal/dorsal ACC.

Although thalamus and temporal-parietal-occipital cortices play a role in the processing of sensory cues that signal danger, few studies probe these regions and interrogate general sensory processing of threat cues across anxiety disorders. Similarly, the VS, part of the basal ganglia, is most consistently implicated in reward response and reward learning, which have be relatively understudied in anxiety disorders; very recent studies implicated striatal abnormalities in SAD in adolescents (Guyer et al., 2012) and adults (Sripada et al., 2013). Lastly, despite strong evidence of their involvement in stress response and fear expression, deep subcortical structures such as the hypothalamus and brainstem have been less investigated in human patients, given methodological constraints. Therefore, a full discussion of their roles in relation to anxiety disorders is beyond the scope of this chapter.

FEAR PROVOCATION AND THE EXPERIENCE OF ANXIETY

Fear, anxiety, and other negative affect states can be evoked by visual-auditory stimulation (images, words, sounds), social interactions (extemporaneous public speaking, social "rejection"), imagery (recall of past events), and pharmacological challenge (drugs). Studies have used these strategies to provoke disorder-specific responses (Etkin and Wager, 2007; Etkin, 2010; Shin and Liberzon, 2010; Hilbert et al., 2014; Ipser et al., 2013; Durant et al., 2010; Hayes et al., 2012; Sartory et al., 2013; Linares et al., 2012; Ramage et al., 2013). Processing and imagery of negative, threating content produces an exaggerated response in the amygdala and INS across a range of anxiety disorders, including SP, SAD, PTSD, and OCD. Of note, some studies have reported *decreased* amygdala responsivity to emotional evocation in PTSD, which has been hypothesized to reflect emotional avoidance or blunting in some patients. Growing evidence suggests that this enhanced amygdala and INS reactivity in anxiety disorders is accompanied by *hypo*-activation in ACC, DMPFC, and VMPFC, which is thought to represent a failure to engage frontal regions during the appropriate appraisal or contextual processing of these evocative stimuli. Once considered specific to PTSD, increasing evidence finds that the VMPFC, DMPFC, and ACC are also underengaged in other anxiety disorders. However, hyperactivation has also been observed in SAD, GAD, and PTSD, suggesting inconsistency, which may reflect cross-study differences in cognitive processing. However, taken as a whole, perturbed amygdala-frontal interactions occur along a range of anxiety disorders. For example, disorders characterized by dysregulated fear to exogenous, sensory stimuli (SP, PD) exhibit amygdala hyperreactivity in the context of prefrontal inhibitory failure, whereas disorders characterized by more pervasive, tonic anxiety (GAD, SAD) are more likely to involve prefrontal hyperactivity. Due to complexity and heterogeneity, PTSD may involve *both* dysfunctional processes. However, no study to date has directly tested amygdala-frontal interactions (e.g., functional connectivity) in the context of emotional/trauma imagery and symptom provocation to elucidate similarities and differences among the anxiety disorders.

Although disgust-eliciting images linked to OCD patients' fears of contamination elicit exaggerated insular and prefrontal responses, OCD has been conceptualized along a distinct pathophysiological brain circuit involving the thalamo-cortico-striatal loop (see Section 6), based on studies that either provoke negative affect or OCD-like symptoms (Menzies et al., 2008; Ferreira and Busatto, 2010). Moreover, although enhanced amygdala, ACC, or INS activation occurs in some research, GAD has been least studied with symptom-induction and anxiety-experience paradigms to reliably evoke worry, in part because the free-floating anxiety in GAD is ill suited for the temporal "phasic" demands typical of fMRI/PET designs.

Panic would be an ideal prototype to interrogate the fear expression network (amygdala to brainstem) alongside entero- and exteroceptive awareness and anticipatory anxiety (INS, BNST). Of the anxiety disorders, PD has been most extensively studied with panic provocation via chemical/pharmacological challenge (Durant et al., 2010; Martin et al., 2010; Kim and Gorman, 2005). Panic induced by sodium lactate infusion has been associated with increased sodium lactate levels in the INS as measured by MRS, and the adrenergic antagonist yohimbine elicits panic concurrent with serum NE concentrations. Panicogens like lactate, yohimbine, CCK, and doxapram change cerebral blood flow to certain areas (prefrontal cortex, ACC, amygdala) in PD patients, but these findings should be interpreted with caution in the context of possible confounding effects of physiological changes. Despite consistent evidence that CCK and procaine can evoke subjective fear and anxiety and increase activation of amygdala, INS, ACC, and brainstem, this evidence comes from healthy volunteers, not patients with anxiety disorders.

Induction of fear and provocation of illness-specific anxiety have been associated with an enhanced limbic-hypothalamic-pituitary-adrenal (LHPA) axis reactivity, likely reflecting acute, phasic response under stress (Pego et al., 2010; Abelson et al., 2007; Martin et al., 2010). Anxiety and fear responses are often preceded by, overlap, and/or interact with stress—particularly the "stress response" the leads to activation of the LHPA axis centrally involving the hypothalamaus, HPC, amygdala, and BNST and secretion of CRF, ACHT, and CORT. However, very few studies have measured dynamic changes in central or peripheral neurotransmitters, neuropeptides, or neurohormones, those reflecting LHPA axis reactivity during functional neuroimaging of symptom provocation, and/or concurrent and acute state of stress/fear in anxiety disorders. ACTH responses to aversive pictures and traumatic imagery covaries with activation of MPFC, ACC and INS in PTSD; MPFC and INS reactivity also predict neuroendocrine responses to traumatic recall (Shin and Liberzon, 2010; Pitman et al., 2012). There also is evidence of decreased central CRF in patients with PTSD watching trauma-related videos. Also, some panicogens such as the CCK-agonist pentagastrin produce elevated ACTH responses in PD. However, interpretations of these findings are limited by the absence of brain-based simultaneous measures. Other findings reveal enhanced ACTH and/or CORT response to symptom provocation paradigms in SAD, enhanced cortisol suppression following dexamethasone challenge in PTSD, and reduced fear, presumably through facilitation of extinction, from CORT during exposure-based treatment in SP. It is noteworthy that (1) elicitation of subjective fear/anxiety does not necessarily activate the LHPA axis; (2) states such as awakening or eating elicit LHPA axis activation without anxiety; and (3) other features of stress, such as novelty or the presence of social support, may more powerfully influence the LHPA axis than levels of subjective fear/anxiety. Although it would be reasonable to expect relationships between the LHPA axis and anxiety, these factors and other methodological issues contribute to inconsistent findings on CRF, ACTH, and CORT differences in "provoked" or basal conditions.

Pharmacological induction of anxiety demonstrates the complexity of the chemistry of anxiety disorders. Serotonin has long been implicated in anxiety disorders, particularly as medications that act on the serotonergic system (e.g., selective serotonin reuptake inhibitors [SSRIs]) are effective treatments (Martin et al., 2010; Maron et al., 2012). However, the existing data support both 5-HT "excess" and "deficiency" theories; for example, serotonin agonists and acute administration of SSRIs are acutely anxiogenic, whereas chronic administration of SSRIs is anxiolytic, and acute tryptophan depletion (which lowers 5-HT), particularly when combined with a panicogenic challenge, potentiates anxiety. Other catecholamines such as NE and DA have also been implicated; improvements in anxiety have been achieved from β blockers and chronic administration of NE and DA reuptake inhibitors, whereas elevated NE levels following stress induction increases anxiety. Similar to 5-HT, acute challenge by adrenergic and dopaminergic agents produce inconsistent results across anxiety disorders. (See the section Basal Conditions: "At Rest" for evidence from patients in unprovoked, basal states.)

FEAR PERCEPTION AND LEARNING

Fear and anxiety can arise in response to environmental danger cues. The ventral/subcortical brain circuit (amygdala, INS) implicated in subjective fear and anxiety is also involved in fear perception, as probed by paradigms requiring the viewing of facial expressions, which are social signals (Costafreda et al., 2008). The amygdala, INS, and ACC also represent threats and neutral conditioned stimuli as produced from Pavlovian fear conditions (Sehlmeyer et al., 2009). Exaggerated amygdala and INS reactivity to angry/fearful faces is arguably the most consistent finding in psychiatric functional neuroimaging observed in highly anxious individuals and across several anxiety disorders including SAD, PTSD, PD, with inconsistent findings in GAD (Etkin and Wager, 2007; Shin and Liberzon, 2010; Binelli et al., 2014; Hilbert et al., 2014; Brühl et al., 2014); of note, some studies suggest that SP and OCD differ from these other conditions (Ipser et al., 2013; Ferreira and Busatto, 2010). In patients with PTSD, exaggerated activation of the amygdala to fearful faces has been observed outside of conscious awareness (e.g., implicitly processed). The amygdala-INS activation to threat faces is also accompanied by hyperreactivity in PFC (ACC and/or VLPFC), particularly in SAD and GAD, whereas *hypo*-activation of PFC has been observed in PTSD. Interestingly, some emerging evidence suggests altered functional connectivity or interactions between amygdala and ACC-VLPFC in SAD, GAD, and PTSD patients when processing threat signals. Acute and chronic administration of catecholamine (e.g., SSRIs), GABAergic and cannaboinoid modulators, and peuropeptides such as OXT can attenuate amygdala and INS reactivity to threat stimuli and modulate amygdala-frontal interactions, but this evidence has been limited to healthy volunteers, with little evidence by extension to anxiety disorders.

Although fear can be adaptive, enhanced learning or "overlearning" of fear is associated with some anxiety disorders such as PTSD (Lissek and van Meurs, 2014; Lissek et al., 2005). Greater amygdala response to phasic fear cues predicts greater levels of trait anxiety, and amygdala-dorsal ACC activation is increased in PTSD during the acquisition of conditioned fear. Although a similar finding was not observed in OCD, no functional neuroimaging studies to date have been published on other anxiety disorders during fear conditioning to compare/contrast against this finding in PTSD. In contrast to cued fear, fear and anxiety in the absence of trauma-related or feared stimuli can represent sensitization or fear generalization, which may better reflect the underlying pathology in GAD. Emerging evidence suggests that fear generalization in GAD is associated with enhanced ventral tegmental activity (VTA), enhanced VTA connectivity to ACC and VS, and impaired VMPFC thickness and connectivity to limbic systems (Cha et al., 2014). Again, no investigations have been extended to other anxiety disorders to determine the specificity of these findings.

Neuroimaging tasks involving threat faces and associating cues with fear are often event-related designs intended to measure the speed (e.g., temporal aspects) of the perceptual and learning processes. Thus, temporal features of these paradigms limit simultaneous assessment of chemicals thought to influence individual differences in fear learning. Therefore, methodological limitations currently prevent scientists from linking chemical responses to fear perception and learning in human imaging research.

FEAR AND ANXIETY REGULATION

Some acute responses to threat signals are adaptive, but poor or inefficient contextualization or regulation of such signals may underlie anxiety psychopathology (Gross and Thompson, 2007). Emotion or fear regulation strategies can be explicit (conscious, intentional) or implicit. For example, instructed cognitive reappraisal (reframing or re-interpreting negative content to neutral or positive terms) and distancing can be learned and deployed volitionally under stress or anxiety provocation. Attention control and fear desensitization or extinction are reflexive, adaptive reactions that can occur outside of awareness or intentionality (Milad and Quirk, 2012; Etkin et al., 2011; Phelps et al., 2004). Growing evidence implicates DLPFC, DMPFC, VLPFC, ACC during the down-regulation of negative affect; ACC and DLPFC during effective disengagement of threat distractors; and VMPFC and HPC during the extinction of previously acquired fear associations (Buhle et al., 2014; Etkin et al., 2011; Milad and Quirk, 2012). Together the engagement of these areas modulates amygdala reactivity. Patients with anxiety disorders commonly have difficulty with controlling negative emotions, shifting attention away from threat signals, and inhibiting fear memories. Most studies have examined one anxiety disorder at a time, using either implicit or explicit regulation tasks. When directly compared, both GAD and SAD show similar deficient engagement of ACC and parietal cortex during both explicit and implicit emotion regulation (Blair et al., 2012). Although promising, too few studies directly compare these and other forms of prefrontal function across *multiple* anxiety disorders.

During cognitive reappraisal, SAD, PTSD, GAD, and PD patients each fail to engage dorsal frontal areas, including dorsal ACC, DLPFC, and DMPFC (Goldin et al., 2009; Rabinak et al., 2014; Ball et al., 2013; Blair et al., 2012). Some studies also link the extent of DLPFC/DMPFC activation during volitional regulation to the intensity of negative affect, as well as amygdala activation (Banks et al., 2007; Buhle et al., 2014). Nevertheless, *how* frontal engagement shapes amygdala activation remains unclear. Failure to engage VMPFC and HPC during fear extinction learning has been observed in many anxiety disorders, including PTSD and OCD. This may reflect impaired retention of extinction memory. Evidence from animal studies suggests that a wide variety of neurotransmitters and neurosteriods, including 5-HT, ALLO, CRF, GABA, Glu, and endocanabinoid, can influence fear and extinction learning (Griebel and Holmes, 2013). Interestingly, glutamatergic and cannabinoid modulators have been shown to attenuate amygdala reactivity to threat, enhance HPC and VMPFC activation during extinction learning, and facilitate success of exposure-based psychotherapy for PTSD and SAD. However, it remains unclear whether the deficiency in these or other neurochemicals in PTSD and anxiety disorders can explain the failure to extinguish fear and/or retain that inhibitory learning.

BASAL CONDITIONS: "AT REST"

Although dynamic processes are disrupted in anxiety disorders, much of what we know about anxiety-disorder biology comes from investigations under basal, unprovoked, "at rest" conditions, as studied by many methodologies, such as PET-based receptor imaging, MRI-based magnetic resonance spectroscopy (MRS), MRI-based volumetric/morphometric structural imaging, MRI-based diffusion tensor imaging (DTI), and MRI-based resting state connectivity studies (Shin and Liberzon, 2010; Brennan et al., 2013; Engel et al., 2009; Karl et al., 2006; Maron et al., 2012; Durant et al., 2010; Martin et al, 2010; Woon and Hedges, 2009; Maddock and Buoconore, 2012; Rosso et al., 2014). Receptor imaging studies have shown (1) reduced $GABA_A$ receptor binding in MPFC, amygdala, INS, and HPC and reduced mu-opioid receptor binding in amygdala in PTSD; (2) reduced $GABA_A$ receptor binding in ACC, MPFC, and amygdala/HPC/temporal lobe and reduced $5\text{-}HT1_A$ receptor binding in PD; (3) reduced $5\text{-}HT1_A$ receptor binding in amygdala, ACC, INS, in SAD; and (4) reduced $5\text{-}HT1_A$ receptor binding in ACC and other frontal areas in OCD. MRS studies have revealed increased lactate in ACC and reduced GABA in occipital cortex (but no difference in ACC, DLPFC, or VLPFC) in PD increased Glu in ACC in SAD, and reduced GABA in INS but not ACC. The alterations could influence how limbic and frontal areas (amygdala, INS, ACC, MPFC) respond under stress/anxiety provocation and/or be central to the pathophysiology of anxiety disorders themselves. The most robust finding of brain volumetric abnormalities involve PTSD in relation to theories of enhanced cortisol release during chronic stress leading to neurotoxicity and atrophy. For example, PTSD is associated with diminished volumes in the amygdala, INS, ACC, and HPC; of note, the origin of HPC atrophy remains unclear as a twin study has shown that hippocampal atrophy may be a familial risk factor for developing PTSD following trauma. In contrast, few structural abnormalities have been reported in SAD and GAD, while ACC volumes have been observed to be decreased in PD and ACC thickness greater in SP. DTI structural studies show altered white matter integrity in the uncinate fasciculus, believed to be the white matter tract connecting amygdala and frontal cortex, in both SAD and GAD. Moreover, recent studies suggest aberrant amygdala-ACC and amygdala-DLPFC resting state connectivity in both SAD and GAD. These latter findings add support to the model of abnormal amygdala-frontal interactions in anxiety disorders.

Studies of patients in basal unprovoked states provide important knowledge on neurotransmitters, neurohormones, neurosteroids, and neuropeptides. The LHPA axis arguably has been the most studied system across anxiety disorders, but its dysfunction remains a controversial topic (Martin et al., 2010; Risbrough and Stein, 2006; Kim and Gorman, 2005; Elnazer and Baldwin, 2014). Central cerebral spinal fluid (CSF) and/or blood measures of CRF have been shown to be elevated in PTSD but not consistently related to PTSD severity, and studies of peripheral measures of LHPA readouts in PTSD have been conflicting. Early studies suggested a paradoxical finding of abnormally low CORT in PTSD, but larger studies have failed to replicate these data; nevertheless, there is little evidence of *increased* tonic levels of CORT in PTSD, as might be expected in a chronically stressed state. Other evidence, again not consistently observed, points to a greater suppression of plasma CORT from dexamethasone challenge in PTSD. These particular findings suggest excessive down-regulation of the LHPA axis due to enhanced sensitivity to negative feedback in PTSD, in contrast to findings in major depression. Given the frequent comorbidity of depression in PTSD, these two opposing, interactive effects on LHPA axis function may contribute to the inconsistency or negative findings in PTSD. With regard to other anxiety disorders, CSF CRF appears normal in GAD and PD, but overnight hypercortisolemia and greater non-suppression following dexamethasone have been observed in PD but not in SAD or GAD, where afternoon CORT levels have been observed to be elevated.

Findings for monoamine and neuropeptide systems are inconsistent (Martin et al., 2010; Kormos and Gaszner, 2013). CSF NE and 24-hour urinary catecholamines have been shown to be tonically elevated, while plasma NPY is lower, in PTSD. Basal blood levels of NE do not appear to differentiate anxiety patients from controls, though PD has been associated with increased cardiac NE spillover. Increased 5-HT turnover has been observed in PD while CSF levels of 5-hydroxyindoleacetic acid (5-HIAA), the main metabolite of serotonin, is decreased in some studies. In GAD, 5-HIAA urinary levels have been reported to be elevated. These diverse findings in the 5-HT system have been hypothesized to reflect different serotonergic pathways that could exert opposite within and across anxiety disorders. DA can be metabolized to NE and homovanillic acid (HVA), and CSF measures of HVA has been observed to be decreased in patients with SAD *and* PD but not PD alone. Lastly, CSF and serum levels of ALLO appear to be low in PTSD. Perhaps the most salient observation is that these systems are understudied across *all* anxiety disorders, and that very few studies demonstrate a correlation to anxiety behavior or symptom severity. Moreover, a number of potentially relevant neurotransmitters (GABA, Glu) and neuropeptides (AVP, OXT) are not investigated because of methodologic constraints or limitations to meaningful interpretation (e.g., limited or no peripheral measurement or reliability; technical difficulty). Thus, inference about the exact or specific role of tonically fluctuating levels of these and other neurochemicals in the etiology or maintenance of anxiety psychopathology remains limited, and a unifying, cohesive model across disorders remains elusive.

CONCLUSION AND FUTURE DIRECTIONS

Neuroimaging informs understanding of fear and anxiety in part because of rapid methodological advances. This work is largely correlational and cross-sectional in nature, thus limiting causal inferences. Nevertheless, available data demonstrate strong, well-replicated cross-species consistency in brain-behavior relationships for fear and anxiety. Future imaging studies will need to increase the recent trend of greater emphasis on circuitry-based interactions (Menon, 2011). For anxiety disorders, more precise delineation of functioning in amygdala-frontal (sub)-network(s) and their emergence during development (Blackford and Pine, 2012; Swartz et al., 2014) appears to be particularly important. This may clarify how biomarkers represent cross-disorder or symptom-specific entities. Lastly, the early state of clinical translational research can be contrasted with the more advanced state of basic neuroscience research. Thus, continued attempts to clinically leverage findings in basic neuroscience hold promise.

REFERENCES

Abelson, J. L., Khan, S., Liberzon, I., and Young, E. A. (2007). HPA axis activity in patients with panic disorder: Review and synthesis of four studies. *Depress Anxiety, 24* (1), 66–76. doi:10.1002/da.20220

Bakermans-Kranenburg, M. J., and van I Jzendoorn, M. H. (2013). Sniffing around oxytocin: Review and meta-analyses of trials in healthy and clinical groups with implications for pharmacotherapy. *Translational Psychiatry, 3,* e258. doi:10.1038/tp.2013.34

Ball T. M., Ramsawh, H. J., Campbell-Sills, L., Paulus, M. P., Stein, M. B. (2013). Prefrontal dysfunction during emotion regulation in generalized anxiety and panic disorders. *Psychol Med, 43* (7):1475–1486. doi: 10.1017/S0033291712002383.

Banks, S. J., Eddy, K. T., Angstadt, M., Nathan, P. J., and Phan, K. L. (2007). Amygdala–frontal connectivity during emotion regulation. *Soc Cog Affect Neurosci, 2* (4), 303–312. doi:10.1093/scan/nsm029

Bechara, A., Damasio, H., and Damasio, A. R. (2000). Emotion, decision making and the orbitofrontal cortex. *Cerebral Cortex, 10* (3), 295–307.

Beer, J. S., John, O. P., Scabini, D., and Knight, R. T. (2006). Orbitofrontal cortex and social behavior: Integrating self-monitoring and emotion-cognition interactions. *J Cog Neurosci, 18* (6), 871–879. doi:10.1162/jocn.2006.18.6.871

Blair K. S., Geraci, M., Smith, B. W., Hollon, N., DeVido, J., Otero M., Blair J. R., Pine D. S. (2012). Reduced dorsal anterior cingulate cortical activity during emotional regulation and top-down attentional control in generalized social phobia, generalized anxiety disorder, and comorbid generalized social phobia/generalized anxiety disorder. *Biol Psychiatry, 72* (6), 476–482. doi: 10.1016/j.biopsych.2012.04.013

Binelli, C., Subirà, S., Batalla, A., Muñiz, A., Sugranyés, G., Crippa, J. A., . . . Martín-Santos, R. (2014). Common and distinct neural correlates of facial emotion processing in social anxiety disorder and Williams syndrome: A systematic review and voxel-based meta-analysis of functional resonance imaging studies. *Neuropsychologia, 64C,* 205–217. doi:10.1016/j.neuropsychologia.2014.08.027

Blackford J. U., Pine D. S. (2012). Neural substrates of childhood anxiety disorders: A review of neuroimaging findings. *Child Adolesc Psychiatr Clin N Am, 21* (3):501–525. doi: 10.1016/j.chc.2012.05.002

Brennan, B. P., Rauch, S. L., Jensen, J. E., and Pope, H. G. (2013). A critical review of magnetic resonance spectroscopy studies of obsessive-compulsive disorder. *Biol Psychiatry, 73* (1), 24–31. doi:10.1016/j.biopsych.2012.06.023

Buhle, J. T., Silvers, J. A., Wager, T. D., Lopez, R., Onyemekwu, C., Kober, H., Weber, J., Ochsner, K. N. (2014). Cognitive Reappraisal of Emotion: A Meta-Analysis of Human Neuroimaging Studies. *Cereb Cortex, 24*(11), 2981–2990.

Brühl, A. B., Delsignore, A., Komossa, K., Weidt. S (2014). Neuroimaging in social anxiety disorder: A meta-analytic review resulting in a new neurofunctional model. *Neurosci Biobehav Rev, 47C,* 260–280.

Bush, G., Luu, P., and Posner, M. I. (2000). Cognitive and emotional influences in anterior cingulate cortex. *Trends Cog Sci, 4* (6), 215–222.

Calder, A. J., Lawrence, A. D., and Young, A. W. (2001). Neuropsychology of fear and loathing. *Nature Rev Neurosci, 2* (5), 352–363. doi:10.1038/35072584

Cha, J., Greenberg, T., Carlson, J. M., Dedora, D. J., Hajcak, G., Mujica-Parodi L. R. (2014). Circuit-wide structural and functional measures predict ventromedial prefrontal cortex fear generalization: implications for generalized anxiety disorder. *J Neurosci, 34* (11):4043–4053. doi: 10.1523/JNEUROSCI.3372-13.2014.

Cortese, B., Phan, K. L.(2005). The role of glutamate in anxiety and related disorders. *CNS Spectrums*, *10* (10):820–830.

Costafreda, S. G., Brammer, M. J., David, A. S., and Fu, C. H. Y. (2008). Predictors of amygdala activation during the processing of emotional stimuli: A meta-analysis of 385 PET and fMRI studies. *Brain Res Rev*, *58* (1), 57–70. doi:10.1016/j.brainresrev.2007.10.012

Craig, A. D. (2002). How do you feel? Interoception: The sense of the physiological condition of the body. *Nature Rev Neurosci*, *3* (8), 655–666. doi:10.1038/nrn894

Damasio, A. R. (1996). The somatic marker hypothesis and the possible functions of the prefrontal cortex. *Philos Trans Royal Soc London, Ser B*, *351* (1346), 1413–1420. doi:10.1098/rstb.1996.0125

Davis, M., and Whalen, P. J. (2001). The amygdala: Vigilance and emotion. *Mol Psychiatry*, *6* (1), 13–34.

Diekhof, E. K., Geier, K., Falkai, P., and Gruber, O. (2011). Fear is only as deep as the mind allows: A coordinate-based meta-analysis of neuroimaging studies on the regulation of negative affect. *NeuroImage*, *58* (1), 275–285. doi:10.1016/j.neuroimage.2011.05.073

Durant, C., Christmas, D., and Nutt, D. (2010). The pharmacology of anxiety. *Curr Top Behav Neurosci*, *2*, 303–330.

Elnazer, H. Y., and Baldwin, D. S. (2014). Investigation of cortisol levels in patients with anxiety disorders: A structured review. *Curr Top Behav Neurosci*. doi:10.1007/7854_2014_299

Engel, K., Bandelow, B., Gruber, O., and Wedekind, D. (2009). Neuroimaging in anxiety disorders. *J Neural Trans* (Vienna, Austria: 1996), *116* (6), 703–716. doi:10.1007/s00702-008-0077-9

Etkin, A. (2010). Functional neuroanatomy of anxiety: A neural circuit perspective. *Curr Top Behav Neurosci*, *2*, 251–277.

Etkin, A., Egner, T., and Kalisch, R. (2011). Emotional processing in anterior cingulate and medial prefrontal cortex. *Trends Cog Sci*, *15* (2), 85–93. doi:10.1016/j.tics.2010.11.004

Etkin, A., and Wager, T. D. (2007). Functional neuroimaging of anxiety: A meta-analysis of emotional processing in PTSD, social anxiety disorder, and specific phobia. *Am J Psychiatry*, *164* (10), 1476–1488. doi:10.1176/appi.ajp.2007.07030504

Ferreira, L. K., and Busatto, G. F. (2010). Heterogeneity of coordinate-based meta-analyses of neuroimaging data: An example from studies in OCD. *Br J Psychiatry*, *197* (1), 76–77; author reply 77. doi:10.1192/bjp.197.1.76a

Fuster, J. M. (2013). Cognitive functions of the prefrontal cortex. In *Principles of Frontal Lobe Function*, edited by D. T. Struss and R. T. Knight (pp. 11–22). New York: Oxford University Press.

Goldin, P. R., Manber, T., Hakimi, S., Canli, T., and Gross, J. J. (2009). Neural bases of social anxiety disorder: emotional reactivity and cognitive regulation during social and physical threat. *Arch Gen Psychiatry*, *66*(2), 170–180. doi: 10.1001/archgenpsychiatry.2008.525.

Griebel, G., and Holmes, A. (2013). 50 years of hurdles and hope in anxiolytic drug discovery. *Nature Rev Drug Discovery*, *12* (9), 667–687. doi:10.1038/nrd4075

Gross, J. J., and Thompson, R. (2007). Emotion regulation: Conceptual foundations. In J. J. Gross (ed.), *Handbook of emotion regulation* (pp. 3–26). New York: Guilford Press.

Guyer, A. E., Choate, V. R., Detloff, A., Benson, B., Nelson, E. E., Perez-Edgar, K., Fox, N. A., Pine, D. S., Ernst, M. (2012). *Striatal functional alteration during incentive anticipation in pediatric anxiety disorders.* Am J Psychiatry, *169* (2), 205–212.

Hattingh, C. J., Ipser, J., Tromp, S., Syal, S., Lochner, C., Brooks, S. J. B., and Stein, D. J. (2013). Functional magnetic resonance imaging during emotion recognition in social anxiety disorder: An activation likelihood meta-analysis. *Frontiers Human Neurosci*, *6*, 347. doi:10.3389/fnhum.2012.00347

Hayes, J. P., Hayes, S. M., and Mikedis, A. M. (2012). Quantitative meta-analysis of neural activity in posttraumatic stress disorder. *Biol. .Mood Anxiety Disorders*, *2* (1), 9. doi:10.1186/2045-5380-2-9

Hilbert, K., Lueken, U., and Beesdo-Baum, K. (2014). Neural structures, functioning and connectivity in generalized anxiety disorder and interaction with neuroendocrine systems: A systematic review. *J Affect Disorders*, *158*, 114–126. doi:10.1016/j.jad.2014.01.022

Ipser, J. C., Singh, L., and Stein, D. J. (2013). Meta-analysis of functional brain imaging in specific phobia. *Psychiatry and Clinical Neurosciences, 67* (5), 311–322. doi:10.1111/pcn.12055

Karl, A., Schaefer, M., Malta, L., Dorfel, D., Rohleder, N., and Werner, A. (2006). A meta-analysis of structural brain abnormalities in PTSD. *Neurosci Biobehav Rev, 30* (7), 1004–1031. doi:10.1016/j.neubiorev.2006.03.004

Kim, J., and Gorman, J. (2005). The psychobiology of anxiety. *Clin Neurosci Res, 4* (5–6), 335–347. doi:10.1016/j.cnr.2005.03.008

Kober, H., Barrett, L. F., Joseph, J., Bliss-Moreau, E., Lindquist, K., and Wager, T. D. (2008). Functional grouping and cortical-subcortical interactions in emotion: A meta-analysis of neuroimaging studies. *NeuroImage, 42* (2), 998–1031. doi:10.1016/j.neuroimage.2008.03.059

Kormos, V., and Gaszner, B. (2013). Role of neuropeptides in anxiety, stress, and depression: From animals to humans. *Neuropeptides, 47* (6), 401–419. doi:10.1016/j.npep.2013.10.014

Linares, I. M. P., Trzesniak, C., Chagas, M. H. N., Hallak, J. E. C., Nardi, A. E., and Crippa, J. A. S. (2012). Neuroimaging in specific phobia disorder: A systematic review of the literature. *Revista Brasileira De Psiquiatria* (São Paulo, Brazil: 1999), *34*(1), 101–111.

Lissek, S., Powers, A. S., McClure, E. B., Phelps, E. A., Woldehawariat, G., Grillon, C., and Pine, D. S. (2005). Classical fear conditioning in the anxiety disorders: A meta-analysis. *Behav Res Ther, 43* (11), 1391–1424. doi:10.1016/j.brat.2004.10.007

Lissek S., and van Meurs, B. (2014). Learning models of PTSD: Theoretical accounts and psychobiological evidence. *Int J Psychophysiol*, Nov 20. pii: S0167-8760(14)01647-X. doi: 10.1016/j.ijpsycho.2014.11.006. [Epub ahead of print] Review.

Maddock, R. J., and Buonocore, M. H. (2012). MR spectroscopic studies of the brain in psychiatric disorders. *Curr Top Behav Neurosci, 11*, 199–251. doi:10.1007/7854_2011_197

Maron, E., Nutt, D., and Shlik, J. (2012). Neuroimaging of serotonin system in anxiety disorders. *Curr Pharmaceut Design, 18* (35), 5699–5708.

Martin, E. I., Ressler, K. J., Binder, E., and Nemeroff, C. B. (2010). The neurobiology of anxiety disorders: Brain imaging, genetics, and psychoneuroendocrinology. *Clin Lab Med, 30* (4), 865–891. doi:10.1016/j.cll.2010.07.006

Menon, V. (2011). Large-scale brain networks and psychopathology: A unifying triple network model. *Trends Cog Sci, 15* (10), 483–506. doi:10.1016/j.tics.2011.08.003

Menzies, L., Chamberlain, S. R., Laird, A. R., Thelen, S. M., Sahakian, B. J., and Bullmore, E. T. (2008). Integrating evidence from neuroimaging and neuropsychological studies of obsessive-compulsive disorder: The orbitofronto-striatal model revisited. *Neurosci Biobehav Rev, 32* (3), 525–549. doi:10.1016/j.neubiorev.2007.09.005

Milad, M. R., and Quirk, G. J. (2012). Fear extinction as a model for translational neuroscience: Ten years of progress. *Annu Rev Psychol, 63*, 129–151. doi:10.1146/annurev.psych.121208.131631

Neumann, I. D., and Landgraf, R. (2012). Balance of brain oxytocin and vasopressin: Implications for anxiety, depression, and social behaviors. *Trends Neurosci, 35* (11), 649–659. doi:10.1016/j.tins.2012.08.004

Paulus, M. P., and Stein, M. B. (2006). An insular view of anxiety. *Biological Psychiatry, 60*(4), 383–387. doi:10.1016/j.biopsych.2006.03.042

Pêgo, J. M., Sousa, J. C., Almeida, O. F. X., and Sousa, N. (2010). Stress and the neuroendocrinology of anxiety disorders. *Curr Top Behav Neurosci, 2*, 97–117.

Pessoa, L., and Adolphs, R. (2010). Emotion processing and the amygdala: From a "low road" to "many roads" of evaluating biological significance. *Nature Rev Neurosci, 11* (11), 773–783. doi:10.1038/nrn2920

Phan, K. L., Wager, T., Taylor, S. F., and Liberzon, I. (2002). Functional neuroanatomy of emotion: A meta-analysis of emotion activation studies in PET and fMRI. *NeuroImage, 16* (2), 331–348. doi:10.1006/nimg.2002.1087

Phelps, E. A., Delgado, M. R., Nearing, K. I., and LeDoux, J. E. (2004). Extinction learning in humans: Role of the amygdala and VMPFC. *Neuron, 43* (6), 897–905. doi:10.1016/j.neuron.2004.08.042

Pitman, R. K., Rasmusson, A. M., Koenen, K. C., Shin, L. M., Orr, S. P., Gilbertson, M. W., . . . Liberzon, I. (2012). Biological studies of post-traumatic stress disorder. *Nature Reviews. Neuroscience, 13* (11), 769–787. doi:10.1038/nrn3339

Rabinak C., MacNamara A., Angstadt A., Kennedy A., Liberzon I., Stein M. B., Phan K.L. (2014). Focal and aberrant prefrontal engagement during emotion regulation in veterans with posttraumatic stress disorder. *Depress Anxiety, 31*(10), 851–861.

Ramage, A. E., Laird, A. R., Eickhoff, S. B., Acheson, A., Peterson, A. L., Williamson, D. E., . . . Fox, P. T. (2013). A coordinate-based meta-analytic model of trauma processing in posttraumatic stress disorder. *Hum Brain Map, 34* (12), 3392–3399. doi:10.1002/hbm.22155

Risbrough, V. B., and Stein, M. B. (2006). Role of corticotropin releasing factor in anxiety disorders: A translational research perspective. *Hormones Behav, 50* (4), 550–561. doi:10.1016/j.yhbeh.2006.06.019

Rosso, I. M., Weiner, M. R., Crowley, D. J., Silveri, M. M., Rauch, S. L., and Jensen, J. E. (2014). Insula and anterior cingulate GABA levels in posttraumatic stress disorder: Preliminary findings using magnetic resonance spectroscopy. *Depress Anxiety, 31*(2), 115–123. doi:10.1002/da.22155

Sabatinelli, D., Fortune, E. E., Li, Q., Siddiqui, A., Krafft, C., Oliver, W. T., . . . Jeffries, J. (2011). Emotional perception: Meta-analyses of face and natural scene processing. *NeuroImage, 54* (3), 2524–2533. doi:10.1016/j.neuroimage.2010.10.011

Sartory, G., Cwik, J., Knuppertz, H., Schürholt, B., Lebens, M., Seitz, R. J., and Schulze, R. (2013). In search of the trauma memory: A meta-analysis of functional neuroimaging studies of symptom provocation in posttraumatic stress disorder (PTSD). *PloS One, 8* (3), e58150. doi:10.1371/journal.pone.0058150

Sehlmeyer, C., Schöning, S., Zwitserlood, P., Pfleiderer, B., Kircher, T., Arolt, V., and Konrad, C. (2009). Human fear conditioning and extinction in neuroimaging: A systematic review. *PloS One, 4* (6), e5865. doi:10.1371/journal.pone.0005865

Sergerie, K., Chochol, C., and Armony, J. L. (2008). The role of the amygdala in emotional processing: A quantitative meta-analysis of functional neuroimaging studies. *Neurosci Biobehav Rev, 32* (4), 811–830. doi:10.1016/j.neubiorev.2007.12.002

Shin, L. M., and Liberzon, I. (2010). The neurocircuitry of fear, stress, and anxiety disorders. *Neuropsychopharmacology, 35* (1), 169–191. doi:10.1038/npp.2009.83

Simmons, A. N., and Matthews, S. C. (2012). Neural circuitry of PTSD with or without mild traumatic brain injury: A meta-analysis. *Neuropharmacology, 62* (2), 598–606. doi:10.1016/j.neuropharm.2011.03.016

Sripada C., Angstadt, M., Liberzon, I., McCabe, K., and Phan, K. L. (2013). Aberrant reward center response to partner reputation during a social exchange game in generalized social phobia. *Depress Anxiety, 30*(4):353–361. doi: 10.1002/da.22091.

Swartz, J. R., Carrasco, M., Wiggins, J. L., Thomason, M. E., Monk, C. S. (2014). Age-related changes in the structure and function of prefrontal cortex-amygdala circuitry in children and adolescents: A multi-modal imaging approach. *Neuroimage, 86*, 212–220. doi: 10.1016/j.neuroimage.2013.08.018.

Woon, F. L., and Hedges, D. W. (2009). Amygdala volume in adults with posttraumatic stress disorder: A meta-analysis. *J Neuropsychiatry Clin Neurosci, 21* (1), 5–12. doi:10.1176/appi.neuropsych.21.1.5

/// 4 /// THE GENETICS OF ANXIETY DISORDERS

JORDAN W. SMOLLER, FELECIA E. CERRATO,
AND SARAH L. WEATHERALL

INTRODUCTION

Anxiety disorders have long been known to run in families, suggesting a genetic contribution to risk. Unlike diseases that have a clear inheritance pattern and are caused by a single gene, such as Huntington disease, multiple genetic and environmental factors contribute to anxiety disorders. This chapter will review the common approaches taken to discover the genetic basis of anxiety disorders, including generalized anxiety disorder (GAD), panic disorder (PD), agoraphobia (AG), social anxiety disorder (SAD), specific phobias, posttraumatic stress disorder (PTSD), and obsessive-compulsive disorder (OCD), as well as the genetics of anxiety-related traits.

The overall goal of psychiatric genetic research is to identify and characterize the genetic basis of psychopathology. The discovery of genes and biological pathways that contribute to disorder risk can provide targets for the development of novel and more effective treatments. Identification of genetic determinants of disease may also aid in refining diagnosis and nosology. In addition, information about genetic susceptibility may provide patients and clinicians with information about disease severity and prognosis.

Anxiety disorders are common, with aggregate lifetime prevalence of up to 29% (Kessler and Wang, 2008). While much evidence indicates that anxiety disorders are influenced by genes, the complexity of anxiety disorder phenotypes has complicated efforts to identify susceptibility loci. The *Diagnostic and Statistical Manual of Mental Disorders*, fifth edition (DSM-5), currently includes seven primary anxiety disorders. The transition from DSM-IV to DSM-5 included several changes in the classification of anxiety disorders, most notably, the addition of separation anxiety disorder and selective mutism, the disaggregation of PD and AG, and the development of separate categories for obsessive-compulsive disorders and trauma-related disorders including PTSD. For historical purposes, we include OCD and PTSD in this chapter. The evolving nature of diagnostic criteria reflects, in part, the difficulty in drawing clear boundaries among anxiety disorders and between pathologic and normative anxiety. As we will see, genetic studies have supported the hypothesis that heritable influences transcend clinically defined categories.

APPROACHES TO STUDYING THE GENETICS OF ANXIETY DISORDERS

The genetic basis of diseases and disorders has traditionally been classified as either "Mendelian" or "complex." Mendelian disorders are typically caused by a single gene in which the causal mutations exhibit a clear inheritance pattern (e.g. dominant, recessive, or X-linked) and are highly penetrant (that is, carrying the mutations is sufficient to cause disease in most or all cases). In contrast, the genetic contributions to complex diseases, which include most common medical illnesses, involve variations in many genes—each of which may confer a small increase in risk and whose penetrance may depend on interactions with other genes or the environment. Anxiety disorders, like others in psychiatry, are complex disorders. Traditionally, efforts to characterize the genetic basis of complex disorders rely on a series of study designs to address a series of questions (as illustrated by Figure 4.1): Does the disorder run in families? If so, how much of this familial component is attributable to genetic variation? What specific genes are involved? What are the biological mechanisms by which these genes lead to disorder?

Family Studies

To determine whether a disorder runs in families, *family studies* compare the prevalence of the disorder among relatives of affected probands (people with the disorder of interest) to the prevalence among relatives of unaffected probands (controls). Family studies of anxiety disorders have shown that the risk of anxiety disorders is approximately 4–6 times higher in first-degree relatives of affected probands compared with relatives of unaffected probands (Hettema, Neale, and Kendler, 2001) (Table 4.1). The familial risk of PTSD has been more difficult to estimate because of the need to match cases and controls on exposure to a traumatic event. Family studies have also demonstrated that anxiety disorders do not "breed true"—that is, familial risk factors overlap. For example, relatives of probands with SAD are at risk of developing PD and specific phobia, and children of parents with PD are at risk of developing agoraphobia and OCD (Smoller, Gardner-Schuster, and Misiaszek, 2008).

Twin Studies

The fact that anxiety disorders run in families does not necessarily imply that genetic variation is involved, since family members share both genes and environment. Twin studies allow us to estimate the contribution of genetic variation by comparing the phenotypic similarity between pairs of monozygotic (MZ, genetically identical) versus dizygotic (DZ, nonidentical) twins. Twin similarity is often measured by concordance rates—the probability of an affected co-twin given that the index twin is affected. When the concordance rates are higher for MZ twin pairs than for DZ twin pairs, we can infer that this greater phenotypic similarity is attributable to the greater genetic similarity between MZ twins. To the extent that the MZ concordance rate is less than 100%, this is evidence that environmental factors are also contributing. Reported concordance rates for anxiety disorders range from 12–26% for monozygotic twins and 4–15% for dizygotic twins (Hettema et al., 2001; Smoller, Block, and Young, 2009).

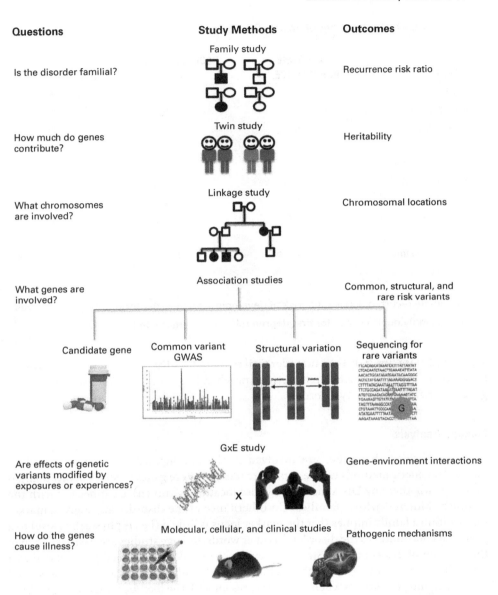

FIGURE 4.1 The "Sequencing" of Psychiatric Genetic Research. This figure depicts the sequence of questions, study methods, and outcomes that are most commonly used to characterize the genetic basis of psychiatric and other complex trait disorders.

The contribution of genetic variation to a disorder or trait can be measured in terms of *heritability*—an estimate of the proportion of individual differences in disease risk that is due to genetic variation in a population. Heritability may range from 0 (no contribution of genetic variation to disease risk) to 100% (disease risk entirely attributable to genetic variation). Heritability estimates from twin studies of anxiety disorders have typically been in the range of 30–50% (McGrath, Weill, Robinson, Macrae, and Smoller, 2012) (Table 4.1) Note that heritability estimates may be inflated by greater epigenetic similarity among identical twins and by methodological issues (e.g., if identical twins

TABLE 4.1 Genetic Epidemiology of Anxiety Disorders

DISORDER	LIFETIME PREVALENCE, %	RECURRENCE RISK RATIO*	HERITABILITY, %
Panic disorder	3.5	5	45
Social anxiety disorder	12	3–10	35
Generalized anxiety disorder	6	2–6	30
Agoraphobia (without panic disorder)	1.5	3.1	30–40
Specific phobias	12.5	3–4	30–50
Obsessive-compulsive disorder	2.3	5	40
Posttraumatic stress disorder	7	N/A	35

*Approximate recurrence risk ratio; risk of developing the disorder for first degree relatives of affected individuals vs. risk for first degree relatives of unaffected individuals.

are treated more similarly than non-identical twins). In addition, these estimates provide little insight into the genetic architecture (number, frequency, or effect size of specific genetic variants) of anxiety disorders.

Linkage Analysis

After establishing that genes are involved in the development of anxiety disorders, molecular genetic methods can be applied to identify these genes or loci. *Linkage analysis* examines whether any DNA markers (whose location is known) are inherited with the disorder of interest within families. Co-inheritance of the disorder and a given marker locus within a family implies that the marker locus is linked (i.e., is physically close) to a gene that contributes to the disorder. In other words, linkage studies are designed to map the location of disease genes. Statistical evidence of linkage is typically calculated as a logarithm of odds (LOD) score that compares the likelihood of detecting the observed genotypes and phenotypes when linkage is present with the likelihood assuming no linkage is present. Linkage studies have successfully mapped loci underlying many Mendelian disorders, in which there is a clear familial inheritance pattern and the disorder is caused by a single gene, such as Huntington disease or cystic fibrosis. However, they have been less powerful for complex disorders because of uncertain inheritance patterns and the modest effect of many contributing loci.

Linkage analyses of anxiety disorders have implicated many chromosomal regions, though results have been inconsistent. A meta-analysis of anxiety disorder linkage studies comprising 162 families found modest, but not genome-wide significant, evidence of linkage at 24 chromosomal regions (Webb et al., 2012). Linkage studies on adults with PD have found varying degrees of evidence for linkage on 16 chromosomes (Maron, Hettema, and Shlik, 2010; Smoller, Gardner-Schuster, and Covino, 2008). In OCD, studies have suggested evidence for linkage on 11 chromosomes, though none of these findings have reached statistical significance and most sample sizes were small (Pauls, Abramovitch, Rauch, and Geller, 2014). Other linkage studies have combined anxiety disorder categories due to evidence (reviewed later) that genetic influences on these disorders overlap. Evidence for linkage of specific phobia on chromosome 14 and SAD on chromosome 16 has been reported, as well as evidence for linkage with a phenotype combining elements of SAD, specific phobia, PD, and AG on chromosome 4 (Smoller, Gardner-Schuster, and Covino, 2008). To date, no linkage studies have been published in PTSD.

Association Analysis

Compared with linkage studies, association studies can be more powerful for identifying loci of modest effect and have become the dominant strategy for genetic studies of complex disorders. Association studies typically utilize a case-control design to determine whether specific genetic variants (alleles) are more common among affected (cases) than among unaffected individuals (controls). For continuous traits, association analysis examines whether specific alleles are associated with quantitative variation in the trait of interest. Association analyses can also be conducted using families. Family-based association studies typically examine parent-child trios to determine whether alleles from heterozygous parents are transmitted to affected offspring significantly more than 50% of the time (which would be expected by chance).

Candidate Gene Association Studies

To date, association studies of anxiety disorders have primarily examined variations in candidate genes—that is, genes hypothesized to be involved in the etiology of a disorder based on prior biological evidence (biological candidates) or physical location within a chromosomal region implicated by linkage analysis (positional candidates). Most candidate gene association studies of anxiety disorders have focused on monoaminergic neurotransmitter pathways that are the putative targets of pharmacotherapies for pathologic anxiety and stress hormone pathways that have been implicated in animal models (e.g., serotonin, norepinephrine, dopamine, and HPA axis related genes). The variants assessed in these studies are typically single nucleotide polymorphisms (SNPs) or variable number tandem repeats (VNTRs). SNPs are variations in a single DNA nucleotide and represent the most common form of variation in the genome. VNTRs are short sequences of nucleotides that vary in number of repeats between individuals.

Hundreds of candidate gene studies of anxiety disorders and related traits have been reported, but few associations have been replicated in independent analyses. Several genes have shown nominal association with one or more anxiety disorders in independent studies including SNPs in catechol-O-methyltransferase (*COMT*), the dopamine receptor (*DRD2*), the serotonin 2A receptor (*HTR2A*), and FK506 binding protein 5 (*FKBP5*) (Smoller, Block, and Young 2009). The most widely studied VNTRs have been variations in the promoter of the monoamine oxidase A gene *MAOA* and the 5-HTTLPR VNTR in the promoter region of the serotonin transporter gene *SLC6A4*. The "short" allele of the 5-HTTLPR variant appears to result in reduced expression of the gene (the target of SSRI medications), making this a popular functional candidate.

Most candidate gene studies of anxiety disorders have been underpowered and therefore prone to both false positive and false negative findings. Consistent with this, few specific associations have been consistently replicated. In some cases, the same variant has received support in more than one study, but the direction of allelic effect has been inconsistent. A recent review of 65 candidate gene studies in anxiety disorders with independent samples of at least 200 cases or nuclear families found no instances of replication (i.e. association of the same allele in the same direction at a significance level of $p < 0.05$) (McGrath et al., 2012). Meta-analyses of commonly studied candidate variants have been performed, but results have again been equivocal. These include negative meta-analyses in PTSD (for 5-HTTLPR; Gressier et al., 2013; Navarro-Mateu, Escamez, Koenen, Alonso, and Sanchez-Meca, 2013), and PD (for 5-HTTLPR, the promoter variant of *MAOA*, and the functional Val158Met SNP rs4680 of *COMT*), although secondary analyses have provided modest support for sex-specific effects of *COMT* and *MAOA* in PD (reviewed in McGrath et al., 2012; see also Reif et al., 2012). For OCD, a meta-analysis of 20 candidate polymorphisms in OCD (Taylor, 2013) found significant associations for two variants (5-HTTLPR and a variant in *HTR2A*) while another meta-analysis, focused on the neuronal glutamate transporter *SLC1A1*, was essentially negative (Stewart, Mayerfeld, et al., 2013).

In some cases, candidate loci have been implicated by convergent studies of anxiety-related phenotypes in animals and humans. For example, a recent study (Smoller et al., 2014) examined the gene encoding ASIC1a (*ACCN2*), an acid-sensing ion channel that had been shown to mediate carbon dioxide (CO_2)-induced fear behavior in mice by amygdala sensing of reduced pH (Ziemann et al., 2009). Heightened sensitivity to CO_2 is an established biological correlate of PD. Inhaled CO_2 triggers panic attacks in a majority of individuals with PD, but only a minority of unaffected controls. Smoller and colleagues (Smoller et al., 2014) observed evidence of association between variants in *ACCN2* and PD that appeared to be stronger in cases with early-onset or the respiratory subtype of PD. In healthy volunteers, PD-associated alleles were also associated with amygdala volume and amygdala reactivity to emotional faces.

Genome-wide Association Studies

Candidate gene studies have inherent limitations. Given our incomplete understanding of the pathogenesis of psychiatric disorders, the prior probability of association for any biological candidate gene is low; this raises the odds that an association with that candidate is a chance (false positive) finding. In addition, by their very nature, association studies of biological candidates can at best validate existing hypotheses rather than identify new risk genes. A decade ago, it became possible instead to conduct *genome-wide association studies* (GWAS). GWAS are possible due to large-scale efforts such as the HapMap Project and 1000 Genomes Project that have cataloged common SNP variation across populations and the development of DNA microarrays ("DNA chips") that interrogate up to one million or more SNPs across the genome. Alleles of many SNPs in a given genomic region are correlated and inherited together (due to linkage disequilibrium, or LD). Therefore, a given SNP in high LD with other SNPs may provide information about other correlated SNPs, so that only a subset of the millions of SNPs in the genome need to be genotyped directly. Unlike candidate gene studies, GWAS offer an "unbiased" approach to gene discovery in that they do not rely on predetermined hypotheses about which genes may be associated with the disorder of interest.

GWAS in psychiatry and other areas of medicine have been successful in identifying thousands of risk loci, but they have also shown that SNPs associated with complex traits have modest effect sizes (odds ratios typically less than 1.20). Because of this and the multiple testing burden entailed by evaluating hundreds of thousands or millions of SNPs, adequately powered GWAS require very large sample sizes. The conventional threshold for "genome-wide significance" is a p value less than 5×10^{-8}, effectively a Bonferroni correction for a million statistical tests.

Although several GWAS of anxiety disorders have been reported (Table 4.2), none have achieved sample sizes that are usually needed to identify robust genome-wide associations (on the order of tens of thousands of subjects). The first GWAS in PD was conducted in 200 Japanese cases and 200 controls (Otowa et al., 2009) and reported genome-wide significant SNPs in the genes encoding transmembrane protein 16B (*TMEM16B*) and plakophilin-1 (*PKP1*), but these findings were not supported by a replication attempt in an independent sample of 558 cases and 556 controls (Otowa et al., 2010). However, more robust support has emerged for transmembrane protein 132D (*TMEM132D*). An initial GWAS found association of a *TMEM132D* SNP (rs7309727) as well as a haplotype combining this and another SNP (rs11060369). Risk genotypes were associated with higher *TMEM132D* mRNA expression in human post-mortem frontal cortex, results that were further supported by a mouse model in which high anxiety-related behavior was associated with a *Tmem132d* SNP and correlated with expression of *Tmem132d* mRNA in the anterior cingulate cortex (Erhardt et al., 2011). In a subsequent meta-analysis of eight independent case-control samples (2,678 cases and 3,262 controls), genome-wide significant associations of rs7309727 and the haplotype of rs7309727–rs11060369 were reported when the analysis was restricted to European ancestry cases with primary PD (Erhardt et al., 2012). TMEM132D is a transmembrane protein highly expressed in the cortical regions of the brain. The function of this gene product is not fully understood, but it has been suggested that this gene plays a role in threat processing (Haaker et al., 2014).

Several recent GWAS in PTSD have pointed to susceptibility loci. Logue et al. (2013) reported a genome-wide significant association between PTSD (discovery sample of 295 cases and 196 controls) and a SNP (rs8042149) in the retinoid-related orphan receptor gene (*RORA*). While this SNP was not significantly associated in two replication samples in the same publication, further analysis of *RORA* SNPs in a subset of the discovery and replication samples from Logue et al. ($N = 540$) reported an association between rs17303244 and a fear component of PTSD (Miller, Wolf, Logue, and Baldwin, 2013). Examination of rs8042149 in a group of individuals of European descent assessed for PTSD symptoms after hurricane exposure ($N = 551$) detected an association with PTSD symptom severity (Amstadter et al., 2013). However, associations between *RORA* SNPs (including rs8042149) were not detected in two larger independent replication samples from the Nurses' Health Study II and a cohort of Iraq and Afghanistan-era US veterans (Guffanti et al., 2014).

Genome-wide significant associations have also been reported with PTSD in the Tolloid-Like 1 gene (*TLL1*), the cordon-bleu WH2 repeat protein gene (*COBL*) (Xie et al., 2013), and in the long intergenic non-coding RNA (lincRNA) gene *AC068718.1*, although the association with *AC068718.1* was observed in a female-only sample (Guffanti et al., 2013). In a sample of 3,215 trauma-exposed individuals, no significant association between the *COBL* SNP rs406001 with PTSD symptoms was found, but a significant interaction between this SNP with childhood trauma was reported ($p = 0.0006$) (Almli et al., 2014). Another GWAS of dissociative symptoms associated with PTSD did not report any genome-wide significant hits, but the strongest signals were observed for

TABLE 4.2 Genome-wide Association Studies in Anxiety Disorders

REFERENCE	DISORDER	SAMPLES (RACE/ETHNICITY)	GENOME-WIDE SIGNIFICANT FINDINGS ($p < 5 \times 10^{-8}$)	ADDITIONAL/FOLLOW-UP FINDINGS
Otowa et al., 2009	Panic disorder	*Discovery:* 200 cases and 200 controls (Japanese) *Replication:* None	rs860554, *PKP1* ($p = 4.6 \times 10^{-8}$); rs12579350, *TMEM16B* ($p = 3.73 \times 10^{-9}$)	The top 32 SNPs did not replicate in a larger sample (Otowa, et al., 2010). No genome-wide significant associations were reported in a meta-analysis with replication samples (Otowa et al., 2012).
Erhardt et al., 2010	Panic disorder	*Discovery:* 216 cases and 222 controls (EU) *Replication 1:* 225 cases and 225 controls (EU) *Replication 2:* 468 cases with expanded anxiety diagnoses (84% comorbidity with other anxiety disorders) and 452 controls (EU)	rs7309727, *TMEM132D* ($p = 4.87 \times 10^{-8}$) in combined discovery sample and replication sample 1	Meta-analysis of 8 samples including Erhardt et al 2010 (total $N = 2,678$ cases and 3,262 controls) supported the association for rs7309727 ($p = 1.05 \times 10^{-8}$, OR 1.45, 95% CI 1.20–1.72) and haplotype rs7309727– rs11060369 (haplotype TA, $p = 1.4 \times 10^{-8}$, OR 1.44, 95% CI 1.20–1.73) but only in an EU subset (Erhardt et al., 2012). Sequencing of *TMEM132D* in 300 cases and 300 controls detected an overrepresentation of putatively functional coding variants in controls as compared with cases (Quast, et al., 2012).
Logue et al., 2012	Posttraumatic stress disorder	*Discovery:* 295 cases and 196 controls (EA) (Trauma-exposed cohort of veterans and partners/spouses) *Replication 1:* 43 cases and 41 controls (AA) *Replication 2:* 100 cases and 421 controls (AA)	rs8042149, *RORA* (G allele, $p = 2.5 \times 10^{-8}$, OR = 2.1) in discovery sample only	The association with rs8042149 was not supported in 2 larger independent samples (Guffanti et al., 2014), but this SNP was nominally associated with PTSD symptoms post-hurricane (Amstadter et al., 2013).

Study	Disorder	Sample	Findings	Comments
Xie et al., 2013	Posttraumatic stress disorder	*Discovery:* 444 cases and 2,322 controls (AA) and 300 cases and 1,278 controls (EA) *Replication 1:* 207 cases and 1692 controls (EA) *Replication 2:* 134 cases and 1,524 controls (EA) *Replication 3:* 89 cases and 655 controls (AA)	rs406001, *COBL* ($p = 3.97 \times 10^{-8}$) in EA discovery sample; rs681289, *TLL1* ($p = 3.1 \times 10^{-9}$) in combined EA discovery sample and replication sample 1	No genome-wide significant associations were reported when comparing cases to trauma-exposed controls only. Main effect of rs406001 was not replicated in an independent sample ($N = 3215$ trauma-exposed, primarily female AA individuals), but GxE interaction of this SNP with childhood trauma reported ($p = 0.0006$) (Almli et al., 2014).
Guffanti et al., 2013	Posttraumatic stress disorder	*Discovery:* 94 cases and 319 controls (all female sample; all controls were trauma-exposed) (86% AA) *Replication:* 578 cases and 1963 controls (EA females)	rs10170218, lincRNA *AC068718.1* ($p = 5.09 \times 10^{-8}$, OR = 2.88, 95% CI 1.97–4.23) in discovery sample only	Nominal support was reported in the replication sample.
Stewart, Yu, et al., 2013	Obsessive-compulsive disorder	*Discovery:* 1,465 cases (1279 EU/EA), 5,557 controls (5,139 EU/EA), and 400 complete trios (299 EU/EA). *Replication:* None	rs6131295, *BTBD3* ($p = 3.84 \times 10^{-8}$, OR 0.51) in trio-only analysis	Top SNPs in the case-control analysis: rs11081062 ($p = 2.49 \times 10^{-6}$) and rs11663827 ($p = 3.44 \times 10^{-6}$), both in the gene *DLGAP1*.
Mattheisen et al., 2014	Obsessive-compulsive disorder	*Discovery:* 5,061 subjects: 1,065 families including 1,406 cases, 192 singleton cases, and 1,984 controls. *Replication:* None	None	Top SNP: rs4401971 ($p = 4.13 \times 10^{-7}$) near *PTPRD*.

Abbreviations: EU, European. AA, African-American. EA, European-American. OR, odds ratio. CI, confidence interval. Race/ethnicity, associated allele, OR, and 95% CIs provided if reported in the original publication.

SNPs in the genes *ADCY8*, which has been implicated in fear-related learning, and *DPP6*, which is involved in synaptic integration (Wolf et al., 2014).

Two GWAS have been reported in OCD. In a study of 1,465 cases, 5,557 controls, and 400 trios, a SNP in *BTBD3* showed genome-wide significant association when the analysis was limited to parent-child trios, but a meta-analysis of all case/control and trio data did not support the association (Stewart, Yu, et al., 2013). A second OCD GWAS found no genome-wide significant associations in a sample of over 5,000 individuals (including 1,065 families, 192 unrelated cases, and 1,984 controls); the smallest p value reported (4.13×10^{-7}) was for a SNP in the gene *PTPRD*, a member of the receptor protein tyrosine phosphatase family involved in the regulation of inhibitory GABAergic synapses (Mattheisen et al., 2014).

The absence of robust associations in GWAS of anxiety disorders does not mean that risk SNPs cannot be found or do not exist. For example, the heritability of OCD attributable to common SNPs was estimated to be 37% based on GWAS data (Davis et al., 2013), close to the estimates of OCD heritability estimate in prior twin studies. In other words, common variants seem to explain most of the genetic liability to OCD even though the individual risk loci have yet to be identified. Experience from large-scale GWAS, such as those reported by the Psychiatric Genomics Consortium (PGC) have proven that risk loci can be found for psychiatric disorders given sufficient power. The most successful example to date has come from a GWAS of nearly 37,000 schizophrenia cases that identified 108 genome-wide significant loci (Schizophrenia Working Group of the Psychiatric Genomics Consortium, 2014). Larger sample sizes will be required to detect loci influencing anxiety disorder at genome-wide significant thresholds.

Copy Number Variation

Copy number variants (CNVs) are duplications, insertions, or deletions of large DNA sequences ranging from thousands to millions of bases. CNVs can span multiple genes and arise through de novo (novel) mutations or are inherited. CNVs have been implicated in a range of psychiatric disorders—particularly de novo CNVs in neurodevelopmental phenotypes including autism spectrum disorder and schizophrenia.

Williams syndrome, a neurodevelopmental disorder caused by a deletion of approximately three megabases on chromosome 7q, is associated with excess rates of GAD and specific phobias, suggesting that one or more genes influencing anxiety may reside in the deleted region (Leyfer, Woodruff-Borden, and Mervis, 2009). The role of CNVs in more common, non-syndromic anxiety disorders has received little attention. A CNV study of PD in a Japanese sample (535 cases and 1,520 controls) found no association of rare CNVs but found a statistically significant excess of common duplications in the 16p11.2 region (Kawamura et al., 2011).

The first genome-wide CNV analysis in OCD found no global increase in CNV burden in OCD cases as compared with controls, but there was a 3.3-fold enrichment of large deletions overlapping deletions previously implicated in neurodevelopmental disorders (McGrath et al., 2014). Five of these deletions were on 16p13.11, which has previously been implicated in intellectual disability, autism, and seizures, although none of the OCD patients had these comorbidities.

Rare Single Nucleotide Variants

One limitation of GWAS is that rare variants, those with allele frequencies less than 1%, or those that arise de novo are typically not assayed. Whole genome sequencing (WGS) and whole exome sequencing (WES) can interrogate every nucleotide in the human genome and in protein-coding regions, respectively. DNA sequencing can also be used to target specific genes or regions of interest. Rare variants detected through these methods may provide more information about the genetic architecture of these disorders and the extent to which less common variation contributes to anxiety disorders.

Following the association of *TMEM132D* in GWAS analyses of PD, the gene was resequenced in 300 anxiety disorder cases (85% with a diagnosis of PD) and 300 healthy controls (Quast et al., 2012). An overrepresentation of putatively functional coding variants in controls as compared with cases was reported, thus suggesting that rare alleles in *TMEM132D* may have a protective effect. This finding awaits further replication and functional analyses. No WGS or WES has been reported in anxiety disorders to date.

Gene-Environment Interactions

Given the moderate heritabilities reported for all anxiety disorders, there are substantial environmental factors that play a role in the development of these disorders. A major focus of research into the etiology of anxiety disorders in recent years has been the interaction between genetic variants and environmental exposures. A gene-environment interaction (GxE) occurs when the effect of genetic risk factors is modified by life experiences or other environmental exposures. Studying GxE interactions could provide information on the type and severity of exposures that affect anxiety disorders in the presence of genetic vulnerability. However, recent reviews of candidate gene GxE studies in psychiatry have shown that these studies are limited in power and replicability. In fact, there is evidence of publication bias toward positive findings, and it has been estimated that >97% of all associations reported in GxE studies conducted in the 1st decade of psychiatric GxE research were false positives (Duncan, Pollastri, and Smoller, 2014).

To date, some of the most compelling evidence regarding candidate gene-environment interaction effects has emerged from studies incorporating epigenetic effects of environmental exposures. *Epigenetics* refers to the study of factors affecting gene expression that do not result from DNA sequence variation. The most widely studied class of epigenetic effects in anxiety disorders has been DNA methylation, which involves the addition of a methyl group to cytosine nucleotides located at CpG sites (where a cytosine nucleotide is next to a guanine). DNA methylation is typically associated with reduced gene transcription. A variety of environmental exposures and experiences have been shown to affect DNA methylation. Of particular relevance to psychopathology, early adversity and trauma have been associated with local and genome-wide profiles of DNA methylation (Oh et al., 2013).

Epigenetically mediated interaction has been reported between childhood adversity and variation in the FK506 binding protein 5 gene, *FKBP5*. FKBP5 reduces glucocorticoid activation of the glucocorticoid receptor, thus altering the HPA axis stress response. Klengel and colleagues (2013) found that an allele of the *FKBP5* SNP rs1360780, previously associated with PTSD and depression, increases *FKBP5* expression by creating an enhancer site near a glucocorticoid response element (GRE) and altering chromatin (DNA-protein complex) structure. Glucocorticoid release in response to early life adversity then drives enhanced *FKBP5* expression among risk allele carriers, causing demethylation of another GRE elsewhere in the gene. This leads to persistently elevated *FKBP5* expression, which can be further amplified by increased glucocorticoid release in response to later-life stress or trauma. The results include increased *FKBP5*-mediated hippocampal glucocorticoid resistance that appears to confer risk of stress-related disorders in adulthood.

The widely studied 5-HTTLPR variant in the promoter of the serotonin transporter gene (*SLC6A4*) has also been investigated in GxE studies of PTSD. A significant interaction between homozygosity for the short allele and childhood adversity for PTSD has been reported, though this association was found only in European-Americans (Xie, Kranzler, Farrer, and Gelernter, 2012). A meta-analysis of 12 studies of the association with 5-HTTLPR and PTSD found no overall association, but further analysis suggested that harboring two copies of the short allele may be a risk factor for PTSD after high trauma exposure (Gressier et al., 2013). Epigenetic studies have also suggested that the effect of adversity on stress-related phenotypes may be mediated by DNA methylation within *SLC6A4*, though the specific nature of the effect remains unclear. Koenen and colleagues (2011) found that *reduced* methylation (in blood samples) at an intron of *SLC6A4* moderated the effect of trauma on PTSD, independent of 5-HTTLPR genotype. Specifically, increasing number of traumatic life events was associated with PTSD in the presence of hypomethylation, while hypermethylation appeared to be protective for high-trauma-exposed individuals. More recently, methylation of the promoter (in both blood and saliva DNA samples) was associated with threat-related amygdala reactivity (a phenotype previously shown to be associated with anxious temperament and anxiety disorders) as well as reduced *SLC6A4* expression in post-mortem amygdala, and these effects were again independent of 5-HTTLPR genotype (Nikolova et al., 2014).

Genetic and epigenetic influences on PTSD risk have also been reported in studies of the pituitary adenylate cyclase-activating polypeptide (PACAP) receptor gene (*ADCYAP1R1*). PACAP, a hypothalamic neuropeptide, has been associated with fear behavior and stress responses in animal models. Ressler and colleagues (2011) reported that variation in *ADCYAP1R1* is associated with PTSD in females. In particular, a SNP (rs2267735) in a putative estrogen response element (ERE) was associated with PTSD risk as both a main effect and a gene-environment interaction with trauma. Further analyses revealed associations between the PTSD risk allele at this SNP and expression of the PACAP receptor in human brain, as well as increased amygdala reactivity to threat stimuli and reduced amygdala/hippocampal connectivity by fMRI (Ressler et al., 2011; Stevens et al., 2014). Methylation (in blood DNA) of *ADCYAP1R1* was also associated with PTSD. While several subsequent association analyses did not support a main effect of rs2267735 with PTSD (Chang et al., 2012), gene-environment interactions for this SNP have been observed with childhood adversity and high levels of lifetime trauma in females (Almli et al., 2013; Uddin et al., 2013).

To date, GxE studies of anxiety disorders have been limited by a focus on candidate genes and relatively small sample sizes. In the coming years, larger scale efforts, including genome-wide GxE studies, may facilitate discoveries in this area.

BEYOND DIAGNOSTIC BOUNDARIES

Family and twin studies have shown that anxiety disorders do not "breed true." That is, genetic influences transcend the diagnostic boundaries defined in the DSM and ICD nosology. Relatives of individuals with a given anxiety disorder are also at increased risk for a range of other anxiety disorders, and twin studies have documented genetic overlap among most if not all anxiety disorders (Hettema, Prescott, Myers, Neale, and Kendler, 2005; Smoller, Gardner-Schuster, and Covino, 2008; Tambs et al., 2009). Factor analyses of twin data show genetic overlap of phobic fears that do not respect DSM boundaries (Loken, Hettema, Aggen, and Kendler, 2014). In fact, the shared genetic component among PD, phobias, GAD, OCD, and PTSD is substantially larger than their disorder-specific genetic components (Tambs et al., 2009). The familial and genetic factors underlying anxiety disorders also overlap substantially with those influencing risk of major depressive disorder (MDD). A meta-analysis of family studies of anxiety disorders showed that the offspring of parents with anxiety have 2.67 higher odds of having depressive disorders than nonpsychiatric control offspring (Micco et al., 2009). Twin studies have found strong genetic correlations between anxiety disorders and depression, as high as 0.77 for PTSD and MDD and 1.0 for GAD and MDD (Kendler, Gardner, Gatz, and Pedersen, 2007; Koenen et al., 2008).

ANXIETY-RELATED TRAITS

The genetic overlap among anxiety disorders may reflect genetic influences on underlying dimensions of anxiety-proneness that confer liability to multiple disorders. Fear and anxiety are universal human experiences with clear adaptive significance, and the precise line between normal and pathological anxiety is often difficult if not impossible to draw. Considering anxiety disorders as a spectrum of quantitative traits, however, avoids the difficulty of drawing arbitrary lines of anxiety diagnoses and may better model the genetic liability of anxiety disorders. In addition, if anxiety disorders, in reality, represent more extreme variations of a continuously distributed set of traits, genetic studies may be more powerful by studying the underlying traits. Studies of the genetics of anxiety-related traits have focused on temperamental and personality traits that have been associated with a liability to develop various anxiety disorders in children and adults, including behavioral inhibition, neuroticism, introversion, and harm avoidance.

Heritability estimates for these anxiety-related traits have been comparable to or greater than those of anxiety disorders themselves (in the range of 40–70%) (Smoller, Gardner-Schuster, and Misiaszek, 2008). Linkage studies of anxiety-related traits have implicated multiple areas of the genome. A recent meta-analysis of eight linkage studies of neuroticism found evidence for linkage on chromosomes 9, 11, 12, and 14 (Webb et al., 2012), while linkage to chromosome 8q has been reported for harm avoidance (Dina et al., 2005).

Much like those focusing on anxiety disorders themselves, candidate gene studies of anxiety-related traits have tended to be underpowered and report conflicting results. However, several loci have received convergent support for association with anxiety traits in studies of temperament, personality and underlying brain circuitry. The most widely studied polymorphism has been the 5-HTTLPR in the serotonin transporter gene promoter. Scores of studies have examined the association of the 5-HTTLPR with a range of anxiety-related traits, but results have been inconclusive. Nevertheless, numerous studies have reported an association between the short allele of the 5-HTTLPR and individual differences in emotion-related circuitry. In particular, a significant though modest effect of the short allele on amygdala reactivity to emotional or threatening stimuli has been supported by a meta-analysis of 34 studies (Murphy et al., 2013). There is also evidence that this allele is associated with reduced top down modulation of the amygdala by the anterior cingulate cortex, an effect associated with increased harm avoidance (Pezawas et al., 2005).

Behavioral and brain anxiety-related traits have also been associated with regulator of G protein signaling 2 (*RGS2*), which modulates G-protein-coupled receptor signaling in response to neurotransmitters such as serotonin and norepinephrine. Mouse studies first implicated this gene as a quantitative trait gene influencing anxious temperament. Subsequently, variants in *RGS2*, including a SNP (rs4606) associated with reduced *RGS2* expression, were associated with behavioral inhibition, a stable tendency to be cautious and behaviorally restrained in novel social and nonsocial situations that is a familial and developmental risk factor for SAD and other anxiety disorders (Smoller, Paulus, et al., 2008). The same alleles were also associated with introversion in adults and amygdala and insular cortex activation in response to emotional faces, brain phenotypes implicated in liability to social and other anxiety disorders.

A third example of convergent evidence involves a functional polymorphism (Val66Met) in the gene encoding brain derived neurotrophic factor (*BDNF*), a growth factor that is important in neurogenesis and synaptic plasticity. Candidate gene studies of this polymorphism have had conflicting results, but Casey and colleagues (Casey, Pattwell, Glatt, and Lee, 2013) have demonstrated that mice engineered to express the human Met allele exhibit increased anxiety-related behaviors and are resistant to SSRI treatment. They further found that the Met allele is associated with impaired fear extinction in mice and humans and amygdala-prefrontal cortical imbalance in humans. Other groups have found that the Val/Met polymorphism is associated with anxiety-related brain structure and function and that epigenetic variation at BDNF is also associated with impairments in fear extinction.

Anxiety-related traits have also been the subject of several GWAS, but no genome-wide significant loci have been established. Indeed, meta-analyses of up to 17,000 subjects have found no genome-wide significant associations for neuroticism or harm avoidance (de Moor et al., 2012; Service et al., 2012). Estimates of heritability from aggregate genome-wide SNP data ("SNP-chip heritability") have been substantially lower than those reported in twin studies: 6% for neuroticism and 1–19% for anxiety-related behaviors as measured by the Anxiety-Related Behaviors Questionnaire (Trzaskowski et al., 2013; Vinkhuyzen et al., 2012). These results suggest that common variants influencing these traits exist, but they have very modest effects, consistent with the hypothesis that anxiety-related personality traits are highly polygenic and that environmental influences play a substantial role.

CHALLENGES AND FRONTIERS IN THE GENETICS OF ANXIETY DISORDERS

Key insights from genetic studies of anxiety disorders are summarized in Box 4.1. Family and twin studies have established that anxiety disorders are familial and heritable. However, efforts to identify the specific DNA variations contributing to the heritability of these disorders have had limited success. Genetic studies of anxiety face a number of obstacles. The first has to do with defining the relevant phenotypes. The line between normal and pathologic anxiety is often unclear, and the phenotypic and genetic boundaries between clinical anxiety syndromes are fuzzy. Second, the discovery of anxiety-related genetic loci has been hampered by the relatively small sample sizes of existing studies. Like other psychiatric disorders, anxiety disorders are likely to be highly polygenic, involving thousands of genetic variants of modest effect. The successful discovery of genetic risk variants for other psychiatric disorders (notably, schizophrenia,

> ### BOX 4.1
> ## SUMMARY OF THE GENETICS OF ANXIETY DISORDERS
>
> - Anxiety disorders run in families. First-degree relatives of affected individuals (probands) have approximately a five-fold increased risk of the proband's anxiety disorder compared to individuals in the general population. Family history remains the most relevant clinical predictor of risk.
> - Anxiety disorders are heritable. Twin studies have shown that 20–40% of the risk of anxiety disorders is attributable to genetic variation in the population.
> - Genetic association studies of anxiety disorders have had limited success to date. Several candidate genes have been implicated in risk of various anxiety disorders, anxiety-related traits, and anxiety-related brain phenotypes, but results have been inconsistent. No specific common or rare variants have been established by genome-wide association studies.
> - Anxiety disorders are likely to be highly polygenic, reflecting hundreds or thousands of variants of individually small effects.
> - Genetic influences are substantially shared across a range of anxiety disorders and depression.
> - Success in identifying risk loci and gene-environment interactions will require much larger samples and should capitalize on insights from animal models and human studies of anxiety-related brain circuitry.

bipolar disorder, and autism) has required sample sizes much larger than any reported to date for the anxiety disorders. While the genetic architecture of anxiety disorders is still unclear, it may be similar to that of MDD, for which even a GWAS mega-analysis comprising nearly 9,500 cases failed to detect any genome-wide significant associations. Progress in defining the genetic architecture of anxiety disorders will require large-scale studies (including meta-analyses) and systematic replication efforts.

Despite these challenges, genetic research on anxiety can make use of several resources that are less well-developed for other psychiatric disorders. In particular, well-established experimental animal models capture key aspects of human anxiety and fear behavior, and neuroimaging studies have made substantial progress in mapping the structural and functional components of anxiety/fear circuitry. These resources create opportunities for focusing genetic studies on relevant biological pathways as well as platforms for evaluating the functional significance of risk loci that may be identified in the future.

REFERENCES

Almli, L. M., Mercer, K. B., Kerley, K., Feng, H., Bradley, B., Conneely, K. N., and Ressler, K. J. (2013). ADCYAP1R1 genotype associates with post-traumatic stress symptoms in highly traumatized African-American females. *Am J Med Genet B Neuropsychiatr Genet, 162B* (3), 262–272. doi: 10.1002/ajmg.b.32145

Almli, L. M., Srivastava, A., Fani, N., Kerley, K., Mercer, K. B., Feng, H., . . . Ressler, K. J. (2014). Follow-up and extension of a prior genome-wide association study of posttraumatic stress disorder: Gene x environment associations and structural magnetic resonance imaging in a highly traumatized African-American civilian population. *Biol Psychiatry, 76*(4), e3–e4. doi: 10.1016/j.biopsych.2014.01.017

Amstadter, A. B., Sumner, J. A., Acierno, R., Ruggiero, K. J., Koenen, K. C., Kilpatrick, D. G., . . . Gelernter, J. (2013). Support for association of RORA variant and post traumatic stress symptoms in a population-based study of hurricane exposed adults. *Mol Psychiatry, 18*(11), 1148–1149. doi: 10.1038/mp.2012.189

Casey, B. J., Pattwell, S. S., Glatt, C. E., and Lee, F. S. (2013). Treating the developing brain: Implications from human imaging and mouse genetics. *Annu Rev Med, 64*, 427–439. doi: 10.1146/annurev-med-052611-130408

Chang, S. C., Xie, P., Anton, R. F., De Vivo, I., Farrer, L. A., Kranzler, H. R., . . . Koenen, K. C. (2012). No association between ADCYAP1R1 and post-traumatic stress disorder in two independent samples. *Mol Psychiatry, 17* (3), 239–241. doi: 10.1038/mp.2011.118

Davis, L. K., Yu, D., Keenan, C. L., Gamazon, E. R., Konkashbaev, A. I., Derks, E. M., . . . Scharf, J. M. (2013). Partitioning the heritability of Tourette syndrome and obsessive compulsive disorder reveals differences in genetic architecture. *PLoS Genet, 9* (10), e1003864. doi: 10.1371/journal.pgen.1003864

de Moor, M. H., Costa, P. T., Terracciano, A., Krueger, R. F., de Geus, E. J., Toshiko, T., . . . Boomsma, D. I. (2012). Meta-analysis of genome-wide association studies for personality. *Mol Psychiatry, 17* (3), 337–349. doi: 10.1038/mp.2010.128

Dina, C., Nemanov, L., Gritsenko, I., Rosolio, N., Osher, Y., Heresco-Levy, U., . . . Ebstein, R. P. (2005). Fine mapping of a region on chromosome 8p gives evidence for a QTL contributing to individual differences in an anxiety-related personality trait: TPQ harm avoidance. *Am J Med Genet B Neuropsychiatr Genet, 132B* (1), 104–108. doi: 10.1002/ajmg.b.30099

Duncan, L. E., Pollastri, A. R., and Smoller, J. W. (2014). Mind the gap: Why many geneticists and psychological scientists have discrepant views about gene-environment interaction (GxE) research. *Am Psychol, 69* (3), 249–268. doi: 10.1037/a0036320

Erhardt, A., Akula, N., Schumacher, J., Czamara, D., Karbalai, N., Muller-Myhsok, B., . . . Binder, E. B. (2012). Replication and meta-analysis of TMEM132D gene variants in panic disorder. *Transl Psychiatry, 2*, e156. doi: 10.1038/tp.2012.85

Erhardt, A., Czibere, L., Roeske, D., Lucae, S., Unschuld, P. G., Ripke, S., . . . Binder, E. B. (2011). TMEM132D, a new candidate for anxiety phenotypes: Evidence from human and mouse studies. *Mol Psychiatry, 16* (6), 647–663. doi: 10.1038/mp.2010.41

Gressier, F., Calati, R., Balestri, M., Marsano, A., Alberti, S., Antypa, N., and Serretti, A. (2013). The 5-HTTLPR polymorphism and posttraumatic stress disorder: A meta-analysis. *J Trauma Stress, 26* (6), 645–653. doi: 10.1002/jts.21855

Guffanti, G., Ashley-Koch, A. E., Roberts, A. L., Garrett, M. E., Solovieff, N., Ratanatharathorn, A., . . . Koenen, K. C. (2014). No association between RORA polymorphisms and PTSD in two independent samples. *Mol Psychiatry, 19*(10), 1056–1057. doi: 10.1038/mp.2014.19

Guffanti, G., Galea, S., Yan, L., Roberts, A. L., Solovieff, N., Aiello, A. E., . . . Koenen, K. C. (2013). Genome-wide association study implicates a novel RNA gene, the lincRNA AC068718.1, as a risk factor for post-traumatic stress disorder in women. *Psychoneuroendocrinology, 38* (12), 3029–3038. doi: 10.1016/j.psyneuen.2013.08.014

Haaker, J., Lonsdorf, T. B., Raczka, K. A., Mechias, M. L., Gartmann, N., and Kalisch, R. (2014). Higher anxiety and larger amygdala volumes in carriers of a TMEM132D risk variant for panic disorder. *Transl Psychiatry, 4*, e357. doi: 10.1038/tp.2014.1

Hettema, J. M., Neale, M. C., and Kendler, K. S. (2001). A review and meta-analysis of the genetic epidemiology of anxiety disorders. *Am J Psychiatry, 158* (10), 1568–1578.

Hettema, J. M., Prescott, C. A., Myers, J. M., Neale, M. C., and Kendler, K. S. (2005). The structure of genetic and environmental risk factors for anxiety disorders in men and women. *Arch Gen Psychiatry, 62*(2), 182–189. doi: 10.1001/archpsyc.62.2.182

Kawamura, Y., Otowa, T., Koike, A., Sugaya, N., Yoshida, E., Yasuda, S., . . . Sasaki, T. (2011). A genome-wide CNV association study on panic disorder in a Japanese population. *J Hum Genet, 56* (12), 852–856. doi: 10.1038/jhg.2011.117

Kendler, K. S., Gardner, C. O., Gatz, M., and Pedersen, N. L. (2007). The sources of co-morbidity between major depression and generalized anxiety disorder in a Swedish national twin sample. *Psychol Med*, 37(3), 453–462. doi: 10.1017/S0033291706009135

Kessler, R. C., and Wang, P. S. (2008). The descriptive epidemiology of commonly occurring mental disorders in the United States. *Annu Rev Public Health*, 29, 115–129. doi: 10.1146/annurev.publhealth.29.020907.090847

Klengel, T., Mehta, D., Anacker, C., Rex-Haffner, M., Pruessner, J. C., Pariante, C. M., . . . Binder, E. B. (2013). Allele-specific FKBP5 DNA demethylation mediates gene-childhood trauma interactions. *Nat Neurosci*, 16 1), 33–41. doi: 10.1038/nn.3275

Koenen, K. C., Fu, Q. J., Ertel, K., Lyons, M. J., Eisen, S. A., True, W. R., . . . Tsuang, M. T. (2008). Common genetic liability to major depression and posttraumatic stress disorder in men. *J Affect Disord*, 105 (1–3), 109–115. doi: 10.1016/j.jad.2007.04.021

Koenen, K. C., Uddin, M., Chang, S. C., Aiello, A. E., Wildman, D. E., Goldmann, E., and Galea, S. (2011). SLC6A4 methylation modifies the effect of the number of traumatic events on risk for posttraumatic stress disorder. *Depress Anxiety*, 28 (8), 639–647. doi: 10.1002/da.20825

Leyfer, O., Woodruff-Borden, J., and Mervis, C. B. (2009). Anxiety disorders in children with Williams syndrome, their mothers, and their siblings: Implications for the etiology of anxiety disorders. *J Neurodev Disord*, 1 (1), 4–14. doi: 10.1007/s11689-009-9003-1

Logue, M. W., Baldwin, C., Guffanti, G., Melista, E., Wolf, E. J., Reardon, A. F., . . . Miller, M. W. (2013). A genome-wide association study of post-traumatic stress disorder identifies the retinoid-related orphan receptor alpha (RORA) gene as a significant risk locus. *Mol Psychiatry*, 18 (8), 937–942. doi: 10.1038/mp.2012.113

Loken, E. K., Hettema, J. M., Aggen, S. H., and Kendler, K. S. (2014). The structure of genetic and environmental risk factors for fears and phobias. *Psychol Med*, 1–10. doi: 10.1017/S0033291713003012

Maron, E., Hettema, J. M., and Shlik, J. (2010). Advances in molecular genetics of panic disorder. *Mol Psychiatry*, 15(7), 681–701. doi: 10.1038/mp.2009.145

Mattheisen, M., Samuels, J. F., Wang, Y., Greenberg, B. D., Fyer, A. J., McCracken, J. T., . . . Nestadt, G. (2014). Genome-wide association study in obsessive-compulsive disorder: Results from the OCGAS. *Mol Psychiatry*. doi: 10.1038/mp.2014.43

McGrath, L. M., Weill, S., Robinson, E. B., Macrae, R., and Smoller, J. W. (2012). Bringing a developmental perspective to anxiety genetics. *Dev Psychopathol*, 24(4), 1179–1193. doi: 10.1017/S0954579412000636

McGrath, L. M., Yu, D., Marshall, C., Davis, L. K., Thiruvahindrapuram, B., Li, B., . . . Scharf, J. M. (2014). Copy number variation in obsessive-compulsive disorder and tourette syndrome: A cross-disorder study. *J Am Acad Child Adolesc Psychiatry*, 53 (8), 910–919. doi: 10.1016/j.jaac.2014.04.022

Micco, J. A., Henin, A., Mick, E., Kim, S., Hopkins, C. A., Biederman, J., and Hirshfeld-Becker, D. R. (2009). Anxiety and depressive disorders in offspring at high risk for anxiety: a meta-analysis. *J Anxiety Disord*, 23 (8), 1158–1164. doi: 10.1016/j.janxdis.2009.07.021

Miller, M. W., Wolf, E. J., Logue, M. W., and Baldwin, C. T. (2013). The retinoid-related orphan receptor alpha (RORA) gene and fear-related psychopathology. *J Affect Disord*, 151(2), 702–708. doi: 10.1016/j.jad.2013.07.022

Murphy, S. E., Norbury, R., Godlewska, B. R., Cowen, P. J., Mannie, Z. M., Harmer, C. J., and Munafo, M. R. (2013). The effect of the serotonin transporter polymorphism (5-HTTLPR) on amygdala function: A meta-analysis. *Mol Psychiatry*, 18(4), 512–520. doi: 10.1038/mp.2012.19

Navarro-Mateu, F., Escamez, T., Koenen, K. C., Alonso, J., and Sanchez-Meca, J. (2013). Meta-analyses of the 5-HTTLPR polymorphisms and post-traumatic stress disorder. *PLoS One*, 8(6), e66227. doi: 10.1371/journal.pone.0066227

Nikolova, Y. S., Koenen, K. C., Galea, S., Wang, C. M., Seney, M. L., Sibille, E., . . . Hariri, A. R. (2014). Beyond genotype: Serotonin transporter epigenetic modification predicts human brain function. *Nat Neurosci*, 17 (9), 1153–1155. doi: 10.1038/nn.3778

Oh, J. E., Chambwe, N., Klein, S., Gal, J., Andrews, S., Gleason, G., . . . Toth, M. (2013). Differential gene body methylation and reduced expression of cell adhesion and neurotransmitter receptor genes in adverse maternal environment. *Transl Psychiatry, 3,* e218. doi: 10.1038/tp.2012.130

Otowa, T., Kawamura, Y., Nishida, N., Sugaya, N., Koike, A., Yoshida, E., . . . Sasaki, T. (2012). Meta-analysis of genome-wide association studies for panic disorder in the Japanese population. *Transl Psychiatry, 2,* e186. doi: 10.1038/tp.2012.89

Otowa, T., Tanii, H., Sugaya, N., Yoshida, E., Inoue, K., Yasuda, S., . . . Sasaki, T. (2010). Replication of a genome-wide association study of panic disorder in a Japanese population. *J Hum Genet, 55* (2), 91–96. doi: 10.1038/jhg.2009.127

Otowa, T., Yoshida, E., Sugaya, N., Yasuda, S., Nishimura, Y., Inoue, K., . . . Okazaki, Y. (2009). Genome-wide association study of panic disorder in the Japanese population. *J Hum Genet, 54* (2), 122–126. doi: 10.1038/jhg.2008.17

Pauls, D. L., Abramovitch, A., Rauch, S. L., and Geller, D. A. (2014). Obsessive-compulsive disorder: An integrative genetic and neurobiological perspective. *Nat Rev Neurosci, 15* (6), 410–424. doi: 10.1038/nrn3746

Pezawas, L., Meyer-Lindenberg, A., Drabant, E. M., Verchinski, B. A., Munoz, K. E., Kolachana, B. S., . . . Weinberger, D. R. (2005). 5-HTTLPR polymorphism impacts human cingulate-amygdala interactions: A genetic susceptibility mechanism for depression. *Nat Neurosci, 8* (6), 828–834. doi: 10.1038/nn1463

Quast, C., Altmann, A., Weber, P., Arloth, J., Bader, D., Heck, A., . . . Binder, E. B. (2012). Rare variants in TMEM132D in a case-control sample for panic disorder. *Am J Med Genet B Neuropsychiatr Genet, 159B*(8), 896–907. doi: 10.1002/ajmg.b.32096

Reif, A., Weber, H., Domschke, K., Klauke, B., Baumann, C., Jacob, C. P., . . . Deckert, J. (2012). Meta-analysis argues for a female-specific role of MAOA-uVNTR in panic disorder in four European populations. *Am J Med Genet B Neuropsychiatr Genet, 159B* (7), 786–793. doi: 10.1002/ajmg.b.32085

Ressler, K. J., Mercer, K. B., Bradley, B., Jovanovic, T., Mahan, A., Kerley, K., . . . May, V. (2011). Post-traumatic stress disorder is associated with PACAP and the PAC1 receptor. *Nature, 470* (7335), 492–497. doi: 10.1038/nature09856

Schizophrenia Working Group of the Psychiatric Genomics, Consortium. (2014). Biological insights from 108 schizophrenia-associated genetic loci. *Nature, 511* (7510), 421–427. doi: 10.1038/nature13595

Service, S. K., Verweij, K. J., Lahti, J., Congdon, E., Ekelund, J., Hintsanen, M., . . . Freimer, N. B. (2012). A genome-wide meta-analysis of association studies of Cloninger's Temperament Scales. *Transl Psychiatry, 2,* e116. doi: 10.1038/tp.2012.37

Smoller, J. W., Block, S. R., and Young, M. M. (2009). Genetics of anxiety disorders: The complex road from DSM to DNA. *Depress Anxiety, 26* (11), 965–975. doi: 10.1002/da.20623

Smoller, J. W., Gallagher, P. J., Duncan, L. E., McGrath, L. M., Haddad, S. A., Holmes, A. J., . . . Cohen, B. M. (2014). The human ortholog of acid-sensing ion channel gene ASIC1a is associated with panic disorder and amygdala structure and function. *Biol Psychiatry, 76*(11), 902–910. doi: 10.1016/j.biopsych.2013.12.018

Smoller, J. W., Gardner-Schuster, E., and Covino, J. (2008). The genetic basis of panic and phobic anxiety disorders. *Am J Med Genet C Semin Med Genet, 148C* (2), 118–126. doi: 10.1002/ajmg.c.30174

Smoller, J. W., Gardner-Schuster, E., and Misiaszek, M. (2008). Genetics of anxiety: Would the genome recognize the DSM? *Depress Anxiety, 25* (4), 368–377. doi: 10.1002/da.20492

Smoller, J. W., Paulus, M. P., Fagerness, J. A., Purcell, S., Yamaki, L. H., Hirshfeld-Becker, D., . . . Stein, M. B. (2008). Influence of RGS2 on anxiety-related temperament, personality, and brain function. *Arch Gen Psychiatry, 65* (3), 298–308. doi: 10.1001/archgenpsychiatry.2007.48

Stevens, J. S., Almli, L. M., Fani, N., Gutman, D. A., Bradley, B., Norrholm, S. D., . . . Ressler, K. J. (2014). PACAP receptor gene polymorphism impacts fear responses in the amygdala and hippocampus. *Proc Natl Acad Sci U S A, 111* (8), 3158–3163. doi: 10.1073/pnas.1318954111

Stewart, S. E., Mayerfeld, C., Arnold, P. D., Crane, J. R., O'Dushlaine, C., Fagerness, J. A., . . . Mathews, C. A. (2013). Meta-analysis of association between obsessive-compulsive disorder and the 3' region of neuronal glutamate transporter gene SLC1A1. *Am J Med Genet B Neuropsychiatr Genet, 162B* (4), 367–379. doi: 10.1002/ajmg.b.32137

Stewart, S. E., Yu, D., Scharf, J. M., Neale, B. M., Fagerness, J. A., Mathews, C. A., . . . Pauls, D. L. (2013). Genome-wide association study of obsessive-compulsive disorder. *Mol Psychiatry, 18* (7), 788–798. doi: 10.1038/mp.2012.85

Tambs, K., Ronning, T., Prescott, C. A., Kendler, K. S., Reichborn-Kjennerud, T., Torgersen, S., and Harris, J. R. (2009). The Norwegian Institute of Public Health twin study of mental health: Examining recruitment and attrition bias. *Twin Res Hum Genet, 12* (2), 158–168. doi: 10.1375/twin.12.2.158

Taylor, S. (2013). Molecular genetics of obsessive-compulsive disorder: A comprehensive meta-analysis of genetic association studies. *Mol Psychiatry, 18*(7), 799–805. doi: 10.1038/mp.2012.76

Trzaskowski, M., Eley, T. C., Davis, O. S., Doherty, S. J., Hanscombe, K. B., Meaburn, E. L., . . . Plomin, R. (2013). First genome-wide association study on anxiety-related behaviours in childhood. *PLoS One, 8* (4), e58676. doi: 10.1371/journal.pone.0058676

Uddin, M., Chang, S. C., Zhang, C., Ressler, K., Mercer, K. B., Galea, S., . . . Koenen, K. C. (2013). Adcyap1r1 genotype, posttraumatic stress disorder, and depression among women exposed to childhood maltreatment. *Depress Anxiety, 30* (3), 251–258. doi: 10.1002/da.22037

Vinkhuyzen, A. A., Pedersen, N. L., Yang, J., Lee, S. H., Magnusson, P. K., Iacono, W. G., . . . Wray, N. R. (2012). Common SNPs explain some of the variation in the personality dimensions of neuroticism and extraversion. *Transl Psychiatry, 2*, e102. doi: 10.1038/tp.2012.27

Webb, B. T., Guo, A. Y., Maher, B. S., Zhao, Z., van den Oord, E. J., Kendler, K. S., . . . Hettema, J. M. (2012). Meta-analyses of genome-wide linkage scans of anxiety-related phenotypes. *Eur J Hum Genet, 20* (10), 1078–1084. doi: 10.1038/ejhg.2012.47

Wolf, E. J., Rasmusson, A. M., Mitchell, K. S., Logue, M. W., Baldwin, C. T., and Miller, M. W. (2014). A genome-wide association study of clinical symptoms of dissociation in a trauma-exposed sample. *Depress Anxiety, 31* (4), 352–360. doi: 10.1002/da.22260

Xie, P., Kranzler, H. R., Farrer, L., and Gelernter, J. (2012). Serotonin transporter 5-HTTLPR genotype moderates the effects of childhood adversity on posttraumatic stress disorder risk: a replication study. *Am J Med Genet B Neuropsychiatr Genet, 159B* (6), 644–652. doi: 10.1002/ajmg.b.32068

Xie, P., Kranzler, H. R., Yang, C., Zhao, H., Farrer, L. A., and Gelernter, J. (2013). Genome-wide association study identifies new susceptibility loci for posttraumatic stress disorder. *Biol Psychiatry, 74* (9), 656–663. doi: 10.1016/j.biopsych.2013.04.013

Ziemann, A. E., Allen, J. E., Dahdaleh, N. S., Drebot, II, Coryell, M. W., Wunsch, A. M., . . . Wemmie, J. A. (2009). The amygdala is a chemosensor that detects carbon dioxide and acidosis to elicit fear behavior. *Cell, 139* (5), 1012–1021. doi: 10.1016/j.cell.2009.10.029

DEVELOPMENT OF FEAR, FEAR PATHWAYS, AND ANXIETY DISORDERS IN CHILDREN AND ADOLESCENTS

5

DEVELOPMENTAL BIOLOGY RELATED TO EMOTION AND ANXIETY

DANIEL S. PINE

INTRODUCTION

Fear and anxiety motivate behaviors across species and are often experienced during childhood. This chapter applies the same terms across species to facilitate translational perspectives on expressions of fear and anxiety across development. Hence, the term "emotion" is used to refer to brain states elicited by stimuli that influence behavior, with rewards eliciting approach, punishments eliciting avoidance, and threats being punishments that are avoided because they are dangerous. The term "fear" refers to the brain state elicited by an immediately present threat; "anxiety" refers to the state elicited by a distal, chronic threat. Humans can richly describe their experiences when threatened, but, given a translational perspective, the current chapter more strongly emphasizes data on behavior, information-processing, and brain functions shared across species than on reported experience. While the chapter broadly considers emotions, it focuses most deeply on fear and anxiety.

Current developmental conceptualizations reflect three research areas reviewed in three chapter sections. First, longitudinal research is described on developmental aspects of anxiety in humans. Second, basic research is described on neural circuitry in rodents and non-human primates. Finally, brain imaging research is described to integrate these two areas.

DEVELOPMENTAL PSYCHOPATHOLOGY

Research in developmental psychopathology charts age-related changes in behavior, emphasizing the mutually informative nature of research on normal and abnormal variations. Current conceptualizations of anxiety are informed by both areas of research.

Two observations on normal fear shape current thinking. First, fear and anxiety are common; many surveys find fear and anxiety to represent one of children's most common concerns (Beesdo, Knappe, and Pine, 2009). Of note, despite consistent findings in this area, there has been disagreement on the point that separates normal and abnormal fear and anxiety: clinicians of today are more likely to view fears and anxieties as signs of pathology than clinicians of earlier times. Second, fear and anxiety exhibit prototypical developmental changes (Kagan, 1994). Infants and toddlers manifest fears of strangers and separation. As children approach school-age, these fears are replaced by fears of small animals or other particular objects. Next, as children begin to approach adolescence, fears about social encounters gain prominence, followed by fears about abstract concepts, such as self-worth or the unknown.

Two complementary observations shape views of abnormal fears. First, anxiety disorders are common in adults, who typically date the onset of their problems to childhood or adolescence (Beesdo et al., 2009). Second, prospective research in children largely confirms these findings (Beesdo et al., 2009). When children are followed prospectively, most anxiety disorders seen in adults are preceded by pediatric anxiety disorders. Moreover, in many cases, adults with prior histories of pediatric anxiety manifest other serious problems, such as major depression.

These and other data on normal and abnormal behavior raise questions on how to balance categorical and dimensional perspectives. Categorical perspectives clearly separate normal from pathological anxiety, which is particularly useful when trying to select patients needing treatment. However, data on the boundaries between normal and abnormal fear suggest that such stark divisions only apply in some contexts, such as when related to treatment. For example, some longitudinal studies stratify individuals based on their levels of anxiety in childhood and follow them longitudinally. In these individuals, the relationship between early anxiety and later psychopathology is continuous, without a stark division between health and illness (Beesdo-Baum et al., 2011; Beesdo et al., 2009; Copeland, Shanahan, Costello, and Angold, 2009; Pine, Cohen, and Brook, 2001). Similarly, other longitudinal work focuses on infant and young children's reactions to mildly threatening scenarios (Kagan, 1994). Children with a specific temperament known as "behavioral inhibition" face a high risk for anxiety, particularly social anxiety (Clauss and Blackford, 2012). This temperament is conceptualized as a normal variant, again suggesting that the boundaries are murky between normal and pathological anxiety.

Data on normal and abnormal anxiety also raise questions on how to balance a focus on general and specific aspects of anxiety. In current nosology, children with prominent separation fears are classified differently from children with prominent social anxiety or pervasive worries. However, longitudinal research demonstrates considerable nonspecificity in outcomes; distinct forms of anxiety broadly predispose a child to many other distinct forms of anxiety as well as mood disorders (Beesdo et al., 2009; Copeland et al., 2009). This pattern, known as "heterotypic continuity," suggests that anxiety states are not easily viewed as discrete. Longitudinal work does find some distinctions at least partially reflected in research on treatment, familial aggregation, and other correlates. As a result, these distinctions inform the fifth edition of the *Diagnostic and Statistical Manual* (DSM-5; American Psychiatric Association, 2013), which divides conditions that had previously been grouped with the anxiety disorders into three relatively broad, separate categories: one associated with obsessive compulsive disorder (OCD) and related syndromes; a second associated with post-traumatic stress disorder (PTSD) and other stress-related syndromes; and a third containing other anxiety disorders.

The current chapter reviews research on the biology of pediatric anxiety disorders as it relates to these three groups. For OCD-related syndromes, the review focuses mostly on OCD per se, due to the lack of research on other conditions in this broader category of conditions. Nevertheless, this review is relevant for body dysmorphic disorder and trichotillomania, which have received limited biological research in children but are grouped with OCD in DSM-5, as well as tic disorders, which appear in a different section of DSM-5. For similar reasons, for PTSD-related syndromes, the review focuses mostly on PTSD per se but is relevant for acute stress disorder and attachment disorders, which also have received limited biological research. Moreover, considerable work focuses on associations with trauma, independent of symptoms. As a result, the current review also summarizes data in this area. Finally, in the third group, the review focuses on social anxiety, separation anxiety, and generalized anxiety disorders.

BASIC NEUROSCIENCE

Developmental biology research can be organized around the same three broad groups of anxiety-related syndromes that appear in DSM-5. One set of studies, largely performed in rodents, defines the neural architecture of goals and habits, as it informs perspectives on OCD-related disorders. A second set, performed in both rodents and primates, defines the neural correlates of stress exposure and their relevance for PTSD; a final set examines other aspects of anxiety. Each set adopts a circuitry-based perspective on dimensional variations in behavior, reflecting the Research Domains of Criteria (RDoC; Insel et al., 2010). From this perspective, variations in neural circuits arising during development are thought to produce risk.

The circuitry associated with these three groups of disorders is depicted in Figure 5.1. Components of these circuits show both shared and particular associations with

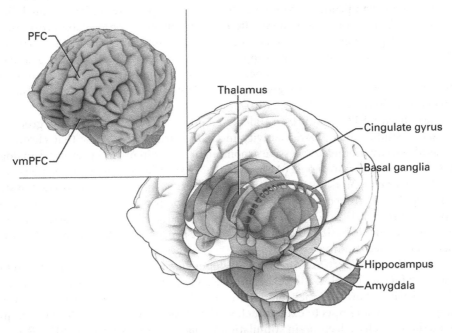

FIGURE 5.1 The neural correlates of anxiety. The basal ganglia and thalamus, relate to OCD. The hippocampus and amygdala, relate to PTSD and other anxiety disorders more strongly than OCD. The prefrontal cortex (PFC), particularly ventro-medial PFC (vmPFC), and cingulate gyrus relate to all types of anxiety.

the three groups of disorders covered in the current chapter. Thus, the basal ganglia, Figure 5.1, exhibit a particularly strong association with OCD-related disorders, whereas trauma-related disorders are associated with all of the circuitry components in Figure 5.1. Finally, other anxiety disorders show particularly strong associations with the amygdala and hippocampus, and sections of the prefrontal cortex and cingulate, shown in green and purple, that interact with the amygdala and hippocampus.

OCD-Related Circuitry

Considerable research relevant to OCD-related syndromes differentiates circuitry that supports goal-based and habit-based learning (Balleine and O'Doherty, 2010). In goal-based learning, behavior changes in tandem with changing outcome-behavior contingencies, whereas in habit-based learning, behaviors persist even when contingencies change. Basic research on rodents in these areas links different components of so-called cortico-striato-thalamo-cortical (CSTC) circuitry to the two sets of phenomena (Balleine and O'Doherty, 2010). This circuitry, depicted in Figure 5.1 connects sectors of the prefrontal cortex (PFC) to the basal ganglia and then the thalamus as part of a closed-loop through which activity can reverberate when thalamic efferents terminate in the PFC.

CSTC circuitry differs in rodents and primates, as primates possess PFC and striatal components that do not exist in rodents, which leads goals and habits to be supported by somewhat different circuitry across species (Balleine and O'Doherty, 2010; Wise, 2008). Interest in understanding these differences follows from the homologies between the human and nonhuman primate circuitry, coupled with the availability of more extensive data in rodents than primates. Moreover, few studies in primates link individual differences in CSTC function to individual differences in behavior. The available cross-species research attempts to emphasize aspects of CSTC circuitry function that are shared. In rodents, some CSTC components support habits, whereas others support goal-based behavior. The components that support habits are thought to relate to stereotyped behaviors, expressed as excessive grooming in rodents and obsessions or compulsions in humans (Balleine and O'Doherty, 2010).

Research on CSTC circuitry in rodents maps the circuitry of excessive grooming. One set of studies manipulates activity in CSTC circuitry to show that chronically increased activity produces excessive grooming behavior in mice, a presumed analogue of OCD-like behaviors in people (Ahmari et al., 2013). Other studies focus on these same set of behavior endpoints but adopt genetically informed approaches; in this set of studies, manipulations in genes encoding transmembrane proteins also produce excessive grooming (Proenca, Gao, Shmelkov, Rafii, and Lee, 2011). Demonstrating the mutually informative nature of basic and clinical work, these genes are implicated in OCD, tic disorders, and related syndromes.

Minimal basic research examines the development biology of OCD-related behaviors. Basic work focuses largely on OCD-related behaviors in mature rodents, with relatively little emphasis on how these behaviors arise from developmental processes in CSTC circuitry. Moreover, attempts to extend such work to humans have drawn heavily on invasive methods, such as deep-brain stimulation (Goodman and Alterman, 2012; Rodman et al., 2012). While this does differentiate circuits involved in OCD-related behaviors from other anxiety-related behaviors, such approaches are not easily applied with children. Nevertheless, as reviewed below, results from brain imaging do extend the work through developmental studies of OCD.

PTSD-Related Circuitry

PTSD and other trauma-related syndromes are unique in DSM-5, based on their causal link to a stressful experience. While stress relates to many syndromes, only in stress-related disorders does stress exposure represent a disorder perquisite. This provides major benefits for basic research, which maps how stress exposure changes brain function and behavior, work which profoundly shapes current thinking (C. Gross and Hen, 2004; Pitman et al., 2012).

In contrast to the sparse developmental research on OCD-related circuitry, extensive developmental research examines the circuitry that supports fear conditioning and related forms of fear-based learning (Casey, Pattwell, Glatt, and Lee, 2013; C. Gross and Hen, 2004; LeDoux, 2000; Meaney, 2001). Figure 5.2 illustrates the procedures in a typical fear conditioning experiment, conducted in rodents, and methods for extending this work to developmental research with humans. In fear conditioning, a neutral conditioned stimulus (CS+) acquires the capacity to elicit fear after it is paired with an aversive, unconditioned stimulus (UCS), depicted in Figure 5.2 as the pairing of a sound with a shock in rodents. The neural circuitry supporting this form of learning has been precisely

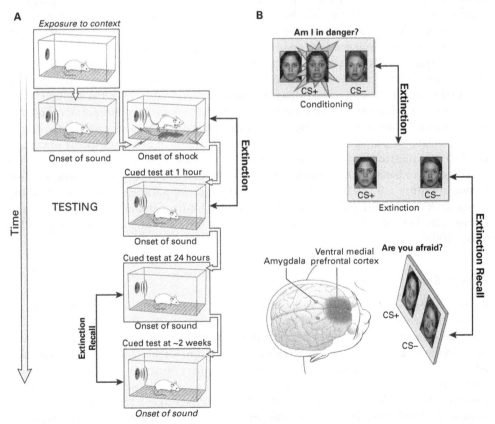

FIGURE 5.2 Procedures for fear conditioning in rodents and children. On the left side of the figure, procedures for studying conditioning, extinction, and extinction recall are illustrated in rodents. On the right side of the figure, procedures for studying these same processes are illustrated in children.

mapped and shown to exhibit marked cross-species similarities. This circuitry depends heavily on the amygdala, a collection of nuclei lying within the medial temporal lobe. In Chapter 6 of this volume, Richardson and colleagues review the developmental neurobiology of this circuitry in greater depth.

The core circuitry interacts with various brain regions to support related forms of fear-based learning. Thus, during conditioning, organisms also learn to fear the contexts where conditioning occurs, and this requires the hippocampus. Similarly, when a CS+ is repeatedly presented without the UCS, organisms respond with less fear to the CS+, a process known as "extinction." Maintaining a memory of extinction requires the ventral PFC (Milad and Quirk, 2012). Figure 5.2 shows how extinction is studied in rodents. In children, ethical factors complicate research on fear conditioning. Thus, shock UCS, the most frequently used stimulus in adults, may not be appropriate for children. Recent work employs facial photograph CS+ stimuli, shown in Figure 5.2, to engage the amygdala and ventral PFC in children.

Two related findings heighten interest in developmental biology. First, as reviewed elsewhere (Casey et al., 2013) and by Richardson and colleagues (Chapter 6) in this volume, age-related changes in neural circuitry occur in tandem with changes in anxiety-related phenomena. For example, PFC maturation is thought to relate to changes in fear in adolescence. Second, early-life experiences have more enduring effects than similar experiences at later points in life. For example, early-life variation in parent-offspring relationships shapes rodent circuitry function (Meaney, 2001), generating interest in extensions to humans in research on brain imaging and trauma.

Major questions arise about clinical translation. One set relates to specificity. As already noted, stress relates to many anxiety disorders, besides the conditions that are grouped with PTSD in DSM-5. Imaging studies, reviewed later in the chapter, have only begun to differentiate neural correlates of PTSD, trauma exposure, and other anxiety disorders. Thus, it remains unclear the degree to which research on fear learning in rodents relates to particular subsets of anxiety disorders or broader aspects of experience. Other questions relate to cross-species extensions. Strong cross-species parallels clearly exist in basic brain-behavior relationships that support fear learning, as illustrated in Figure 5.2 (LeDoux, 2000). Nevertheless, the parallels appear less striking in research on individual differences. For example, findings in nonhuman primates fail to replicate key aspects of research in rodents (Lyons, Parker, and Schatzberg, 2010; Wise, 2008).

Anxiety-Related Circuitry

Compelling studies in rodents and nonhuman primates extend research on fear learning to other aspects of anxiety-related behavior. Of particular clinical relevance, some such work examines how naturally occurring individual differences in anxiety relate to individual differences in circuitry function; other such relevant work examines effects of clinically anxiolytic treatments on circuitry function (C. Gross and Hen, 2004). In both areas, the implicated neural circuits strongly overlap with the circuit implicated in fear learning. Such overlaps led scientists to use the term "fear circuit" to describe PFC-amygdala connections implicated in both fear learning and naturally occurring individual differences in fear-related behaviors.

Some such individual differences are expressed stably throughout development. In rodents, such differences have been studied in selective breeding experiments (Flint, 2010). In primates, such differences have been studied in research on a fearful temperament, which involves a tendency to exhibit wariness in laboratory settings when confronted with novel or mildly threatening scenarios. Monkeys with a fearful temperament tend to freeze and emit distress vocalizations in such scenarios, reflecting functional aspects of the fear circuit (Kalin, 2004). As described later in the chapter, imaging studies extend this work to humans.

Studies of naturally occurring individual differences tend to aggregate fear-related behaviors expressed in diverse contexts to quantify general levels of fearfulness. However, other studies in rodents suggest that such general levels of fearfulness occur in tandem with other variations (C. T. Gross and Canteras, 2012). These other variations reflect more particular forms of fear, which appear to have unique neural signatures, including fear of social threats or threats involving other particular features. This creates tension in research on general and specific forms of fear, reminiscent of tension in clinical, longitudinal research on developmental variations in human fears. Moreover, consistent with such work in humans, emerging basic data suggest that specific and general forms of fear coexist but also may exhibit unique developmental neurobiology (Pine, Helfinstein, Bar-Haim, Nelson, and Fox, 2009).

A final set of studies in rodents and primates examines relationships among stressful rearing conditions, functioning in the fear circuit, and fear-related behaviors. This raises questions on whether stress-related disorders truly can be differentiated from other anxiety disorders. Thus, various stressors, particularly in early development, profoundly shape an organism's tendency to manifest fear (C. Gross and Hen, 2004; Meaney, 2001; Suomi, 2003). These stressors include exposure to chronically unpredictable or threatening environments as well as briefer exposures to other factors that lead to mobilization of stress-related brain systems.

TRANSLATIONAL NEUROSCIENCE

Translational neuroscience research on pediatric anxiety disorders uses three sets of measures. These comprise (1) indirect measures of brain function, as reflected in performance on psychological tasks or measures of peripheral physiology, (2) measures of brain structure derived from structural magnetic resonance imaging (MRI), and (3) measures of brain function derived from either functional MRI (fMRI) or event-related potentials (ERP). A fourth set of studies relies on measures brain chemistry, such as magnetic resonance spectroscopy or positron emission tomography. Results from such studies are not reviewed, since fewer studies rely on these methods compared to the other three sets of methods.

OCD-Related Disorders

From a clinical perspective, OCD-related disorders differ from trauma-related and other anxiety disorders based on their longitudinal course, familial aggregation, and treatment response. OCD-related disorders generally show particularly strong associations with tic disorders and ADHD. Findings in translational neuroscience generally reflect these same trends, in that the patterns reveal similarities among OCD, tic disorders, and ADHD (Pauls, Abramovitch, Rauch, and Geller, 2014). Nevertheless, such conclusions remain tentative, since few studies directly contrast brain structure or function in multiple, distinct groups of children with various disorders. Rather, conclusions follow by comparing findings across individual studies, in distinct groups of children, each focused on one particular pediatric mental disorder.

In terms of indirect measures of brain function, patterns in OCD-related disorders generally reflect broad signs of perturbed functioning, paralleling findings in adults with OCD-related disorders. At all ages, such patterns are thought to reflect more specific involvement of CSTC circuitry in OCD-related disorders than in PTSD-related or other anxiety disorders (Pauls et al., 2014). In children and adolescents, such dysfunction appears to manifest in tests of motor fluency, visual organization, and executive functions. Some scientists consider the association between OCD and motor dysfunction to provide particularly strong evidence of shared dysfunction with tic disorders and ADHD, suggesting basal ganglia involvement in the three groups of syndromes. Finally, interest in pediatric autoimmune neuropsychiatric disorders associated with streptococcal infections (PANDAS) also reflects a focus on CSTC circuitry, which is through to be perturbed by such infections (Brimberg et al., 2012). This also has led to research on peripheral inflammatory markers. As with studies of motor and cognitive performance, findings do differentiate healthy subjects from subjects with OCD-related disorders, but more research is needed in other disorders to evaluate specificity.

Sufficient MRI data exist on brain structure in OCD to support quantitative meta-analysis. These data generally confirm basic science research and findings from indirect measures of brain function on involvement of CSTC circuitry (Radua et al., 2014; Radua, van den Heuvel, Surguladze, and Mataix-Cols, 2010). Moreover, such structural perturbations appear to occur in a relatively broad expanse of the brain in OCD, encompassing diverse gray matter structures as well as white matter tracts that connect these structures. Relatively few cross sectional studies compare findings in OCD-related disorders occurring at distinct ages, and no longitudinal studies exist. Nevertheless, some data suggest that age-related differences in cortical or striatal volumes could contribute to changing clinical expression (de Wit et al., 2014).

Findings in functional imaging research generally replicate patterns in other translational studies. Thus, evidence of relatively broad dysfunction exists in fMRI and ERP studies of OCD-related disorders, which occurs on many cognitive tasks and in many brain regions (Blackford and Pine, 2012; Pauls et al., 2014). The breadth of dysfunction in OCD-related disorders does appear to be greater than occurs in many other anxiety disorders, though findings in PTSD-related disorders are also quite broad, as described below. At least in adults, sufficient data exist to support meta-analysis of fMRI data, and this demonstrates hyperactivity in key components of CSTC circuitry (Rotge et al., 2008). However, while fewer studies examine children and adolescents, those that exist do not always replicate patterns seen in adults. Perhaps the most consistent finding is for increased error-related negativity (ERN) in OCD, an ERP measure implicated in both pediatric and adult OCD (Pauls et al., 2014). Research on ERN extends basic science work on cognitive control and error monitoring in monkeys, as illustrated in Figure 5.3. Thus, striatal and PFC neurons of monkeys respond when a monkey makes an error on a task (Figure 5.3). These responses are thought to parallel responses in humans on cognitive control tasks also depicted in the figure. Of note, this measure differentiates patients with OCD from patients with ADHD, but no differences are found between patients with ADHD or other anxiety disorders, thus raising questions on specificity.

Trauma-Related Disorders

Much like OCD-related disorders, trauma-related disorders display a unique course, familial aggregation, and treatment response. Comorbidity is generally greater than in all other pediatric anxiety disorders, and risk tends to aggregate with risks for many other

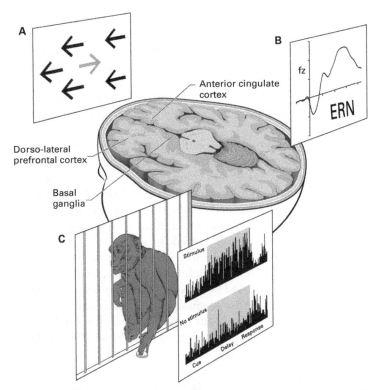

FIGURE 5.3 Procedures for studying event-related negativity (ERN), which extend work in non-human primates. Thus, (A) depicts a cognitive-control task, where a research subject must indicate the direction in which a central gray arrow points, appearing amid distractors. This engages the depicted neural circuitry, which is thought to generate the ERN as depicted in electrophysiologic data in (B). This experiment in humans extends data from an experiment in nonhuman primates shown in (C). In the primate experiment, the monkey must learn to respond to a select group of stimuli to obtain a reward while activity in neurons is recorded, as depicted in the associated graphs.

adversities, since traumatic exposures tend to occur in families living under conditions of adversity. This raises largely unanswered questions on the degree to which findings reflect adversity per se or anxiety symptoms in children exposed to adversity.

For indirect measures of brain function, broad perturbations occur in traumatized children or children with PTSD-related disorders, as they do in OCD-related disorders. For example, in both sets of disorders, dysfunction occurs in executive functions where patients with other anxiety disorders generally show no such dysfunction (Pitman et al., 2012). PTSD-related disorders also show signs of dysfunction that are not found in OCD-related disorders. Thus, reduced intelligence may occur in PTSD, though this could reflect the above-noted more general effects of adversity (De Bellis, Hooper, Woolley, and Shenk, 2010; De Bellis, Spratt, and Hooper, 2011). Similarly, PTSD-related disorders also involve biased or distorted processing of threats and other stimuli that evoke memories of traumatic exposures (Pitman et al., 2012). Finally, PTSD-related disorders involve perturbations in autonomic and hormonal systems that are acutely responsive to stress (Pitman et al., 2012). These include measures of cardiovascular responses, hypothalamic-pituitary-adrenal (HPA) axis activity, and startle regulation. Of note, studies in other anxiety disorders also find signs of dysfunction in these systems. However, the consistency and pervasiveness of dysfunction appears greater in traumatized children and PTSD-related disorders than in other anxiety disorders. Moreover, when perturbations occur in other anxiety disorders, they usually involve enhanced responsiveness. Patients with PTSD-related disorders exhibit enhanced responsiveness in some studies or for some indices, but reduced responsiveness in other studies or for other indices.

As in OCD-related disorders, considerable MRI data compare brain structures in traumatized and non-traumatized children, and signs of widespread perturbations emerge in this work. Thus, reduced brain volume occurs in many structures in traumatized relative to nontraumatized children, with some additional evidence of the greatest reductions in the subset of traumatized children who also manifest psychopathology, including PTSD-related and other anxiety symptoms (De Bellis et al., 2011). Findings do not fully replicate the patterns found in adults with PTSD-related disorders or in adults with histories of traumatic childhoods. Thus, perturbations occur in a broader array of structures among children than adults. Moreover, findings in adults demonstrate consistent evidence of reduced volume in the hippocampus among individuals with history of chronic trauma either in childhood or later in life (C. Gross and Hen, 2004; Pitman et al., 2012); this is a brain region consistently implicated in research on rodents and non-human primates examining aspects of PTSD-related disorders. Evidence in children linking the hippocampus to trauma or PTSD appears less consistent than in adults or basic research.

Findings in fMRI and ERP research suggest that brain dysfunction in PTSD-related disorders encompass the types of dysfunction that occurs in OCD-related disorders and other anxiety disorders. Thus, as in OCD-related disorders, fMRI research finds dysfunction on executive function tasks (Pitman et al., 2012). Patients with other anxiety disorders besides OCD typically do not exhibit dysfunction on these tasks. Similarly, as in other anxiety disorders, fMRI research finds signs of threat hypersensitivity in the amygdala in PTSD-related disorders, tasks where OCD-related disorders show less consistent signs of dysfunction. Some suggest that the particular sets of findings in traumatized children or in PTSD-related disorders can be separated based on the nature of traumatic exposures (McLaughlin et al., 2014). Exposures that involve neglect are thought to predict perturbations in executive and other cognitive functions, similar to those that occur in OCD-related disorders as opposed to other anxiety disorders. Traumatic exposures that are extremely frightening for the child are thought to predict perturbations in the amygdala and other circuitry implicated in other anxiety disorders as opposed to OCD-related disorders.

Anxiety Disorders

Patients with OCD, PTSD, MDD, and many other emotional disorders frequently also exhibit features of other anxiety disorders, particularly social anxiety disorder/social phobia (SoPh), separation anxiety disorder (SAD), and generalized anxiety disorder (GAD). The current section reviews translational neuroscience findings on these three anxiety disorders. In general, relative to OCD and PTSD, these three anxiety disorders exhibit lower rates of comorbidity, better outcomes, and higher responses to treatment. Moreover, findings in translational neuroscience research reveal more restricted perturbations in SoPh, SAD, and GAD, relative to in OCD and PTSD.

In terms of indirect measure of brain function, patients with SoPh, SAD, or GAD typically exhibit normal functioning on many of the cognitive tasks where patients with either OCD-related or PTSD-related disorder show signs of dysfunction. For example, while perturbed executive function occurs in OCD and PTSD, executive function is typically intact in these three anxiety disorders and sometimes appears even better than in healthy subjects (Henderson, Pine, and Fox, 2015). Patients with SoPh, SAD, or GAD do show biased processing of threat-related stimuli on tests of attention and appraisal, similar to what has been found in children exposed to trauma (Pine et al., 2009). Such children also show enhanced responding in the HPA axis and autonomic systems in some threat-response paradigms. Few studies of such indirect measures find consistent differences among patients with SoPh, SAD, and GAD. Nevertheless, studies do more consistently find perturbations in respiratory function among pediatric patients with SAD than with either SoPh or GAD (Pine, 2007); this generally replicates patterns in adults with panic disorders. Similarly, other studies more consistently find biased processing of social information among pediatric patients with SoPh or SAD, consistent with findings in adults with SoPh. Finally, data on behavioral inhibition generally parallel data in pediatric anxiety disorders.

Less MRI data exist on brain structure in SoPh, SAD, and GAD than in either OCD-related or PTSD-related disorders. Moreover, the few studies that do exist generally find perturbations in a more narrow range of brain structures than in OCD-related or PTSD-related disorders (Blackford and Pine, 2012). The most consistent findings in SoPh, SAD, and GAD reveal perturbed amygdala volumes in pediatric anxiety patients, consistent with a wealth of basic research implicating this medial temporal lobe structure in developmental models of anxiety. However, some studies document elevated amygdala volume in pediatric anxiety disorders, whereas others document the reverse, differences that may reflect inconsistencies in the subject characteristics and technical aspects of the brain-imaging approaches. A growing number of fMRI and ERP studies examine the neural correlates of SoPh, SAD, and GAD, as well as behavioral inhibition, the early-child temperament most consistently related to pediatric anxiety disorders. These studies rely on various techniques, as reviewed elsewhere (Blackford and Pine, 2012). Stronger evidence of anxiety-related perturbations emerges from these fMRI and ERP studies relative to the structural MRI studies. The most consistent perturbations appear in the amygdala and PFC, consistent with basic science research reviewed above implicating amygdala-PFC circuitry in behavioral reactions to threat. In general, findings document increased activations within this circuitry, among subjects with SoPh, SAD, GAD, or behavioral inhibition, relative to comparison subjects free of these conditions. However, the precise nature of the findings varies as a function of the particular fMRI technique that is used and brain region that is examined across the many studies.

CONCLUSIONS

Three major sets of discoveries support developmental perspectives. Research in developmental psychopathology establishes the early age at which anxiety begins and divides disorders into three groups: OCD-related, PTSD-related, and other anxiety disorders. Basic research delineates the neural architecture that might contribute to each of these groups. Finally, brain imaging studies have begun to define the neural circuits in which functional perturbations may arise, accounting for both shared and unique features of the three main groups of pediatric anxiety disorders. Due to the complex nature of development and translational neuroscience, advances are likely to accrue relatively slowly over the coming decades in each of the three major areas covered in this chapter. Nevertheless, as such integrative approaches mature, translational neuroscience is likely to become increasingly relevant for the diagnosis and care of individual patients with anxiety disorders.

ACKNOWLEDGMENT

Supported by the NIMH Intramural Research Program.

REFERENCES

Ahmari, S. E., Spellman, T., Douglass, N. L., Kheirbek, M. A., Simpson, H. B., Deisseroth, K., . . . Hen, R. (2013). Repeated cortico-striatal stimulation generates persistent OCD-like behavior. *Science, 340* (6137), 1234–1239.

American Psychiatric Association. (2013). *Diagnostic and Statistical Manual of Mental Disorders (5th ed.).* Arlington, VA: American Psychiatric Association.

Balleine, B. W., & O'Doherty, J. P. (2010). Human and rodent homologies in action control: Corticostriatal determinants of goal-directed and habitual action. *Neuropsychopharmacology, 35* (1), 48–69.

Beesdo-Baum, K., Winkel, S., Pine, D. S., Hoyer, J., Hofler, M., Lieb, R., and Wittchen, H. U. (2011). The diagnostic threshold of generalized anxiety disorder in the community: A developmental perspective. *J Psychiatr Res, 45* (7), 962–972.

Beesdo, K., Knappe, S., and Pine, D. S. (2009). Anxiety and anxiety disorders in children and adolescents: Developmental issues and implications for DSM-V. *Psychiatr Clin North Am, 32* (3), 483–524.

Blackford, J. U., and Pine, D. S. (2012). Neural substrates of childhood anxiety disorders: A review of neuroimaging findings. *Child Adolesc Psychiatr Clin N Am, 21* (3), 501–525.

Brimberg, L., Benhar, I., Mascaro-Blanco, A., Alvarez, K., Lotan, D., Winter, C., . . . Joel, D. (2012). Behavioral, pharmacological, and immunological abnormalities after streptococcal exposure: A novel rat model of Sydenham chorea and related neuropsychiatric disorders. *Neuropsychopharmacology, 37* (9), 2076–2087.

Casey, B. J., Pattwell, S. S., Glatt, C. E., and Lee, F. S. (2013). Treating the developing brain: implications from human imaging and mouse genetics. *Annu Rev Med, 64,* 427–439.

Clauss, J. A., and Blackford, J. U. (2012). Behavioral inhibition and risk for developing social anxiety disorder: A meta-analytic study. *J Am Acad Child Adolesc Psychiatry, 51* (10), 1066–1075 e1061.

Copeland, W. E., Shanahan, L., Costello, E. J., and Angold, A. (2009). Childhood and adolescent psychiatric disorders as predictors of young adult disorders. *Arch Gen Psychiatry, 66* (7), 764–772.

De Bellis, M. D., Hooper, S. R., Woolley, D. P., and Shenk, C. E. (2010). Demographic, maltreatment, and neurobiological correlates of PTSD symptoms in children and adolescents. *J Pediatr Psychol, 35* (5), 570–577.

De Bellis, M. D., Spratt, E. G., and Hooper, S. R. (2011). Neurodevelopmental biology associated with childhood sexual abuse. *J Child Sex Abus, 20* (5), 548–587.

de Wit, S. J., Alonso, P., Schweren, L., Mataix-Cols, D., Lochner, C., Menchon, J. M., . . . van den Heuvel, O. A. (2014). Multicenter voxel-based morphometry mega-analysis of structural brain scans in obsessive-compulsive disorder. *Am J Psychiatry, 171* (3), 340–349.

Flint, J., Greenspan, R. J., Kendler, K. S. (2010). *How Genes Influence Behavior.* Oxford, United Kingdom: Oxford University Press.

Goodman, W. K., & Alterman, R. L. (2012). Deep brain stimulation for intractable psychiatric disorders. *Annu Rev Med, 63,* 511–524.

Gross, C., & Hen, R. (2004). The developmental origins of anxiety. *Nat Rev Neurosci, 5* (7), 545–552.

Gross, C. T., & Canteras, N. S. (2012). The many paths to fear. *Nat Rev Neurosci, 13*(9), 651–658.

Henderson, H. A., Pine, D. S., and Fox, N. A. (2015). Behavioral inhibition and developmental risk: A dual-processing perspective. *Neuropsychopharmacology, 40,* 207–224. doi: 10.1038/npp.2014.189

Insel, T., Cuthbert, B., Garvey, M., Heinssen, R., Pine, D. S., Quinn, K., . . . Wang, P. (2010). Research domain criteria (RDoC): Toward a new classification framework for research on mental disorders. *Am J Psychiatry, 167* (7), 748–751.

Kagan, J. (1994). *Galen's prophecy.* New York, NY: Basic Books.

Kalin, N. H. (2004). Studying non-human primates: A gateway to understanding anxiety disorders. *Psychopharmacol Bull, 38* (1), 8–13.

LeDoux, J. E. (2000). Emotion circuits in the brain. *Annu Rev Neurosci, 23,* 155–184.

Lyons, D. M., Parker, K. J., and Schatzberg, A. F. (2010). Animal models of early life stress: Implications for understanding resilience. *Dev Psychobiol, 52* (7), 616–624.

McLaughlin, K. A., Sheridan, M. A., Winter, W., Fox, N. A., Zeanah, C. H., and Nelson, C. A. (2014). Widespread reductions in cortical thickness following severe early-life deprivation: A neurodevelopmental pathway to attention-deficit/hyperactivity disorder. *Biol Psychiatry, 76,* 629–638.

Meaney, M. J. (2001). Maternal care, gene expression, and the transmission of individual differences in stress reactivity across generations. *Annu Rev Neurosci, 24,* 1161–1192.

Milad, M. R., and Quirk, G. J. (2012). Fear extinction as a model for translational neuroscience: Ten years of progress. *Annu Rev Psychol, 63,* 129–151.

Pauls, D. L., Abramovitch, A., Rauch, S. L., and Geller, D. A. (2014). Obsessive-compulsive disorder: An integrative genetic and neurobiological perspective. *Nat Rev Neurosci, 15* (6), 410–424.

Pine, D. S. (2007). Research review: A neuroscience framework for pediatric anxiety disorders. *J Child Psychol Psychiatry, 48* (7), 631–648.

Pine, D. S., Cohen, P., and Brook, J. (2001). Adolescent fears as predictors of depression. *Biol Psychiatry, 50* (9), 721–724.

Pine, D. S., Helfinstein, S. M., Bar-Haim, Y., Nelson, E., and Fox, N. A. (2009). Challenges in developing novel treatments for childhood disorders: Lessons from research on anxiety. *Neuropsychopharmacology, 34* (1), 213–228.

Pitman, R. K., Rasmusson, A. M., Koenen, K. C., Shin, L. M., Orr, S. P., Gilbertson, M. W., . . . Liberzon, I. (2012). Biological studies of post-traumatic stress disorder. *Nat Rev Neurosci, 13* (11), 769–787.

Proenca, C. C., Gao, K. P., Shmelkov, S. V., Rafii, S., and Lee, F. S. (2011). Slitrks as emerging candidate genes involved in neuropsychiatric disorders. *Trends Neurosci, 34* (3), 143–153.

Radua, J., Grau, M., van den Heuvel, O. A., Thiebaut de Schotten, M., Stein, D. J., Canales-Rodriguez, E. J., . . . Mataix-Cols, D. (2014). Multimodal voxel-based meta-analysis of white matter abnormalities in obsessive-compulsive disorder. *Neuropsychopharmacology, 39* (7), 1547–1557.

Radua, J., van den Heuvel, O. A., Surguladze, S., and Mataix-Cols, D. (2010). Meta-analytical comparison of voxel-based morphometry studies in obsessive-compulsive disorder vs other anxiety disorders. *Arch Gen Psychiatry, 67* (7), 701–711.

Rodman, A. M., Milad, M. R., Deckersbach, T., Im, J., Chou, T., and Dougherty, D. D. (2012). Neuroimaging contributions to novel surgical treatments for intractable obsessive-compulsive disorder. *Expert Rev Neurother, 12* (2), 219–227.

Rotge, J. Y., Guehl, D., Dilharreguy, B., Cuny, E., Tignol, J., Bioulac, B., . . . Aouizerate, B. (2008). Provocation of obsessive-compulsive symptoms: A quantitative voxel-based meta-analysis of functional neuroimaging studies. *J Psychiatry Neurosci, 33* (5), 405–412.

Suomi, S. J. (2003). Gene-environment interactions and the neurobiology of social conflict. *Ann N Y Acad Sci, 1008,* 132–139.

Wise, S. P. (2008). Forward frontal fields: phylogeny and fundamental function. *Trends Neurosci, 31* (12), 599–608.

6

THE DEVELOPMENT OF FEAR AND ITS INHIBITION: KNOWLEDGE GAINED FROM PRECLINICAL MODELS

BRIDGET L. CALLAGHAN AND
RICK RICHARDSON

INTRODUCTION

Fear is fundamental to our survival. When appropriately expressed, fear allows us to respond to danger signals in the environment and to protect ourselves from harm. However, fear that is expressed excessively or inappropriately (i.e., in situations which do not predict danger) can have debilitating consequences and is characteristic of all anxiety disorders. For this reason, understanding the conditions under which fear becomes maladaptive, as well as developing strategies to effectively inhibit fear responses, remains at the forefront of research in psychology and psychiatry.

To date, much of the empirical research modeling anxiety disorder development and treatment has utilized Pavlovian fear conditioning and extinction procedures. These procedures have direct clinical relevance: the most widely employed and empirically-validated treatment for anxiety disorders, exposure therapy, is based on the process of extinction (Milad and Quirk, 2012). In addition, these procedures lend themselves very well to translational models of analysis as the neural circuitry underlying fear conditioning and extinction has been exceptionally well-preserved across species (Milad and Quirk, 2012). However, while we know a considerable amount about the anatomy and physiology of fear and extinction circuits in the adult brain, our understanding of how these circuits develop across the lifespan is relatively limited. This is despite the fact that early life has long been believed to function as a "critical period" for the establishment of life-long mental health. Indeed, the fact that many anxiety disorders first emerge in childhood or adolescence has led to the suggestion that trajectories of mental health are established early in development and, therefore, that prevention and treatment of mental health problems should be targeted to the early years (Kessler et al., 2007). In this chapter we examine what is known about fear and its inhibition through the perspective of developmental neuroscience, and we explore the possibility that early alterations in the developmental trajectory of fear circuits may lead to increased risk for anxiety disorders across the lifespan.

EARLY FEAR AND EXTINCTION CIRCUITS

Considering the significant structural and functional changes taking place in the developing brain, it is perhaps not surprising that fear is expressed and inhibited differently in infancy than in adulthood. In this section we outline some of the behavioral, structural, neurochemical, and molecular differences in fear expression and extinction which have been reported across development. While these developmental dissociations have largely been documented in rodent models, we make reference to human research where appropriate.

Behavioral differences in fear and extinction. One of the major behavioral differences in fear expression that occurs across development is that infants forget much faster than adults—a phenomenon called *infantile amnesia.* This rapid forgetting in early development is a robust effect and occurs in all altricial species, including humans (Callaghan et al., 2014; Hayne, 2004; Josselyn and Frankland, 2012). In the first demonstration of infantile amnesia in the rodent, rats trained at postnatal day (P) 18 (infants) and P100 (adults) were equally apt at forming an association between the black side of a black-white shuttle box and foot shock, and passively avoiding the black side when tested immediately after training. When tested at longer intervals, however, the performance of adults and infants differed; adults exhibited excellent retention for as long as 42 days after training whereas infants forgot within a week (Campbell and Campbell, 1962). While the exact fate of these forgotten memories remains elusive, studies in both rats and humans have shown that forgetting in infancy is not always permanent, as infantile amnesia can be alleviated if individuals are exposed to appropriate reminder cues prior to testing (Campbell and Jaynes, 1966; Hayne, 2004; Li et al., 2014).

Developmental differences are not only observed in fear expression but have also been reported to occur in fear extinction procedures. For example, while adult rodents exhibit relapse following fear extinction (Bouton, 2002), fear responses extinguished during infancy are relapse-resistant; that is, infant rodents do not show renewal, reinstatement, or spontaneous recovery of extinguished fear (Gogolla et al., 2009; Kim and Richardson, 2010). In other words, fear appears to be permanently inhibited following extinction training in infancy (but see Revillo et al., 2013). Considering that the occurrence of relapse after extinction training in adults is taken as evidence that extinction involves the formation of a new inhibitory conditioned stimulus (CS)–no unconditioned stimulus (US) association, which competes with the original CS–US association for expression, the fact that relapse does not occur in infancy has been taken as evidence that extinction at that age may involve some form of fear memory erasure.

Structural differences in fear and extinction circuits. These behavioral findings are supported by studies demonstrating developmental differences in the neural circuitry underlying the expression and inhibition of conditioned fear. For example, in a recent study P16 and P23 rats were conditioned and then tested for fear responding after the prelimbic prefrontal cortex (PL) was inactivated (via infusion of the gamma-aminobutyric acid [GABA] agonist muscimol) or not (saline infusion; Li et al., 2012). It was shown that while temporary inactivation of the PL impaired the expression of fear in P23 rats (like what has been reported in adults; Corcoran and Quirk,

Adult fear and extinction
circuit

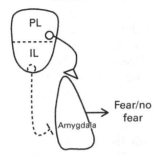

Infant fear and extinction
circuit

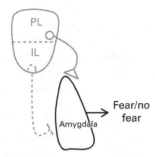

FIGURE 6.1 Simplified depiction of the neural circuitry involved in fear expression and extinction learning in adult and infant rats. While adult rodents store fear memories across multiple neural sites (i.e., PL and amygdala) and utilize the IL to inhibit fear memory expression during extinction, infant rats appear to use a much simpler, amygdala-only, circuit during both fear expression and extinction learning.

2007), infant rats exhibited good fear expression regardless of whether the PL was inactivated or not. These data suggest that infant fear memories are acquired using a much simpler circuit than in adulthood (i.e., amygdala only; see Figure 6.1) and raise the interesting possibility that reduced storage sites for infant fear memories may contribute to more rapid forgetting at that age.[1]

An amygdala-only circuit also appears to support extinction learning in infant rodents (see Figure 6.1). For example, inactivation of the amygdala before extinction training impairs extinction retention 24 hours later in both P17 and P23 rats (see Kim and Richardson, 2010). Interestingly, if rats were given a second conditioning episode and then re-extinguished under amygdala inactivation, extinction retention was impaired only in P17 rats. These findings suggest that the initial extinction occurring on P23 involved "new learning" which could then be retrieved without amygdala activity during the re-extinction session. On the other hand, initial extinction at P17 appeared to cause erasure because re-extinction remained amygdala-dependent; that is, there was no previous extinction memory to retrieve.

In contrast to the amygdala, which is involved in initial extinction across development, the infralimbic region of the prefrontal cortex (IL) appears to have a developmentally dissociated role in extinction across development. Specifically, extinction retention is impaired when the IL is inactivated before extinction training in P23 (and adult) but not in P17 rats (Kim and Richardson, 2010). These data suggest that IL activity is not required to regulate amygdala output during the expression of extinction in infancy, in contrast to adult and juvenile animals.

Although neural activity during fear and extinction learning has not yet been examined in the developing human, recent studies indicate significant developmental changes in functional activity within amygdala-prefrontal circuitry during both a passive face viewing task and at rest. Specifically, when compared to responses toward a "neutral" face, a passively viewed "fearful" face elicited amygdala-prefrontal responses which switched from being positively coupled in childhood (<10 years) to negatively coupled in adolescence (11 years +; Gee et al., 2013b). Similarly, resting state functional connectivity between the amygdala and prefrontal cortex changed from zero to positive coupling at the transition into adolescence (i.e., 10–11 years; Gabard-Durnam et al., 2014). These studies point toward substantial maturation of connectivity in the amygdala-prefrontal circuit across human development, and raise the exciting possibility that fear and extinction learning, which rely on this circuitry, might also differ across those ages.

Neurochemical differences in fear and extinction. While developmental studies on the neurochemistry of emotional learning are limited, the work so far has demonstrated both similarities and differences in the neurotransmitter systems involved in fear learning and extinction across development. For instance, N-methyl-d-aspartate (NMDA) appears to be involved in the consolidation of fear memories across development because NMDA receptor antagonists impair fear acquisition in both infant (Langton et al., 2007) and adult rats (Miserendino et al., 1990). GABA also appears to be involved in memory retention regardless of age; benzodiazepines (which increase the efficiency of GABA) cause amnesia in adults and antagonizing GABA receptors with the drug FG7142 alleviates infantile amnesia (Kim et al., 2006).

In contrast to fear conditioning, however, NMDA and GABA appear to be differentially involved in fear extinction across development. Injection of the NMDA receptor antagonist MK-801 before extinction training had no effect on infant rats whereas the same treatment resulted in poor extinction retention in both juveniles and adults (Baker and Azorlosa, 1996; Langton et al., 2007). Similarly, GABA is not involved in infant extinction because reduction of GABAergic inhibition at test (via FG7142) had no effect in infants but recovered extinguished fear memories in juveniles and adults (Harris and Westbrook, 1998; Kim and Richardson, 2010). Nevertheless, there is at least one similarity between the infant and the adult extinction systems as a pre-extinction injection of the opioid antagonist naloxone impairs extinction acquisition in both infants (see Kim and Richardson, 2010) and adults (McNally and Westbrook, 2003). Considering that endogenous opioid signaling is hypothesized to code for "erasure" of fear during extinction in adult rats (McNally et al., 2004), the fact that infant extinction appears to involve only the opioids, and not NMDA or GABA, supports the possibility that extinction during infancy is dominated by erasure.

Molecular differences in fear and extinction. To date, only a few studies have investigated the molecular underpinnings of fear and extinction in the developing rat. In one of those studies, phosphorylated mitogen activated protein kinase (pMAPK) was measured in the PL, IL, and amygdala of P16 and P23 rats that had been conditioned and then tested for CS-elicited fear 48 hours later (Kim et al., 2012). The authors found that juvenile rats remembered the fear association at test whereas infants had forgotten. Interestingly, pMAPK in the amygdala was higher in trained rats (relative to an unpaired control group), regardless of age, suggesting that amygdala pMAPK is associated with conditioning history rather than fear expression per se. In contrast, pMAPK in the PL/IL was higher in the trained P23 rats than in the trained P17 rats, suggesting that levels of pMAPK in the mPFC was positively correlated with the behavioral expression of fear. In addition, pMAPK activity in the BLA and the mPFC after test was significantly correlated in P23 rats but not in P16 rats, suggesting that only the P23 rats exhibited coordinated activity between the amygdala and mPFC during the retention test.

Similar to the findings in fear retention, pMAPK expression is also differentially expressed in the mPFC following fear extinction at different ages (Kim et al., 2009). In that study, pMAPK was assessed in the amygdala and mPFC one hour after extinction at P16 or P23. While extinction training resulted in increased pMAPK expression in the amygdala at both ages, pMAPK expression in the IL was increased only in the P23 extinguished rats, suggesting that the IL was active during extinction only in the older animals.

Another recent study demonstrated that a particular molecular signal may be critical for the expression of adult-like extinction. Specifically, the developmental emergence of the adult-like extinction system was correlated with the formation of perineuronal nets (PNNs) around neurons in the basolateral amygdala (BLA; Gogolla et al., 2009). PNNs appear to stabilize circuits and regulate the excitability of the neurons which they surround (for a review see Hensch, 2005). Interestingly, Gogolla and her colleagues demonstrated that adult rats could show infant-like extinction when PNNs were degraded in the BLA (via intra-amygdala injection of chondroitinase ABC; chABC). That is, adults treated with chABC did not exhibit renewal or reinstatement effects after extinction. This study is exciting as it is the first demonstration that infant-like extinction can be reactivated in adulthood, which has interesting implications for the treatment of anxiety.

In summary, the data to date support the notion that the outcomes of emotional learning during early development (infantile amnesia and infant-like extinction) reflect the rapidly maturing, and therefore extremely plastic, nature of the underlying circuitry. When viewed from this perspective, the brain and behavior of infant rodents are particularly interesting as many pharmacological treatments for anxiety disorders are known to enhance plasticity, which may be important for their therapeutic action (Duman, 2002). Hence, understanding the plasticity inherent within the infant fear and extinction systems may help to inform the treatment of anxiety disorders across the lifespan.

WHY MIGHT DEVELOPMENTAL DIFFERENCES IN NEUROCIRCUITRY AND NEUROCHEMISTRY EXIST?

The findings described highlight the fact that infants are not merely underdeveloped adults. Rather, at each stage of development, individuals are exquisitely adapted to their distinctive environmental niche. It is now well-established that early "limitations" in functioning may, in fact, serve to facilitate the organization of developing neural circuits. Neural networks typically develop in a staggered fashion, and it has been hypothesized that this allows neural structures and circuits to develop in the absence of interference from competing input (Turkewitz and Kenny, 1985). As such, alterations to the prescribed developmental trajectory of a given circuit are likely to result in impairments both within that circuit as well as within other circuits which are developing at the same time. This idea has been supported by many empirical studies in the domain of sensory functioning. For example, early visual stimulation of the quail embryo results in accelerated development of visual functioning but at the cost of auditory responsiveness (reviewed in Lickliter and Banker, 1994). Also, excessive noise experienced by preterm infants in the neonatal intensive care unit (NICU) has been shown to negatively affect cardiovascular and respiratory development (Wachman and Lahav, 2011).

Not surprising, hierarchical brain development is also proposed to be important for the proper maturation of circuits which support emotional functioning. For example, neurodevelopmental disorders, such as autism and schizophrenia, are characterized by early disruptions to structures which may then compromise the foundations of complex emotional behaviors and circuits by upsetting their developmental trajectory, or by making them vulnerable to future challenges (Thompson and Levitt, 2010). Mood and anxiety disorders have traditionally been excluded from the category of neurodevelopmental disorders. However, it is now increasingly recognized that anxiety too may have a neurodevelopmental origin, highlighting the need for a developmental approach when studying this phenomenon. Specifically, anxiety disorders manifest early in development, and are associated with a genetic risk and with many environmental risk factors which are specific to early development (e.g., adverse rearing). Further, future risk for anxiety disorders can be predicted from early emerging emotional traits such as behavioral inhibition (see Leonardo and Hen, 2007 for a review of these findings). When considered from this perspective, understanding the development of emotional learning systems (e.g., fear and extinction) becomes even more important for our understanding of anxiety pathogenesis. An appreciation for how early life risk factors for anxiety interact with developing fear and extinction systems is required. In the next section we review what is known about one early risk factor for anxiety (disruption of the infant-caregiver relationship) on the developing fear and extinction systems.

THE EFFECTS OF STRESS ON THE DEVELOPMENT OF FEAR AND EXTINCTION CIRCUITS

Childhood adversities related to the early rearing environment (e.g., parental mental illness, physical abuse, neglect, and parent criminality) have been associated with increased risk for anxiety disorder onset and persistence (Green et al., 2010; McLaughlin et al., 2010). It is possible that this association exists because of the effects of these early rearing stressors on the development of emotion regulation systems. Indeed, we now have evidence from both rodent and human studies which supports the view that the developmental trajectory of systems which regulate fear and extinction learning are significantly altered by rearing stress. In the first study to investigate the role of rearing stress on fear retention in the infant rat, Callaghan and Richardson (2012) exposed rats to repeated bouts of maternal-separation (MS; 3 hours per day from P2-14) and compared their fear retention to a group of standard-reared (SR) infant laboratory rats. They found that when infants were trained at P17 and then tested 1 day later, there were no differences in memory between the different rearing conditions; both MS and SR rats exhibited high levels of fear responding. If, however, infants were tested 10 days following training, then fear behavior differed according to rearing condition; while the MS infants exhibited high levels of fear responding (indicating that they remembered), SR infants exhibited age-appropriate infantile amnesia (i.e., their freezing at the 10 day test was low). In other words, MS appeared to have accelerated the emergence of the adult-like fear memory system. Interestingly, a recent study in humans reported a similar outcome in that the offset of infantile amnesia was found to occur earlier in individuals from separated families (Artioli and Reese, 2014).

Similarly, MS also accelerates the emergence of the adult-like extinction system (Callaghan and Richardson, 2011). In that study MS and SR infants were compared on two relapse phenomena after extinction training. In the first comparison it was shown that MS infants exhibited the renewal effect, i.e., an increase in fear responding when test occurs in a different context to where extinction took place (an effect which was not observed in SR infants). In the second comparison it was shown that MS infants, but not SR infants, exhibited the reinstatement effect (i.e., a return in fear when animals are given a post-extinction stressor). In both cases, the behavior of infant MS rats was similar to that of adults from previous studies (Myers and Davis, 2002). Interestingly, it was not only the extinction behavior of infants that was altered by the rearing stress because MS infants were also shown to use a neurotransmitter during extinction learning that is not involved in the infant extinction system but that is involved in the adult extinction system: GABA. Together, these studies show that rearing stress significantly alters the developmental trajectory of fear and extinction systems, leading to an early transition between the infant- and adult-like phenotypes.

Accelerated developmental transitions following rearing stress also appear to occur in humans. As mentioned earlier, fear and extinction learning in the adult are supported by amygdala-prefrontal circuitry, and functional connectivity in this circuit differs across development (Gabard-Durnam et al., 2014; Gee et al., 2013b). A recent study has shown that the developmental trajectory of functional connectivity during a passive face viewing task is significantly affected by rearing stress—previous institutionalization in an overseas orphanage (PI; a naturally occurring model of maternal deprivation in humans; Gee et al., 2013a). In that study, it was shown that PI children were more likely to exhibit the adult-like pattern of amygdala-prefrontal connectivity (i.e., negatively coupled) compared to typically reared children (the typically reared children exhibited the immature, positively coupled, pattern). These data suggest that the development of mature connectivity in this circuit had been accelerated following PI (see Tottenham et al., 2011, for a similar result but in amygdala reactivity). Animal studies also suggest accelerated development of fear circuitry following rearing stress. For example, rats that were weaned from maternal care a week earlier than normal exhibited accelerated myelination specifically in the basolateral amygdala (Ono et al., 2008).

Taken together these findings indicate that early adverse events alter the trajectory of the developing fear and extinction systems, resulting in the expression of adult-like functioning earlier in development. It is possible that early rearing stress may be associated with anxiety disorder emergence through its disruptive effects on the developing fear and extinction circuitry. Indeed, many of the early rearing stressors known to affect the developing fear and extinction systems also result in adult anxiety (Bos et al., 2011; Kalinichev et al., 2002), suggesting that there may be a link between these early emerging emotional learning outcomes and the disordered adult state. This link between early disruptions to fear and extinction circuits and adult anxiety could occur through multiple pathways. For example, it is possible that accelerated development causes increased neural competition, negatively impacting structures and functions which develop over a similar time frame. Alternately, hastened development of fear and extinction systems may have compromised their functional integrity, destabilizing the foundations upon which more complex emotional responding skills are based (see Figure 6.2). Whatever the mechanism, these rodent and human data are consistent with the conceptualization of anxiety as a developmental disorder and provide exciting new insights into early-emerging phenotypic and biological markers for anxiety risk, as well as suggesting potential early treatments for anxiety disorders. The next section will discuss some these novel avenues for anxiety treatments.

TREATING ANXIETY: INSIGHTS FROM NEURODEVELOPMENT

Perhaps the most consistent message to emerge from studies in developmental affective neuroscience is the need for early intervention. However, one of the difficulties associated with early interventions is knowing when and how to intervene. The studies discussed in this chapter suggest that it may be possible to identify children at risk for anxiety by examining the early characteristics of fear and extinction or by examining the functional connectivity of the amygdala-prefrontal circuitry. Yet knowing how to treat early emerging deficits, once identified, remains elusive. One possibility is that treatments could aim to reopen infant-like plasticity and functioning in adult circuitry, effectively reverting accelerated trajectories back to a typical developmental pattern. Indeed, this approach would be useful across the lifespan because adults with anxiety may well benefit from treatments which increase forgetting of fear associations and decrease relapse after fear inhibition.

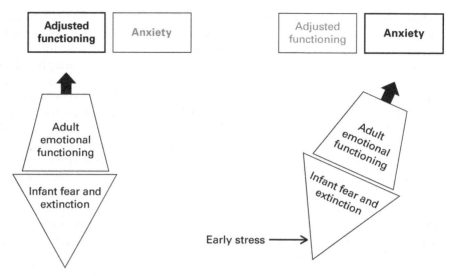

FIGURE 6.2 Adjusted functioning in the adult is probably achieved on the basis of strong foundations in early emotional learning systems, namely, fear and extinction. Exposure to early life stress may affect adult emotional responding by destabilizing the foundation processes upon which mature emotional functioning is based, resulting in increased risk of anxiety disorders.

Infant-like plasticity in fear extinction circuits has been successfully reactivated in several recent studies. For example, it has been shown that acute exogenous manipulations of the neurotrophic factor fibroblast growth factor-2 (FGF2), either injected systemically or infused directly into the amygdala, significantly reduced renewal and reinstatement of extinguished fear in juvenile and adult rats (Graham and Richardson, 2011a; Graham and Richardson, 2011b). In other words, infant-like extinction was reactivated in older rats. In a subsequent study it was shown that, similar to infant rats, erasure mechanisms appear to be the dominant process involved in extinction in juveniles injected with FGF2 (see Graham and Richardson, 2011a for a review).

Other studies have demonstrated a causal role for particular molecular structures in limiting infant-like plasticity. As mentioned earlier, degrading PNNs in the adult amygdala resulted in the expression of the infant extinction phenotype (i.e., the chABC-treated adult mice did not show renewal or spontaneous recovery of extinguished fear; Gogolla et al., 2009). Hence, the infant profile of extinction learning could be reactivated in adulthood by removal of a structural brake on plasticity—PNNs. Degrading PNNs from the adult amygdala can also be achieved through antidepressant administration. For example, Karpova et al. (2011) chronically exposed adult mice to the antidepressant fluoxetine in their drinking water before fear conditioning and extinction. They showed that the fluoxetine-exposed mice had a lower proportion of PNNs in the BLA and behaved like infant mice in past studies (Gogolla et al., 2009), showing less post-extinction relapse than the vehicle-treated mice. These findings suggest that combining antidepressants like fluoxetine with psychological treatments for anxiety (e.g., cognitive behavioral therapy; CBT) may result in enhanced fear inhibition and less fear relapse. However, studies which have examined this interaction have reported very mixed results (for a review of this issue see Graham et al., 2014). A greater understanding of how antidepressants regulate infant-like extinction learning in the adult brain is required.

SUMMARY

In this chapter we have reviewed evidence demonstrating developmental dissociations in fear and extinction behaviors, as well as in the neurochemistry and neurocircuitry supporting those behaviors. Importantly, we have also reviewed evidence demonstrating that the developmental trajectory of fear and extinction learning and associated neurocircuitry is not static (i.e., maturation of these behaviors and circuits can be accelerated by early life rearing stress). Considering that enhanced fear learning and disrupted extinction learning are implicated in the emergence and maintenance of anxiety disorders, and that our best evidence-based treatments for anxiety (i.e., exposure therapy) are modeled on the process of extinction, understanding how these forms of emotional learning develop is likely to yield information which can be used to enhance anxiety disorder treatment and prevention. Indeed, the studies reviewed here fit well with the emerging evidence supporting the categorization of anxiety disorders as having a neuro-developmental origin and suggest that alterations in the developmental trajectory of fear and extinction learning may be fundamental in establishing risk for anxiety disorders. In light of this evidence, it would seem that in order to truly understand how anxiety disorders emerge, and therefore, how they can be prevented, a greater understanding of the development of emotional learning is required.

CLINICAL VIGNETTE

While the studies examining fear and extinction learning in rats and humans have clear translational potential, the application of these preclinical studies to clinical practice remains an important goal for the future. However, some principles to emerge from this work should be considered both when treating anxiety disorders and when designing studies examining anxiety emergence, prevention, and treatment in human populations. These principles are discussed next.

Developmental trajectories are not set in stone. While the mapping of typical developmental trajectories has been useful in identifying the skills and functions which can be expected of children at different ages, the research discussed in this chapter suggests that at least some developmental trajectories are malleable and can change in response to different early-life experiences. It may be worth considering (both in treatment and research) that children with a history of early stress are at a very different emotional age than their typically developing peers.

Documenting early events is essential in research examining treatment efficacy. The importance of early experiences in mental health across the lifespan is well-established (Green et al., 2010; McLaughlin et al., 2010). The studies described in this chapter show that the development of fear and extinction systems is affected by exposure to early-life stress, which may have implications for the effectiveness of anxiety treatments which utilize the fear and extinction circuits. We know that our best treatments for anxiety (exposure therapy) do not work for all patients, suggesting that there should be a greater focus on individual difference factors in treatment trials. We suggest that exposure to early-life stress, and the age of that exposure, are two individual difference factors which will be important to consider when studying treatment efficacy. Therefore, we would encourage the routine examination of these factors in future anxiety treatment trials or preclinical studies examining fear learning and extinction.

Early-life events may need to be considered in choice of pharmacotherapy. The studies described in this chapter show that early life stress affects the involvement of certain neurotransmitter systems in extinction. Specifically, GABA is involved in extinction earlier following stressful rearing (see Callaghan and Richardson, 2013). These studies raise the interesting possibility that early experiences may play an important role in determining the effectiveness of anxiety pharmacotherapies and pharmacological adjuncts to extinction. Also, developmental studies have opened the exciting possibility that infant-like plasticity may be induced pharmacologically in adults (e.g., through fluoxetine) which might aid in better extinction retention. Continued exploration of this issue is required.

DISCLOSURE STATEMENT

Neither author has any financial interests or potential conflicts of interest to declare.

ACKNOWLEDGMENTS

Preparation of this chapter was supported by grants from the Australian Research Council (DP120104925) and the National Health and Medical Research Council (APP1031688) to RR.

NOTE

1. Chan et al. (2011) have reported that a simpler neural circuit is also involved in the expression of innate fear.

REFERENCES

Artioli, F., and Reese, E. (2014). Early memories in young adults from separated and non-separated families. *Memory, 22*, 1082–1102.

Baker, J. D., and Azorlosa, J. L. (1996). The NMDA antagonist MK-801 blocks the extinction of Pavlovian fear conditioning. *Behav Neurosci, 110*, 618–620.

Bos, K., Zeanah, C. H., Fox, N. A., Drury, S. S., McLaughlin, K. A., and Nelson, C. A. (2011). Psychiatric outcomes in young children with a history of institutionalization. *Harvard Rev Psychiatry, 19*, 15–24.

Bouton, M. E. (2002). Context, ambiguity, and unlearning: Sources of relapse after behavioral extinction. *Biological Psychiatry, 52*, 976–986.

Callaghan, B., and Richardson, R. (2012). The effect of adverse rearing environments on persistent memories in young rats: Removing the brakes on infant fear memories. *Translat Psychiatry, 2*, e138.

Callaghan, B. L., Li, S., and Richardson, R. (2014). The elusive engram: What can infantile amnesia tell us about memory? *Trends Neurosci, 37*, 47–53.

Callaghan, B. L., and Richardson, R. (2011). Maternal separation results in early emergence of adult-like fear and extinction learning in infant rats. *Behav Neurosci, 125*, 20–28.

Callaghan, B. L., and Richardson, R. (2013). Early experiences and the development of emotional learning systems in rats. *Biol Mood Anxiety Disorders, 3*.

Campbell, B. A., and Campbell, E. H. (1962). Retention and extinction of learned fear in infant and adult rats. *J Comp Physiol Psychol, 55*, 1–8.

Campbell, B. A., and Jaynes, J. (1966). Reinstatement. *Psychol Rev, 73*, 478–480.

Chan, T., Kyere, K., Davis, B. R., Shemyakin, A., Kabitzke, P. A., Shair, H. N., et al. (2011). The role of the medial prefrontal cortex in innate fear regulation in infants, juveniles, and adolescents. *J Neurosci, 31*, 4991–4999.

Corcoran, K. A., and Quirk, G. J. (2007). Activity in prelimbic cortex is necessary for the expression of learned, but not innate, fears. *J Neurosci, 27*, 840–844.

Duman, R. (2002). Synaptic plasticity and mood disorders. *Molec Psychiatry, 7*, S29–S34.

Gabard-Durnam, L. J., Flannery, J., Goff, B., Gee, D. G., Humphreys, K. L., Telzer, E., et al. (2014). The development of human amygdala functional connectivity at rest from 4 to 23 years: A cross-sectional study. *NeuroImage, 95*, 193–207.

Gee, D., Gabard-Durnam, L. J., Flannery, J., Goff, B., Humphreys, K. L., Telzer, E. H., et al. (2013a). Early developmental emergence of mature human amygdala-prefrontal phenotype following maternal deprivation: Evidence of stress-induced acceleration. *Proc Natl Acad Sci, 110*, 15638–15643.

Gee, D. G., Humphreys, K. L., Flannery, J., Goff, B., Telzer, E. H., Shapiro, M., et al. (2013b). A developmental shift from positive to negative connectivity in human amygdala–prefrontal circuitry. *J Neurosci, 33*, 4584–4593.

Gogolla, N., Caroni, P., Lüthi, A., and Herry, C. (2009). Perineuronal nets protect fear memories from erasure. *Science, 325*, 1258–1261.

Graham, B., and Richardson, R. (2011a). Memory of fearful events: The role of fibroblast growth factor-2 in fear acquisition and extinction. *Neuroscience, 189*, 156–169.

Graham, B. M., Callaghan, B. L., and Richardson, R. (2014). Bridging the gap: Lessons we have learnt from the merging of psychology and psychiatry for the optimisation of treatments for emotional disorders. *Behav Res Ther, 62*, 3–16.

Graham, B. M., and Richardson, R. (2011b). Intraamygdala infusion of fibroblast growth factor 2 enhances extinction and reduces renewal and reinstatement in adult rats. *J Neurosci, 31*, 14151–14157.

Green, J. G., McLaughlin, K. A., Berglund, P. A., Gruber, M. J., Sampson, N. A., Zaslavsky, A. M., et al. (2010). Childhood adversities and adult psychiatric disorders in the national comorbidity survey replication I: Associations with first onset of DSM-IV disorders. *Arch Gen Psychiatry, 67*, 113–123.

Harris, J. A., and Westbrook, R. F. (1998). Evidence that GABA transmission mediates context-specific extinction of learned fear. *Psychopharmacology, 140*, 105–115.

Hayne, H. (2004). Infant memory development: Implications for childhood amnesia. *Dev Rev, 24*, 33–73.

Hensch, T. K. (2005). Critical period plasticity in local cortical circuits. *Nature Rev Neurosci, 6*, 877–888.

Josselyn, S. A., and Frankland, P. W. (2012). Infantile amnesia: A neurogenic hypothesis. *Learning and Memory, 19*, 423–433.

Kalinichev, M., Easterling, K. W., Plotsky, P. M., and Holtzman, S. G. (2002). Long-lasting changes in stress-induced corticosterone response and anxiety-like behaviors as a consequence of neonatal maternal separation in Long–Evans rats. *Pharmacol Biochem Behav, 73*, 131–140.

Karpova, N. N., Pickenhagen, A., Lindholm, J., Tiraboschi, E., Kulesskaya, N., Ágústsdóttir, A., et al. (2011). Fear Erasure in Mice Requires Synergy Between Antidepressant Drugs and Extinction Training. *Science, 334*, 1731–1734.

Kessler, R. C., Amminger, G. P., Aguilar-axiola, S., Alonso, J., Lee, S., and Ustun, T. B. (2007). Age of onset of mental disorders: a review of recent literature. *Curr Opinion psychiatry, 20*, 359–364.

Kim, J. H., Hamlin, A. S., and Richardson, R. (2009). Fear extinction across development: The involvement of the medial prefrontal cortex as assessed by temporary inactivation and immunohistochemistry. *J Neurosci, 29*, 10802–10808.

Kim, J. H., Li, S., Hamlin, A. S., McNally, G. P., and Richardson, R. (2012). Phosphorylation of mitogen-activated protein kinase in the medial prefrontal cortex and the amygdala following memory retrieval or forgetting in developing rats. *Neurobiol Learning Memory, 97*, 59–68.

Kim, J. H., McNally, G. P., and Richardson, R. (2006). Recovery of fear memories in rats: Role of gamma-amino butyric acid (GABA) in infantile amnesia. *Behav Neurosci, 120*, 40–48.

Kim, J. H., and Richardson, R. (2010). New findings on extinction of conditioned fear early in development: Theoretical and clinical implications. *Biol Psychiatry, 67*, 297–303.

Langton, J. M., Kim, J. H., Nicholas, J., and Richardson, R. (2007). The effect of the NMDA receptor antagonist MK-801 on the acquisition and extinction of learned fear in the developing rat. *Learning and Mem, 14*, 665–668.

Leonardo, E. D., and Hen, R. (2007). Anxiety as a developmental disorder. *Neuropsychopharmacology, 33,* 134–140.

Li, S., Callaghan, B. L., and Richardson, R. (2014). Infantile amnesia: Forgotten but not gone. *Learning Mem, 21,* 135–139.

Li, S., Kim, J. H., and Richardson, R. (2012). Differential involvement of the medial prefrontal cortex in the expression of learned fear across development. *Behav Neurosci, 126,* 217–225.

Lickliter, R., and Banker, H. (1994). Prenatal components of intersensory development in precocial birds. In *The development of intersensory perception: Comparative perspectives,* edited by D. J. Lewkowicz and R. Lickliter (pp. 59–80). New Jersey: Lawrence Earlbaum Associates.

McLaughlin, K. A., Green, J. G., Gruber, M. J., Sampson, N. A., Zaslavsky, A. M., and Kessler, R. C. (2010). Childhood adversities and adult psychiatric disorders in the national comorbidity survey replication II: associations with persistence of DSM-IV disorders. *Arch Gen Psychiatry, 67,* 124–132.

McNally, G. P., Pigg, M., and Weidemann, G. (2004). Opioid receptors in the midbrain periaqueductal gray regulate extinction of Pavlovian fear conditioning. *J Neurosci, 24,* 6912–6919.

McNally, G. P., and Westbrook, R. F. (2003). Opioid receptors regulate the extinction of Pavlovian fear conditioning. *Behav Neurosci, 117,* 1292–1301.

Milad, M. R., and Quirk, G. J. (2012). Fear extinction as a model for translational neuroscience: Ten years of progress. *Annu Rev Psychol, 63,* 129–151.

Miserendino, M. J. D., Sananes, C. B., Melia, K. R., and Davis, M. (1990). Blocking of acquisition but not expression of conditioned fear-potentiated startle by NMDA antagonists in the amygdala. *Nature, 345,* 716–718.

Myers, K. M., and Davis, M. (2002). Behavioral and neural analysis of extinction. *Neuron, 36,* 567–584.

Ono, M., Kikusui, T., Sasaki, N., Ichikawa, M., Mori, Y., and Murakami-Murofushi, K. (2008). Early weaning induces anxiety and precocious myelination in the anterior part of the basolateral amygdala of male Balb/c mice. *Neuroscience, 156,* 1103–1110.

Revillo, D., Molina, J., Paglini, M., and Arias, C. (2013). A sensory-enhanced context allows renewal of an extinguished fear response in the infant rat. *Behav Brain Res, 253,* 173–177.

Thompson, B. L., and Levitt, P. (2010). The clinical-basic interface in defining pathogenesis in disorders of neurodevelopmental origin. *Neuron, 67,* 702–712.

Tottenham, N., Hare, T., Millner, A., Gilhooly, T., Zevin, J., and Casey, B. (2011). Elevated amygdala response to faces following early deprivation. *Dev Sci, 14,* 190–204.

Turkewitz, G., and Kenny, P. A. (1985). The role of developmental limitations of sensory input on sensory/perceptual organization. *J Dev Behav Pediatrics, 6,* 302–306.

Wachman, E. M., and Lahav, A. (2011). The effects of noise on preterm infants in the NICU. *Arch Dis Childhood-Fetal Neonat Ed, 96,* F305–F309.

7

INVOLVING THE FAMILY IN TREATMENT

KAREN LYNN CASSIDAY

INTRODUCTION

This chapter is designed to help clinicians approach the task of involving parents, stepparents, and caretakers in the process of effective therapy for an identified child, adolescent, or young adult patient. It assumes the therapist has a working knowledge of exposure-based therapies and other cognitive-behavioral interventions for children and teens (Davis, Whiting and May, 2012; Kendall, 2012). It also assumes that the therapist, like many child and adolescent therapists, really enjoys the interactions with younger clients. Some child and adolescent therapists might feel less comfortable working with parents and caretakers because their training was specialized toward working with kids and they spent relatively less time learning how to motivate and work with parents and caretakers.

Therapists working with children and teens can face many dilemmas that arise from the misinformed efforts of their parents and caretakers to decrease child distress or to motivate their child to overcome anxiety. Treatment outcome can be greatly improved when parents and caretakers are successfully involved (Reynolds, Wilson, Austin and Hooper, 2012; Podell and Kendall, 2011; Ginsburg, Siqueland, Masia-Warner and Hedtke, 2004). Therapists who fail to adequately involve parents and caretakers risk undermining their treatment, whether it is cognitive behavioral or pharmacological. They also overlook important scientific literature indicating that family-based risk factors influence the expression and maintenance of child and teen anxiety. These factors include overprotection, perfectionism, provision of reassurance, negative reinforcement, role modeling through the presence of parental anxiety disorders, and lack of awareness of the child's symptoms (Beesdo, Knappe and Pine, 2009; Marikangas, 2005). Moreover, successful treatment requires more than educating a parent or caretaker about their child's disorder(s) and treatment. Parents need as much practice at managing their child's anxiety disorder as does their child or teen. Successful treatment often involves the entire family to create an exposure-based lifestyle, designed to improve behavior management skills and create appropriate expectations of the child.

THE CULTURE OF ANXIETY IN FAMILIES

It helps to first understand the culture behind parents who seek treatment for their children who have anxiety disorders. Such parents often know anxiety well due to their own or their relatives' experiences with an anxiety disorder. This can increase sympathy toward their child's desire to avoid anxiety-provoking situations. If the parent or relative has never attempted cognitive behavioral therapy, then one or both parents may actively endorse avoidance behaviors and provide reassurance to the child because negative reinforcement has worked to quickly alleviate the adult's anxiety.

Several psychological factors may make it difficult for parents to respond to their children's anxiety effectively. Parents may feel guilty about having transmitted or taught the disorder to their child; this can make discussions about treatment or any evidence of distress in the child an intolerable reminder of the parents' limitations. Parental worry can lead parents to respond to their child's distress in ways that increase anxiety in the child. For example, parents might make statements such as, "If you don't stop doing that, you are going to give me a heart attack!" or "You will never be able to go to college or marry or hold a job if you don't get better!" In addition, parents can develop sleep-deprivation due to their child's nighttime behavior, which can complicate parents' attempts to regulate their own emotions or think clearly when interacting with their children.

Cultural factors may also impede effective parenting. For example, the popular parenting culture of the past 20 years has emphasized the value of strong parental attachment and the adverse consequences of attachment problems. Well-intentioned parents of anxious children can misinterpret this as indicating that they should use talking and discussion in place of effective discipline or use hugging and "I love you" statements when time-outs would be best applied. Families of middle and upper-middle class children and teens can feel pressure to have their children experience unrealistic levels of success in order to gain a college entry with scholarships. This can lead parents to begin enrichment activities as early as the toddler years and to create other circumstances in which the entire family experiences pressure to achieve and excel in comparison to other families.

Lastly, since many parents are not experts in child development, they often misunderstand which skills are age-appropriate. For example, parents may unrealistically expect an eight-year-old child to want to complete all of his exposure homework because he has said that he hates his anxiety. Similarly, other parents may prevent a 12-year-old from attending a party or other event due to their own inappropriate concerns about the safety of the event.

In summary, parents and caretakers of anxious children and teens often are tired, worried, afraid of making mistakes, and incompletely equipped to fully engage in cognitive behavioral therapy. However, parents who manage to come to treatment also clearly are highly invested in helping their child and being good parents. Successful treatment can follow when the therapist effectively shows parents how to tolerate uncertainty, embrace mistakes, face fear, and confront difficult tasks by repeating them until they become easy. The nature of this involvement varies with the age of the child. For children through age 12 to 13, parents usually should attend therapy sessions in their entirety, unless an exposure task requires their absence. This creates opportunities for the therapist to model appropriate behavior with an anxious child and to actively coach the parent/caretakers while they coach their child. For older teens, parents usually should be present only at the beginning and end of each session, as well as for the initial exposure sessions in order to be able to model and coach.

ASSESSMENT OF PARENTAL ACCOMMODATION AND OVERPROTECTION

Therapists can administer The Family Accommodation Scale—Anxiety (Liebowitz et al., 2013) to quantify parental behaviors that promote the child's anxiety. Therapists also can ask several simple questions of both the parent and child.

Questions for the Parent

1. What do you do when your child gets anxious?
2. What are you afraid will happen if you do not do this?
3. What is the worst thing that could happen if your child has an out-of-control episode of panic, worry, obsession, compulsion, or if your child feels socially outcast?
4. What do you do when your child has tantrums about things other than their anxiety? (to assess general parenting discipline skills)
5. Describe your family's method of discipline. Do you use rewards and/or negative consequences? What kind? Do you ever forget to give earned rewards?
6. Give me an example of how you would praise your child.
7. What is your opinion about rewarding your child for doing exposure practice? Why?

Questions for the Child or Teen

Parental worry can lead parents to attend to possible negative outcomes for their child and fail to realize that parental worry impedes the child's healthy functioning. Therapists can pose questions to children and teens to assess children's anxiety and the subsequent parental influence on it through parental overprotection and worry.

1. What happens to your anxiety when your parent/caretaker gives you reassurance? Lets you avoid? Does something for you, for example, a compulsion, finishing your homework, doing your chores, calling you in sick to school? Do you like this?
2. Which makes you feel more proud of yourself—when you do something really difficult by yourself or when mom or dad does it for you?
3. What do you think would happen to you if mom or dad did not get so upset or worried when you get anxious?
4. What happens inside of you when mom and dad keep talking to you when you are mad or anxious or panicking?
5. How do you feel when mom or dad is worrying about you and your anxiety?

GETTING-STARTED: ROLE PLAYING

Therapists should help parents appreciate the ways in which their attempts at reassurance, facilitated avoidance, and worry can negatively impact their children. This can be accomplished through role playing.

One role-playing strategy requires the parent to play-act their typical response to their child while the child play acts his or her typical behavior when they are extremely anxious and out-of-control. Many children and teens enjoy the opportunity to publically humiliate their parents and eagerly participate. In the context of such play-acting, the therapist can suggest ways for parents to adopt different response patterns than typically employed in these contexts. This play-acting is followed by a discussion in which the therapist may ask the child if parents' unique responses made it easier for the child to stop the tantrum or encouraged the child to make it increase. Similarly, the therapist may ask the parent to reflect on how their child's behavior changes with different parenting approaches.

Next, this initial role-play can be repeated with the child or teen repeating his or her behavior and having the therapist play the role of calm parent. In this context, when the child or teen becomes anxious, the therapist-parent simply states, "Looks like you are really anxious. Of course this is difficult because your fear is telling you that you cannot do your exposure practice. It will just take practice." The therapist then may offer a forced choice based upon the child's or teen's concerns. "You can either do _____ for exposure practice or _____ for exposure practice." As with the first instance of role-playing, this second instance also is followed by a discussion. The child or teen can compare his or her experiences in the two instances. If the parent is slow to observe the difference in effect between the two styles of responding, repeating the role-play a third time may be helpful. This time, the parent might play the part of the child or teen, with the therapist delivering the two corresponding responses so that the parent can directly experience the effects of varying methods for responding to their child or teen. Typically, the parent then readily learns the ways in which parental behavior markedly influences anxiety in the child.

REINFORCE PARENTS, NOT JUST IDENTIFIED PATIENTS

Many therapists forget that parents and caretakers long for praise and recognition not just from the therapist, but also from their children. Remembering to find and praise parental effort is crucial. An effective therapist should begin each session with the caretaker present and describe at least one way that the parent helped the child move toward improvement. The therapist can also have the child acknowledge this contribution, possibly by giving parents a smiley face or "A" letter grade in instances where parents facilitated successful response to an exposure task. It is not unusual for children and teens to assign their parents either a frowny face or an "F" in early sessions. The therapist can normalize this experience by informing parents that this is the expected response early in treatment, as quantified by scientists who have studied many children with anxiety disorders.

The therapist can use other questions to acknowledge effective parenting—"What smiley face, or grade, do you give your parent since we last met for not listening to your anxiety, not giving in and not talking back to your anxiety?" Therapists also can give their own evaluation to call attention to success, for example, noting: "I would give you an 'A+' today because even though you lost your temper, you tried most of the time not to reassure and to ignore your child's tantrum. That is really hard to do for most parents. No one gets it right without lots of practice." Parents and caretakers find these positive evaluations fun and motivating because they demonstrably reveal concrete areas of improvement. Unsuccessful attempts at therapy often are characterized by reports from parents about lack of clarity regarding expectations for parental behavior. Direct feedback to parents addresses the need to provide clear expectations.

ANXIETY MANAGEMENT VERSUS ABSENCE

The parents' desire to eliminate their child's anxiety creates a two-fold dilemma: therapists can teach patients to manage anxiety, but they cannot fully eliminate anxiety from their patients' entire lives. In fact, successful therapy typically requires a desperate parent to *deliberately provoke* and endure the very symptoms for which the parent is seeking help. This means that therapists must help parents adjust their expectations and their role.

This process can be facilitated by using an analogy. The parent's role can be compared to that of a master sergeant leading a platoon in a battle that is suddenly ambushed with crossfire and rockets. A good master sergeant directs his platoon to locate and fire their weapons because it is the best chance of surviving the battle. What would happen if the master sergeant responded in a fashion frequently observed by parents of anxious children? "Oh My God! We are all going to die! I cannot believe how big those rockets are! This is just too much—I cannot believe how scared you are! I didn't see this one coming! Don't get mad at me—I told you this would happen?!" The parental equivalent of competent master sergeant behavior involves coaching the child to use the skills that they learn in therapy on the battlefield of anxiety. Parents also should be taught to welcome each episode in which their child or teen becomes visibly anxious because that means that their child or teen has an opportunity to become an expert at managing anxiety.

It is also helpful to have parents list their own concerns about treatment with a side-by-side list of helpful cognitive reframes. The parents can then be asked to read through this list each day for homework to help prime their ability to counter thoughts that undermine their compliance with treatment. Here are some examples of unhelpful parental thoughts and cognitive reframes:

> Unhelpful parent belief: My child will feel abandoned/unloved if I do not comfort her when she is anxious.
> Reframe: My child will see that I believe that she is strong and capable to manage her fear if I redirect her to cope by doing exposure practice.
> Unhelpful parent belief: He will never be able to sleep and neither will anyone else if I do not reassure him.
> Reframe: Going in to reassure my child/teen will only prolong the problem of sleep deprivation. I might as well make this anxiety worth something by doing exposure practice. Going into his room and sleeping with him has kept this problem alive. I might as well start now to help him learn to overcome his anxiety.
> Unhelpful parent belief: She is just too young to have to do exposure therapy. Maybe I should wait until she is ready and wants to do treatment.
> Reframe: Why would I want to put off recovery or guarantee further anxiety for my child by delaying what science shows will help? This really is my best choice. Kids who recover are stronger and grateful to no longer be suffering. Since my child has an anxiety disorder, the best gift that I can give her is learning how to overcome it. My child's fear of exposure is just normal for having an anxiety disorder. That is why we are here in the first place!

KEEPING ON TRACK

Therapists and parents both should expect problems as a typical part of successful treatment. Several simple steps can reduce the impact of these problems and prepare families to confront them when they arise. One helpful step is to provide families with written copies of expectations for the week. With this guide, nobody needs to be reminded of homework assignments. Another helpful step is to also write out the list of practices, including encouragements for previous successes. For example, write out, "Way to go, mom, with just walking away after you dropped Susie at day care—you are being a fantastic exposure mom!" or "Dad, keep up the good work by continuing to refuse to write your son's papers. You are helping him overcome his OCD." Is also is important for the therapist to do everything possible to provide an absent caretaker the opportunity to attend sessions via videoconference or telephone and to ensure that the absent caretaker receives copies of written material.

CONSENT AND OPEN COMMUNICATION

Parents and caretakers who are overprotective frequently fear harming their children. This might lead them to avoid conversation about diagnosis, prognosis, treatment, parental concerns, or issues in the family. The unintended outcome is to increase anxiety for everyone, along with a sense of shame. Things that are made unmentionable are at high risk to become the things that shame parents, caretakers, children and teens. This also robs from families the sense of self-esteem that follows when an individual overcomes significant challenges and obstacles, such as an anxiety disorder.

Having the preteen or teen's assent/consent for open communication among parents, therapist, and patient facilitates recovery. This creates an opportunity for helpful feedback and prevents oppositional patients from holding treatment hostage by refusing to allow open communication about areas of difficulty with respect to exposure practice or other skills training. Therapists should state that effective treatment requires open communication so that everyone in the family can develop an improved system for managing the patient's anxiety disorder. Therapists should strive to teach everyone how to be an expert at fighting anxiety and how to avoid common mistakes that interfere with this goal. This might require open communication with parents about the ways in which they accidentally interfere with recovery or open communication with patients about how they are accidentally interfering with their parents' attempts to help them recover. If circumstances necessitate a private conversation with one member of the family, other members of the family should be informed about the conversation, and every effort should be made to insure that all members of the family are made aware of the issues discussed. This effectively models open communication about anxiety-related topics in a matter of fact, accepting and neutral manner. If a teen is reluctant to agree to an open communication policy, it helps to offer an analogy such as, "What would you do if you had a serious disease and the doctor told you to take pills that would help you recover but taste bad? Would you ask the doctor for the pills that taste good but do not work? Or wouldn't you want to make sure that any medicine you take is really going to help you get better?" The therapist should then explain that failing to agree to an open communication policy is akin to guaranteeing that treatment will be less effective and that it would be foolish to knowingly enter into such an agreement.

Appropriate communication is critical to overcoming a pattern of overprotection and mistake intolerance that can interfere with treatment. Such communication requires the therapist to tell even preschoolers the name of their disorder and the treatment plan in age-appropriate language. This models calm and optimistic communication. This may necessitate some private conversation with a parent who believes that it would be harmful to tell their child that they have a mental health diagnosis or that they are taking their child to see a mental health professional. Parents can be told that their child certainly already knows that something is wrong, because they are experiencing symptoms that brought them to the attention of adults. The child will also surmise that something is terribly wrong if no one can talk about it. Parents can also be told that prior experience establishes the benefits that accrue from such an open approach to communication. Lastly, parents can be encouraged to show their child how to be brave in the face of adversity by talking openly and hopefully about the problem.

DECREASING PARENTAL SELF-BLAME AND SHAME

Language can profoundly impact parents' and caretakers' willingness to accept feedback. This includes language that acknowledges parents' good intentions, willingness to love lavishly, and that accepts mistakes as a normal part of life. A therapist might point out parental mistakes by saying, "You are accidentally making it difficult for your kid to recover when you _____," or "It looks like you are really trying hard to help your child. In fact you are even trying too hard. How about we come up with some ways for you to not have to do so much?" or "I can tell how much you love your kid. You are willing to do anything to help him, even to lose sleep or miss work. I would love for you to learn how to show your love in a way that keeps you from burning out and helps your kid to recover at the same time." Therapists might normalize a parent's experience by giving examples of how other parents and caretakers make the same mistakes in promoting avoidance, worrying aloud, losing their temper or giving reassurance. The therapist should highlight the immense value of any parental attempt to change behavior. Parents should be taught to consider their efforts to change as being evidence of parental greatness because they are rising to the challenge of helping their child.

It is also very helpful to point out that the parent's task in treatment is to become a more effective parent and not to produce a perfect child who is symptom-free. For parents of young children and elementary-aged children, this will mean being willing to help the child do exposure homework, keep track of rewards earned, and help the child manage mistakes made by using corrective exposure. For preteens and teens this may mean a similar level of involvement if the teen's symptoms are severe or developmental delays are present. Parents of teens who are more self-sufficient may simply need help and coaching in coordination and delivery of rewards, noticing their child's progress, and promoting more independent exposure practice.

Parents can be encouraged to consider mistakes as the best opportunities for learning and to welcome situations that are unexpected, whether it be an anxiety trigger, a child's refusal to cooperate with exposure tasks, a parental mistake in providing reassurance, or just a rough day. Therapists can explain that no one has ever been a perfect parent and note that successful parenting follows from a willingness to identify and learn from mistakes.

PRIORITIZING SYMPTOMS—WHAT TO TREAT FIRST

Typical exposure therapy protocol dictates that treatment begins with low anxiety-provoking exposure tasks. Starting at the low end of the exposure hierarchy is not always the best strategy when a child's anxiety symptoms have interfered with sleep. A sleep-deprived patient or family will have less capacity to tolerate distress or understand new information. Therefore, it is often important to address sleep problems early in treatment. This may mean making arrangements for one parent and the siblings to sleep at another house while the other parent is "on duty" and then alternating sleeping in a restful setting so that neither parent (nor the siblings) becomes hopelessly sleep-deprived. Symptoms that interfere with healthy eating also should be tackled early, possibly by encouraging nutritional supplementation to address the child's food avoidance symptoms. Symptoms that result in school refusal should be targeted after the previous two symptom categories in order to restore normalcy to the child's life as quickly as possible. Targeting symptoms in the usual ascending order follows this.

COACHING PARENTS DURING EXPOSURE

Parents and caretakers will learn best when they can both observe the therapist prompting the child to do exposure and when they can be observed in the act of coaching their child. This includes office-based observation and coaching as well as coaching in the community or family home. Prior to exposure, the therapist can explain the procedures to parents and ask them to observe as the therapist instructs and praises the child during exposure. The therapist should note the importance of specificity in this communication to the child, avoiding global statements of praise, e.g. "You touched the toilet seat and that is going to help you overcome your OCD" versus "Way to go!" The therapist also should explain procedures for reframing anxiety as the definitive sign of successful exposure, e.g., "You are scared? Of course you are because you are doing good exposure practice! That means that you are right on track in treatment." Parents also should be reminded to keep a friendly calm manner to communicate faith in their child's ability to cope.

Once exposure begins and the child is successfully encountering difficult situations, parents and caretakers can be encouraged to give feedback in a fashion similar to the therapist, e.g., "Mom, what do you think of how Johnny is asking the counter clerk for ice cream?" The therapist also can suppress parental concerns about the child's evident anxiety if they begin to express worry or doubt, e.g., "Dad, when you tried to hug your son while he was crying instead of redirecting him to do exposure, you accidentally showed him that you did not think he could do exposure. Let's try that again. How can you be the strong master sergeant leading your son through the battlefield of anxiety?" The therapist may ask the child, "How strong did that make you feel when Dad just tried to make you feel better but did not ask you to keep doing exposure?"

Therapists also must encourage parents, even when difficulties arise in an exposure session, e.g., "It looks like you are trying really hard to stop reassuring Susie and you did it way less than last session. Let's see if you can catch yourself before you say anything reassuring and just tell Susie, 'Doctor's orders—I cannot talk about that to you because it will only make you feel more scared in the long run.'" Therapists also should elicit the child's feedback during the session, asking, "How do you think your mom is doing at not giving you reassurance and helping you to do exposure practice?" Additionally, play acting the management of tantrums and prediction and preparation for worst-case home situations can be helpful. This involves asking the family to predict all the things that could go wrong once they leave the therapist's office or to describe all the obstacles that make it difficult to complete exposure practice at home. The entire family is asked to develop solutions in advance of the anticipated obstacles before leaving the therapist's office. A parent who can demonstrate child management skills in the office is more likely to be helpful outside your office.

MANAGING HOSTILE PARENTS

Sometimes parents become alarmed when their child experiences high levels of anxiety during an exposure session and mistakenly assume that the therapist is asking too much of their child. No matter how carefully therapists construct an exposure hierarchy, it is impossible to ensure that children or teens can readily manage all of their exposure tasks. More than likely, children will express more distress at home than in the office because they have had the frequent past experience of negative reinforcement. Overprotective parents and caretakers believe that their child is emotionally fragile. This can result in the parent getting angry and then verbally attacking and blaming the therapist for their child's distress. When this occurs, it is critical to address this rupture in the therapeutic alliance by remembering that it is a great opportunity to role model how to manage someone's unexpected distress.

Defensive therapist responses generally do not address these problems. Such commonly used defensive responses include attempting to justify the exposure practice, responding with anger by criticizing the unjustified verbal attack, or responding with shaming tactics by pointing out how other parents have been more effective at handling exposure. The best response is to disarm the angry parent by agreeing with the parent that the exposure task was very difficult—it alarmed both the parent and the kid—and to apologize for the fact that exposure therapy can be so difficult and upsetting. Then point out how fortunate the patient is to have a parent who cares so much as to want to make sure that the treatment the child is receiving really is the very best.

The therapist might then ask the parents to explain the factors that led them to believe that this was an impossible task for their child. Parents also might be asked for real proof that an exposure task was impossible (such as evidence of a terrible mental breakdown vs. an anxiety meltdown). Parents should be taught that they would actually have to see prolonged repeated exposure with no evidence of habituation in anxiety in order to conclude that their child was a rare case in which exposure would not work. They should be told that this has not yet been the case with their child, who had not experienced repeated prolonged exposure, and should be encouraged to count all the past times when they have given in to the child's anxiety. Parents then can be reminded that clearly this had not been helpful, given the patient's ongoing problems with anxiety. Finally, parents can be told that they have nothing to lose by trying this new approach, which can be viewed as an experiment that tests whether or not a prolonged crying meltdown or tantrum really destroys the child's mental health or instead just makes everyone tired. In such situations, the real enemy is not exposure therapy, or a mean therapist, but the willingness to believe that nothing is worse than getting really anxious. Parents should be challenged to become stronger than their overprotection or their child's fears by learning to reframe a high level of anxiety as their child's best opportunity for getting better. Next, they can be asked to try again, to see how well they can manage, providing a great opportunity for practice. It is preferable to make such interventions quickly so that the parents can discover, along with their child, that they can manage a difficult situation. Waiting until the next session can increase anticipatory anxiety and incorrectly suggest that the exposure task really was too difficult.

In short, parent oppositional behavior and distress can be treated in the same manner as child oppositional behavior and distress—by not taking it personally, understanding it as an expression of anxiety, using motivational interviewing, and reengaging in the therapeutic task of exposure.

SUMMARY

Getting parents and caretakers successfully involved in treatment can accelerate and secure good treatment outcomes. The therapist's willingness to fully include parents facilitates effective therapy. It makes is easier for parent and caretakers to improve their anxiety management skills when therapists use the same role modeling, coaching, and corrective feedback skills that are effective with children. This also conveys the message that the therapist values parental participation and good intentions while building an alliance toward the shared goal of alleviating the suffering caused by anxiety disorders.

REFERENCES

Beesdo, K., Knappe, S., and Pine, D. S. (2009). Anxiety and anxiety disorders in children and adolescents: Developmental issues and implications for DSM-V. *Psychiatr Clin North Am*, 32 (3), 483–524.

Davis, T., Whiting, S. E., and May, A. C. (2012). Exposure therapy for anxiety disorders in children. In *Exposure therapy: Rethinking the model—refining the method,* edited by P. Neudeck, H. Wittchen (pp. 111–125). New York, NY: Springer Science + Business Media.

Kendall, P. C. (2012). *Child and adolescent therapy: Cognitive-behavioral procedures (4th ed.).* New York, NY: Guilford Press.

Liebowitz, E., Woolsten, J., Bar-Haim, Y., Calvocoressi, L., Dauer, C., Warnick, E., . . . Leckman, J. (2013). Family accommodation in pediatric anxiety disorders. *Depress Anxiety*, 30: 47–54.

Merikangas, K. (2005). Vulnerability factors for anxiety disorders in children and adolescents. *Child Adolesc Psychiatr Clin North Am*, 14 (4), 649–679.

Podell, J. L., and Kendall, P. C. (2011). Mothers and fathers in family cognitive-behavioral therapy for anxious youth. *J Child Fam Studies*, 20 (2), 182–195.

Ginsburg, G. S., Siqueland, L., Masia-Warner, C., and Hedtke, K. A. (2004). Anxiety disorders in children: Family matters. *Cog Behav Pract*, 11 (1), 28–43.

Reynolds, S., Wilson, C., Austin, J., and Hooper, L. (2012). Effects of psychotherapy for anxiety in children and adolescents: A meta-analytic review. *Clin Psychol Rev*, 32 (4), 251–262.

/// 8 /// TREATING THE COLLEGE-AGE PATIENT

LISA R. HALE AND
KATHRYN D. KRIEGSHAUSER

INTRODUCTION

Perhaps more so than covering clinical issues for any other life stage, a discussion of treating college-age patients requires at least a cursory review of shifting viewpoints in how society has conceptualized young adulthood. While providing extensive historical context for the college mental health system is beyond the scope or intent of the current chapter (see Prescott, 2008 in its entirety for a review), where helpful we will note its evolution as a contributor or contrast to the current climate. According to the 2013 Annual Survey of the Association for University and College Counseling Center Directors (AUCCCD), the primary mental health concerns of college students include anxiety (46.2%), depression (39.3%), and relationship problems (35.8%). An important aspect of treating today's college-age population is that as access to higher education has expanded, student bodies have become more representative of the general population, including similar epidemiological rates of mental health diagnoses with greater chronicity and severity (Locke, Bieschke, Castonguay, and Hayes, 2012; Mitchell, Kader, Haggerty, Bakhai, and Warren, 2013; Schwartz, 2011). Individuals now enter college with a wider range of background experiences, needs, and expectations. Careful consideration of these factors when patients are presenting for care, and facilitating a path for young adults becoming voluntarily engaged in services in the first place, are seen as primary challenges (Hunt and Eisenberg, 2010).

The following sections offer a framework for considering a number of developmental and societal challenges pertinent to work with this population. A variety of existing evidence-based pharmacological and psychosocial treatments are recognized as safe and appropriate for this age group. As such, rather than a discussion of specific disorders or detailed descriptions of interventions themselves (many which are covered elsewhere in this volume) we will focus on ways access and delivery for young adults may affect clinical response, and how systems are evolving to meet the needs of this demographic (Eisenberg, Hunt, and Speer, 2012).

Student Mental Health: Focus and Policy

University programs targeting "mental hygiene" arose in response to changing campus populations following the world wars. The Group for the Advancement of Psychiatry, formed in 1946, focused on prevention and awareness of mental health programming for schools and colleges, and received broad political and public policy support. In particular, these curriculums were seen as an investment in ensuring the stability of young men poised to take on active roles as business and community leaders. Rapid societal shifts occurred, moving further away from early campus climates that attempted to control and closely chaperone most areas of a student's life away from home. By the 1960s and 70s, more independent student bodies of both genders were successfully lobbying for greater personal privacy protections and a voice in the direction of campus health care, including services for contraception, mental health, and sexual assault (Prescott, 2008). Some campuses sought to become models of more comprehensive services, integrating mental health and primary care (American College Health Association, 2010). A majority of programs, however, have seen staff and services expand or contract in response to institutional, state, and federal budgets. In many respects, college mental health services have functioned as background aspects of academia; working closely among themselves, but burdened by a lack of resources or ties to broader networks of psychiatry and psychology (Locke et al., 2012). In the years following a number of incidents of campus and student shootings, particularly those occurring at Virginia Tech in 2007, the topic of student mental health became a heightened focus of public and political scrutiny. It is important to note these were not the first occurrences of student violence (Prescott, 2008) and to stress the overall weak connection between violence and mental illness, with rates in the United States only at 4% (Fazel and Grann, 2006). Yet the dialogues that arose from this period highlighted a number of neglected issues, particularly the limitations of screening and early warning systems, and at times conflicting legal and ethical guidelines for clinicians charged with responsibilities for alerting authorities to potentially violent patients. Subsumed under larger, ongoing conversations about the governance of mental health issues, a new era of collaborative research has been accelerated for examining both the service needs and economics of modern student mental health (Eisenberg et al., 2012).

Characterizing Today's College-age Patient

Compared to wider options for post high-school employment in earlier generations, jobs in the current economy tend to require at least some level of formal higher education. Even for vocations that have typically been viewed as suitable to on the job training (e.g., retail, restaurant, hospitality) substantial advancement opportunities in those fields may be limited without a college degree. As such, rates of pursuing some level of college are now estimated at over 60%, and the makeup of students increasingly heterogeneous (e.g., Stebleton, Soria, and Huesman, 2014). College mental health systems have made concerted efforts to keep up with the needs of diverse groups, including tracking action steps and programming for minority and international students, disability diagnoses, gender, sexual orientation, and student athletes (Reetz, Barr, and Krylowicz, 2014; Stebleton, Soria, and Huesman, 2014; Woodford, Han, Craig, Lim, and Matney, 2014). Similar to the rise in veterans attending college seen following the world wars, a record number are now taking advantage of the Post-9/11 GI Bill passed in 2008, with attention being drawn to their academic and mental health needs (Hart and Thompson, 2013; Zinger and Cohen, 2010). And while college environments vary in progressive programming and are not "stigma free," today's systems are a strong contrast to past generations where a uniform response to students experiencing significant mental health challenges was to withdraw from school. It is now becoming more typical to assist the student and their family in resuming academics or otherwise engaging in alternative activities during the recovery period. Recent, innovative frameworks include the partnership of college mental health organizations and prominent psychiatric and academic settings, such as the College Mental Health Program (CMHP) created at Harvard (Pinder-Amaker and Bell, 2012). The impact of these developments is already promising in improved coordination of access to resources and new abilities for evaluating services and policies (Hunt and Eisenberg, 2010).

Developmental Stage and Maturation

Taking a cue from Johnson et al. (2009), "maturity" is best defined not as implying a particularly defined or measured endpoint to development but as a milestone at which an individual is considered to hold adultlike capacities and privileges. A concept of wide variability across time and culture, modern day expectations of maturity may be seen as particularly conflictual. Given that most "adult" markers come to be accepted despite being rather arbitrarily tied to age (e.g., driving, voting, drinking, holding political office), it can be overlooked that we may not have credible or uniform ways of defining or assessing readiness. Handling new responsibilities and stressors for which the young adult, their family, or society may wish to assume they are ready for does not always go smoothly. It may be particularly difficult to discern readiness for those who have struggled with mental health problems in childhood or earlier adolescence, perhaps leaving that individual particularly vulnerable to the stressors of early adulthood. Advances in neuroscience have established that the human brain continues rapid maturation well into the 20s, yet researchers caution that interpretation of how this data ties to daily functioning, as well as its application to clinical meaning for the individual patient, would be premature uses of the science (Farah and Gillihan, 2012; Insel, 2010; Johnson, Blum, and Giedd, 2009). Beyond factors of physiology, there are an even greater number of environmental influences viewed as impactful to an individual's deficits and potential. When approaching work with patients in late adolescence, it is beneficial to remember that marked differences exist in baseline levels of maturity and capabilities.

Assessment and Initial Protocol Planning

Completing a truly comprehensive assessment of the young adult across broad areas of psychosocial functioning can be difficult for a variety of reasons. Individuals may be reticent to disclose details of prior treatment or involve their support system even when helpful to do so. Conversely, some families may be overinvolved, dealing with challenges themselves, or otherwise serving as barriers to treatment. Determining why, when, and how to seek corroborative contacts and discussing this with the patient can seem an especially delicate task. Healthcare providers standardly receive training in disclosure privacy laws of the Health Insurance Portability and Accountability Act of 1996 (HIPAA); those working with students and campus health programs should also familiarize themselves with any institutional policies as well as the Family Educational Rights and Privacy Act (FERPA) for awareness of how areas of regulation may intersect (more specifics of which are discussed in a later section).

The clear assessment of a person's premorbid functioning, apart from any symptom complaints first presenting in college, helps to limit the risk of overpathologizing what may be situational stressors or self-limiting symptoms. If background information confirms a history of otherwise healthy and adaptive coping experiences, there is increased likelihood that a number of transitional complaints would respond well to conservative early intervention. Schwartz (2011) highlights the importance of weighing both selection and timing of particular therapeutics, even beyond first ensuring the use of evidence based practices. For example, considering if a short-term trial of anxiolytic medication for a student presenting with new onset panic attacks in the weeks before final exams may be more sensible than prescribing SSRI medication, with its potential of greater initiatory side effects and lengthier course of therapy. Further, an increasing number of counseling centers have begun offering specific preventive and early intervention programs adapted from evidence-based practices, averaging four to eight sessions but with some as brief as one meeting paired with self-help follow-up. A review and meta-analysis conducted by Regehr, Glancy, and Pitts (2013) found that brief trials of cognitive behavioral and mindfulness strategies significantly reduced symptoms of student stress (viz., anxiety, depression, and cortisol levels). These findings are in line with data that many well-established therapies are considered both effective and appropriate for use with college-age patients and that university mental health settings are increasingly integrating resources for research-based practices (Eisenberg et al., 2012; Locke et al., 2012). Efforts to increase the ease of access and appeal of mental health programs, such as online or smart-phone technologies, show promise in targeting dissemination efforts to youth (Boydell et al., 2014). As noted, however, the diverse growth of the college system has brought with it challenges of responding to needs of more ill students. Selecting a course of evidence-based care known to work for a given diagnosis is therefore considered a necessary, yet possibly insufficient, step. Intervention choice or possible adjustments to the structure of treatment can impact the accessibility, adherence, and ultimate effectiveness of an intervention.

Besides the need to orient students to psychotherapy offerings on campus, prescribing practices for college-age patients is an area that warrants particularly judicious oversight. An estimated 25% of students present to college with already prescribed psychotropic medications (Reetz et al., 2014); given their new environment, considerations may arise for their ability to adhere to taking medications, as well as possible risks of abuse. Noted misuse has become increasingly common not only with those pharmacological treatments more traditionally targeted for monitoring due to addiction risks (e.g. benzodiazepines), but also in students sharing clinically unnecessary stimulants and antidepressants in ways not necessarily recreational, but rather in trying to garner a performance advantage—that is, thinking of these types of substances as "mental steroids" (Arria and DuPont, 2010; Kadison, 2005). Such issues are of course not uncommon or new to the psychiatric management concerns for this age group, where behavioral changes considered normative cross-culturally (even cross-species!) include heightened novelty seeking, risk taking, and stronger peer influences (Johnson et al., 2009). Cognitive dissonance may also strongly feature in behavioral choices surrounding self-care. For example, research on smoking practices has found that students discount facts about harmfulness when considering their own hookah usage (Sidani et al., 2014), and resist labeling themselves "cigarette smokers" (despite regular acts of smoking) through selective rules and definitions (Levinson et al., 2007). These factors understandably drive concerns surrounding choice of therapies, as well as in deliberating how "hands off" healthcare can effectively be for some patients. Especially in cases where delays in the developmental trajectory had already been noted with symptom challenges in earlier adolescence, greater over-sight or support system involvement, at least for a time, may prove necessary for realistic clinical gains.

Privacy Concerns and Constraints: The Basics

FERPA dictates that when a student turns 18 years old, *or* enters a post-secondary insti-tution (at any age), rights to privacy and review of records transfer from parents to the student. However, exceptions are noted, including a 1998 amendment to the law that allows institutions to disclose to parents violations of alcohol or drug policies if the stu-dent is under the age of 21. A school may also disclose records to parents if a student of any age is considered their dependent for tax purposes (United States Department of Education, n.d.). In most health care settings, HIPAA will be of primary focus, and regulations dictate that even adolescents who are minors have rights to protection of con-fidentiality in areas of reproductive health, substance abuse, and mental health. These laws were designed with the understanding that some youth would avoid seeking care if disclosure to parents was automatic, risking not only their own health but larger societal consequences as well (English and Ford, 2004). Even when services are provided within a university or college student health system, ordinarily HIPAA will override FERPA, unless state or local laws apply.

Lending additional confusion to these matters are debates surrounding the adequacy of current laws for breaking confidentiality, which naturally arise in the aftermath of a mental health tragedy. Whether it is a shooting capturing national attention or a suicide with quieter local coverage, as with most news, the most fervent levels of media and com-munity attention tends to dissipate within weeks or months, wearied by the realities that there are rarely satisfying answers. Nevertheless, a close review of the policies, proce-dures, and steps taken by the academic institutions and professionals involved are under-taken in hopes of shedding light on both what went wrong, and ways to prevent future occurrences. While most professionals would consider a stance of "there's nothing to be done" as unacceptable, it is equally acknowledged that the vast number, size, and com-plexity of services that impact college students requires careful and far-reaching plan-ning. Lead psychiatric institutions have taken the charge of creating dedicated programs for evaluating existing service networks and developing improvements in policy and col-laborative care, particularly in supporting students with more severe mental health diag-noses (Locke et al., 2012; Pinder-Amaker and Bell, 2012).

Privacy Concerns and Constraints: Pragmatics in Clinical Application

Approaching a situation in which a patient age 18 or older expresses reluctance in signing a release of information (ROI) allowing corroborative information from family or other providers may be handled in a variety of ways, dependent upon the presenting clinical problem, and the setting and nature of services being offered. Most instances where there is consideration of imminent harm will automatically allow a justification of such breaches (Baker, 2005; Ford and English, 2002; May, 2006; Stefkovich, 2006). Outside of these most dire circumstances, providers may find themselves needing to respond to this patient impasse as a focus of clinical attention in its own right. For some individuals, the college healthcare encounter may be one of the first times they have been directly presented with such a degree of control over their care, apart from their parents. In these instances, simply allowing additional service time for fully discussing the request, answering questions, and explaining how the information will be used (as well as not used) may alleviate concerns. Particularly when students ask a provider not to involve family in any way, yet list parents as the responsible party for payment or insurance, the rationale for coming to an agreement in obtaining at least a limited release should be emphasized. This explanation can be effectively positioned as minimizing the student's risk of additional stressors or family conflict that may arise from possible misunderstandings about the nature of services or payment policies, since the occurrence of treatment may inevitably be conveyed through billing or insurance paperwork sent to parents.[1]

Additional strategies may include further exploring concerns about family involvement during sessions using motivational interviewing, or MI (Rollnick, Miller, and Butler, 2007). A collaborative counseling style that has been widely adapted across areas of health, MI was originally developed out of substance abuse research targeting ambivalence to change. Inarguably, the first line and most desirable approach for orienting and engaging an individual to appropriate treatment is in drawing upon their own aspirations for change. Once these initial attempts have been made, however, what further steps may be taken? The patient who continues to restrict levels of collaboration yet displays levels of clinical need that demand greater structure and accountability places the provider in an untenable situation. Ethically and legally established avenues available to the provider in this dilemma would include termination or transfer of care to an alternate referral. These actions require careful preparation; both reasonable steps in establishing viable referral avenues and for considering additional elements in ending the therapeutic alliance (Klumpp, 2010). While these choices should not be made prematurely, and may not be appropriate in all instances, candid conversation about clinical concerns and limitations of the current status of treatment best communicates the reality of the situation. In some instances, the very act of setting these boundaries and reviewing alternative options may more saliently highlight for the patient areas for which they have degrees of choice and empowerment for changing their situation. Some clinicians may feel squeamish about stopping treatment, particularly those working from an orientation that places therapeutic rapport as the primary agent of change. We would argue that, if truly at an impasse in the ability to design and deliver an appropriate course of care, continuing with what isn't working, or seeking ongoing adjustments or dilution of procedures could be considered an ethical breach in its own right. While a modest number of sessions specifically aimed at building trust and credibility for the proposed treatment step, i.e., a "foot in the door" psychological approach, may be warranted, continual attempts to appease patients to prevent them from leaving treatment rarely results in meaningful or lasting treatment gains. For some interventions, such as exposure-based therapies, providing treatment in a manner that restricts the level and momentum of delivery can be argued as particularly clinically problematic in its risks of reinforcing symptoms (Meyer, Farrell, Kemp, Blakey, and Deacon, 2014).

Active Treatment Phases

In the more fortunate situation where a collaborative relationship with a young adult patient is in place (or ultimately reached) there are a number of possibilities for bolstering clinical efforts and/or reducing treatment interfering behaviors for this population. In our own setting (an anxiety specialty cognitive behavioral center), the architecture of a clinical plan is evaluated in terms of what additional treatment readiness activities or adjunct therapies may facilitate the core intervention indicated for their presentation. Degree of adherence for baseline homework assignments (e.g., symptom monitoring) can help ascertain if higher degrees of oversight and behavioral contingencies will likely be needed for effectively approaching more active and difficult strategies later in treatment. For patients exhibiting reluctance, resistance, or greater impairment due to overall severity of symptoms, first steps will often focus on functional analysis and behavioral strategies.

As an example, consider a situation where a patient with chronic panic disorder and co-occurring depressive symptoms also notes difficulties consistently taking their SSRI medication. Initial protocol phases could be structured with behavioral strategies and contingencies to build reminders and accountability for taking medication as prescribed, as well as reinforcing behavioral activation to target low motivation and mood. Starting behavioral plans aim for implementing the least intrusive/least restrictive strategies and structure necessary for building adherence and momentum. Methods of monitoring with increasing oversight could include a variety of steps (although some of which may not be appropriate to policies of the clinical setting). These can include symptom monitoring forms and calendars, use of smart phones and apps, email check-ins with clinician, text message check-ins, phone or tele-video sessions or check-ins, training a support person coach to monitor/confirm activity to therapist, or therapist or other professional staff directly monitoring an activity. Increasing intensity of the overall protocol itself may be another consideration, titrating level of care from outpatient to intensive outpatient, to partial hospital or day program, to inpatient psychiatric options for the most acute and highest level of need, or targeted residential treatment programs if stable for active treatment but in need of heightened environmental support (e.g., Osgood-Hynes, Riemann, and Björgvinsson, 2003).

Choosing a Helpful Degree of Parent Involvement

Assuming a patient is exhibiting basic levels of help-seeking behaviors, i.e., in presenting for initial treatment planning sessions, a forward course of treatment might proceed in a number of different ways. Again highlighting diverse degrees of independence and maturity for this age group, it is certainly sometimes the case where a college-age student manages treatment activities and ownership of their care independently. Among those students with more chronic or longstanding mental health concerns, new environmental or situational issues may be viewed as contributors to exacerbated symptoms. An optimistic but not uncommon scenario might be found for the patient with a past positive response to treatment; a brief protocol revisiting therapy concepts and relapse prevention skills or reevaluating current medication needs may be all that is required to aid their adjustment to this new stage of life.

In some instances, an initial parent or family feedback meeting or phone call may be warranted, particularly if determined this would be helpful for assisting the student in communicating their level of need (whether it is heightened or otherwise provides reassurance to the family the young adult is appropriately seeking care). This initial contact serves to provide basic psychoeducation as well as establish communication boundaries surrounding questions that may arise during treatment or for aftercare needs. For some college students, this level of parent involvement in treatment will suffice. On occasion, parents may initiate contact prior to the identified patient presenting for treatment or may even accompany the patient to the first appointment, warranting clinicians to prepare to address the issue of parent involvement in this population. Patients who are particularly ill, have had past struggles with prior treatment, or those still living at home may be among those likely to benefit from higher degrees of support system involvement, including participation in at least a portion of sessions. As with other oversight steps, we attempt to discern the most conservative starting level of family involvement anticipated for effective progression, then adjust throughout stages of treatment dependent upon response.

In our own facility, coordination of family service elements may be addressed in a number of ways: (1) provided directly by the patient's primary therapist and integrated into core protocol sessions, (2) provided by our marriage and family therapist in separate sessions, either joined by or with planning input from the patient's primary therapist, or (3) referred to an outside provider with our center taking on a consultant role in determining when resuming an individual protocol for active CBT/ERP may be appropriate. Typically the latter option is more common in the treatment of younger children and adolescents, where primary responsibility for home structure and accountability for the patient requires a parent-driven approach. For college-age patients, a focus remains on the individual patient, using the support system to increase plan accountability, thus accelerating levels of self-sufficiency and independence in forming healthier habits.

A number of college-age students seen in our specialty center have been considered "treatment refractory," with extensive histories by the time they reach late adolescence. Past interventions often include seeing multiple therapists for supportive counseling, play therapy, or limited elements of CBT (e.g., breath retraining and relaxation, thinking errors). There may or may not be a history of pharmacotherapy as managed by either a psychiatrist, a primary care provider, or pediatrician; typically, more severe patients will also have an extensive list of medication trials. More rarely, they may have also participated in family therapy focused on patterns and influences of that system. As with individually-focused therapy, the theoretical orientation and structure of activities for family therapy can widely vary. Across all services, more structured treatment that utilizes measurable assessment tools and provides session-by-session feedback and monitoring has been found to yield more effective clinical results than does more loosely structured treatment, independent of theoretical orientation or presenting problem (Mead, 2013). While this chapter focuses on issues of particular impact to college students, descriptions of evidence-based pharmacotherapy and psychotherapy protocols appropriate to specific disorders are included elsewhere in this volume, and we advocate delivering evidenced-based care to college students within this framework.

Unfortunately there are a number of patients who, despite extensive intervention histories, could still be considered "treatment naive" to evidence-based care. These situations are in fact some of those most likely to require more extensive orientation and psychoeducation efforts in order to address concomitant factors of skepticism, treatment fatigue, or misconceptions about diagnoses or treatment procedures. Even for patients and families presenting with past individual or family treatments that were evidence-based, a collaborative reevaluation detailing both acute symptom needs as well as any residual or altered patterns contributing to relapse should be adjusted to the present course of treatment. For example, when past family therapy goals were concentrated on problem-solving skills for open communication, but current challenges are instead observed to be difficulties with separation and family overaccommodation, redirecting the focus towards adaptive coping and boundaries would best support the patient's individual treatment plan (Meade, 2013).

At first glance, a heavy utilization of behavioral techniques may appear ill-targeted for a population often characterized as having a resistance to authority. A framework offered to patients is that a period of heightened "external" structure (e.g., behavioral contingencies, monitoring by therapist or family) assists them during times their abilities at "internal structure" may be compromised. This approach helps mitigate concerns voiced by patients, families, even some professionals, that college-age students are "too old" for behavior plans. Certainly, ease of success in engaging patients of any age lies in partnering to assist them in making changes they see as important to their own viewpoints and values. Again, heavily incorporating MI techniques and language, initial treatment targets will attempt to find consensus with a number of salient short and longer-term goals. For those situations where symptom levels and accompanying behavioral features impair abilities to engage more fully and independently in treatment, it is sometimes helpful to return to basics of behavioral theory, practice elements that are sometimes neglected in our desired goals of most quickly targeting cognitive change. For some situations, cognitive elements of treatment may appear stalled because we have gotten ahead of ourselves and the patient! As functioning and adherence goals are observed as stable for a period of time (we often work towards guidelines requiring 80% adherence over two to four weeks), behavioral contingencies and monitoring are faded out. Simultaneously, more active challenges of the core treatment plan are added in, i.e., the therapeutic effectiveness of formal cognitive work, exposure exercises, or consideration of possible medication changes are able to be more clearly evaluated at this juncture.

Summary and Future Directions

Pinpointing exact characterizations of "the college-age student" is increasingly difficult, reflecting the broader makeup of this demographic than years past. Nevertheless, common challenges in providing mental health care for young adults can be identified (see Figure 8.1). Considering adjustments in communication, structure, and monitoring in applying an intervention may increase the effectiveness of standard therapies within this population.

From a systems perspective, changing expectations for better targeting both the acute and long-term recovery concerns of college-age patients point to the need for an integrated, multi-disciplinary approach. As opposed to more insular levels of treatment of the young adult within college mental health programs or outside community or hospital referrals, newer initiatives promote active collaboration and communication among referral networks and a deliberate assessment of the effectiveness of policies and procedures. For example, Harvard's College Mental Health Program has proposed a framework of "bioecological systems" to help discern areas of impact for the college cohort, spanning factors from within the individual to broad environmental influences. Analyses and development stemming from this conceptual model has already generated a number of improvements, including content and focus for therapy groups across psychiatric units of the hospital system, establishing formal visitation exchange programs between hospital and campus personnel, and developing and maintaining a contact database for streamlining communication across care units and colleges (Pinder-Amaker and Bell, 2012).

Fitting to the history of campus activism, peer-driven support also continues as impactful, including the rapid expansion of *Active Minds* (http://activeminds.org), a nonprofit organization targeted to students and campus leaders speaking openly about mental health and encouraging help-seeking behaviors. Parent support has become better developed in recent years, as well, with resource materials and educational programs created to their needs of navigating these complex systems.

Finally, for a population expanding in mental health severity, up to 25% of colleges report no access to psychiatry services except as off-campus referrals (Reetz et al., 2014). Within increased awareness of the overlap of settings and referral sources beyond campus health care, collaborations with practicing psychiatrists, emergency rooms, and

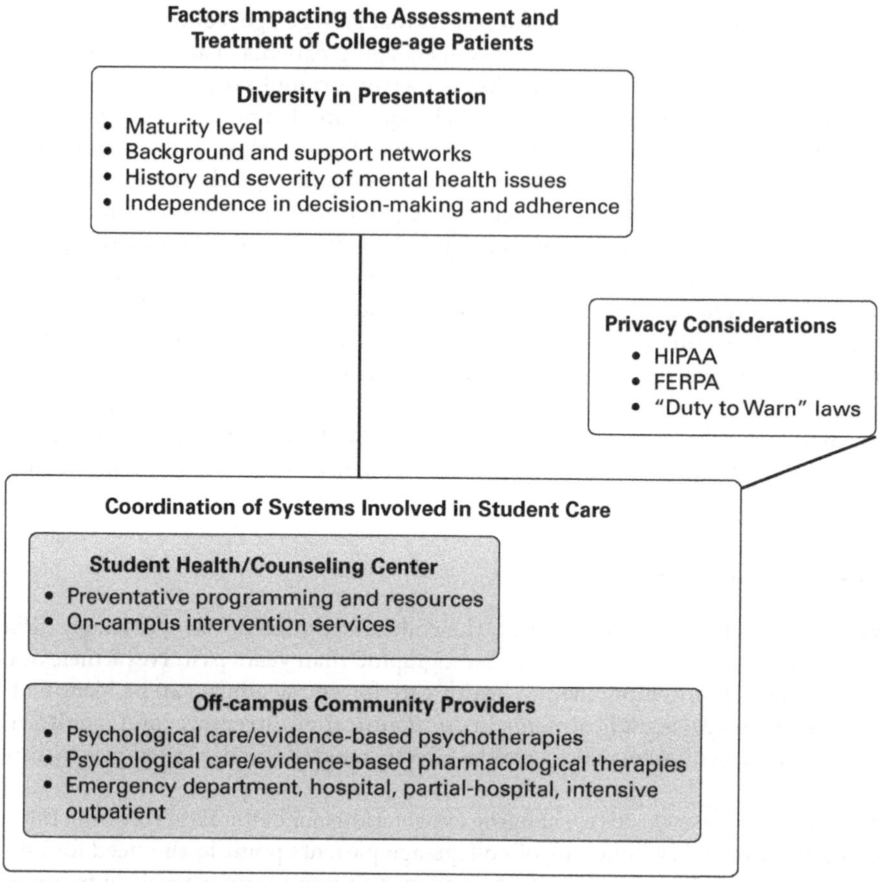

Factors Impacting the Assessment and
Treatment of College-age Patients

Diversity in Presentation
- Maturity level
- Background and support networks
- History and severity of mental health issues
- Independence in decision-making and adherence

Privacy Considerations
- HIPAA
- FERPA
- "Duty to Warn" laws

Coordination of Systems Involved in Student Care

Student Health/Counseling Center
- Preventative programming and resources
- On-campus intervention services

Off-campus Community Providers
- Psychological care/evidence-based psychotherapies
- Psychological care/evidence-based pharmacological therapies
- Emergency department, hospital, partial-hospital, intensive outpatient

FIGURE 8.1 Factors impacting the assessment and treatment of college-age patients.

psychiatry training programs local to academic settings are additional ways of improving outreach and management for young adult mental health (Mitchell, et al., 2013). Given substantial variation in the scope and needs of students, the systems approach may be particularly important in promoting rigorous evaluation and resource standards. Treatment at the individual level can only benefit from better coordination of services, which in the past may have progressed mostly in parallel.

CLINICAL CASE EXAMPLE: MOLLY

Molly presented to services at the anxiety disorders clinic with longstanding difficulties of social anxiety and panic attacks. Now 22, symptoms had been present since childhood, with frequent stomachaches and reluctance to join activities and social gatherings. Although a good student, she experienced test anxiety and nervousness when speaking to teachers and peers. Upon high school graduation, Molly was excited to attend a large university a few hours from home. At the time of evaluation, she had been enrolled in college for five years, having withdrawn from so many classes that she was classified a sophomore. Molly optimistically approached each semester but would quickly experience difficulties attending class. Following the required year of living in a dorm, Molly had lived alone in an apartment. She attempted online classes, but found even the required blog postings anxiety provoking. Her primary social relationship had been dating a classmate for several months. Initially socializing was easier when with him, but eventually her symptoms strained the relationship. As symptoms worsened over the last semester, she again withdrew from classes. She also failed to return to her job after spring break, giving no notice and avoiding calls from work. She had quit a previous job in a similar manner, and she reported employers and instructors praised her work but considered her unreliable. Overwhelmed and embarrassed, Molly mostly stayed in bed for the last weeks of the term, missing final exams. It was then that she and her parents decided she would move back home.

Molly had seen numerous providers since starting college, first being treated for inattentive-type ADHD and prescribed a stimulant and given an undifferentiated diagnosis of "anxiety." She was currently prescribed two benzodiazepine medications; several other medications, including SSRIs, had been tried but discontinued within weeks due to stomach distress. She participated in general talk therapy, as well as eye movement desensitization and reprocessing (EMDR), reported as minimally helpful in resuming driving. Her parents were especially alarmed by the severity of her recent withdrawal symptoms and were desperate for help. Her father read a self-help book promoting diagnostic use of single photon emission computed tomography (SPECT), and the family traveled for evaluation at a clinic offering this approach. She was diagnosed with anxiety and depression NOS, social phobia, and panic disorder. Recommendations consisted of adding nutritional supplements and an SSRI medication to her current prescriptions.

Assessment at our center included semistructured interviews, review of records, consultation with prior providers, and a battery of standardized questionnaires. Molly met criteria for social phobia and major depressive disorder, single past episode. Current depressive symptoms were less severe and pervasive, with withdrawal and avoidance secondary to severity of social symptoms. Panic attacks were exclusive to targeted worry and social stimuli. Social symptoms included excessive concerns of feeling on the spot or embarrassed before and during contact with others, and avoidance of numerous social situations including attending parties, participating in meetings/classes, being in groups, speaking formally, using public restrooms, initiating conversations, dating, being assertive, staying in conversations, e-mailing, talking on the phone, and driving during the day ("when more people are out"). Panic attack symptoms in these situations included pounding heart, trembling/shaking, shortness of breath, stomach distress, dizziness, tingling sensations, and crying.

Molly's treatment at the center lasted approximately a year, consisting of 22 active treatment sessions over the first six months, followed by monthly maintenance/relapse prevention boosters. Specific components following evaluation included six treatment readiness sessions (psychoeducation, behavior plan construction, self-monitoring, behavioral activation, home evaluation session), four cognitive-behavioral skill building sessions (cognitive restructuring, interoceptive assessment, hierarchy building), five sessions of office-based exposure and response prevention (ERP); six sessions of community-based ERP, and six relapse prevention and maintenance sessions. Molly also attended the young adult support group and successfully titrated off benzodiazepines and began SSRI medication once better management of side effects was accomplished through interoceptive exposures.

Following assessment, Molly and her parents attended a feedback and education session, where the therapist explained her diagnoses through the cognitive behavioral model and provided education about evidence-based approaches, including feedback as to the extraneous nature of SPECT. Molly voiced good motivation for treatment, and relief she "was not out of options." Parents expressed understanding, although a high level of symptom accommodation was noted. Given symptom severity and the fact Molly was living at home, the proposed treatment plan included family involvement and a formal behavioral support plan. Symptoms immediately impacted starting treatment; Molly became so distressed attempting to drive to the next appointment that her mother called to reschedule. The therapist then requested at least one parent accompany Molly to sessions. Beginning goals were to reinforce Molly for treatment-consistent behaviors (e.g., practice leaving the house, running errands, completing exercises, and tracking forms). Difficulties were experienced at this stage, with parents inconsistent with rewards and requesting behaviors premature to the plan, and Molly complaining parents were too harsh and the plan felt "babyish." To reduce tension, the therapist conducted a home visit to assess environmental structure and designed nightly family meetings with checklists outlining progressive expectations tied to rewards and independence. Consistency was stressed for reducing intermittent reinforcement, viewed as contributory to Molly's symptoms.

With improved behavioral adherence, Molly was able to engage in more active protocol elements. Good response was noted for interoceptive exposures targeting panic and ERP targeting social concerns, first creating scenarios in-office and progressing to community exposures. As Molly experienced symptom relief, the formal behavioral plan and degree of family involvement was faded out. Final months of treatment focused on generalization of skills and improved independence, with Molly contributing goals, which included improving sleep schedule and organization and timelines for finding a job, reenrolling in school, and obtaining an apartment. With continued success, Molly has enjoyed increased freedom, better relationships with family and peers, and the ability to engage in work and college classes without symptom interference.

DISCLOSURE STATEMENT

Authors have no conflicts to disclose.

ACKNOWLEDGMENTS

Grant Support through the National Institute of Mental Health (1R43MH098470-01).

NOTE

1. Authorization is generally not required to disclose basic information tied to purposes of payment or health care operations. The Department of Health and Human Services purposefully left some areas of regulation open to "provider discretion" in considering if disclosure may contribute to either benefit or risk for the patient, and for future adjustments to the law. Practice settings are advised to consult with health care attorneys to review or establish procedures and policies applicable to their location and service type (Ford & English, 2002).

REFERENCES

American College Health Association. (2010). *Considerations for Integration of Counseling and Health Services on College and University Campuses*. Linthicum, MD: American College Health Association.

Arria, A. M., and DuPont, R. L. (2010). Nonmedical prescription stimulant use among college students: Why we need to do something and what we need to do. *J Addict Dis, 29*(4), 417–426. doi:10.1 080/10550887.2010.509273

Baker, T. R. (2005). Notifying parents following a college student suicide attempt: A review of case law and FERPA, and recommendations for practice. *NASPA J, 42*(4). doi:10.2202/1949-6605.5043

Boydell K. M., Hodgins M., Pignatiello A., Teshima, J., Edwards, H., and Willis, D. (2014). Using technology to deliver mental health services to children and youth: a scoping review. *Journal of the Canadian Academy of Child and Adolescent Psychiatry, 23* (2), 87–99.

Eisenberg, D., Hunt, J. B., and Speer, N. (2012). Help-seeking for mental health on college campuses: Review of evidence and next steps for research and practice. *Harvard Review of Psychiatry, 20* (4), 222–232. doi:10.3109/10673229.2012.712839

English, A., and Ford, C. A. (2004). The HIPAA privacy rule and adolescents: Legal questions and clinical challenges. *Perspect Sexual Repro Health, 36*(2), 80–86. Retrieved from https://www.guttmacher. org/pubs/journals/3608004.html

Farah, M. J., and Gillihan, S. J. (2012). Diagnostic brain imaging in psychiatry: Current uses and future prospects. *Virtual Mentor: VM, 14*(6), 464–471. doi:10.1001/virtualmentor.2012.14.6.s tas1-1206

Fazel, S., and Grann, M. (2006). The population impact of severe mental illness on violent crime. *Am J Psychiatry, 163* (8), 1397–1403. doi:10.1176/appi.ajp.163.8.1397

Ford, C. A., and English, A. (2002). Limiting confidentiality of adolescent health services: what are the risks? *J Am Med Assoc, 288* (6), 752–753. doi:10.1001/jama.288.6.752

Hart, D. A., and Thompson, R. (2013). *"An ethical obligation": Promising practices for student veterans in college writing classrooms* (Results of a 2011 CCCC Research Grant). Retrieved from the National Council of Teachers of English website: http://www.ncte.org/library/nctefiles/groups/cccc/anethi-calobligation.pdf

Hunt, J., and Eisenberg, D. (2010). Mental health problems and help-seeking behavior among college students. *J Adolesc Health, 46* (1), 3–10. doi:10.1016/j.jadohealth.2009.08.008

Insel, T. (2010, October 7). Brain scans: Not quite ready for prime time. [Web log post] Retrieved from http://www.nimh.nih.gov/about/director/2010/brain-scans-not-quite-ready-for-prime-time. shtml

Johnson, S. B., Blum, R. W., and Giedd, J. N. (2009). Adolescent maturity and the brain: The promise and pitfalls of neuroscience research in adolescent health policy. *J Adolesc Health, 45* (3), 216–221. doi:10.1016/j.jadohealth.2009.05.016

Kadison, R. (2005). Getting an edge: Use of stimulants and antidepressants in college. *New Engl J Med,* 353(11), 1089–1091. doi:10.1056/NEJMp058047

Klumpp, E. (2010). Terminating the treatment relationship. *Psychiatry, 7* (1), 40–42. Retrieved from http://europepmc.org/articles/pmc2848460

Levinson, A. H., Campo, S., Gascoigne, J., Jolly, O., Zakharyan, A., and Tran, Z. V. (2007). Smoking, but not smokers: Identity among college students who smoke cigarettes. *Nicotine Tobacco Res, 9* (8), 845–852. doi:10.1080/14622200701484987

Linthicum, M. D. (2010). American College Health Association considerations for integration of counseling and health services on college and university campuses. *American College Health Association,* 58, 583–96. Retrieved from http://www.acha.org/publications/docs/Considerations_for_ Integration_of_Counseling_White_Paper_Mar2010.pdf

Locke, B. D., Bieschke, K. J., Castonguay, L. G., and Hayes, J. A. (2012). The Center for Collegiate Mental Health: Studying college student mental health through an innovative research infrastructure that brings science and practice together. *Harvard Rev Psychiatry, 20* (4), 233–245. doi:10.3109/106732 29.2012.712837

May, R. (2006). Legal and ethical issues. In P. Grayson and P. Meilman (Eds.), *College mental health practice* (pp. 43–58). New York, NY: Routledge.

Mead, E. (2013). *Becoming a marriage and family therapist: From classroom to consulting room.* Malden, MA: John Wiley & Sons.

Meyer, J. M., Farrell, N. R., Kemp, J. J., Blakey, S. M., and Deacon, B. J. (2014). Why do clinicians exclude anxious clients from exposure therapy? *Behav Res Ther, 54*, 49–53. doi:10.1016/j.brat.2014.01.004

Mitchell, S. L., Kader, M., Haggerty, M. Z., Bakhai, Y. D., and Warren, C. G. (2013). College student utilization of a comprehensive psychiatric emergency program. *J College Counsel, 16* (1), 49–63. doi:10.1002/j.2161-1882.2013.00026.x

Osgood-Hynes, D., Riemann, B., and Bjorgvinsson, T. (2003). Short-term residential treatment for obsessive-compulsive disorder. *Brief Treat Crisis Interven, 3* (4), 413. Retrieved from http://btci.edina.clockss.org/cgi/reprint/3/4/413

Pinder-Amaker, S. and Bell, C. (2012). A bioecological systems approach for navigating the college mental health crisis. *Harvard Rev Psychiatry, 20* (4), 174–188. doi:10.3109/10673229.2012.712842

Prescott, H. M. (2008). College mental health since the early twentieth century. *Harvard Rev Psychiatry, 16* (4), 258–266. doi:10.1080/10673220802277771

Reetz, D. R., Barr, V., and Krylowicz, B. (2014). *The Association for University and College Counseling Center Directors Annual Survey* (AUCCD 2013 annual survey). Retrieved from http://files.cmc-global.com/AUCCCD_Monograph_Public_2013.pdf

Regehr, C., Glancy, D., and Pitts, A. (2013). Interventions to reduce stress in university students: A review and meta-analysis. *J Affect Disord, 148* (1), 1–11. doi:10.1016/j.jad.2012.11.026

Rollnick, S., Miller, W. R., and Butler, C. C. (2008). *Motivational interviewing in health care.* New York: Guilford Press.

Schwartz, V. I. (2011). College mental health: How to provide care for students in need. *Current Psychiatry, 10* (12), 22–29. Retrieved from http://www.currentpsychiatry.com/the-publication/past-issue-single-view/college-mental-health-how-to-provide-care-for-students-in-need/e24485d21b38247215e23164f0718162.html

Sidani, J. E., Shensa, A., Barnett, T. E., Cook, R. L., and Primack, B. A. (2014). Knowledge, attitudes, and normative beliefs as predictors of hookah smoking initiation: A longitudinal study of university students. *Nicotine Tobacco Res, 16* (6), 647–654. doi:10.1093/ntr/ntt201

Stebleton, M. J., Soria, K. M., and Huesman, R. L. (2014). First generation students' sense of belonging, mental health, and use of counseling services at public research universities. *Journal of College Counseling, 17* (1), 6–20. doi:10.1002/j.2161-1882.2014.00044.x

Unites States Department of Education. (n.d.) *Laws and guidance.* Retrieved from http://www2.ed.gov/policy/landing.jhtml?src=ln

Woodford, M. R., Han, Y., Craig, S., Lim, C., and Matney, M. M. (2014). Discrimination and mental health among sexual minority college students: The type and form of discrimination does matter, *J Gay Lesbian Ment Health, 18* (2) 142–163. doi:10.1080/19359705.2013.833882

Zinger, L. and Cohen, A. (2010). Veterans returning from war into the classroom: How can colleges be better prepared to meet their needs. *Contemp Issues Educ Res, 3* (1), 39–51. Retrieved from http://www.cluteinstitute.com/ojs/index.php/CIER/article/view/160/153

POSTTRAUMATIC STRESS AND THE NEUROBIOLOGY OF TRAUMA

9

NEUROBIOLOGY AND TRANSLATIONAL APPROACHES TO POSTTRAUMATIC STRESS DISORDER

SHEILA A. M. RAUCH, JAMES L. ABELSON,
ARASH JAVANBAKHT, AND ISRAEL LIBERZON

INTRODUCTION

Considerable research over the past 20 years has examined biological factors involved in the development and maintenance of posttraumatic stress disorder (PTSD). Understanding of the neurobiological processes that contribute to this complex and often devastating disorder is expanding rapidly, but understanding of the specific stages of development involved (i.e., risk, onset, course and outcome) remains inadequate, and there is a need for better treatments and preventive measures. Many comprehensive reviews of PTSD neurobiology recently have been published. This chapter provides a relatively selective review to meet two goals: (1) To provide an overview that is accessible to a general audience with broad interests in the neurobiology of anxiety and (2) To synthesize neurobiological data, to move forward toward deeper understanding and better treatments.

We first present a heuristic model of the biological stages involved in the development and maintenance of PTSD (see Figure 9.1). Growing evidence implicates pre-, peri-, and posttraumatic factors in shaping the processes that lead to the "PTSD phenotype." Historically, neurobiological work has focused on the fully expressed phenotype, studying people who already have PTSD. This work has revealed that (1) genetic factors contribute to risk (Skelton, Ressler, Norrholm, Jovanovic, and Bradley-Davino, 2012); (2) the PTSD phenotype involves neurobiological systems that orchestrate and regulate threat and stress responses, most notably the hypothalamic–pituitary–adrenal (HPA) axis and the autonomic/catecholaminergic system (Roger K. Pitman et al., 2012); and (3) the PTSD phenotype is characterized by altered function in brain circuits connecting the amygdala, insula, dorsal anterior cingulate, rostral and ventral medial prefrontal cortex (mPFC) and

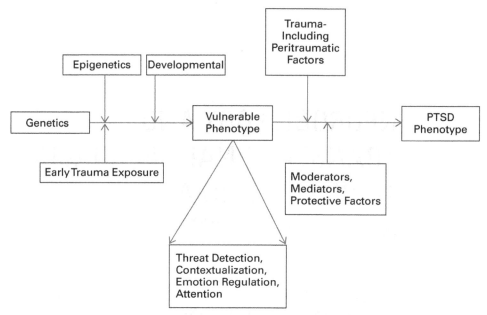

FIGURE 9.1 Model of biological factors in PTSD development and maintenance.

hippocampus, which participate in networks that generate emotion and regulate fear associated learning processes. The emerging model (Figure 9.1) suggests that genetic factors interact with early stress/trauma exposure to shape (via epigenetic processes) developing stress reactivity and fear processing circuits. These potential "intermediate phenotypes" reflecting several potential system vulnerabilities, such as HPA axis reactivity, can transform into a full-blown PTSD phenotype in response to an "index" trauma, influenced by peri-traumatic factors. Additional posttraumatic factors maintain or modify symptom expression over time. This process creates etiological complexity, with many pathways, involving different genetic loadings, interacting with different developmental experiences, triggering various peri- and posttraumatic responses culminating in complexly unfolding processes. Further complexity is created by an interacting balance between activating and modulatory control systems. Similar "abnormalities" can likely arise from either hyperactivity in the activating components, or hypo-activity in the regulatory components, with some evidence of potential disruption of both in PTSD.

We organize this review by focusing first on the stress/threat response systems most consistently related to PTSD (HPA axis and catecholaminergic systems); we then summarize data on neural circuitry abnormalities. We end with a synthesis designed to shape future work.

STRESS AND THREAT RESPONSE SYSTEMS

PTSD develops in response to clear and identifiable traumatic exposures in a subgroup of people so exposed. Risk is influenced by individual vulnerability factors and the nature and context of the trauma. Risk is higher when the trauma involves physical injury (Breslau, Chilcoat, Kessler, and Davis, 1999; Kessler, Sonnega, Bromet, Hughes, and Nelson, 1995), is interpersonal (Kessler et al., 1995), and particularly when it involves assaultive violence (Breslau et al., 1999). Regarding individual risk, many studies have focused on the HPA axis and the catecholaminergic/autonomic system. Studies of PTSD have revealed abnormalities in both systems.

HYPOTHALAMIC–PITUITARY–ADRENAL (HPA) AXIS

Evidence of reduced HPA-axis activity provided some of the earliest data showing neurobiological abnormalities in PTSD (Mason, Giller, Kosten, Ostroff, and Podd, 1986). However, subsequent replication failures suggest that PTSD involves more than simple hypo- or hypercortisolemia (Mason et al., 2002). This is not surprising in light of this system's complex functions and intricately regulated physiology. Cortisol release is influenced by interactions among numerous brain regions involved in cognitive, emotional and behavioral control processes, including input from the amygdala, hippocampus, and prefrontal cortex (King et al., 2009) which shape the release of corticotrophin releasing hormone (CRH) from the hypothalamus. Cortisol levels are influenced by experience-regulated receptor sensitivities at the level of the pituitary (where adrenocorticotropic hormone [ACTH] is released in response to CRH), and the level of the adrenal (where cortisol is released in response to ACTH). The system is influenced by specific psychosocial factors like novelty, lack of control or access to coping responses in the face of perceived threat, and an absence of social support (Dickerson and Kemeny, 2004). Moreover, such influences may vary across the sexes (Stroud, Salovey, and Epel, 2002). Environmentally sensitive reactivity of this system is essential for survival, but inhibitory feedback processes constrain it to prevent over activity, which can be damaging. It acutely helps allocate internal resources in the context of challenge, but also has slower effects on learning and memory that shape future behavior, and plays a role in long-term epigenetic programming that shapes lifelong responses to later challenges (Ladd et al., 2000). Given the importance and complexity of this system, it is not surprising that it is clearly involved in PTSD in ways that we do not fully understand.

PTSD phenotype. Patients with PTSD have repeatedly been shown to have HPA axis abnormalities, primarily enhanced glucocorticoid (GC) receptor sensitivity leading to enhanced negative feedback and, less consistently, hypocortisolemia (Elzinga, Schmahl, Vermetten, van Dyck, and Bremner, 2003; Israel Liberzon, Abelson, Flagel, Raz, and Young, 1999; Rachel Yehuda, Yang, Buchsbaum, and Golier, 2006) and flattened diurnal cortisol rhythms (Rachel Yehuda, Morris, Labinsky, Zemelman, and Schmeidler, 2007). Enhanced GC receptor sensitivity has been demonstrated via direct measurement on peripheral leukocytes (Rachel Yehuda, Golier, Yang, and Tischler, 2004) and as reflected in hypersuppression of cortisol using a low-dose dexamethasone suppression test (Rachel Yehuda, 2006). There is evidence of increased CRH levels in cerebrospinal fluid (Bremner, Licinio, Darnell, and Krystal, 1997) and plasma (de Cloet, Vermetten, Rademaker, Geuze, and Westenberg, 2012). The corresponding literature is vast but inconsistent; important reviews (Rachel Yehuda, 2006) highlight influences of methodological variation, sample characteristics (e.g., combat vs. civilian trauma; nature of comparison subjects), and time since trauma exposure. It remains unclear precisely what is dysregulated, how it came to be that way, and whether phenotypic abnormalities represent preexisting risk factors or biomarkers of the disorder itself; but general consensus implicates the HPA axis and the brain regions that control it in the development and course of PTSD (van Zuiden, Kavelaars, Geuze, Olff, and Heijnen, 2013).

Risk and vulnerability. The fact that a minority of people exposed to a trauma develop PTSD implicates individual risk factors. Data in rodents suggest that the HPA axis, genetics, and early experience interact to alter sensitivities within this system and shape psychopathology-relevant behavior across development (Meaney, Szyf, and Seckl, 2007).

Genetic risk factors for PTSD appear to confer risk in the context of stress exposure during early life (Mehta et al., 2013). The best documented of these is an HPA regulatory gene, *FKBP5*, which contains the only HPA-related risk allele that has been replicated in more than one large cohort and shows no negative findings (Liberzon et al., 2014; Roger K. Pitman et al., 2012). This gene codes for a GC receptor chaperone protein with important regulatory influences on GC receptor internalization, which helps regulate GC signaling in cells. Two FKBP5 polymorphisms interact with childhood trauma to predict severity of PTSD (Roger K. Pitman et al., 2012; Vermetten and Lanius, 2012). They are also linked to peri-traumatic dissociation and enhanced suppression of cortisol in response to challenge (Binder et al., 2008). Other HPA-related genes have been implicated, including a GC receptor gene, NR3C1, and a CRH receptor gene, CRHR1, but have not been replicated in large cohorts (Liberzon et al., 2014; Roger K. Pitman et al., 2012).

These interactions between genes and early life stress implicate epigenetic processes, through which environmental exposures shape gene expression, in risk development. The nature and timing of environmental events, and the genetic context in which they occur, determines how they influence risk. Salient events range from prenatal exposures (e.g., elevated maternal stress hormones) to early abuse, loss or neglect, or later traumas. Childhood trauma increases PTSD risk following adult trauma (for a review see Vermetten and Lanius, 2012), and emerging models suggest that age and exposure type interact in shaping risk (Fonzo et al., 2010; Martin, Ressler, Binder, and Nemeroff, 2009) and adult HPA axis functioning (Carpenter, Shattuck, Tyrka, Geracioti, and Price, 2011), specifically in PTSD patients (Kellner et al., 2010; Van Voorhees, Dennis, Calhoun, and Beckham, 2013). Various developmental models of PTSD have been proposed (Delahanty and Nugent, 2006; Koenen, 2006), but more empirical work is needed to better define how genetic and environmentally driven genomic processes interact to alter adult HPA axis functioning and contribute to PTSD.

Intermediate vulnerability. If genes create risk endophenotypes, biomarkers might predict PTSD risk in a way that informs prevention. The strongest data for pretrauma HPA axis abnormalities in people who develop PTSD focus on GC receptors. Both the number and sensitivities of these receptors, as measured on peripheral immune cells, can predict PTSD symptom levels after trauma (van Zuiden et al., 2013), but additional study is necessary before the work can be considered clinically relevant. A recent study (Rothbaum et al., in press) found that an early intervention delivered in the emergency room seemed to mitigate a genetic risk for PTSD (Rothbaum et al., 2014).

Trauma/PTSD acquired changes. Though HPA factors may shape risk and mark vulnerability, the "classic" HPA abnormality of PTSD (low cortisol) may develop over time as a consequence of trauma (Roger K. Pitman et al., 2012). Low cortisol is not present prior to trauma in those at risk, though low cortisol in the immediate aftermath of trauma predicts risk (van Zuiden et al., 2013). Recent hair cortisol studies support these results, with evidence that low cortisol is a consequence of trauma exposure rather than presence of the disorder and is linked to accumulated number of traumatic exposures (Steudte et al., 2013). A prospective study confirmed that hair cortisol is not elevated prior to trauma in those who subsequently develop PTSD and that low cortisol in association with PTSD evolves slowly over time following trauma exposure (Luo et al., 2012).

CATECHOLAMINE SYSTEMS

Sympathetic–adrenal–medullary (SAM) and catecholaminergic systems (epinephrine and norepinephrine) play major roles in arousal regulation, immediate threat detection and response, and in memory systems. They were an obvious early target for research on PTSD neurobiology, given that it is a disorder of heightened arousal, hypervigilance for threat, and intense/intrusive memory (de Quervain and Yehuda, 2006). Recent genetic work supports a potential role for this system in the etiology of PTSD (Liberzon et al., 2014).

PTSD phenotype. Hyperarousal-related symptoms in PTSD suggest SAM activation, and abnormalities in norepinephrine regulation are widely replicated (Roger K. Pitman et al., 2012). The locus coeruleus (LC)—the major source of central norepinephrine activity—projects to regions of interest in PTSD, including the amygdala, hippocampus, prefrontal cortex and hypothalamus, where it contributes to activation of the HPA axis (T. O'Donnell, Hegadoren, and Coupland, 2004).

There is replicated evidence for long term hyperactivity of the SAM in PTSD. High levels of norepinephrine have been detected in cerebrospinal fluid, urine, and blood of PTSD patients, and elevated heart rate and blood pressure have been reported (Pace and Heim, 2011). Meta-analysis has also documented reduced heart rate variability, which may reflect sympathetic over parasympathetic dominance in cardiac "traffic" from the brain (Chalmers, Quintana, Abbott, and Kemp, 2014). Psychophysiological research has consistently indicated that PTSD patients, compared to healthy and trauma controls, display exaggerated fear potentiated startle (Pineles et al., 2013; Pole, 2007). However, this measure reflects much more than simple SAM activity.

Risk and vulnerability. Two genetic studies suggest that the catecholaminergic system contributes to PTSD risk. A deletion variant in the ADRA2B gene, which codes for the alpha2b-adrenergic receptor, predicts enhanced emotional memory in trauma survivors (de Quervain and Yehuda, 2006). More recently, a SNP in the ADRB2 gene, which codes for the beta2-adrenergic receptor, was shown to interact with trauma exposure to predict presence of PTSD in a large cohort of military personnel, with replication in a larger cohort of African Americans with high levels of trauma exposure. The greatest risk appeared in those with the risk allele and exposure to at least two different types of trauma during childhood (Liberzon et al., 2014). These studies support the idea that preexisting alterations in catecholaminergic neurotransmission can create risk for PTSD following trauma exposure.

Intermediate vulnerability. If preexisting alterations in sympathetic or catecholaminergic activity influence risk, then such alterations may represent vulnerability factors. Existing data support this possibility. For example, elevated heart rate at the time of trauma or in its immediate aftermath predicts subsequent PTSD symptoms (Blanchard et al., 1996; M. L. O'Donnell, Creamer, Elliott, and Bryant, 2007). High-catecholaminergic activity mediates memory enhancing effects of emotional arousal (de Quervain and Yehuda, 2006), contributes to memory consolidation (R. K. Pitman and Delahanty, 2005), and may play a role in the intense, intrusive memories seen in PTSD. High norepinephrine may therefore directly contribute to symptom development, perhaps particularly in the context of low cortisol (Delahanty and Nugent, 2006) through impact on fear learning processes (R. Yehuda, McFarlane, and Shalev, 1998). Trauma memories may be strongly encoded in the context of high norepinephrine, and trauma reminders might produce an escalating cycle as they repeatedly elicit noradrenergic arousal and subsequent strengthening of the recalled traumatic memory trace (T. O'Donnell et al., 2004).

Trauma/PTSD acquired changes. While some of the changes noted may reflect risk, others may be consequences of trauma exposure or manifestations of the disorder itself. The limited data from co-twin studies suggest that exaggerated fear-potentiated startle in PTSD occurs after trauma (Roger K. Pitman et al., 2012).

OTHER SYSTEMS

Rapid expansion of biological studies implicates multiple brain systems. For example, genome-wide association studies (GWAS) search for genetic risks across the whole genome. Such studies on PTSD implicate a retinoid-related orphan receptor alpha gene (*RORA*) and a Tolloid-like 1 gene (*TLL1*). Other biological pathways linked to PTSD include GABAergic and serotoninergic neurotransmission, neurosteroids (e.g., allopregnenolone, dehydroepiandrosterone [DHEA] / dehydroepiandrosterone sulfate [DHEAS]), neuropeptide Y (NPY), endogenous cannabinoids, and endogenous opioids. For example, PTSD symptom severity is linked to low levels of NPY in cerebrospinal fluid and blunted NPY response to sympathetic activation (Roger K. Pitman et al., 2012). NPY reduces anxiogenic effects of CRH during sympathetic activation—so it is a modulator that interacts with both the HPA and SAM systems. Serotonin and GABAergic transmission both modulate amygdala firing, and polymorphisms in promoter regions of both the serotonin transporter gene and the GABA Alpha-2 receptor gene have been linked to risk for PTSD, in interaction with environmental stress (Roger K. Pitman et al., 2012). Finally, endogenous cannabinoids likely play a role in extinction learning and retention by modifying activation and connectivity in prefrontal-amygdala pathways; and DHEA and allopregnenolone might play a role in emotional regulation by modulating hippocampal, mPFC and amygdala connectivity (Roger K. Pitman et al., 2012). More studies are needed to integrate these additional factors into PTSD models.

NEUROCIRCUITRY OF POSTTRAUMATIC STRESS DISORDER

Research on PTSD neurorcircuitry implicates brain circuits involved in fear associated learning, emotion generation, and emotion regulation processes. Next we describe neural circuits associated with the PTSD phenotype, and then describe initial findings relevant to the role of these abnormalities in PTSD development.

PTSD phenotype. One consistent finding in PTSD is hyperactive emotional response to threat cues. Animal models suggest that threat response circuits involve the amygdala, bed nucleus of stria terminalis, nucleus accumbens, hippocampus, periaqueductal gray, thalamic nuclei, insular cortex, and infralimbic cortex (L. Shin and Liberzon, 2010). The emerging human model suggests that the amygdala plays a key role in threat detection, expression of fear response, and fear-associated learning; dorsal anterior cingulate (dACC, a potential human homolog of the rat prelimbic cortex) facilitates expression of conditioned fear in concert with the amygdala (Milad et al., 2009); insula interacts with both in acquisition of fear learning and is implicated in threat anticipation and introspective somatic sensation of emotions (Linnman, Rougemont-Bücking, Beucke, Zeffiro, and Milad, 2011). The amygdala and dACC process incoming stimuli, with outputs to hypothalamus, basal ganglia, and brainstem to induce threat related adaptive behaviors and activate HPA axis (see Figure 9.2). Structurally, both increased and decreased the amygdala volumes have been reported in PTSD (Woon and Hedges, 2009). However, fMRI studies on threat sensitivity in PTSD consistently have shown the amygdala hyperactivity and dACC responses (Hayes, Hayes, and Mikedis, 2012). The amygdala activity

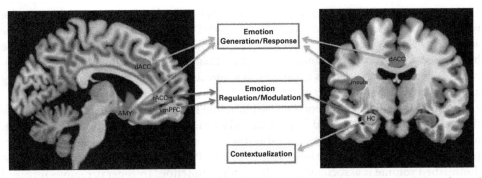

FIGURE 9.2 Heuristic model of the neurocircuitry of PTSD. vmPFC: ventromedial prefrontal cortex; rACC: rostral anterior cingulate cortex; dACC: dorsal anterior cingulate cortex; HC: hippocampus; AMY: amygdala. Dark gray areas are hyperactive/hyperresponsive. Light gray areas are hypoactive/hyporesponsive.

correlated with symptom severity and self-reported anxiety (Britton, Phan, Taylor, Fig, and Liberzon, 2005). Insular cortical volume is reduced in PTSD, but insula is hyperactive in symptom provocation tasks, perhaps reflecting detection of bodily arousal (Shvil, Rusch, Sullivan, and Neria, 2013). These abnormalities, however, may not be PTSD-specific, perhaps reflecting general brain phenomena associated with strong emotional reactivity (Etkin and Wager, 2007).

While not necessarily specific to PTSD alone, important abnormalities in fear associated learning circuitry are now being revealed in studies of anxiety. Recall of extinction leaning is impaired in PTSD (Milad et al., 2009), and this impairment is coupled with hypoactivity in the hippocampus (Admon, Milad, and Hendler, 2013) and mPFC (Garfinkel et al., 2014). In contrast, amygdala and dACC are *hyper*active during extinction recall (Milad et al., 2009), as is insula (Garfinkel et al., 2014). Brain-based problems in extinction recall suggest difficulty in acquiring new learning about the safety of a cue that has previously been conditioned to indicate threat, resulting in a failure to update adaptive behavior to the new contexts in which extinction occurred.

PTSD patients also demonstrate deficits in *regulation* of emotional responses, studied using emotion provocation paradigms (Hayes et al., 2012). Findings indicate diminished activation in rostral ACC and vmPFC in PTSD patients during emotion regulation tasks (Hayes et al., 2012), findings that also appear to be more PTSD-specific than amygdala hyperactivation though studies with non-PTSD anxiety control groups are needed (Etkin and Wager, 2007). Volumetric differences might also be present in these regions in PTSD, with low mPFC volume consistently reported in PTSD and linked to symptom severity or illness progression (Thomaes et al., 2014). Volume changes in ACC and vmPFC seem to be associated with PTSD phenotype rather than risk, and there is evidence for improvement in vmPFC function after successful treatment (Thomaes et al., 2014). Hypoactivity in vmPFC—seen in a variety of emotion-provocation, emotion-regulation, and fear-inhibition studies—is often linked to the amygdala hyperactivity, perhaps due to reduced functional connectivity between these structures (L. Shin and Liberzon, 2010).

Finally, hippocampus plays a role in contextual learning, including fear learning and extinction. Failure to recall extinction is related to lower hippocampal activation (Milad et al., 2009). Research finds diminished volume, neuronal integrity, and functional integrity of hippocampus in PTSD suggesting a mechanism involved in over overgeneralization of fear learning (L. M. Shin, Rauch, and Pitman, 2006). While smaller hippocampal volume appears to be a preexisiting risk factor for PTSD following trauma exposure, there may also be additional changes in structure and function that occur posttrauma based on the neurotoxic effects of chronic stress as noted about. Specifically, deficits in extinction learning appear to be acquired (Milad et al., 2008).

In summary, evidence supports altered function in a network of interconnected emotion generation, regulation and fear associated learning regions, including the amygdala, insula, dorsal anterior cingulate, rostral and ventral mFC and hippocampus. Some structural findings, especially in the hippocampus and mPFC, are consistent with the idea that diminished volume is associated with diminished function. In general, regions involved in emotion generation—i.e., the amygdala, insula and dACC—appear to be hyperactive, while emotion regulatory and extinction recall/retention regions (i.e., rostral mPFC, vmPFC and hippocampus) usually demonstrate hypo-activation patterns, potentially associated with diminished volume and lower functional connectivity to the amygdala.

Risk and vulnerability. Genetic studies have identified potential PTSD risk factors among the abnormalities in structure or function of the amygdala, insula, medial prefrontal cortex and hippocampus. A recent review of co-twin studies concludes that small hippocampal volume is likely a predisposing risk factor for PTSD, although additional hippocampal loss also probably occurs with PTSD development (Kremen, Koenen, Afari, and Lyons, 2012; Woon and Hedges, 2009). Evidence for treatment-related reversal of the volume changes further supports a link to PTSD symptom development (Thomaes et al., 2014).

Some initial evidence suggests that exaggerated reactivity of the amygdala and/or of dACC predicts risk for PTSD, though this may not be PTSD-specific. Combined genetic-imaging studies have been equivocal when examining the potential association between the short allele of 5-HTTLPR (serotonin transporter) gene and increased amygdala responsivity in affective disorders (Bastiaansen et al., 2014). The relationship has been demonstrated in subjects with PTSD though additional replication is warranted (Skelton et al., 2012). Further, if specific to PTSD, amygdala responsivity might either constitute a vulnerability factor or develop in association with genetic risk factors. A twin study found higher dACC activation during a non-emotional interference task in twins who do not have PTSD but may be at genetic risk (Mehta and Binder, 2012).

Intermediate vulnerability. While one might expect "downstream" brain changes based on neurotoxic effects of chronic stress exposure, studies have not examined the interaction of PTSD and early childhood adversity on brain structure or function. However, in a longitudinal study of children focused on development of major depressive disorder, greater early life stress was related to increased amygdala activation in response to emotional faces (Suzuki et al., 2014). Further, in depressed children, greater left hippocampal activity in response to sad faces increased with the number of early life stress/trauma events (Suzuki et al., 2014). Stress-induced epigenetic changes in orbitofrontal cortex, amygdala and hippocampus might create risk for PTSD with later trauma exposure (Blanchard et al., 1996). Though such changes may create functional adaptations within high-stress early environments, they may create future risk through impact on executive function and emotion regulation areas of the brain (Koenen, 2006).

Trauma/PTSD acquired changes. Theoretically, findings in the PTSD phenotype not detected in studies of risk are likely acquired following trauma exposure or PTSD development. Findings in this category include insula hyperactivity, and rostral ACC and mPFC hypoactivation, although one can argue that sufficient work has not yet been done to exclude roles as potential risk or intermediate vulnerability factors. There is also some evidence that hypoactivation of mPFC and hippocampus in extinction recall studies may be acquired (Milad et al., 2008). As noted, however, brain regions contributing risk (e.g., smaller hippocampal volume) may also change in structure and function posttrauma, perhaps adding to prior neurotoxic effects of stress exposure that helped create risk. Pre- and posttrauma changes may thus be intertwined and together contribute to the diminished volume, and altered neuronal and functional integrity seen in hippocampus in PTSD, suggesting a mechanism for overgeneralization of fear learning (L. Shin and Liberzon, 2010).

SUMMARY

Much has been learned about the biology of PTSD, but more remains to be discovered. It is clear that processes related to fear learning and extinction play critical roles in the development and maintenance of PTSD. Brain regions involving emotional activation (amygdala, dACC, insula) and emotion regulation and fear extinction (rostral mPFC, vmPFC, hippocampus) are involved. The HPA axis and SAM/catecholaminergic systems are also players. Somehow, these brain regions and systems accumulate "information" and create behavioral propensities over time, as a genetically shaped brain interacts with challenging environments to shape functional networks involving stress and threat response systems in ways that create risk for PTSD in response to subsequent trauma exposure. Continued investigation is needed to clarify how these systems function and interact through many pathways leading to PTSD. Much work is needed to identify the precise pathways and to utilize our understanding of them to develop clinically useful new approaches to prevention and treatment. Identifying and overcoming some of the systematic limitations in the current literature will be critical to make this on-going work successful. We also need to continue to look for the organizing and integrating principles that will ultimately allow us to assemble large volumes of data into a coherent neurobiological picture. Though highly preliminary, we will conclude this review with our own attempt at a partial synthesis.

PRELIMINARY SYNTHESIS

PTSD arises from multiple, complex pretraumatic vulnerability factors, which interact with exposure and postexposure processes. Given the complexity of this developmental process, there are likely to be numerous different "entry points" and contributing factors that can lead to PTSD. A comprehensive neurobiological and developmental framework will be necessary to understand both the adaptive and maladaptive processes that can unfold in response accumulating stress exposures and acute exposure to threat and safety information.

In all organisms, exposure to threat signals *activates* a host of detection, salience determination, immediate response systems, and learning processes. These are followed by complex adaptations that *regulate* immediate responses and attune them to the nature of the threat, based on a more granular analysis that also takes into account experience with prior threats. These processes are followed by longer-term adaptation processes. This postexposure process refines future response tendencies by "tweaking" the various components of response, regulation, and adaptation systems to allow more "prepared" responses in the future and improve long-term adaptation to the environment.

From a circuitry perspective, immediate-reactivity networks encompassing amygdala, insula, and dACC may detect threats, identify salience, and initiate immediate responses to preserve safety. Other, regulatory/modulatory regions, including PFC and hippocampus, may disambiguate the detected threat vs. safety cues by integrating contextual information that helps the organism select the most appropriate responses. This allows similar signals to have different meanings, depending upon context. Functioning of these two threat detection/learning and regulatory/modulatory control systems are mediated and modulated by major neurotransmitter and hormonal systems, the SAM-catecholaminergic system and the HPA axis, respectively. The HPA axis and SAM/catecholaminergic systems reviewed earlier have key functional roles both in threat detection regions, like the amygdala and insula, and in regulatory regions, like the mPFC and hippocampus, with the ability to up- or down-regulate different components of these systems based on the level of immediate threat (catecholamines), longer term needs (GCs), and their interaction. These interacting systems create an adaptive integration of cue (immediate threat) and context information (which includes the "surround" in which the cue occurs and past experience with similar cues and contexts) and shapes appropriate responding, facilitating true, long-term adaptation. This process is dependent upon complex interactions between the amygdala, insula, dACC, mPFC, and hippocampus, and it is tuned and regulated by catecholaminergic and GC inputs.

PTSD clearly involves immediate threat detection and response systems, as well as the systems that have evolved to regulate and modulate these systems to facilitate longer term adaptations. It may be possible to develop PTSD symptoms with deficits in either component, but full-blown disorder may evolve only in the context of multiple "hits," with disrupted functioning in both the immediate threat detection and response systems and in the slower reacting, regulatory/modulatory adaptation systems. For example, amygdala hypersensitivity (perhaps due to 5-HTTPRP risk-alleles) may produce general risk for psychopathology and produce some PTSD symptoms in the context of trauma exposure; and inadequate activity in regulatory regions (perhaps due to smaller hippocampi) might also lead to symptoms in the context of trauma exposure. But emergence of full-blown chronic PTSD over the days, weeks and months following a trauma exposure may require abnormalities in both components.

Consistent evidence of a role in PTSD for the HPA axis and GCs on one hand, and of mPFC abnormalities on the other, may organize future work designed to refine emerging models. The hippocampus and mPFC, both rich in GC receptors, may shape context-dependent learning, which supports nuanced understanding of a given cue's meaning. In animal models, up-regulation of GC receptors in both regions in response to stress exposure supports PTSD-like fear associational learning deficits. In these same models, abnormal noradrenergic activity in the hippocampus has been reported (Roger K. Pitman et al., 2012). Catecholaminergic signals from the LC to the hippocampus are critical for synaptic depotentiation and plasticity within the hippocampus, which are critical aspects of its functioning. Thus altered catecholaminergic and GC signaling may contribute to alter hippocampal/prefrontal functioning in ways that impact contextual processing and modulation, which may be abnormal in PTSD. In a recent study, we have demonstrated that patients with PTSD do in fact have a specific deficit in contextualization processes, which is more general than just a failure to detect safety signals (Garfinkel et al., 2014). This supports an integrative model in which a proposed general context processing deficit may be central and focuses attention on the mPFC-hippocampal circuits that subserve this function.

The emerging picture is complex. Long-term, healthy adaptation to threat and safety requires a finely tuned balance within activation and regulation circuits and well-tuned catecholaminergic and GC systems regulating these circuits. Disruptions in many different components of this carefully constructed system can create dysregulations that have behavioral consequences. The complexity creates the possibility of many different types of potentially disruptive "hits" within different places within this system and in a variety of brain regions that could ultimately impact its functioning detrimentally and create a "final common outcome" of a deficit in capacity for contextualization. Diminished capacity for contextualization, which is required for nuanced responding to threat and for long term adaptations needed to regulate threat and safety systems in ways that allow healthy recovery from trauma exposure, may be a fundamental element in the evolution of PTSD. It, in a sense, "brings together" many of the neurobiological elements we have discussed in this chapter. This model also illuminates the way in which accumulating "hits" to components of this system, through recurrent exposure to stress or trauma, could contribute to accumulating "weaknesses" that, over time, build escalating risk for breakdown and emergence of PTSD.

By focusing on context processing deficits as a conceptual framework for organizing and integrating the vast array of physiological, neuroanatomical, and clinical PTSD data that has been generated in the past few decades, we might be able to more clearly see the roles of the various systems and processes that are critical to this function and perhaps critical to the development of PTSD. This may help us integrate information on circuits, transmitters, and hormones within a more unified theoretical framework and move us a few steps closer to being able to utilize our vast and growing body of research to more concretely improve treatment, and perhaps prevention, of this devastating disorder.

DISCLOSURE STATEMENT

The authors have no conflicts to disclose. The authors are funded by National Institutes of Health, Veterans Health Administration, and Department of Defense.

REFERENCES

Admon, R., Milad, M. R., and Hendler, T. (2013). A causal model of post-traumatic stress disorder: Disentangling predisposed from acquired neural abnormalities. *Trends Cog Sci, 17* (7), 337–347.

Bastiaansen, J. A., Servaas, M. N., Marsman, J. B. C., Ormel, J., Nolte, I. M., Riese, H., and Aleman, A. (2014). Filling the gap: Relationship between the serotonin-transporter-linked polymorphic region and amygdala activation. *Psych Sci, 25,* 2058–2066. doi: 10.1177/0956797614548877

Binder, E. B., Bradley, R. G., Liu, W., Epstein, M. P., Deveau, T. C., Mercer, K. B., . . . Ressler, K. J. (2008). Association of FKBP5 polymorphisms and childhood abuse with risk of posttraumatic stress disorder symptoms in adults. *J Am Med Assoc, 299* (11), 1291–1305.

Blanchard, E. B., Hickling, E. J., Buckley, T. C., Taylor, A. E., Vollmer, A., and Loos, W. R. (1996). Psychophysiology of posttraumatic stress disorder related to motor vehicle accidents: Replication and extension. *J Consult Clin Psychol, 64* (4), 742–751.

Bremner, J. D., Licinio, J., Darnell, A., and Krystal, J. H. (1997). Elevated CSF corticotropin-releasing factor concentrations in posttraumatic stress disorder. *The American Journal of Psychiatry, 154* (5), 624–629.

Breslau, N., Chilcoat, H. D., Kessler, R. C., and Davis, G. C. (1999). Previous exposure to trauma and PTSD effects of subsequent trauma: results from the Detroit Area Survey of Trauma. *Am J Psychiatry, 156* (6), 902–907.

Britton, J. C., Phan, K. L., Taylor, S. F., Fig, L. M., and Liberzon, I. (2005). Corticolimbic blood flow in posttraumatic stress disorder during script-driven imagery. *Biol Psychiatry*, *57* (8), 832–840.

Carpenter, L., Shattuck, T., Tyrka, A., Geracioti, T., and Price, L. (2011). Effect of childhood physical abuse on cortisol stress response. *Psychopharmacology (Berlin)*, *214*, 367–375.

Chalmers, J. A., Quintana, D. S., Abbott, M. J., and Kemp, A. H. (2014). Anxiety disorders are associated with reduced heart rate variability: A meta-analysis. *Front Psychiatry*, *5*, 80. doi: 10.3389/fpsyt.2014.00080

de Cloet, C. S., Vermetten, E., Rademaker, A. R., Geuze, E., and Westenberg, H. G. M. (2012). Neuroendocrine and immune responses to a cognitive stress challenge in veterans with and without PTSD. *Eur J Psychotraumatology*, *3* (http://dx.doi.org/10.3402/ejpt.v3i0.16206).

de Quervain, D. J. F., and Yehuda, R. (2006). Glucocorticoid-induced inhibition of memory retrieval: Implications for posttraumatic stress disorder. *Psychobiol Posttraumatic Stress Disorders*, *1071*, 216–220.

Delahanty, D. L., and Nugent, N. R. (2006). Predicting PTSD prospectively based on prior trauma history and immediate biological responses. *Ann NY Acad Sci*, *1071*, 27–40.

Dickerson, S. S., and Kemeny, M. E. (2004). Acute stressors and cortisol responses: A theoretical integration and synthesis of laboratory research. *Psychol Bull*, *130* (3), 355–391.

Elzinga, B. M., Schmahl, C. G., Vermetten, E., van Dyck, R., and Bremner, J. D. (2003). Higher cortisol levels following exposure to traumatic reminders in abuse-related PTSD. *Neuropsychopharmacology*, *28* (9), 1656–1665.

Etkin, A., and Wager, T. (2007). Functional neuroimaging of anxiety: A meta-analysis of emotional processing in PTSD, social anxiety disorder, and specific phobia. *Am J Psychiatry*, *164* (10), 1476–1488.

Fonzo, G. A., Simmons, A. N., Thorp, S. R., Norman, S. B., Paulus, M. P., and Stein, M. B. (2010). Exaggerated and disconnected insular-amygdalar blood oxygenation level-dependent response to threat-related emotional faces in women with intimate-partner violence posttraumatic stress disorder. *Biol Psychiatry*, *68* (5), 433–441.

Garfinkel, S. N., Abelson, J. L., King, A. P., Sripada, R. K., Wang, X., Gaines, L. M., and Liberzon, I. (2014). Impaired contextual modulation of memories in PTSD: An fMRI and psychophysiological study of extinction retention and fear renewal. *J Neurosci*, *34* (40), 13435–13443. doi: 10.1523/jneurosci.4287-13.2014

Hayes, J., Hayes, S., and Mikedis, A. (2012). Quantitative meta-analysis of neural activity in posttraumatic stress disorder. *Biol Mood Anxiety Disorders*, *2* (1), 9.

Kellner, M., Muhtz, C., Peter, F., Dunker, S., Wiedemann, K., and Yassouridis, A. (2010). Increased DHEA and DHEA-S plasma levels in patients with post-traumatic stress disorder and a history of childhood abuse. *J Psychiatric Res*, *44* (4), 215–219.

Kessler, R. C., Sonnega, A., Bromet, E., Hughes, M., and Nelson, C. B. (1995). Posttraumatic stress disorder in the National Comorbidity Survey. *Arch Gen Psychiatry*, *52* (12), 1048–1060.

King, A., Abelson, J., Britton, J., Phan, K., Taylor, S., and I. L. (2009). Medial prefrontal cortex and right insula activity predict plasma ACTH response to trauma recall. *Neuroimage*, *47*, 872–880.

Koenen, K. C. (2006). Developmental epidemiology of PTSD: Self-regulation as a central mechanism. *Ann NY Acad Sci*, *1071*, 255–266.

Kremen, W. S., Koenen, K. C., Afari, N., and Lyons, M. J. (2012). Twin studies of posttraumatic stress disorder: Differentiating vulnerability factors from sequelae. *Neuropharmacology*, *62* (2), 647–653.

Ladd, C. O., Huot, R. L., Thrivikraman, K. V., Nemeroff, C. B., Meaney, M. J., and Plotsky, P. M. (2000). Long-term behavioral and neuroendocrine adaptations to adverse early experience. *Prog Brain Res* *122*, 81–103.

Liberzon, I., Abelson, J. L., Flagel, S. B., Raz, J., and Young, E. A. (1999). Neuroendocrine and psychophysiologic responses in PTSD: A symptom provocation study. *Neuropsychopharmacology*, *21* (1), 40–50.

Liberzon, I., King, A. P., Ressler, K. J., Almli, L. M., Zhang, P., Ma, S. T., . . . Galea, S. (2014). Interaction of the ADRB2 gene polymorphism with childhood trauma in predicting adult symptoms of post-trauamtic stress disorder. *J Am Med Assoc Psychiatry.* doi: 10.1001/jamapsychiatry.2014.999

Linnman, C., Rougemont-Bücking, A., Beucke, J. C., Zeffiro, T. A., and Milad, M. R. (2011). Unconditioned responses and functional fear networks in human classical conditioning. *Behav Brain Res, 221* (1), 237–245.

Luo, H., Hu, X., Liu, X., Ma, X., Guo, W., Qiu, C., . . . Li, T. (2012). Hair cortisol level as a biomarker for altered hypothalamic-pituitary-adrenal activity in female adolescents with posttraumatic stress disorder after the 2008 Wenchuan earthquake. *Biol Psychiatry, 72,* 65–69.

Martin, E. I., Ressler, K. J., Binder, E., and Nemeroff, C. B. (2009). The neurobiology of anxiety disorders: Brain imaging, genetics, and psychoneuroendocrinology. *Psychiatric Clin of North Am, 32* (3), 549–575.

Mason, J. W., Giller, E. L., Kosten, T. R., Ostroff, R. B., and Podd, L. (1986). Urinary free-cortisol levels in posttraumatic stress disorder patients. *J Nervous and Mental Dis, 174* (3), 145–149.

Mason, J. W., Wang, S., Yehuda, R., Lubin, H., Johnson, D., Bremner, J. D., . . . Southwick, S. (2002). Marked lability in urinary cortisol levels in subgroups of combat veterans with posttraumatic stress disorder during an intensive exposure treatment program. *Psychosom Med, 64* (2), 238–246.

Meaney, M. J., Szyf, M., and Seckl, J. R. (2007). Epigenetic mechanisms of perinatal programming of hypothalamic-pituitary-adrenal function and health. *Trends Mol Med, 13* (7), 269–277.

Mehta, D., and Binder, E. B. (2012). Gene x environment vulnerability factors for PTSD: the HPA-axis. *Neuropharmacology, 62* (2), 654–662.

Mehta, D., Klengel, T., Conneely, K. N., Smith, A. K., Altmann, A., Pace, T. W., . . . Binder, E. B. (2013). Childhood maltreatment is associated with distinct genomic and epigenetic profiles in posttraumatic stress disorder. *Proc Natl Acad Sci US, 110* (20), 8302–8307.

Milad, M. R., Orr, S. P., Lasko, N. B., Chang, Y., Rauch, S. L., and Pitman, R. K. (2008). Presence and acquired origin of reduced recall for fear extinction in PTSD: Results of a twin study. *J Psychiatric Res, 42* (7), 515–520.

Milad, M. R., Pitman, R. K., Ellis, C. B., Gold, A. L., Shin, L. M., Lasko, N. B., . . . Rauch, S. L. (2009). Neurobiological basis of failure to recall extinction memory in posttraumatic stress disorder. *Biol Psychiatry, 66* (12), 1075–1082.

O'Donnell, M. L., Creamer, M., Elliott, P., and Bryant, R. (2007). Tonic and phasic heart rate as predictors of posttraumatic stress disorder. *Psychosom Med, 69* (3), 256–261.

O'Donnell, T., Hegadoren, K., and Coupland, N. (2004). Noradrenergic mechanisms in the pathophysiology of post-traumatic stress disorder. *Neuropsychobiology, 50* (4), 273–283.

Pace, T. W. W., and Heim, C. M. (2011). A short review on the psychoneuroimmunology of posttraumatic stress disorder: From risk factors to medical comorbidities. *Brain, Behav Immun, 25* (1), 6–13. doi: http://dx.doi.org/10.1016/j.bbi.2010.10.003

Pineles, S. L., Suvak, M. K., Liverant, G. I., Gregor, K., Wisco, B. E., Pitman, R. K., and Orr, S. P. (2013). Psychophysiologic reactivity, subjective distress, and their associations with PTSD diagnosis. *J Abnorm Psychol, 122* (3), 635–644.

Pitman, R. K., and Delahanty, D. L. (2005). Conceptually driven pharmacologic approaches to acute trauma. *CNS Spectrums, 10* (2), 99–106.

Pitman, R. K., Rasmusson, A. M., Koenen, K. C., Shin, L. M., Orr, S. P., Gilbertson, M. W., . . . Liberzon, I. (2012). Biological studies of post-traumatic stress disorder. *Nature Rev Neurosci, 13,* 769–787. doi: 10.1038/nrn3339

Pole, N. (2007). The psychophysiology of posttraumatic stress disorder: A meta-analysis. *Psychol Bull, 133* (5), 725–746.

Rothbaum, B. O., Kearns, M. C., Reiser, E., Davis, J. S., Kerley, K. A., Rothbaum, A. O., . . . Ressler, K. J. (2014). Early intervention following trauma may mitigate genetic risk for PTSD in civilians: A pilot prospective emergency department study. *J Clin Psychiatry, 75,* 1380–1387.

Shin, L., and Liberzon, I. (2010). The neurocircuitry of fear, stress, and anxiety disorders. *Neuropsychopharmacology, 35* (1), 169–191.

Shin, L. M., Rauch, S. L., and Pitman, R. K. (2006). Amygdala, medial prefrontal cortex, and hippocampal function in PTSD. *Ann NY Acad Sci, 1071,* 67–79.

Shvil, E., Rusch, H., Sullivan, G., and Neria, Y. (2013). Neural, psychophysiological, and behavioral markers of fear processing in PTSD: A review of the literature. *Curr Psychiatry Rep, 15* (5), 1–10. doi: 10.1007/s11920-013-0358-3

Skelton, K., Ressler, K. J., Norrholm, S. D., Jovanovic, T., and Bradley-Davino, B. (2012). PTSD and gene variants: New pathways and new thinking. *Neuropharmacology, 62* (2), 628–637.

Steudte, S., Kirschbaum, C., Gao, W., Alexander, N., Schonfeld, S., Hoyer, J., and Stalder, T. (2013). Hair cortisol as a biomarker of traumatization in healthy individuals and posttraumatic stress disorder patients. *Biol Psychiatry, 74,* 639–646.

Stroud, L. R., Salovey, P., and Epel, E. S. (2002). Sex differences in stress response: Social Rejection versus achievement stress. *Biological Psychiatry, 52,* 318–327.

Suzuki, H., Luby, J. L., Botteron, K. N., Dietrich, R., McAvoy, M. P., and Barch, D. M. (2014). Early life stress and trauma and enhanced limbic activation to emotionally valenced faces in depressed and healthy children. *J Am Acad Child Adolescent Psychiatry, 53* (7), 800–813.

Thomaes, K., Dorrepaal, E., Draijer, N., Jansma, E., Veltman, D., and van Balkom, A. J. (2014). Can pharmacological and psychological treatment change brain structure and function in PTSD? A systematic review. *J Psychiatric Res, 50,* 1–15.

Van Voorhees, E. E., Dennis, M. F., Calhoun, P. S., and Beckham, J. C. (2013). Association of DHEA, DHEAS, and cortisol with childhood trauma exposure and post-traumatic stress disorder. *Int Clin Psychopharmacol, 29* (1), 56–62.

van Zuiden, M., Kavelaars, A., Geuze, E., Olff, M., and Heijnen, C. J. (2013). Predicting PTSD: Pre-existing vulnerabilities in glucocorticoid-signaling and implications for preventive interventions. *Brain Behav Immun, 30,* 12–21.

Vermetten, E., and Lanius, R. A. (2012). Biological and clinical framework for posttraumatic stress disorder. *Handb Clin Neurol, 106,* 291–342.

Woon, F., and Hedges, D. (2009). Amygdala volume in adults with posttraumatic stress disorder: A meta-analysis. *J Neuropsychiatry Clin Neurosci, 21* (1), 5–12.

Yehuda, R. (Ed.) (2006). Psychobiology of posttraumatic stress disorders: A decade of progress (Vol. 1071), *Annals of the New York Academy of Sciences,* Malden: Blackwell Publishing, New York, NY, xxiii–547.

Yehuda, R., Golier, J. A., Yang, R.-K., and Tischler, L. (2004). Enhanced sensitivity to glucocorticoids in peripheral mononuclear leukocytes in posttraumatic stress disorder. *Biol Psychiatry, 55* (11), 1110–1116.

Yehuda, R., McFarlane, A. C., and Shalev, A. Y. (1998). Predicting the development of posttraumatic stress disorder from the acute response to a traumatic event. *Biol Psychiatry, 44* (12), 1305–1313.

Yehuda, R., Morris, A., Labinsky, E., Zemelman, S., and Schmeidler, J. (2007). Ten-year follow-up study of cortisol levels in aging Holocaust survivors with and without PTSD. *J Traumatic Stress, 20* (5), 757–762. doi: 10.1002/jts.20228

Yehuda, R., Yang, R.-K., Buchsbaum, M. S., and Golier, J. A. (2006). Alterations in cortisol negative feedback inhibition as examined using the ACTH response to cortisol administration in PTSD. *Psychoneuroendocrinology, 31* (4), 447–451. doi: 10.1016/j.psyneuen.2005.10.007

10

CLINICAL ASPECTS OF TRAUMA-RELATED ANXIETY AND POSTTRAUMATIC STRESS DISORDER

ANDREW A. COOPER, NORAH C. FEENY, AND BARBARA O. ROTHBAUM

INTRODUCTION

The publication of the fifth edition of the *Diagnostic and Statistical Manual of Mental Disorders* (DSM-5; American Psychiatric Association, 2013) signals the most dramatic changes to the definition and diagnosis of posttraumatic stress disorder (PTSD) since it was first included in DSM-III. Departing the anxiety disorders to join the newly created trauma- and stressor-related disorders category, PTSD also sees changes in some of its core diagnostic elements, including reorganization of symptom clusters to capture a broader range of negative emotions. These changes (and the accompanying controversy; e.g., Galatzer-Levy and Bryant, 2013) are perhaps a byproduct of the incredible expansion of research on the epidemiology and treatment of PTSD in the past two decades in particular.

In reviewing this literature, we aim to provide a concise and general summary of the key clinical aspects of PTSD, providing references to the most recent, focused reviews and meta-analyses on specific subjects when they exist. We begin by discussing the epidemiology of PTSD, including its associated impairments and conditions. We then describe contemporary psychological models and treatments before reviewing evidence of their efficacy. We conclude by highlighting key problems and future directions for the field, including several promising interventions that may prove influential in the next two decades of clinical research on PTSD.

EPIDEMIOLOGY OF TRAUMA AND PTSD

As in prior iterations of the DSM, a diagnosis of PTSD is contingent on trauma exposure. In DSM-5, this is defined by actual or threatened sexual violence, serious injury, or death that an individual experienced directly, by witnessing, by being informed about (in the case of violent or unexpected injury or death of a loved one), or by way of repeated exposure to aversive details (e.g., first responders). The four clusters of symptoms include intrusive symptoms (e.g., flashbacks; one required), avoidance behaviors (e.g., avoiding trauma reminders; one required), negative trauma-related alterations in cognitions and mood (e.g., persistent self-blame; two required), and trauma-related alterations in reactivity and arousal (e.g., hypervigilance; two required). Distress and enduring symptoms (i.e., greater than one month) round out the core diagnostic features. Notably, the majority of the research reviewed in this chapter is based on earlier DSM diagnostic criteria; it is unclear how changes introduced in the DSM-5 may influence diagnostic estimates in the years to come (e.g., Galatzer-Levy and Bryant, 2013; Hoge, Riviere, Wilk, Harrell, and Weathers, 2014).

Trauma exposure is common in the United States, with an estimated 80% of the general population having experienced at least one lifetime trauma (Breslau, 2009). Nevertheless, development of PTSD is relatively infrequent, with an overall estimate around 10% in trauma-exposed individuals (Breslau, 2009), reflecting the tendency for symptoms to increase around trauma exposure and drop off precipitously thereafter in most cases (Rothbaum, Foa, Riggs, Murdock, and Walsh, 1992). Large national samples have reported rates of 6.4–7.8% (Pietrzak, Goldstein, Southwick, and Grant, 2011; Kessler, Sonnega, Bromet, Hughes, and Nelson, 1995), with sub-syndromal or partial PTSD estimated at around 8.6%. In longitudinal studies of PTSD, approximately 40% of individuals with the diagnosis continue to report significant symptoms and impairment 10 years after trauma exposure (Kessler et al., 1995). In summary, while trauma exposure is far from rare, most individuals experience only transient symptoms, with full diagnostic PTSD resulting in a minority of cases.

PROSPECTIVE RISK FACTORS

Several demographic and clinical characteristics have been identified as predictors of increased risk of PTSD; however, study population and methods appear to moderate the strength of these relationships, resulting in some inconsistencies across studies and meta-analytic reviews (Brewin, Andrews, and Valentine, 2000; Ozer, Best, Lipsey, and West, 2003). Female gender is frequently identified as a risk factor, with some studies reporting PTSD in women at rates twice as high as men. Rates of exposure to different trauma types also vary by sex, with men more likely to experience combat or physical assault, and women more likely to report sexual assault (Breslau, 2009; Kessler et al., 1995; Pietrzak et al., 2011). There is mixed evidence of trauma-specific risks for developing PTSD, although rape and sexual assault appear to be particularly high-risk regardless of gender. In general, individuals with PTSD are more likely to report directly experienced events (e.g., being a victim of assault) as their worst trauma experience versus indirect events (e.g., witnessing an accident), and directly experienced traumas are also associated with greater duration of symptoms (Pietrzak et al., 2011).

Among other clinical characteristics that have been shown to predict odds of PTSD, personal psychiatric history, family psychiatric history, and early abuse are the most stable across method and population variance (Brewin et al., 2000; Ozer et al., 2003). Posttrauma social support appears to have a protective effect in reducing risk of subsequent PTSD diagnosis; however, estimates of its effect size have varied across meta-analytic reviews ($r = .40$, Brewin et al., 2000; $r = .28$, Ozer et al., 2003). Prior trauma exposure (Brewin et al., 2000; Ozer et al., 2003) and peritraumatic dissociation have been shown to predict risk of PTSD (Ozer et al., 2003), but the findings are more nuanced than straightforward (Breslau, 2009). Regarding psychological factors, pretrauma measures of lower cognitive ability, neuroticism, negative affect, and a range of negative coping styles (e.g., avoidance or rumination) have been associated with development of PTSD (DiGangi, Gomez, Mendoza, Jason, Keys, and Koenen, 2013). At present, the literature on predictors of PTSD has identified several consistently predictive variables; however, there is a critical need for further study to identify individual risk factors that can be used to predict risk prospectively.

COMORBIDITY, FUNCTIONING, AND COSTS

Individuals with PTSD are at elevated risk for a number of comorbid psychiatric diagnoses, with lifetime estimates around 80% (Kessler et al., 1995). The most commonly reported comorbid conditions are mood disorders, particularly major depression, as well as anxiety disorders, substance use disorders, and increased suicidal behavior (Kessler et al., 1995; Pietrzak et al., 2011). Personality disorders also frequently co-occur in about 35% of patients with PTSD (Friborg, Martinussen, Kaiser, Overgard, and Rosenvinge, 2013). PTSD has substantial negative effects and costs at both the individual and societal level. PTSD worsens occupational, family, marital and interpersonal functioning and is associated with poorer subjective and objective ratings of quality of life (QOL) (see Rodriguez, Holowka, and Marx, 2012). Individuals with PTSD have greater odds of general health symptoms, medical conditions, higher and more frequent pain, and cardio-respiratory and gastrointestinal symptoms (Pacella, Hruska, and Delahanty, 2013). In terms of impairment, hospitalizations and health visits, PTSD has been estimated as the most costly anxiety disorder at the societal level (Greenberg et al., 1999), with personal medical costs rising in proportion to severity of PTSD symptoms (Walker, Katon, Russo, Ciechanowski, Newman, and Wagner, 2003). In summary, PTSD is associated with elevated rates of psychiatric and general health problems, increased medical costs, and substantial impairments in many domains of life functioning.

PSYCHOLOGICAL THEORIES OF PTSD

We focus our review of psychological theories on contemporary cognitive-behavioral models of the development and maintenance of PTSD, elaborating on emotional processing theory (Foa, Huppert, and Cahill, 2006; Rothbaum, 2006) as an example of how these models account for natural recovery and differential susceptibility to PTSD, and the established efficacy of cognitive behavioral treatments. We conclude with a brief discussion of a contemporary behavioral model emphasizing inhibitory learning and fear extinction. We omit solely biological theories, repeats colleagues, happy to revise to something like "as described in Chapter 9 by Rauch and colleagues".

EARLY BEHAVIORAL MODELS OF FEAR

Mowrer's two-factor conditioning theory (Mowrer, 1947) provided a framework for early behavioral theories of PTSD, emphasizing the role of classical and operant conditioning in the acquisition and maintenance of pathological anxiety. Classical conditioning explains the acquisition of such anxiety by the pairing of a neutral conditioned stimulus (CS) with an aversive unconditioned stimulus (UCS), such that the CS thereafter evokes a conditioned fear response (CR). This accounts for the anxiety-provoking effects of previously neutral stimuli that are connected to the traumatic experience in PTSD (Foa et al., 2006). Operant conditioning explains maintenance of avoidance behaviors in PTSD. Efforts to avoid anxiety-provoking CSs reduce anxiety and are therefore negatively reinforcing, with the added deleterious effect of depriving the individual from learning that the CS itself is not truly dangerous (i.e., extinction training).

COGNITIVE AND SCHEMA THEORIES

Cognitive theories suggest that interpretations give rise to emotional and behavioral reactions. In the case of anxiety disorders specifically, inaccurate assessment of danger drives inflated perceptions of risk and promotes avoidance behaviors, with disproportionate or unrealistically negative interpretations maintaining long term pathological states (Beck, Emery, and Greenberg, 1985). Schema-based cognitive models of PTSD suggest that trauma exposure leads to enduring changes in thoughts and beliefs that are critical to determining emotional and behavioral responses to reminders of the trauma (e.g., Ehlers and Clark, 2000; Foa et al., 2006). In general, these theories posit that trauma exposure violates assumptions about the safety and benevolence of the world, the trustworthiness of others, and one's own worthiness or competence, or confirms existing negative assumptions. Contemporary cognitive models of PTSD vary somewhat in their relative emphasis on appraisals, schemas, memory, and their correspondence with cognitive or information-processing models of normal emotion and perception (for a review, see Dalgleish, 2004); we highlight such differences in our discussion of two important cognitive models.

According to Ehlers and Clark's (2000) model, negative trauma-related appraisals and beliefs about the world provoke and maintain symptoms of fear. Dysfunctional appraisals of the meanings of PTSD symptoms (e.g., interpreting hypervigilance as a sign of personal weakness) may maintain the disorder. Poor integration of trauma memories into autobiographical memory serves as a second maintaining factor, with the isolation of these memories enhancing already strong connections to trauma-related stimuli and responding, increasing the potential for intrusive reexperiencing. This model provides the conceptual foundation for cognitive therapy for PTSD (Ehlers, Clark, Hackmann, McManus, and Fennell, 2005), including its active focus on changing negative trauma-related cognitions.

Dual representation theory (DRT; for a recent review, see Brewin, 2014) characterizes PTSD as a hybrid disorder reflecting pathological effects related to the storage of trauma memories in two separate but parallel memory systems. A conscious, episodic form, dubbed contextualized representations (C-reps), contains verbal and episodic memories, whereas an automatic, inflexible form, called sensation-near representations (S-reps), is linked to traumatic or intrusive experiences, such as flashbacks. Consolidation of the latter form of sensory memory is enhanced during the trauma, with a decrease in C-rep encoding and connections between the two systems. C-reps can be intentionally remembered but may be disorganized or underdeveloped, whereas S-reps are automatically triggered by a variety of trauma-related reminders, leading to distressing intrusive experiences. Per DRT, repeatedly rehearsing trauma images—a practice common to many efficacious therapies (described in the section on Empirically Supported Psychotherapies for PTSD)—results in strengthening of C-reps and reduced S-reps, thereby reducing PTSD symptoms.

EMOTIONAL PROCESSING THEORY

Foa and colleagues' emotional processing theory (EPT) provides a comprehensive framework for understanding the development, maintenance and treatment of pathological fear in PTSD and other anxiety disorders. First described in detail by Foa and Kozak (1986), EPT has been elaborated upon and expanded in numerous publications and books (Foa, Hembree, and Rothbaum, 2007; Foa, Steketee, and Rothbaum 1989; Rothbaum, 2006). EPT integrates learning and cognitive theories within an information-processing framework, specifically Lang's bioinformational model of fear (Lang, 1977). This model characterizes the representation of fear in memory (or "fear structure") as a network of associated representations of fear stimuli, responses to fear, and the meanings of these stimuli and responses. The attribution of a threat meaning to a stimulus and response gives rise to fear and fear-driven responding. This process applies equally to objectively unsafe scenarios in which fear would be a normal reaction (e.g., being confronted by a tiger) as to trauma-related triggers and situations (e.g., tires squealing for a car accident victim). EPT postulates that trauma memories are more likely to be disorganized and impoverished, due in part to disrupted information processing during the trauma itself.

The pathological level of fear seen in PTSD occurs when a traumatic event's representation in memory includes excessive response elements (e.g., hyperarousal), inaccurate associations between stimuli and responses (e.g., physiological and emotional distress cued by being out at night), and more globally inaccurate interpretations (e.g., "The world is an unsafe place"). Trauma memories have many stimulus-danger associations, resulting in fears of danger being evoked by a broad range of stimuli that may be only tangentially related to the trauma itself. The emotional and physiological effects of intrusive symptoms and evoked fear promote avoidance, which is negatively reinforced by reduction of fear, maintaining PTSD symptoms and the fear structure itself (Foa et al., 2006). That is, by avoiding feared stimuli that are objectively safe, including the memory of the trauma itself, individuals with PTSD never have the opportunity to learn that these situations are not dangerous, interrupting the natural recovery process. Negative trauma-related beliefs play a critical role in the development and maintenance of PTSD symptoms. Individual differences in pre-trauma schemas mean that trauma exposure may violate existing beliefs for some, and affirm them for others; critically, the rigidity and extremity of these responses is what impairs one's ability to cope. This helps to explain differential susceptibility to PTSD, and outlines a pathway whereby cognitive appraisals can generate or affirm schematic views of self and the world that maintain symptoms (particularly avoidance) and interfere with natural recovery (Foa et al., 2006). Consider, for example, a woman with PTSD stemming from a sexual assault by a colleague at an office party. She may experience chronic hypervigilance, and avoid returning to work or being around her co-workers, even in objectively safe situations, because of overwhelming feelings of fear (i.e., excessive response elements). She may become extremely upset in the presence of men, even those who do not resemble the perpetrator (i.e., inaccurate associations), leading to further avoidance and withdrawal. And she may come to hold beliefs reflecting self-blame and mistrust of all other people (i.e., inaccurate beliefs), resulting in social isolation and further emotional distress.

According to the EPT model, successful resolution of PTSD involves changes in both trauma memory records and schemas, along with a reduction in trauma-related fear. Changing the trauma memory involves activation of the fear structure and provision of disconfirming information, by way of repeated exposures to the fear memory. Fear memories are not erased or rewritten by successful treatment; rather, the individual develops a new association/structure, based on more accurate information and associated with less fearful responding, which may be activated in place of the trauma memory depending on context. The exposure process is thought to facilitate learning and schema change, by way of incorporating information about safety and personal mastery, as well as promoting extinction of fear responses (Foa, et al., 2007; Foa et al., 2006).

FEAR EXTINCTION AND INHIBITORY LEARNING

Recent translational models of fear extinction has resulted in a model emphasizing inhibitory learning (see chapter 25, this volume) as a mechanism of exposure therapies that is consistent with contemporary work on memory and neurobiology (for reviews, see Milad and Quirk, 2012; Vervliet, Craske, and Hermans, 2013). This transdiagnostic model applies broadly to all anxiety disorders and exposure treatments. Convergent findings from animal paradigms, clinical interventions, and analogue samples indicate that fears are fairly readily extinguished using exposure techniques, but extinction effects are difficult to maintain in the long-term. Extinguished fears can recur under a variety of conditions resulting in a return of symptoms and clinical relapse. Deficits in inhibitory learning may underlie differential susceptibility to developing anxiety disorders in general, and also explain treatment failures (Craske, Treanor, Conway, Zbozinek, and Vervliet, 2014). Because inhibitory associations developed during exposure can reduce the likelihood of fear recurrence, this model contends that exposure therapies should focus on strengthening these processes. An extensive animal and analogue literature provides fodder for specific, testable hypotheses as to how to enhance inhibitory learning, as outlined by Craske and colleagues (Craske et al., 2014), including varying stimuli and contexts and maintaining attentional focus. For example, a man with PTSD stemming from a motor vehicle accident might be encouraged to complete exposure exercises in a variety of vehicles and driving contexts (e.g., highway, night time, rush hour) to maximize the durability and strength of inhibitory learning and reduce the risk of spontaneous fear recurrence.

EMPIRICALLY SUPPORTED PSYCHOTHERAPIES FOR PTSD

We begin this section by describing several of the most well-studied psychotherapies for PTSD, before reviewing empirical findings concerning their efficacy. For a more comprehensive review of psychotherapeutic options not deemed to have empirical support at this time, as well as group/couples therapy options and emerging techniques see Youngner, Rothbaum, and Friedman (2014).

EXPOSURE THERAPY/PROLONGED EXPOSURE

Exposure therapies are first-line treatments for many anxiety disorders and are based on the general principle of approaching, rather than avoiding, feared but objectively safe stimuli for a therapeutic exposure. Prolonged exposure (PE) is among the most well-established and studied treatments for PTSD and is rooted in EPT as described in the preceding section (Foa et al., 2007). Standard PE includes psychoeducation about common responses to trauma, breathing relaxation training, emotional processing of traumatic material, and two kinds of exposure techniques: in vivo exposure and imaginal exposure. In vivo exposure involves repeatedly approaching external situations, places or activities that are objectively safe but that trigger trauma-related anxiety and fear in the patient. During between-session practices, patients are encouraged to remain in each exposure for a prolonged period of time, typically resulting in reduced anxiety within and across practices. In vivo exposures result in extinction of fear, are thought to provide disconfirming evidence to erroneous perceptions of danger, and foster a sense of competence. During imaginal exposure, patients are asked to retell repeatedly the story of their trauma, providing vivid detail about the events, thoughts and feelings that they experienced, and processing this exercise with their therapist afterward. By repeating the memory, patients learn that nothing bad happens when they think about their trauma, that they can tolerate the distress, and that their distress typically reduces across repetitions. In line with EPT, retelling their story also facilitates reorganization of the trauma memory and promotes changes to unhelpful trauma-related beliefs about the world, others and themselves (Foa et al., 2006; Foa et al., 2007).

COGNITIVE THERAPY/COGNITIVE PROCESSING THERAPY

Cognitive therapy for PTSD is aimed at helping patients to recognize the influence of their distorted beliefs and perceptions in maintaining PTSD symptoms, to identify trauma-related thoughts that can provoke negative emotional states, and to challenge these thoughts with more realistic and rational perspectives. Patients work in session and between sessions to identify automatic thoughts that are tied to strong emotional states, to consider alternative explanations and objective evidence, and to experiment with modifying their own behavior to test out or challenge negative beliefs (Ehlers et al., 2005). Cognitive processing therapy (CPT; Resick and Schnicke, 1993) is a particular cognitive approach originally developed for use with female sexual trauma victims. CPT begins with psychoeducation about PTSD, along with identification of unhelpful beliefs related to the trauma dubbed "stuck points." A second phase of treatment consists of the development of a narrative, written exposure aimed at challenging these negative beliefs; followed by a third phase involving cognitive restructuring techniques aimed at modifying "stuck points" into more reasonable ways of thinking. Recent studies of CPT have dropped the written narrative phase of treatment after a dismantling study suggested that its inclusion did not improve outcomes (Resick, 2013). Like other cognitive therapies, CPT emphasizes the need to change underlying negative beliefs. In particular, recovery from trauma is thought to reflect the need to respond to information that is inconsistent with previously held beliefs, by appropriately updating existing schemas to incorporate new information (accommodation), versus adopting overgeneralized negative views (over-accommodation) or struggling to accept the new information without changing one's beliefs (assimilation; Resick, and Schnike, 1993). For instance, a man who was the victim of a daylight robbery in a public, low-crime area must integrate this information with his prior beliefs (e.g., "Sometimes crimes can happen even under relatively safe circumstances"). He may have difficulties if he adopts overly negative views (e.g., "I can never be safe again") or comes to blame himself (e.g., "It was a safe neighborhood, so I must have done something foolish to make them target me.").

EYE MOVEMENT DESENSITIZATION AND REPROCESSING

Eye movement desensitization and reprocessing (EMDR) is typically classified as a cognitive behavioral treatment for PTSD because it includes CBT elements such as a focus on exposure to the trauma memory and cognitive restructuring (for a detailed review, see Shapiro, 2012). Like other CBT treatments described in this chapter, the EMDR protocol is structured and reflects a focus on processing of emotional memories and thoughts. However, in addition to CBT techniques, a core element of treatment and distinguishing feature of EMDR is the use of rapid saccadic eye movements or bilateral stimulation during retelling of a traumatic memory. These movements are typically achieved by having the patient track a therapist's finger, which is waved back and forth in front of her face. Such movements are theorized to override obstruction or neural blockage (Shapiro, 2012); however, this particular aspect of the treatment is controversial, as some studies find that EMDR may be efficacious even without the inclusion of these eye movements. We refer the interested reader to more detailed discussions of this controversy (e.g., Lee and Cuijpers, 2013; Spates and Rubin, 2012).

OTHER FORMS OF COGNITIVE-BEHAVIOR THERAPY AND EMPIRICALLY SUPPORTED TREATMENTS

Several other variants of CBT-based treatments have been shown to have some degree of empirical support for efficacy in the treatment of PTSD. Stress inoculation training (SIT) focuses on training patients to handle anxious feelings when confronted with trauma-related stimuli. SIT has received comparatively little attention as a monotherapy in randomized clinical trials. Combined CBT treatments have been investigated, commonly consisting of variants of the more well-established protocols (i.e., PE, CPT, EMDR) being evaluated in the context of dismantling studies aimed at identifying the "active ingredients" of these treatments. Recently, a meta-analysis of five studies showed efficacy for present-centered therapy (PCT), a psychological control condition originally developed to provide nonspecific psychotherapeutic elements minus the putative active ingredients of cognitive therapy (e.g., trauma-focus) as a comparison for RCTs (Frost, Laska, and Wampold, 2014). PCT outperformed other control conditions, and did not differ from other active treatments. However, as this is a recent publication, PCT has not generally been separated from other control conditions in major meta-analytic reviews, but further study is warranted.

SUMMARY OF EFFICACY AND EMPIRICAL SUPPORT FOR COGNITIVE-BEHAVIOR THERAPY TREATMENTS OF POSTTRAUMATIC STRESS DISORDER

Meta-analytic reviews of randomized clinical trials (RCTs) have consistently found that several different cognitive behavioral treatments (i.e., PE, CPT, CT, EMDR) achieve good outcomes. The average effect size for pretreatment to posttreatment PTSD symptom change in a recent meta-analysis including 54 studies of CBT treatments with 2,585 patients was $g = 1.26$ (95% C.I. 1.09–1.44; Watts, Schnurr, Mayo, Young-Xu, Weeks, and Friedman, 2013). Accordingly, most treatment guidelines for PTSD (e.g., IOM, 2008) recommend trauma-focused cognitive behavioral treatment for PTSD (Jonas et al., 2013), with some variability in strength of recommendation for specific treatments (see Table 10.1). The most recent comprehensive meta-analytic review (Jonas et al., 2013) reported effect sizes as well as strength of evidence for each treatment based on 101 published RCTs. Moderate strength of evidence was found for improvement in PTSD symptoms and loss of diagnosis with CPT, CT, EMDR, and mixed-CBT treatments, with higher evidence for exposure therapy. The overall effect size for pre–post symptom change was estimated at $d = 1.27$, and number needed to treat (NNT) to achieve one loss of PTSD diagnosis was four or less for many of these treatments. We briefly review evidence for the most commonly studied kinds of psychotherapy outlined here; Figures 10.1 and 10.2 depict outcomes from several large RCTs involving direct comparisons between one or more of these treatments.

Exposure therapy/PE. Exposure therapy (including PE) is considered the gold standard, first-line psychotherapy for PTSD, and it was the only treatment to demonstrate sufficient evidence for efficacy in the Institute of Medicine's (2008) treatment recommendations. Jonas et al. (2013) also concluded that exposure-based treatments had the best evidence of efficacy, with high strength of evidence in reduction of PTSD symptoms (standardized mean difference = -1.27) and depressive symptoms and moderate evidence for loss of PTSD diagnosis. Notably, PE has shown efficacy in treating a variety of populations and trauma types, including men and women, civilians and veterans, and populations with heterogeneous primary traumas (Powers, Halpern, Ferenschak, Gillihan, and Foa, 2010), and was numerically superior to other forms of exposure therapy (e.g., narrative exposure) in a recent meta-analysis (Watts et al., 2013). A meta-analysis focusing specifically on studies of PE ($k = 13$, $n = 675$) showed a large effect for PE versus control conditions on primary outcome measures at the end of acute treatment, with PE-treated patients improving better than 86% of those assigned to control conditions at posttreatment, and significant advantages maintained over follow-up (Powers et al., 2010). However, PE did not significantly outperform other active treatments (i.e., CPT, EMDR, CT or SIT), a finding that is consistent with results of other meta-analyses with broader inclusion criteria (e.g., Jonas et al., 2013; Watts et al., 2013). Recent variations of PE include virtual reality exposure therapy in which patients are asked to recount the memory of the traumatic event as in PE but with their eyes open and the therapist matching what they describe in virtual reality. A recent study found six sessions of virtual reality exposure therapy effective for veterans with PTSD (Rothbaum et al., 2014). Another recent variation is using exposure therapy within hours of trauma exposure in the emergency room. A recent trial found that it reduced the development of PTSD by half, even mitigating the genetic risk for PTSD (Rothbaum et al., in press).

Cognitive therapies/CPT. Cognitive therapies for PTSD are also supported by considerable empirical evidence and are recommended as a first level psychological treatment for PTSD by recent treatment guidelines. Although some prior studies have collapsed across all cognitive-based approaches, Jonas et al. (2013) separated studies based on those involving CPT (n = 4) versus non-CPT cognitive therapy (e.g., Ehlers et al., 2005; $n = 3$), with a third category for mixed-CBT treatments, including SIT ($n = 7$). Comparable effects with a moderate strength of evidence were reported across all three of these categories for change in PTSD and depressive symptoms as well as loss of PTSD diagnosis; Watts et al. (2013) also reported comparable pre–post effect sizes between CPT and other cognitive therapies. Concerning CPT in particularly, early empirical support was primarily for female sexual assault survivors, as this was the population for which it was developed; however, subsequent studies have been conducted with veterans, refugee populations, and in non-Western countries (see Resick, 2013, for a review).

EMDR. Meta-analytic reviews suggest that EMDR is an efficacious treatment for PTSD that is generally found to be comparable to other CBT approaches (e.g., Jonas

TABLE 10.1 Recommendation Status of Key Empirically Supported Psychotherapies for PTSD per Leading Clinical Guidelines

GUIDELINE	VA/DOD	APA	NICE	NHMRC	ISTSS	IOM
Publication Year and Country	2004, USA	2004, USA	2005, UK	2007, Australia	2008, International	2008, USA
Description of Level 1 Recommendation	A strong recommendation that the intervention is always indicated and acceptable	Recommended with substantial clinical confidence	At least one RCT as part of a body of literature of overall good quality and consistency	Body of evidence can be trusted to guide practice	Based on randomized, well-controlled clinical trials	Evidence is sufficient to conclude efficacy
Description of Level 2 Recommendation	A recommendation that the intervention may be useful/effective	Recommended with moderate clinical confidence	Well-conducted clinical studies but no RCT . . . or extrapolated from RCT evidence	Body of evidence can be trusted to guide practice in most situations	Based on well-designed clinical studies, without randomization or placebo comparison	Evidence is suggestive but not sufficient to conclude efficacy

STATUS OF TREATMENTS

	VA/DOD	APA	NICE	NHMRC	ISTSS	IOM
TFCBT	Level 1	Level 1	Level 1	Level 1	Level 1	Level 1
EMDR	Level 1	Level 2	Level 1	Level 1[a]	Level 1	Level 2
SIT	Level 1	Level 2	—	Level 2	Level 1	—

[a]Level 1 recommendation when combined with *in vivo* exposure.

Note: TFCBT = trauma-focused CBT (includes exposure and cognitive therapies); EMDR = eye movement desensitization and reprocessing; SIT = stress inoculation therapy; VA/DoD = Veterans Affairs/Department of Defense; APA = American Psychiatric Association; NICE = National Institute of Clinical Excellence; NHMRC = National Health and Medical Research Council; ISTSS = International Society for Traumatic Stress Studies; IOM = Institute of Medicine; RCT = randomized controlled trial. Citations for clinical guidelines can be found in Forbes et al., (2010).

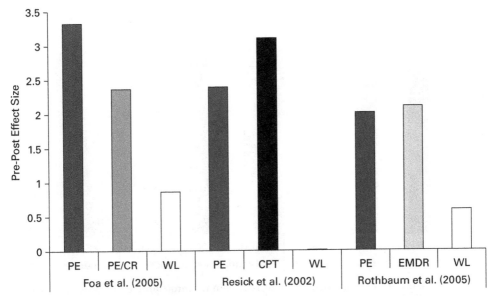

FIGURE 10.1 Pre–post effect size of PTSD symptom change by condition for three large RCTs.

Note: CPT = cognitive processing therapy; EMDR = eye movement desensitization and reprocessing; PE = pro-longed exposure; PE/CR = prolonged exposure plus cognitive restructuring; WL = wait-list; PTSD = posttrau-matic stress disorder. Effect size represents change in primary PTSD symptom measure (clinician-rated) among treatment completers in Foa et al. (2005) (PTSD Symptom Scale—Interview [PSS-I]; N = 120), Resick et al. (2002) (Clinician Administered PTSD Scale [CAPS]; N = 121), and Rothbaum et al. (2005, cited in Forbes et al., 2010) (CAPS; N = 60). Effect size calculated after Foa et al. (2005, cited in Forbes et al., 2010) as $ES = (M_{pre} - M_{post})/SD_{pooled}$ where $SD_{pooled} = \sqrt{((SD_{pre}^2 + SD_{post}^2)/2)}$.

et al., 2013; Watts et al., 2013). Accordingly, most treatment guidelines identify EMDR as a first-line psychotherapeutic option (Jonas et al., 2013), but this is not uniformly the case (see Table 10.1); for instance, the IOM report (2008) failed to find adequate criteria by which to support EMDR versus other treatments. A recent review of seven EMDR studies showed clear evidence of superiority to control conditions, with mixed but gener-ally comparable findings versus exposure (Spates and Rubin, 2012). Controversy remains regarding the necessity of the eye saccade component of EMDR, as some studies have shown that it may be efficacious without their inclusion. A recent meta-analysis includ-ing clinical and experimental samples (Lee and Cuijpers, 2013) concluded there was a modest effect on outcome based on the inclusion of saccadic movements but the effect in clinical samples was small ($d = .27$).

CURRENT ISSUES AND FUTURE DIRECTIONS

Despite evidence that multiple forms of psychotherapy are efficacious in the treatment of PTSD, many individuals fail to respond to treatment or are lost to attrition. Nonresponse rates in RCTs or open clinical trials have been as high as 50%, with attrition or drop-out rates reaching comparable levels in some samples (Schottenbauer, Glass, Arnkoff, Tendick, and Gray, 2008). In a recent meta-analysis of RCTs for PTSD, the average dropout rate was 18%, with estimates varying substantially across studies but no sig-nificant differences between active treatments (Imel, Laska, Jacupcak, and Simpson,

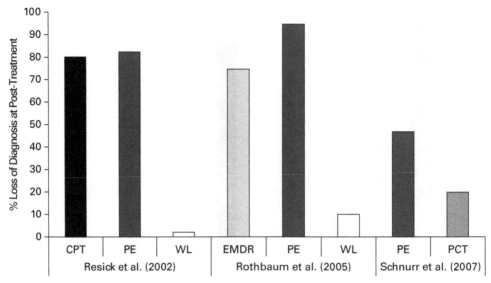

FIGURE 10.2 Loss of PTSD diagnosis at posttreatment for three large RCTs. *Note:* CPT = cognitive processing therapy; EMDR = eye movement desensitization and reprocessing; PCT = present-centered therapy; PE = prolonged exposure; WL = wait-list; PTSD = posttraumatic stress disorder; RCT = randomized clinical trial. PTSD diagnostic status assessed at posttreatment among treatment completers using primary PTSD symptom measure (clinician-rated) in Resick et al. (2002) (CAPS; N = 121), and Rothbaum et al. (2005) (CAPS; N = 60) and Schnurr et al. (2007) (CAPS; N = 194) (cited in Forbes et al., 2010).

2013). Predictors of nonresponse and dropout are not consistent across studies, although motivational issues, symptom severity and comorbidity are commonly identified factors across treatments for anxiety disorders (Taylor, Ambramowitz, and McKay, 2012). Concerns about these issues are superimposed on the larger pragmatic challenge of disseminating and ensuring access to empirically supported treatments, with complicated barriers such as lack of clinician training in these techniques, as well as resistance and opposition to the use of empirically supported therapies in general (Foa, Gillihan, and Bryant, 2013). Persistent misconceptions about inherent risk to patients or providers resulting from trauma-focused approaches remain a continual challenge to efforts to disseminate, even in the face of evidence that treatment-related PTSD symptom worsening is, to quote a recent paper, "nonexistent" (Jayawickreme et al., 2014).

Therapeutic nonresponse, attrition, and relapse all pose substantial challenges to the existing treatments, leading to a variety of efforts to augment or modify conventional therapies in the aim of improving outcome. Dismantling studies or modified protocols offer the prospect of refining existing treatments, such as efforts to identify sufficient duration of imaginal exposure techniques in PE (Foa and McLean, 2014) or utility of written narratives in CPT (Resick, 2013). There is a growing literature on emerging techniques aimed at enhancing outcomes of first-line psychotherapy treatments (see Youngner et al., 2014). Studies of medication-enhanced psychotherapy combine pharmacological and psychotherapeutic interventions have recently been the focus of considerable attention, particularly with pharmacological interventions (dubbed *cognitive enhancers*) targeting agents to enhance exposure-based therapies, in line with the fear inhibition learning and neurobiological models described earlier. Several compounds show promise in translational studies, early clinical research, and a few RCTs (Rothbaum et al., 2014), with the most evidence for d-cycloserine, and emerging lines of research for other compounds (e.g., yohimbine and methylene blue; Youngner et al., 2014).

Alternative methods of treatment delivery modify how patients can participate in treatment (e.g., via internet; in group or family format). For example, virtual reality exposure therapy uses conventional exposure techniques augmented with virtual environments to enhance the impact of exposures. This approach has primarily been used with veterans, with a focus on facilitating more vivid, multi-sensory exposures to combat-related trauma scenarios (Youngner et al., 2014). There are also ongoing efforts to evaluate early interventions with trauma victims to prevent development of PTSD (see Kearns, Ressler, Zatzick, and Rothbaum, 2012) as described earlier.

CONCLUSIONS

An incredible expansion of clinical research on PTSD in the last two decades has resulted in substantial advances in our understanding of its etiology, development, maintenance and effective treatment. Nevertheless, critical areas remain in need of continued study, including symptom heterogeneity and conceptual overlap between PTSD and other disorders. Contemporary psychological models of PTSD offer insights into the potential active ingredients of efficacious trauma-focused cognitive behavioral treatment, and the need for improved clinical outcomes (particularly in terms of engagement, nonresponse, dropout, and relapse) drives development of promising novel treatments. The next decade of PTSD research offers incredible potential to reduce trauma's impact on individuals and society.

DISCLOSURE STATEMENT

Dr. Rothbaum is a consultant to and owns equity in Virtually Better, Inc. that creates virtual environments; however, Virtually Better did not create the Virtual Iraq environment described in this chapter. The terms of this arrangement has been reviewed and approved by Emory University in accordance with its conflict-of interest policies.

REFERENCES

American Psychiatric Association. (2013). *Diagnostic and statistical manual of mental disorders (5th ed.).* Arlington, VA: American Psychiatric Publishing.

Beck, A.T., Emery, G., and Greenberg, R.L. (1985). *Anxiety disorders and phobias: A cognitive perspective.* New York, NY: Basic Books.

Breslau, N. (2009). The epidemiology of trauma, PTSD, and other posttrauma disorders. *Trauma Violence Abuse, 10,* 198–210.

Brewin, C.R. (2014). Episodic memory, perceptual memory and their interaction: Foundations for a theory of posttraumatic stress disorder. *Psychol Bull, 140,* 69–97.

Brewin, C. R., Andrews, B., and Valentine, J. D. (2000). Meta- analysis of risk factors for posttraumatic stress disorder in trauma-exposed adults. *J Consult Clin Psychol, 68,* 748–766.

Craske, M. G., Treanor, M., Conway, C. C., Zbozinek, T., and Vervliet, B. (2014). Maximizing exposure therapy: An inhibitory learning approach. *Behav Res Ther, 58,* 10–23.

Dalgleish, T. (2004). Cognitive approaches to posttraumatic stress disorder: The evolution of multirepresentational theorizing. *Psychol Bull, 130,* 228–260.

DiGangi, J. A., Gomez, D., Mendoza, L., Jason, L. A., Keys, C. B., and Koenen, K. C. (2013). Pretrauma risk factors for posttraumatic stress disorder: A systematic review of the literature. *Clin Psychol Rev, 33,* 728–744.

Ehlers, A., and Clark, D. M. (2000). A cognitive model of posttraumatic stress disorder. *Behav Res Ther*, 38, 319–345.

Ehlers, A., Clark, D. M., Hackmann, A., McManus, F., and Fennell, M. (2005). Cognitive therapy for post-traumatic stress disorder: Development and evaluation. *Behav Res and Ther*, 43, 413–431.

Foa, E. B., Gillihan, S. J., and Bryant, R. A. (2013). Challenges and successes in dissemination of evidence-based treatments for posttraumatic stress: Lessons learned from prolonged exposure therapy for PTSD. *Psychol Sci Public Interest*, 14, 65–111.

Foa, E. B. Hembree, E. A., and Rothbaum, B. O. (2007). *Prolonged exposure therapy for PTSD: Emotional processing of traumatic experiences*. New York, NY: Oxford University Press.

Foa, E. B., Huppert, J. D., and Cahill, S. P. (2006). Emotional processing theory: An update. In B. O. Rothbaum (Ed.), *Pathological anxiety: Emotional processing in etiology and treatment* (pp. 3–24). New York, NY: Guilford.

Foa, E., and Kozak, M. (1986). Emotional processing of fear: Exposure to corrective information. *Psychol Bull*, 99, 20–35.

Foa, E.B. and McLean, C.P. (2014). Therapeutic recovery. In L.A. Zoellner and N.C. Feeny (Eds.), *Facilitating resilience and recovery following trauma* (pp.41–66). New York, NY: Guilford.

Foa, E. B., Steketee, G., and Rothbaum, B. O. (1989). Behavioral/cognitive conceptualizations of post-traumatic stress disorder. *Behav Ther*, 20 (2), 155–176.

Forbes, D., M. Creamer, J. I. Bisson, J. A. Cohen, B. E. Crow, E. B. Foa, ... R. J. Ursano. (2010). A guide to guidelines for the treatment of PTSD and related conditions. *J Traumatic Stress*, 23(5):537–552.

Friborg, O., Martinussen, M., Kaiser, S., Øvergård, K. T., and Rosenvinge, J. H. (2013). Comorbidity of personality disorders in anxiety disorders: A meta-analysis of 30 years of research. *J Affect Disorders*, 145, 143–155.

Frost, N. D., Laska, K. M., and Wampold, B. E. (2014). The evidence for present-centered therapy as a treatment for posttraumatic stress disorder. *J Trauma Stress*, 27, 1–8.

Galatzer-Levy, I. R., and Bryant, R. A. (2013). 636,120 ways to have posttraumatic stress disorder. *Perspect Psychol Sci*, 50, 161–180.

Greenberg, P. E., Sisitsky, T., Kessler, R. C., Finkelstein, S. N., Berndt, E. R., Davidson, J. R., ... and Fyer, A. J. (1999). The economic burden of anxiety disorders in the 1990s. *J Clin Psychiatry*, 60, 427–435.

Hoge, C. W., Riviere, L. A., Wilk, J. E., Herrell, R. K., and Weathers, F. W. (2014). The prevalence of post-traumatic stress disorder (PTSD) in US combat soldiers: A head-to-head comparison of DSM-5 versus DSM-IV-TR symptom criteria with the PTSD checklist. *Lancet Psychiatry*. Advance online publication. DOI: 10.1016/S2215-0366(14)70235-4

Jonas, D. E., Cusack, K., Forneris, C. A., Wilkins, T. M, Sonis J., Middleton J. C., ...Gaynes, B. N. (2013). Psychological and pharmacological treatments for adults with posttraumatic stress disorder (PTSD). *Comparative Effectiveness Review No. 92*. Rockville, MD: Agency for Healthcare Research and Quality.

Imel, Z. E., Laska, K., Jakupcak, M., and Simpson, T. L. (2013). Meta-analysis of dropout in treatments for posttraumatic stress disorder. *J Consult Clin Psychol*, 81, 394–404.

Institute of Medicine (IOM). (2008). *Treatment of posttraumatic stress disorder: An assessment of the evidence*. Washington, DC: The National Academies Press.

Jayawickreme, N., Cahill, S. P., Riggs, D. S., Rauch, S. A., Resick, P. A., Rothbaum, B. O., and Foa, E. B. (2014). Primum non nocere (first do no harm): Symptom worsening and improvement in female assault victims after prolonged exposure for PTSD. *Depress Anxiety*, 31, 412–419.

Kearns, M. C., Ressler, K. J., Zatzick, D., and Rothbaum, B. O. (2012). Early interventions for PTSD: A review. *Depress Anxiety*, 29, 833–842.

Kessler, R. C., Sonnega, A., Bromet, E., Hughes, M., and Nelson, C. B. (1995). Posttraumatic stress disorder in the National Comorbidity Survey. *Arch Gen Psychiatry*, 52, 1048–1060.

Lang, P. J. (1977). Imagery in therapy: An information processing analysis of fear. *Behav Therapy*, 8, 862–886.

Lee, C. W., and Cuijpers, P. (2013). A meta-analysis of the contribution of eye movements in processing emotional memories. *J Behav Ther Exp Psychiatry*, 44, 231–239.

Milad, M. R., and Quirk, G. J. (2012). Fear extinction as a model for translational neuroscience: Ten years of progress. *Ann Rev Psychol*, *63*, 129–151.

Mowrer, O. (1947). On the dual nature of learning—A re-interpretation of "conditioning" and "problem-solving." *Harvard Ed Rev*, *17*, 102–148.

Ozer, E. J., Best, S. R., Lipsey, T. L., and Weiss, D. S. (2003). Predictors of posttraumatic stress disorder and symptoms in adults: A meta-analysis. *Psychol Bull*, *129*, 52–73.

Pacella, M. L., Hruska, B., and Delahanty, D. L. (2013). The physical health consequences of PTSD and PTSD symptoms: A meta-analytic review. *Journal of Anxiety Disorders*, *27*, 33–46.

Pietrzak, R. H., Goldstein, R. B., Southwick, S. M., and Grant, B. F. (2011). Prevalence and Axis I comorbidity of full and partial posttraumatic stress disorder in the United States: Results from Wave 2 of the National Epidemiologic Survey on Alcohol and Related Conditions. *Journal of Anxiety Disorders*, *25*, 456–465.

Powers, M. B., Halpern, J. M., Ferenschak, M. P., Gillihan, S. J., and Foa, E. B. (2010). A meta-analytic review of prolonged exposure for posttraumatic stress disorder. *Clinical Psychology Review*, *30*, 635–641.

Resick, P. A. (2013, Fall). Cognitive processing therapy. *APA Division 56 Trauma Psychology Newsletter*, 11–14.

Resick, P. A., and Schnicke, M. K. (1993). *Cognitive processing therapy for sexual assault victims: A treatment manual*. Newbury Park, CA: Sage Publications.

Rodriguez, P., Holowka, D. W., and Marx, B. P. (2012). Assessment of posttraumatic stress disorder-related functional impairment: A review. *Journal of Rehabilitation Research and Development*, *49*, 649–666.

Rothbaum, B. O., Editor. (2006). *Pathological anxiety: Emotional processing in etiology and treatment of anxiety*. Guilford: New York.

Rothbaum, B. O., Foa, E. B., Riggs, D. S., Murdock, T., and Walsh, W. (1992). A prospective examination of post-traumatic stress disorder in rape victims. *Journal of Traumatic Stress*, *5*, 455–475.

Rothbaum, B. O., Kearns, M. C., Reiser, E., Davis, J., Kerley, K. A., Rothbaum, A. O., . . . and Ressler, K. J. (in press). Early intervention following trauma mitigates genetic risk for PTSD in civilians: A prospective, emergency department study. Accepted for publication in *Journal of Clinical Psychiatry*.

Rothbaum, B. O., Price, M., Jovanovic, T., Norrholm, S., Gerardi, M., Dunlop, B., . . . Ressler, K. (2014). A randomized, double-blind evaluation of d-cycloserine or alprazolam combined with virtual reality exposure therapy for posttraumatic stress disorder (PTSD) in OEF/OIF war veterans. *American Journal of Psychiatry*, *171*(6), 640–648.

Schottenbauer, M. A., Glass, C. R., Arnkoff, D. B., Tendick, V., and Gray, S. H. (2008). Nonresponse and dropout rates in outcome studies on PTSD: Review and methodological considerations. *Psychiatry: Interpersonal and Biological Processes*, *71*, 134–168.

Shapiro, F. (2012). EMDR therapy: An overview of current and future research. *European Review of Applied Psychology*, *62*, 193–195.

Spates, C. R., and Rubin, S. (2012). Empirically supported psychological treatments: EMDR. In J. G Beck, and D. M. Sloan (Eds.), *The Oxford handbook of traumatic stress disorders*. (pp. 449–462). New York, NY: Oxford University Press.

Taylor, S., Abramowitz, J. S., and McKay, D. (2012). Non-adherence and non-response in the treatment of anxiety disorders. *Journal of Anxiety Disorders*, *26*, 583–589.

Vervliet, B., Craske, M. G., and Hermans, D. (2013). Fear extinction and relapse: State of the art. *Annual Review of Clinical Psychology*, *9*, 215–248.

Walker, E. A., Katon, W., Russo, J., Ciechanowski, P., Newman, E., and Wagner, A. W. (2003). Health care costs associated with posttraumatic stress disorder symptoms in women. *Archives of General Psychiatry*, *60*, 369–374.

Watts, B. V., Schnurr, P. P., Mayo, L., Young-Xu, Y., Weeks, W. B., and Friedman, M. J. (2013). Meta-analysis of the efficacy of treatments for posttraumatic stress disorder. *Journal of Clinical Psychiatry*, *74*, e541–e550.

Youngner, C. G., Rothbaum, B. O., and Friedman, M. J. (2014). PTSD. In G. Gabbard (Ed.), *Gabbard's treatments of psychiatric disorders* (5th ed., pp. 539–566). Washington, DC: American Psychiatric Press.

OBSESSIVE COMPULSIVE AND DISORDERS OF CORTICAL-STRIATAL PROCESSING

/// 11 /// DISSECTING OCD CIRCUITS: FROM ANIMAL MODELS TO TARGETED TREATMENTS

SUSANNE E. AHMARI AND
DARIN D. DOUGHERTY

INTRODUCTION

Obsessive compulsive disorder (OCD) is a chronic, severe mental illness with up to 2–3% prevalence worldwide (Kessler, Berglund, et al., 2005). In fact, the World Health Organization has classified OCD as one of the world's 10 leading causes of illness-related disability, largely because of the chronic nature of disabling symptoms (Koran, 2000). Despite the severity and high prevalence of OCD, there is still relatively limited understanding of its pathophysiology. However, this is rapidly changing due to development of powerful technologies that can be used to dissect the neural circuits underlying pathologic behaviors. In this chapter, we will describe recent technical advances that have allowed neuroscientists to start identifying circuits underlying complex repetitive behaviors using animal model systems. We also review current surgical and stimulation-based treatments for OCD that target circuit dysfunction; pharmacotherapeutic and psychotherapeutic treatments will be covered in a companion chapter (chapter 12, Simpson and Foa). Finally, we discuss how findings from animal models may be applied in the clinical arena to help inform and refine targeted brain stimulation-based treatment approaches.

CLINICAL FEATURES OF OCD

Despite recent changes to the *Diagnostic and Statistical Manual* (DSM-5), core clinical features of OCD remain the same. Specifically, OCD is characterized by obsessions, which are recurrent intrusive thoughts, images, or impulses; and compulsions, which are repetitive mental or behavioral rituals. Obsessions and compulsions cause significant distress, are time-consuming, and interfere with patients' ability to function. Though OCD is no longer classified as an anxiety disorder in DSM-5, obsessions are frequently associated with significant distress, and compulsions are often performed with conscious intent to reduce obsession-associated anxiety. Further details are provided in chapter 12, but an example is an intrusive thought about the house burning down leading to ritualized checking to make sure the stove is off. While rituals can provide temporary anxiety relief, it is important to note that performing compulsions is actually believed to strengthen dysfunctional neural circuits that underlie OCD, leading to persistence of symptoms and overall long-term increased anxiety.

Though clinical presentation is covered in detail in chapter 12, several key features are important for understanding OCD neurobiology. Specifically, both clinical and neurobiological evidence indicates that OCD is a heterogeneous disorder, though different metrics for subdividing the illness have been proposed and this is an active area of research. First, there is evidence that tic-related OCD is a biologically distinct entity, with increased prevalence in males, different neurochemical features, distinct striatal pathophysiology, and earlier age of onset (Baxter, Schwartz, et al., 1988). Similarly, there have been suggestions that some childhood-onset OCD may correspond to a distinct subtype with different genetic and environmental underpinnings. In addition, there is significant variation in level of insight both between different OCD patients and within patients throughout their illness course (Leckman, Denys, et al., 2010); specifiers are now included in DSM-5 to reflect this spectrum. Finally, there are indications that differences in specific content of obsessions and compulsions may reflect distinct neurobiological substrates. This is most clearly demonstrated for hoarding, which is therefore now considered a separate disorder in DSM-5.

ETIOLOGY OF OCD

Though our understanding of OCD's etiology is limited, current evidence implicates both genetic and environmental factors. In the next section, we will briefly describe some of the genetic factors and pharmacological approaches that have links to circuit dissection in animal models.

Genetic Dissection

Evidence from both twin and family studies supports a role for genetics in OCD. Genetic vulnerability may be even greater in pediatric-onset OCD, since there is more heritability in this group (Pauls, 2008). Candidate gene studies have focused on serotonin, glutamate, and dopamine-associated genes, because of the hypothesized roles of these neurotransmitters in OCD. More recently, genome-wide linkage and association studies have provided several candidates, although in general OCD genome-wide association studies have been underpowered; definitive genome-wide candidates therefore have yet to be fully elucidated (Taylor, 2013).

SLC1A1. To date, the only consistently replicated genetic finding in OCD is an association with the neuronal glutamate transporter *SLC1A1* (protein: EAAT3 or EAAC1) (Wu, Hanna, et al., 2012). Findings cluster in the 3′ region, with most evidence for association with the rs301430C allele. In cell models and brain tissue, this allele is associated with increased *SLC1A1* expression, suggesting that overexpression contributes to OCD susceptibility. Coding variants are very rare (3/1400 subjects screened) and do not clearly segregate with OCD. Thus, noncoding polymorphisms most likely account for the association of *SLC1A1* with OCD.

Though SLC1A1 knockout mice do not demonstrate clear OCD-relevant phenotypes, they have not yet been screened in targeted behavioral tests. In addition, it is likely that brain-wide deletion is less relevant to OCD pathophysiology than targeted alteration of expression. Ongoing studies are therefore investigating whether tissue-specific manipulations of *SLC1A1* may be more relevant to the human clinical phenotype. Examining the outcome of targeted expression changes in specific neural circuits will allow us to directly address the molecular, cellular, and behavioral impact of this OCD candidate gene.

GRIN2B. Less consistently, association studies have implicated *GRIN2B*, which encodes the NR2B subunit of the NMDA glutamate receptor (Arnold, Rosenberg et al., 2004; Wu, Hanna, et al., 2012), in OCD. Further support for its role in OCD is provided by magnetic resonance spectroscopy studies in OCD patients showing an association between GRIN2B polymorphisms and glutamatergic concentrations in anterior cingulate cortex (ACC). NR2B is an important mediator of synaptic plasticity, since its incorporation into NMDA receptors renders them more calcium-permeable. However, even partial NR2B deficits throughout the brain lead to significant abnormalities in global functioning, since NMDA receptors are essential for basic neurobiological functions necessary for learning and memory. In fact, constitutive NR2B knockout mice have an early postnatal lethal phenotype due to impaired suckling (Kutsuwada, Sakimura, et al., 1996). It is therefore likely that NR2B functional abnormalities in specific brain regions account for the genetic association with OCD; this can now be tested using tissue-specific transgenic mouse models combined with OCD-relevant behavioral tasks.

Pharmacologic Dissection

Serotonin-1B Receptor (5-HT1B). Several lines of evidence suggest that abnormalities in 5-HT1B receptor function (5-HT1D in human literature) play a role in OCD (Hemmings & Stein, 2006), including pharmacological challenge studies and some genetic association studies that provide tentative aggregate support. In addition, studies in mice demonstrate that administration of a 5-HT1B agonist leads to OCD-relevant perseverative locomotion and prepulse inhibition deficits, both of which are reversed with chronic, but not acute, fluoxetine treatment. Further studies have localized the responsible receptors to the orbitofrontal cortex (OFC), demonstrating the utility of pharmacological dissection of neural circuits for understanding OCD pathophysiology.

NEURAL CIRCUITS ASSOCIATED WITH OCD

Despite the need for further studies regarding genetic and environmental causes of OCD, we have a relatively good sense of the involved neural circuits through application of modern neuroimaging technology. Over the past 20 years, functional and structural imaging has led to discovery of aberrant neural circuits in OCD. Despite some discrepancies, particularly regarding directionality of findings (which may be dependent on developmental stage assessed), there is remarkable convergence of neuroanatomy, circuit function, and OCD neurochemistry findings collectively implicating cortico–striato–thalamo–cortical (CSTC) circuits in OCD pathophysiology. We describe this evidence in detail.

Cortico-striato-thalamo-cortical circuit function. CSTC circuits have been implicated in many higher order cognitive functions, including inhibition of impulsive behavior, action selection/modulation of motor activity, and attentional allocation. Anatomical studies in humans and nonhuman primates demonstrate that CSTC circuits are composed of multiple parallel and interconnected loops that connect frontocortical and subcortical brain areas (Parent and Hazrati, 1995). These loops are composed of (1) glutamatergic corticostriatal projections synapsing onto striatal spiny projection neurons and/or interneurons, (2) GABAergic spiny projection neurons targeting basal ganglia output structures (globus pallidus pars internalis [GPi] and substantia nigra pars reticulata [SNr]), (3) GABAergic output neurons from GPi/SNr projecting to thalamic regions, and (4) glutamatergic neurons from thalamus projecting back to cortex. Within striatum, spiny projection neurons can connect to GPi/SNr through either the direct (striatonigral) or indirect (striatopallidal) pathways. In a simplified framework, these anatomically distinct pathways have been thought to oppose each other, resulting in net inhibition of thalamus via activation of the indirect pathway, or net disinhibition (i.e. overall excitation) by activation of the direct pathway (Figure 11.1). However, recent data have suggested this picture is more complex, indicating that (a) direct and indirect basal ganglia pathways may both be simultaneously active during sequence initiation (Jin, Tecuapetla, et al., 2014), and (b) bridging collaterals between direct and indirect pathways may permit modulation of information transmission through CSTC circuits (Cazorla, de Carvalho, et al., 2014).

In general, it is thought that different CSTC loops may be responsible for dictating particular motor and cognitive functions. Evidence from functional imaging studies suggests that selectivity is determined by the specific frontocortical area included in the loop (Pennartz, Berke, et al., 2009). Multiple models have been proposed suggesting that interplay between frontocortical areas and the basal ganglia determines which actions

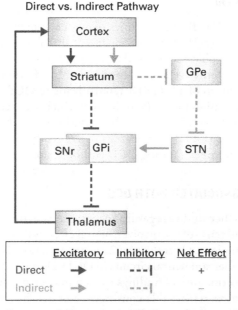

FIGURE 11.1 Schematic diagram of direct versus indirect pathway. The simplified diagram shows the direct and indirect pathways through the cortex and basal ganglia; thalamo-striatal projections and reciprocal connections between striatum and cortex are not shown for simplicity. Direct pathway is represented by dark grey; indirect pathway is represented by light grey. Direct pathway exerts a net excitatory effect on thalamic output to the cortex, while indirect pathway exerts a net inhibitory effect. GPi: globus pallidus interna; GPe: globus pallidus externa; STN: subthalamic nucleus; SNr: substantia nigra pars reticulata.

are selected, and which are screened out as maladaptive. A popular model suggests that changing the balance of activity between direct and indirect pathways can either promote or inhibit the selection of appropriate behavior sequences (Jin, Tecuapetla, et al., 2014). According to this theory, both excessive selection of actions or dysfunction in screening out maladaptive behavior sequences could potentially lead to OCD symptoms.

Structural neuroimaging, Although exact findings have varied across studies, structural abnormalities in CSTC circuits involving orbitofrontal cortex (OFC), anterior cingulate cortex (ACC), and striatum have been repeatedly demonstrated in OCD (Pittenger, Bloch, et al., 2011; Rodman, Milad, et al., 2012). The largest structural MRI study to date reported reduced OFC gray matter and increased gray matter in the highly connected ventral striatum. In addition, a recent meta-analysis reported reduced volumes of left ACC and bilateral OFC, and increased thalamic volumes bilaterally, but no differences in basal ganglia volumes relative to control samples. However, another meta-analysis demonstrated changes in basal ganglia (i.e. increased bilateral caudate gray matter volume) as well as decreased bilateral ACC volume, in OCD patients. Thus, structural imaging studies in OCD have collectively demonstrated changes in ACC, OFC, and striatal volume despite some inconsistencies across studies.

Functional neuroimaging, Similar to findings from structural studies, OFC, ACC, and caudate (specifically the head) have likewise been implicated in OCD using functional PET and fMRI; functional studies also highlight anterior thalamus. These brain regions are linked by well-described neuroanatomical connections (Pittenger, Bloch, et al., 2011). Notably, OCD subjects demonstrate hyperactivity in these areas both at rest and with symptom provocation, though OFC shows the most robust activation. In further support of the role of this regional hyperactivity in symptom generation, most studies have found that successful SRI or cognitive behavioral therapy treatment was associated with reduced activity in OFC or caudate, with decreased ACC activity being less prominent.

Cognitive activation studies, Based on the theory that circuit dysfunction in particular mental illnesses may only be unmasked during performance of neurocognitive tasks, there has been a recent shift toward performing OCD imaging studies during cognitive activation paradigms. Many tasks have been used, though executive functions have been particularly emphasized (Maia, Cooney, et al., 2008). First, several studies have shown hyperactivity of dorsal ACC (dACC) in OCD patients during performance of tasks involving error monitoring and/or conflict resolution, suggesting that dACC and connected regions might function differently in OCD (Milad and Rauch, 2012); these findings correlate well with baseline functional studies. In addition, other studies have used Go/NoGo tasks to assess inhibitory control in OCD, and though the directionality of results is in conflict, both studies report altered activation of OFC (Elliott, Agnew, et al., 2010: increased; Roth, Saykin, et al., 2007: decreased). Similarly, greater frontostriatal activation has been demonstrated in unmedicated OCD patients during engagement of control and conflict resolution on the Simon task (Marsh, Maia, et al., 2009). Overall, these findings support the idea that cortical-basal ganglia circuits are dysfunctional in OCD, and may contribute to symptom generation.

WORKING MODELS OF OCD PATHOPHYSIOLOGY

By synthesizing the studies reviewed, several models of OCD pathophysiology have been proposed (Saxena, Bota, et al., 2001; Ting and Feng, 2011). Though models differ in details, they consistently share the idea that obsessions and compulsions somehow result from malfunctioning neural circuits that include OFC, ACC, caudate, and anterior thalamus (Figure 11.2). The specific regions involved may depend on the particular OCD subtype. For example, based on PET studies, it has been proposed that different OCD symptom dimensions (e.g., symmetry/ordering vs. washing/cleaning) may have different underlying neural substrates within CSTC circuits (Mataix-Cols, Rosario-Campos, et al., 2005). Thus, different OCD subtypes could have distinct core neurobiologic deficits leading to differences in both neuroimaging findings and neurocognitive task performance.

In line with this vein of thinking, evidence from recent human studies suggests that OCD patients have dysfunction in core neural processes mapped onto CSTC circuits, such as response inhibition(van Velzen, Vriend, et al., 2014) and sensorimotor gating (Ahmari, Risbrough, et al., 2012). In addition, a group of studies that examined the balance between goal-directed versus habitual behavior in OCD patients is particularly interesting. Although the ways in which goal-directed and habitual performance cooperate and/or interfere with each other in healthy subjects is still an area of active investigation (see Balleine and O'Doherty, 2010, for comprehensive review), there is growing evidence that patients with OCD are biased to perform habits, sometimes at the expense of goal-directed actions (Gillan, Papmeyer, et al., 2011). Interestingly, this bias toward increased habit formation in OCD not only applies to appetitive habits, it also extends to avoidant habits that may be more relevant to the clinical symptoms seen in patients. Though it is challenging in general to make direct links between dysfunctional neural

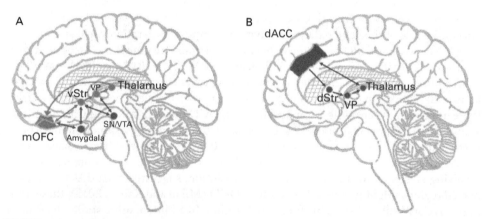

FIGURE 11.2 Cortical-basal ganglia circuits implicated in OCD pathophysiology. Both structural and functional imaging studies provide evidence that orbitofrontal cortex (OFC), anterior cingulate cortex (ACC), caudate, and anterior thalamus are involved in OCD pathophysiology. (A) A circuit linking medial OFC (mOFC), ventral striatum (vStr), ventral pallidum (VP), and thalamus is thought to be involved in OCD pathology. This circuit has classically been associated with attribution of value to the outcome of particular actions to facilitate reward learning. Evidence from both stereotactic ablation and deep brain stimulation (DBS) studies indicates that interrupting this dysfunctional circuit can decrease symptoms in OCD patients. Links between this circuit and amygdala provide opportunities for regulation of activity by affect. Dopaminergic projections from substantia nigra/ventral tegmental area (SN/VTA) provide critical modulatory input. (B) Although the role of ACC in OCD symptomatology is unclear, a circuit linking dorsal ACC (dACC), dorsal striatum (dStr), VP (ventral pallidum), and thalamus is critical for action selection. Abnormalities in this loop could therefore contribute to perseverative behaviors in OCD.

processes and symptoms in patients (highlighted by the finding of Gillan et al., 2011, that avoidance habits did not correlate with the YBOCS compulsion subscale), the possibility that impaired regulation of the goal-directed behavior/habit balance contributes to symptom generation is intriguing.

As described briefly earlier, another pathophysiologic model that is not mutually exclusive proposes that different populations of striatal spiny projection neurons differentially regulate the direct and indirect basal ganglia pathways, ultimately leading to stereotypic motor behaviors. Given the known functions of the direct pathway (i.e. striatum, globus pallidus interna, substantia nigra) and indirect pathway (i.e. striatum, globus pallidus externa, subthalamic nucleus) in modulating thalamic input to cortex and in generating motor patterns, this has led to the hypothesis that OCD symptoms result from excess activity in direct versus indirect OFC-subcortical pathways. This imbalance could lead to OCD symptoms in a variety of ways. For example, increased direct pathway activity would lead to decreased inhibition of thalamus, which in turn could decrease filtering of intrusive thoughts and images to cortex, triggering compulsions. Another model suggests that OCD symptoms stem from increased glutamatergic activity in OFC and ACC, which generates intrusive thoughts and images that override other sensorimotor input. In turn, this could trigger ritualistic compulsions driven by striatum through persistent activation of the direct pathway. As described later, studies in rodents can be used to test these models.

OTHER CANDIDATE REGIONS

Though current models suggest that dysfunctional CSTC circuits are important in generation and/or maintenance of OCD symptoms, evidence for involvement of other structures is beginning to accumulate (Milad and Rauch, 2012). For example, while CSTC models do not provide a satisfying explanation for increased anxiety observed in OCD, exaggerated responses in amygdala observed after presentation of OCD-specific stimuli could be responsible. Furthermore, although dACC has been classically linked to conflict monitoring/obsessions in OCD, there is recent evidence that it also plays a role in expression of fear responses. dACC hyperactivation could therefore explain increased anxiety observed in OCD patients. Finally, recent studies have demonstrated that OCD patients have impaired extinction recall in a fear-conditioning paradigm, with accompanying alterations in cerebellum, posterior cingulate, and putamen activity during extinction recall, and reduced hippocampus and caudate activation during fear extinction (Milad, Furtak et al., 2013). Integration of other brain structures may therefore be necessary to generate a satisfying explanatory model of OCD.

TRANSLATING CIRCUIT FINDINGS FROM HUMANS TO ANIMAL MODELS

Though there is strong evidence from human studies that dysfunction in CSTC circuits is linked to OCD symptoms, it is difficult (and perhaps impossible) to test causality in humans. Researchers have therefore turned to animal models to (1) test the causal role of specific circuits in generation and resolution of OCD-like symptoms; and (2) determine precise localization of neurochemical abnormalities that lead to abnormal repetitive behaviors. In this section, we will review new technologies that allow precise dissection of neural circuits involved in repetitive behaviors, and discuss recent studies in the OCD animal literature that exploit these techniques.

OCD Rodent Models

Since valid animal models are essential for identifying molecular and cellular events that lead to pathology, substantial effort has gone toward establishing rodent models of OCD (Wang, Simpson, et al., 2009). Though it is generally accepted that no one animal model will be able to recreate all aspects of any complex neuropsychiatric disorder, including OCD, powerful models can nevertheless be generated to recreate particular aspects of a clinical disorder. However, it is important for models to be carefully assessed to ensure relevance to the human disorder in question, typically by examining the extent of predictive and construct validity. In this section, we will provide an overview of established OCD animal models, and discuss associated circuit abnormalities.

Symptom modeling. OCD animal models have classically emphasized the presence of stereotyped and compulsive behaviors, although reliance on face validity may lead to discrepancies in the field since identical phenotypes can result from different underlying biological processes (Wang, Simpson, et al., 2009). These include barbering (repetitive hair biting and pulling), acral paw-lick (repetitive canine paw-licking), zoo-related stereotypies, and marble burying. In addition to these models of spontaneously generated behaviors, many groups have studied induced repetitive behaviors, including (1) perseverative lever-pressing in the absence of reward; (2) persistent revisiting of unrewarded arms in a T-maze; and (3) pharmacologically induced compulsive checking and perseverative locomotion. All of these models can be used to dissect circuits underlying stereotyped behaviors via either targeted lesions or drug injections through stereotactically placed cannulae. For example, pharmacologic studies in wild-type rats have shown that striatal NMDA-antagonist injections led to increased perseveration on a T-maze delayed alternation task. similarly, *in vivo* microdialysis in corticostriatal projections in deer mice demonstrated increased glutamate directly preceding stereotypic behaviors.

Genetic modeling. There has been a recent explosion in the use of transgenic technology to generate animal models of neuropsychiatric disorders, due to increasing sophistication of available techniques. These strategies allow investigators to upregulate or downregulate genes of interest in specific brain regions at particular developmental timepoints, with temporal and spatial precision that has not previously been achievable (Donaldson, Nautiyal, et al., 2013). Thus, circuit-specific function of candidate genes identified in human studies can now be directly tested in mice. However, generation of targeted transgenics relevant to OCD is still in its infancy, largely due to the difficulty of identifying candidate genes because of lack of replication in genetic studies.

Although targeted transgenics based on OCD candidate genes are therefore still in development, serendipitously generated OCD models have advanced the field in the meantime. In several recent cases, OCD-like behaviors have emerged following disruption of genes not previously implicated in OCD (Ting and Feng, 2011). For example, knockout of the developmentally expressed $Hoxb8^{lox}$ gene leads to perseverative grooming, which is surprisingly reversed by bone marrow transplant from wild-type mice. In another example, disruption of the serotonin 2C receptor leads to perseverative chewing. However, the link between these genes and human OCD remains unclear.

Two other recently generated knockout mice have stronger evidence for relevance to OCD and related disorders. First, in an elegant study, Welch et al. (2007) created a transgenic knockout of SAPAP3, a corticostriatal postsynaptic density protein. Mutant mice demonstrated both anxiety and perseverative grooming that was so severe it led to facial lesions, calling to mind OCD patients with contamination obsessions and corresponding washing rituals. Interestingly, these investigators also discovered a synaptic mechanism that correlated with the OCD-related behaviors; that is, abnormal glutamate signaling at striatal synapses corresponding with a "juvenile" developmental stage (increased NMDA-dependent and decreased AMPA-dependent fEPSPs). Both behavioral and electrophysiological changes were rescued after either lentiviral-mediated SAPAP3 expression broadly throughout striatum or acute treatment with low-dose fluoxetine. Further characterization of these mice has demonstrated that electrophysiological abnormalities are specifically localized to corticostriatal, and not thalamostriatal, synapses (Wan, Ade, et al., 2014).

In a more recent study, (Shmelkov, Hormigo, et al., 2010) inactivated *Slitrk5*, a member of a gene family implicated in obsessive-compulsive spectrum disorders and Tourette's Syndrome, which encodes a postsynaptic density transmembrane protein. *Slitrk5* KOs demonstrate increased anxiety and perseverative grooming that are reversed by chronic treatment with fluoxetine, again demonstrating relevance to human OCD. Interestingly, *Slitrk5* KO mice also have OFC overactivation, as measured with baseline c-fos staining, paralleling findings from human neuroimaging studies.

Current efforts from the groups who made the SAPAP3 and *Slitrk5* KO mice are focused on the challenge of linking these mechanistic observations back to the human disorder. For example, a recent human genetics study found no association of SAPAP3 single nucleotide polymorphisms with OCD, but did find associations with OCD and grooming disorders such as pathologic skin picking, trichotillomania, and/or nail biting. In addition, though preliminary evidence from *Slitrk5* genetic studies is promising, identifying rare *Slitrk5* genetic variants in OCD patients, these findings must still be validated (F. Lee, personal communication). Regardless, both models clearly link molecular changes at corticostriatal synapses with abnormal repetitive behaviors, and therefore yield new insight into potential molecular and cellular pathologic mechanisms in OCD.

Circuit modeling. Recent technologic advances now permit both acute and chronic manipulation of activity in specific neural circuits, allowing direct simulation of human neuroimaging findings in mice. This approach was first elegantly applied to OCD research using a transgenic line that expresses the active subunit of cholera toxin under control of the D1 receptor promoter (D1CT-7 transgenic mice; Campbell, de Lecea, et al., 1999). Expression of this stimulatory subunit yields constitutive hyperactivation of a subset of D1-positive neurons, leading to strong overactivation of prefrontal-cortex and striatal neurons as observed in OCD imaging studies. At baseline, D1CT-7 mice demonstrate perseverative climbing, leaping, and biting behaviors that are exacerbated by increased NMDA-dependent glutamatergic transmission, demonstrating strong construct validity.

Other new technologies can also be used to mimic circuit abnormalities from human imaging studies (Rogan and Roth, 2011). For example, recently developed chemogenetic technology can generate sustained activation and inhibition in specific circuits. This is achieved by expressing mutated G-protein coupled receptors known as DREADDs (designer receptors exclusively activated by designer drugs) in specific cell-types, and then activating the DREADDs by oral, intraperitoneal, or intracranial administration of inert small molecules. Though this technology has not yet been used to directly investigate OCD, it has already been used to probe circuits underlying complex neuropsychiatric disorders such as schizophrenia and major depressive disorder. Furthermore, chemogenetic studies have demonstrated the importance of OFC in switching between goal-directed behaviors and habits, a process that may be disrupted in OCD (Gremel and Costa, 2013).

In addition, the recent development of optogenetics allows precise modulation of neural circuit activity using light-activated microbial ion channels. Though optogenetics initially focused on channelrhodopsin-2 (ChR2), an excitatory sodium channel gated by 473 nm blue light; and halorhodopsin, an inhibitory chloride pump gated by 593 nm yellow light; many opsin variants have now been synthesized to yield a wider range of activation wavelengths, kinetics, and open-channel current strengths. Through tissue-specific expression and local stimulation of light-activated proteins, distinct neural circuits can therefore be rapidly activated or inhibited without affecting neighboring cells.

Optogenetics has recently been applied to the study of OCD pathology and treatment in two back-to-back studies. Using the SAPAP3 KO mice to investigate treatment mechanisms, Burguiere et al. (2013) demonstrated impaired response inhibition in a conditioned grooming task. By selectively stimulating projections from the lateral OFC to the striatum, they were able to restore normal response inhibition, likely by compensating for SAPAP3 KO deficits in fast-spiking interneurons. In contrast, Ahmari et al. (2013) directly tested whether hyperstimulating OFC-ventral striatal projections, thus simulating hyperactivity seen in OCD patients, would lead to OCD-like behaviors in wild-type mice. While acute stimulation did not generate repetitive behaviors, repeated hyperactivation for multiple days in a row led to a progressive and persistent increase in grooming that correlated with an increased evoked-firing rate at OFC-VMS synapses. Increased grooming and evoked firing were both reversed by chronic fluoxetine treatment. Ongoing studies are attempting to synthesize these two sets of findings.

Though this review is focused on studies explicitly examining pathophysiology of OCD, optogenetic approaches have also been applied to the study of neurocognitive domains that are relevant to OCD, particularly the switch from goal-directed behaviors to habits. Briefly, these studies implicate the infralimbic cortex and the sensorimotor striatum in the development of habitual behavior, and suggest that modulation of these circuits may serve as a targeted treatment for disorders with excessive habit formation (Smith, Virkud, et al., 2012; Smith and Graybiel, 2013). As cumulative evidence begins to highlight abnormalities of particular neurocognitive functions in OCD, such as sensorimotor gating, response inhibition, goal-directed versus habitual behavior, and fear-extinction, we will be able to apply findings from the rich literature investigating the basic neurobiology of these core neural processes to gain improved understanding of circuit dysfunction in OCD.

Limitations of Animal Models

The examples given clearly demonstrate the utility of animal models for investigation of pathologic processes in OCD. However, critical evaluation of models to determine their relevance to OCD is crucial. Translatable probes of neural circuits that are reliably abnormal in OCD patients can be used for validation, helping ensure that dissection of molecular and cellular abnormalities will ultimately yield information relevant for treatment development (Ahmari, Eich, et al., 2014).

CIRCUIT-BASED TREATMENTS IN OCD PATIENTS

Evidence from both patients and animal models converges on the idea that dysfunction in CSTC circuits leads to OCD symptoms. Significant efforts have recently been made to develop new therapeutic approaches that directly target dysfunctional circuits. We will discuss these developments in this chapter; current pharmacologic and psychotherapeutic OCD treatments are reviewed in the following chapter by Simpson and Foa (chapter 12).

Stereotactic lesions. Paralleling the neuroimaging findings described earlier, disruption of CSTC loops via multiple different surgical procedures has been found to decrease symptom severity in OCD (Rodman, Milad, et al., 2012). Though many of these procedures were developed empirically, they are all consistent with the theory that interrupting hyperactive connections and/or severing tracts between key circuit nodes with excess connectivity will lead to decreased abnormal transmission and fewer symptoms. Specific ablation procedures used to treat refractory OCD unresponsive to medications and psychotherapy include anterior cingulotomy, capsulotomy, subcaudate tractotomy, and limbic leucotomy (Greenberg, Rauch, et al., 2010). In anterior cingulotomy, bilateral lesions in the cingulum bundle are thought to disrupt hyperactive connections between frontocortical and subcortical areas; likewise, capsulotomy is thought to sever white matter bundles in the anterior limb of the internal capsule connecting OFC with mediodorsal thalamus. Similarly, both subcaudate tractotomy, which relies on a lesion made below and immediately anterior to the head of the caudate, and limbic leucotomy, which is a combination of subcaudate tractotomy and cingulotomy, are thought to employ a similar mechanism of action—that is, interruption of hyperactive frontothalamic circuits leading to symptom relief. Although, in aggregate, stereotactic lesions are moderately efficacious, with success rates ranging from 27 to 86% depending on criteria used to measure improvement, gauging success of these procedures is complicated by the lack of double-blind studies, which cannot ethically be performed, and the utilization of these approaches in only the most severe, treatment-refractory patients.

Deep brain stimulation (DBS). Following its success as a relatively safe, efficacious, adjustable, and reversible treatment for many movement disorders, including Parkinson's disease, DBS has recently emerged as an investigative treatment for several neuropsychiatric disorders, including OCD. Multiple studies and research groups worldwide have attempted to build on the success of ablative procedures by performing targeted tunable stimulation that avoids the permanence and possible degeneration associated with lesions. Although there are caveats—for example, the sham-control multicenter trial for DBS in OCD is still under way (ClinicalTrials.gov: NCT00640133A), and various groups have different criteria for patient inclusion and treatment efficacy—many independent studies have indicated that DBS for OCD is a promising approach for treatment-resistant patients. DBS currently has a Humanitarian Device Exemption from the FDA, so that severe patients can obtain treatment before completion of the multi-center trial. We briefly describe current DBS targets and theories of mechanism of action; for meta-analysis see (Kisely, Hall, et al., 2014).

Targets. Optimizing brain targets for DBS in OCD remains an area of active investigation. Based on the success of stereotactic capsulotomy procedures, initial DBS cases broadly targeted the anterior limb of the internal capsule, with resulting clinical improvement and decreased frontal cortical activity on PET scan. Subsequent studies by Greenberg and colleagues focused in on a smaller region, the ventral aspect of the anterior limb of the ventral capsule/ventral striatum (VC/VS). These studies demonstrated clinical efficacy, with responders showing 35% reduction in symptoms on average, and some patients showing evidence for decreased OFC, ACC, and thalamus activity on PET. Other groups have also reported positive outcomes when targeting this region (Greenberg, Rauch, et al., 2010; Aronson, Katnani, et al., 2014).

Based in part on the fact that shifting the electrode toward the VS led to improved efficacy and need for lower voltage stimulation, multiple groups have now focused on targeting nucleus accumbens (NAc), a structure classically involved in reward processing that lies within the VS and has extensive connectivity with both prefrontal cortical and thalamic regions. Particularly promising results have been reported by Denys and colleagues, who have performed open-label treatment trials demonstrating efficacy up to two years following surgery.

Though multiple groups are now converging on targets in VC/VS and NAc, research to find new targets with increased efficacy and decreased side effects is still ongoing. One of the most promising additional targets is the subthalamic nucleus (STN), which was initially targeted in OCD patients with comorbid Parkinson's Disease. Based on encouraging findings in this comorbid population, a subsequent study in primary OCD patients demonstrated significant response rates following bilateral STN DBS (Mallet, Polosan, et al., 2008).

Mechanism of action. Although results from clinical studies are promising, the mechanism of action for effective DBS treatment is still unknown (Greenberg, Gabriels, et al., 2010). Even in the more mature field of DBS for movement disorders, questions regarding mechanism remain, including importance of orthodromic versus antidromic propagation of stimulation. However, recent studies in OCD are beginning to reveal clues. Though initial theories partly based on animal models suggested that DBS has an overall inhibitory effect on CSTC network transmission, effectively interrupting hyperactive circuits in a manner similar to stereotactic ablation, accumulation of clinical data suggests a potentially more complicated picture. For example, studies from Greenberg and colleagues indicate that acute VC/VS DBS leads to activation in OFC, ACC, striatum, globus pallidus, and thalamus (Rauch, Dougherty, et al., 2006), while chronic internal capsule activation has been shown to resolve OFC and ACC hyperactivity (Abelson, Curtis, et al., 2005), as has been observed following effective pharmacologic treatment or exposure therapy. Activity normalization in mPFC and OFC has also been observed following effective STN DBS (Le Jeune, Verin, et al., 2010).

Other mechanistic studies of NAc DBS from the Denys group have used neuroimaging in humans combined with neurocognitive tasks to identify possible circuit-based mechanisms underlying symptom resolution. A recent study demonstrated decreased D2/3 receptor availability in putamen following both acute and chronic NAc DBS, suggesting that effective DBS induced striatal dopamine release (Figee, de Koning et al., 2014). Another elegant study showed normalization of NAc activity accompanied by a decrease in excessive PFC-NAc connectivity following DBS (Figee, Luigjes, et al., 2013). Future studies combining DBS with neuroimaging, high resolution EEG, and neurocognitive tasks will be necessary to further define mechanism of action.

Transcranial magnetic stimulation (TMS). Despite promising initial results from DBS studies, it will be challenging to put this treatment into large-scale use if it continues to prove efficacious, due to barriers and risks associated with any neurosurgical procedure. Therefore, attempts have recently been made to determine if TMS, a targeted, less invasive method of circuit stimulation, is effective in decreasing OCD symptoms. The most promising results to date target the supplementary motor area (SMA), which exhibits resting state hyperexcitability in functional imaging studies; this suggests potential impairments in either excitatory or inhibitory activity within SMA (Richter, de Jesus et al., 2012). Based on these findings, multiple studies have applied low frequency TMS in SMA to reverse its hyperactivity with promising results, including two sham-controlled trials (Mantovani, Simpson, et al., 2010; Mantovani, Rossi, et al., 2013). In addition, a single-blind sham-control trial of TMS in left OFC showed decreased symptoms after 3 months despite not showing efficacy at 3 weeks, which raises interesting questions about possible plasticity changes induced by neural stimulation. In contrast, sham-controlled trials of TMS in DLPFC demonstrated no benefit (Lapidus, Stern, et al., 2014). Notably, though TMS is currently limited to superficial brain structures, targeting of deep structures is now being attempted in an ongoing clinical trial (NCT01343732). If efficacious, deep TMS could greatly expand potential treatment targets for this noninvasive procedure.

SUMMARY: THE FUTURE: APPLYING FINDINGS FROM ANIMAL MODELS TO OCD TREATMENT

Though findings from studies involving stereotactic ablation, DBS, and TMS are all highly suggestive that targeted disruption of hyperactive CSTC circuits is therapeutic in OCD, several caveats remain in addition to those already described. First, although the area of intervention is known (e.g., the stereotactic coordinates of the lesion or electrode implant), the specific cell populations affected by the intervention are unknown. For example, although DBS in VC/VS likely stimulates VS projections originating in OFC, it also affects striatal projections from other cortical areas, as well as fibers of passage. Similarly, TMS in the SMA may stimulate both excitatory projections going broadly to all SMA target areas, as well as local inhibitory networks. Thus, the exact circuits and cell-types targeted by these interventions remain unclear. Studies in animal models using optogenetic and chemogenetic approaches may help delineate the specific circuit-based mechanisms underlying therapeutic efficacy of these procedures.

In the short-term, understanding these mechanisms of action could assist in improved targeting of stimulation-based treatments. Though far in the future, mechanistic animal studies may also ultimately provide the foundation for either activation or inhibition of specific neural circuits for the treatment of neuropsychiatric illness. Specifically, variability in treatment response and side effects may be due to the fact that DBS and TMS broadly stimulate cortical projections, striatal cell bodies, and fibers of passage; conversely, specific stimulation of particular cell types could potentially lead to more targeted symptom reduction. Although minimal success has been achieved to date, several groups are currently investing significant resources in using optogenetics to generate behavioral changes in nonhuman primates. This is the first step in the process of performing cell-type specific interventions in people, which may have superior efficacy and fewer side effects compared to the more general stimulation afforded by DBS and TMS.

DISCLOSURE STATEMENT

No specific funding was received for this work. Dr. Dougherty reports the following potential conflicts of interest: grants and honoraria from Medtronic, Inc.; grants from Cyberonics, grants from Eli Lilly, grants and personal fees from Roche, honoraria from Insys, and honoraria from J&J. Dr. Ahmari has no conflicts of interest to disclose.

REFERENCES

Abelson, J. L., G. C. Curtis, et al. (2005). Deep brain stimulation for refractory obsessive-compulsive disorder. *Biol Psychiatry* 57 (5): 510–516.

Ahmari, S. E., T. Eich, et al. (2014). Assessing neurocognitive function in psychiatric disorders: A roadmap for enhancing consensus. *Neurobiol Learn Mem 115*, 10–20.

Ahmari, S. E., T. Spellmann, et al. Repeated cortico-striatal stimulation generates persistent OCD-like behavior. *Science, 340*: 1234–1239, doi:10.1126/science.1234733340/6137/1234 [pii] (2013).

Ahmari, S. E., V. B. Risbrough, et al. (2012). Impaired sensorimotor gating in unmedicated adults with obsessive-compulsive disorder. *Neuropsychopharmacology* 37 (5): 1216–1223.

Arnold, P. D., D. R. Rosenberg, et al. (2004). Association of a glutamate (NMDA) subunit receptor gene (GRIN2B) with obsessive-compulsive disorder: A preliminary study. *Psychopharmacology (Berl)* 174 (4): 530–538.

Aronson, J. P., H. A. Katnani, et al. (2014). Neuromodulation for obsessive-compulsive disorder. *Neurosurg Clin N Am* 25 (1): 85–101.

Balleine, B. W. and J. P. O'Doherty (2010). Human and rodent homologies in action control: corticostriatal determinants of goal-directed and habitual action. *Neuropsychopharmacology* 35 (1): 48–69.

Baxter, L. R., Jr., J. M. Schwartz, et al. (1988). Cerebral glucose metabolic rates in nondepressed patients with obsessive-compulsive disorder. *Am J Psychiatry* 145 (12): 1560–1563.

Burguiere, E., Monteiro, P., et al. Optogenetic stimulation of lateral orbitofronto-striatal pathway suppresses compulsive behaviors. *Science* 340: 1243–1246, doi:10.1126/science.1232380340/6137/1243 [pii] (2013).

Campbell, K. M., L. de Lecea, et al. (1999). OCD-like behaviors caused by a neuropotentiating transgene targeted to cortical and limbic D1+ neurons. *J Neurosci* 19 (12): 5044–5053.

Cazorla, M., F. D. de Carvalho, et al. (2014). Dopamine D2 receptors regulate the anatomical and functional balance of basal ganglia circuitry. *Neuron* 81 (1): 153–164.

Donaldson, Z. R., K. M. Nautiyal, et al. (2013). Genetic approaches for understanding the role of serotonin receptors in mood and behavior. *Curr Opin Neurobiol* 23 (3): 399–406.

Elliott, R., Z. Agnew, et al. (2010). Hedonic and informational functions of the human orbitofrontal cortex. *Cereb Cortex* 20 (1): 198–204.

Figee, M., P. de Koning, et al. (2014). Deep brain stimulation induces striatal dopamine release in obsessive-compulsive disorder. *Biol Psychiatry* 75 (8): 647–652.

Figee, M., J. Luigjes, et al. (2013). Deep brain stimulation restores frontostriatal network activity in obsessive-compulsive disorder. *Nat Neurosci* 16 (4): 386–387.

Gillan, C. M., M. Papmeyer, et al. (2011). Disruption in the balance between goal-directed behavior and habit learning in obsessive-compulsive disorder. *Am J Psychiatry* 168 (7): 718–726.

Greenberg, B. D., L. A. Gabriels, et al. (2010). Deep brain stimulation of the ventral internal capsule/ventral striatum for obsessive-compulsive disorder: Worldwide experience. *Mol Psychiatry* 15 (1): 64–79.

Greenberg, B. D., S. L. Rauch, et al. (2010). Invasive circuitry-based neurotherapeutics: stereotactic ablation and deep brain stimulation for OCD. *Neuropsychopharmacology* 35 (1): 317–336.

Gremel, C. M. and R. M. Costa (2013). Orbitofrontal and striatal circuits dynamically encode the shift between goal-directed and habitual actions. *Nat Commun* 4: 2264.

Hemmings, S. M. and D. J. Stein (2006). The current status of association studies in obsessive-compulsive disorder. *Psychiatr Clin North Am* 29 (2): 411–444.

Jin, X., F. Tecuapetla, et al. (2014). Basal ganglia subcircuits distinctively encode the parsing and concatenation of action sequences. *Nat Neurosci* 17 (3): 423–430.

Kessler, R. C., P. Berglund, et al. (2005). Lifetime prevalence and age-of-onset distributions of DSM-IV disorders in the National Comorbidity Survey Replication. *Archives of General Psychiatry* 62 (6): 593–602.

Kisely, S., K. Hall, et al. (2014). Deep brain stimulation for obsessive-compulsive disorder: a systematic review and meta-analysis. *Psychol Med* 44 (16), 3533–42.

Koran, L. M. (2000). Quality of life in obsessive-compulsive disorder. *Psychiatric Clinics of North America* 23 (3): 509–517.

Kutsuwada, T., K. Sakimura, et al. (1996). Impairment of suckling response, trigeminal neuronal pattern formation, and hippocampal LTD in NMDA receptor epsilon 2 subunit mutant mice. *Neuron* 16 (2): 333–344.

Lapidus, K. A., E. R. Stern, et al. (2014). Neuromodulation for obsessive-compulsive disorder. *Neurotherapeutics* 11 (3): 485–495.

Le Jeune, F., M. Verin, et al. (2010). Decrease of prefrontal metabolism after subthalamic stimulation in obsessive-compulsive disorder: a positron emission tomography study. *Biol Psychiatry 68* (11): 1016–1022.

Leckman, J. F., D. Denys, et al. (2010). Obsessive-compulsive disorder: a review of the diagnostic criteria and possible subtypes and dimensional specifiers for DSM-V. *Depress Anxiety 27* (6): 507–527.

Maia, T. V., R. E. Cooney, et al. (2008). The neural bases of obsessive-compulsive disorder in children and adults. *Dev Psychopathol 20* (4): 1251–1283.

Mallet, L., M. Polosan, et al. (2008). Subthalamic nucleus stimulation in severe obsessive-compulsive disorder. *N Engl J Med 359* (20): 2121–2134.

Mantovani, A., S. Rossi, et al. (2013). Modulation of motor cortex excitability in obsessive-compulsive disorder: an exploratory study on the relations of neurophysiology measures with clinical outcome. *Psychiatry Res 210* (3): 1026–1032.

Mantovani, A., H. B. Simpson, et al. (2010). Randomized sham-controlled trial of repetitive transcranial magnetic stimulation in treatment-resistant obsessive-compulsive disorder. *Int J Neuropsychopharmacol 13* (2): 217–227.

Marsh, R., T. V. Maia, et al. (2009). Functional disturbances within frontostriatal circuits across multiple childhood psychopathologies. *Am J Psychiatry 166* (6): 664–674.

Mataix-Cols, D., M. C. Rosario-Campos, et al. (2005). A multidimensional model of obsessive-compulsive disorder. *Am J Psychiatry 162* (2): 228–238.

Milad, M. R., S. C. Furtak, et al. (2013). Deficits in conditioned fear extinction in obsessive-compulsive disorder and neurobiological changes in the fear circuit. *JAMA Psychiatry 70* (6): 608–618; quiz 554.

Milad, M. R. and S. L. Rauch (2012). Obsessive-compulsive disorder: Beyond segregated cortico-striatal pathways. *Trends Cog Sci 16* (1): 43–51.

Parent, A. and L. N. Hazrati (1995). Functional anatomy of the basal ganglia. I. The cortico-basal ganglia-thalamo-cortical loop. *Brain Res Brain Res Rev 20* (1): 91–127.

Pauls, D. L. (2008). The genetics of obsessive compulsive disorder: A review of the evidence. *Am J Med Genet C Semin Med Genet 148C* (2): 133–139.

Pennartz, C. M., J. D. Berke, et al. (2009). Corticostriatal Interactions during Learning, Memory Processing, and Decision Making. *J Neurosci 29* (41): 12831–12838.

Pittenger, C., M. H. Bloch, et al. (2011). Glutamate abnormalities in obsessive compulsive disorder: neurobiology, pathophysiology, and treatment. *Pharmacol Ther 132* (3): 314–332.

Rauch, S. L., D. D. Dougherty, et al. (2006). A functional neuroimaging investigation of deep brain stimulation in patients with obsessive-compulsive disorder. *J Neurosurg 104* (4): 558–565.

Richter, M. A., D. R. de Jesus, et al. (2012). Evidence for cortical inhibitory and excitatory dysfunction in obsessive compulsive disorder. *Neuropsychopharmacology 37* (5): 1144–1151.

Rodman, A. M., M. R. Milad, et al. (2012). Neuroimaging contributions to novel surgical treatments for intractable obsessive-compulsive disorder. *Expert Rev Neurother 12* (2): 219–227.

Rogan, S. C. and B. L. Roth (2011). "Remote control of neuronal signaling." *Pharmacol Rev 63* (2): 291–315.

Roth, R. M., A. J. Saykin, et al. (2007). Event-related functional magnetic resonance imaging of response inhibition in obsessive-compulsive disorder. *Biol Psychiatry 62* (8): 901–909.

Saxena, S., R. G. Bota, et al. (2001). Brain-behavior relationships in obsessive-compulsive disorder. *Semin Clin Neuropsychiatry 6* (2): 82–101.

Shmelkov, S. V., A. Hormigo, et al. (2010). Slitrk5 deficiency impairs corticostriatal circuitry and leads to obsessive-compulsive-like behaviors in mice. *Nat Med 16* (5): 598–602, 591p following 602.

Smith, K. S. and A. M. Graybiel (2013). A dual operator view of habitual behavior reflecting cortical and striatal dynamics. *Neuron 79* (2): 361–374.

Smith, K. S., A. Virkud, et al. (2012). Reversible online control of habitual behavior by optogenetic perturbation of medial prefrontal cortex. *Proc Natl Acad Sci USA 109* (46): 18932–18937.

Taylor, S. (2013). Molecular genetics of obsessive-compulsive disorder: a comprehensive meta-analysis of genetic association studies. *Mol Psychiatry 18* (7): 799–805.

Ting, J. T. and G. Feng (2011). Neurobiology of obsessive-compulsive disorder: insights into neural circuitry dysfunction through mouse genetics. *Curr Opin Neurobiol 21* (6): 842–848.

van Velzen, L. S., C. Vriend, et al. (2014). Response inhibition and interference control in obsessive-compulsive spectrum disorders. *Frontiers in Human Neuroscience 8*: 419.

Wan, Y., K. K. Ade, et al. (2014). Circuit-selective striatal synaptic dysfunction in the Sapap3 knockout mouse model of obsessive-compulsive disorder. *Biol Psychiatry 75* (8): 623–630.

Wang, L., H. B. Simpson, et al. (2009). Assessing the validity of current mouse genetic models of obsessive-compulsive disorder. *Behav Pharmacol 20* (2): 119–133.

Welch, J. M., J. Lu, et al. (2007). Cortico-striatal synaptic defects and OCD-like behaviours in Sapap3-mutant mice. *Nature 448*: 894–900, doi:nature06104 [pii]10.1038/nature06104.

Wu, K., G. L. Hanna, et al. (2012). The role of glutamate signaling in the pathogenesis and treatment of obsessive-compulsive disorder. *Pharmacol Biochem Behav 100* (4): 726–735.

12

CLINICAL ASPECTS OF OBSESSIVE-COMPULSIVE DISORDER

H. BLAIR SIMPSON AND EDNA B. FOA

INTRODUCTION

Obsessive-compulsive disorder (OCD) is characterized by recurrent intrusive thoughts, images, or urges (obsessions) that typically cause anxiety or distress, and repetitive mental or behavioral acts (compulsions). With a lifetime prevalence of up to 2–3% (i.e., two to three times more common than schizophrenia), OCD is an important cause of illness-related disability: it typically starts in childhood or adolescence, persists throughout a person's life, and produces substantial impairment in functioning. Early detection and proper treatment of OCD can alleviate individual suffering and reduce the public health burden of this disease.

This chapter reviews the clinical phenotype of OCD and discusses evidence-based treatment strategies. A companion chapter (chapter 11, Ahmari and Dougherty) describes the etiology and pathophysiology of the disorder. Both chapters reveal how our understanding of and treatments for OCD are evolving.

CLINICAL FEATURES OF OCD

Clinical phenotype: The criteria for OCD in the Diagnostic and Statistical Manual of Mental Disorders (DSM-5; American Psychiatric Association, 2013) are shown in Box 12.1. The core symptoms of OCD are obsessions and compulsions. Most OCD patients have both (Foa, Kozak et al. 1995, Shavitt, de Mathis et al. 2014). Obsessions include repetitive and persistent thoughts (e.g., fear of being contaminated), images (e.g., of committing violent or horrific acts), or urges (e.g., to stab someone) that are intrusive, unwanted, and cause marked distress or anxiety in most patients with OCD. Compulsions (or rituals) are repetitive behaviors (e.g., washing, checking) or mental acts (e.g., counting, repeating special prayers silently) that the patient feels driven to perform. Compulsions are not done for pleasure, although patients can experience relief from anxiety or distress by performing them. OCD patients often report a functional relationship

BOX 12.1
CRITERIA FOR OBSESSIVE-COMPULSIVE DISORDER

A. Presence of obsessions, compulsions, or both:

Obsessions are defined by (1) and (2):

1. Recurrent and persistent thoughts, urges, or images that are experienced, at some time during the disturbance, as intrusive and unwanted, and that in most individuals cause marked anxiety or distress

2. The individual attempts to ignore or suppress such thoughts, urges, or images, or to neutralize them with some other thought or action (i.e., by performing a compulsion)

Compulsions are defined by (1) and (2):

1. Repetitive behaviors (e.g., hand washing, ordering, checking) or mental acts (e.g., praying, counting, repeating words silently) that the individual feels driven to perform in response to an obsession or according to rules that must be applied rigidly

2. The behaviors or mental acts are aimed at preventing or reducing anxiety or distress, or preventing some dreaded event or situation; however, these behaviors or mental acts are not connected in a realistic way with what they are designed to neutralize or prevent, or are clearly excessive (Note: Young children may not be able to articulate the aims of these behaviors or mental acts.)

B. The obsessions or compulsions are time-consuming (e.g., take more than 1 hour per day) or cause clinically significant distress or impairment in social, occupational, or other important areas of functioning.

C. The obsessive-compulsive symptoms are not attributable to the direct physiological effects of a substance (e.g., a drug of abuse, a medication) or another medical condition.

D. The disturbance is not better explained by the symptoms of another mental disorder (e.g., excessive worries, as in generalized anxiety disorder; preoccupation with appearance, as in body dysmorphic disorder; difficulty discarding or parting with possessions, as in hoarding disorder; hair pulling, as in trichotillomania [hair pulling disorder]; skin picking, as in excoriation [skin picking] disorder; stereotypies, as in stereotypic movement disorder; ritualized eating behavior, as in eating disorders; preoccupation with substances or gambling, as in substance-related and addictive disorders; preoccupation with having an illness, as in illness anxiety disorder; sexual urges or fantasies, as in paraphilic disorders; impulses, as in disruptive, impulse-control, and conduct disorders; guilty ruminations, as in major depressive disorder; thought insertion or delusional preoccupations, as in schizophrenia spectrum and other psychotic disorders; or repetitive patterns of behavior, as in autism spectrum disorder).

Specify if:

- With good or fair insight: The individual recognizes that obsessive-compulsive disorder beliefs are definitely or probably not true, or that they may or may not be true.

- With poor insight: The individual thinks obsessive-compulsive disorder beliefs are probably true.

- With absent insight/delusional: The individual is completely convinced that obsessive-compulsive disorder beliefs are true.

Specify if:

Tic-related: The individual has a past or current history of a tic disorder.

between their obsessions and compulsions (e.g., I wash my hands in order to prevent being contaminated).

Although all OCD patients have obsessions and/or compulsions, the specific content of the obsessions and the exact nature of the compulsive behaviors vary among patients. Certain themes, however, are common, including: forbidden or taboo thoughts (e.g., aggressive, sexual, or religious obsessions and related compulsions); contamination (fears of contamination and related cleaning rituals); harm (fears of harm to oneself or others and checking compulsions); and symmetry (symmetry obsessions and repeating, ordering, and counting compulsions). Some patients also have difficulty discarding, and they accumulate or hoard objects as a consequence of their OCD symptoms, such as their fears of harming others (Pertusa, Frost et al. 2010). These themes, also known as symptom dimensions, have been described across different cultures and are associated with different neural substrates (Leckman, Denys et al. 2010). Individuals often have symptoms in more than one dimension.

OCD patients differ from each other in other important ways. For example, patients can have a range of affective responses when confronted with situations that trigger obsessions and compulsions: although many experience marked anxiety that can include panic attacks, others report strong feelings of disgust or a distressing sense of "incompleteness" until things look, feel, or sound "just right." Patients also differ in their degree of insight about the irrationality of their obsessions and compulsions (Phillips, Pinto et al. 2012): although many patients recognize that their symptoms are not or probably not rational (reflecting good or fair insight), a subset are convinced that their obsessive beliefs are likely or definitely true (reflecting poor or absent insight). That there is a range of insight is now explicit in the DSM-5's revised criteria for OCD (Leckman, Denys et al. 2010), and degree of insight is now a specifier (Box 12.1). Insight can fluctuate over the course of illness, and poor or absent insight can complicate treatment (Leckman, Denys et al. 2010).

The frequency and severity of obsessions and compulsions also vary among patients. Some have mild to moderate symptoms, spending a few hours per day obsessing or ritualizing. Others have near constant intrusive thoughts or compulsions. It is also common for patients to avoid people, places, and things that trigger their obsessions and compulsions. Both the time spent obsessing and ritualizing, as well as the avoidance of situations that trigger their symptoms, can lead to various problems in work, family, and social functioning (Markarian, Larson et al. 2010). Therefore, OCD is a disabling illness.

Onset and course: Both genders develop OCD, at comparable rates. Onset usually occurs in adolescence or early adulthood; however, about 25% of OCD patients, a majority of them male, have onset in childhood (Ruscio, Stein et al. 2010).

If untreated, the course of OCD is usually chronic, often with waxing and waning symptoms (Ravizza, Maina et al. 1997, Skoog and Skoog 1999). Some patients have an episodic course; a minority have a deteriorating course. Without treatment, remission rates in adults are low (e.g., 20% for those reevaluated 40 years later; Skoog and Skoog 1999). Onset in childhood or adolescence can lead to a lifetime of OCD. On the other hand, 40% of individuals with childhood onset may remit by early adulthood (Stewart, Geller et al. 2004). The course of OCD is often complicated by the co-occurrence of other disorders.

Comorbidity: OCD is often comorbid with other psychiatric disorders. Adults with OCD often have a lifetime diagnosis of an anxiety disorder (76%, e.g., panic disorder, social anxiety disorder, generalized anxiety disorder, specific phobia) or a mood disorder (63% for any mood disorder, with the most common being major depressive disorder, 41%). Comorbid obsessive-compulsive personality disorder is also common (e.g., range of 23–32%; Pinto, Eisen et al. 2008), and up to 30% of OCD patients have a lifetime tic disorder (including Tourette's disorder). OCD patients with comorbid tic disorder may be biologically distinct, with earlier age of onset, greater prevalence in males, different neurochemical and neurobiological features, and distinct treatment response (Leckman, Denys et al. 2010). Rates of OCD are also much higher than would be expected (based on its prevalence in the general population) in schizophrenia or schizoaffective disorder, eating disorders (i.e., anorexia nervosa and bulimia nervosa), and Tourette's disorder (American Psychiatric Association, 2013; Ruscio, Stein et al. 2010).

Differential diagnosis: Repetitive thoughts and behaviors occur in disorders other than OCD (Ameringen, Patterson et al. 2014). These include body dysmorphic disorder (where the repetitive thoughts and behaviors focus on perceived defects in appearance), trichotillomania (where the repetitive behaviors are limited to hair pulling in the absence of obsessions), hoarding disorder (where the focus is on the excessive accumulation of objects and the persistent difficulty discarding them), eating disorders (where the focus is on food, weight, and exercise), tic disorders (where the repetitive motor movements are not aimed at preventing or reducing anxiety triggered by an obsession), illness anxiety disorder (where the repetitive thoughts are focused on having an illness), and obsessive-compulsive personality disorder (where the repetitive behaviors are typically ego-syntonic and driven by excessive perfectionism and rigid control and are not in response to intrusive thoughts). Whether there are shared or distinct neural correlates of repetitive thoughts and behaviors across these disorders is an area of active study.

WHAT CAUSES OCD

A companion chapter (chapter 11, Ahmari and Dougherty) reviews in detail the etiology and pathophysiology of OCD. In brief, human and animal data suggest that dysregulation of cortico–striatal–thalamo–cortical (CSTC) circuits leads to OCD symptoms, although other brain circuits (e.g., fear circuitry) are also implicated (Milad and Rauch 2012). Multiple neurotransmitter systems are likely involved, including serotonin, dopamine, glutamate, and GABA. The working model is that dysregulation of these brain circuits leads to dysfunction in core neural processes, such as response inhibition (van Velzen, Vriend et al. 2014), sensorimotor processing (Ahmari, Risbrough et al. 2012), goal-directed versus habitual behavior (Gillan, Papmeyer et al. 2011), and/or extinction of fear (Milad, Furtak et al. 2013). Dysfunction in these core processes then leads to the characteristic symptoms of OCD.

What causes dysregulation in these brain circuits, however, remains unclear. The etiology of OCD is presumed to be a mixture of genetic vulnerability, environmental factors, and developmental trajectory. Indeed, the rate of OCD is about two-fold higher in first-degree relatives of adults with OCD than in those without first-degree relatives with OCD; the rate of OCD is 10-fold higher among first-degree relatives of those with childhood-onset OCD (Pauls 2010). Twin studies indicate that familial transmission is due to both genetic and environmental factors (e.g., a concordance rate of 0.57 for monozygotic versus 0.22 for dizygotic twins; Pauls 2010).

TREATMENT OF OCD

Practice guidelines for treating OCD recommend as first-line treatments: cognitive-behavioral therapy (CBT) consisting of exposure and response prevention (EX/RP), pharmacotherapy with serotonin reuptake inhibitors (SRIs), or their combination (Koran, Hanna et al. 2007, Koran and Simpson 2013). We describe these treatments along with other strategies for when first-line treatments do not succeed. A treatment algorithm is presented that summarizes these treatment options (Figure 12.1).

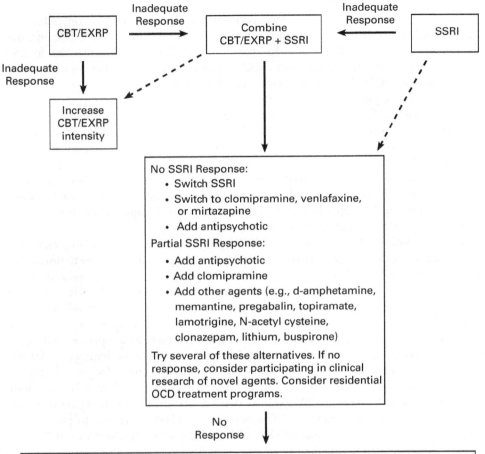

CBT/EXRP

Inadequate Response →

Combine
CBT/EXRP + SSRI

← Inadequate Response

SSRI

Inadequate Response ↓

Increase
CBT/EXRP
intensity

No SSRI Response:
- Switch SSRI
- Switch to clomipramine, venlafaxine, or mirtazapine
- Add antipsychotic

Partial SSRI Response:
- Add antipsychotic
- Add clomipramine
- Add other agents (e.g., d-amphetamine, memantine, pregabalin, topiramate, lamotrigine, N-acetyl cysteine, clonazepam, lithium, buspirone)

Try several of these alternatives. If no response, consider participating in clinical research of novel agents. Consider residential OCD treatment programs.

No
Response ↓

If treatment refractory despite trying treatments above and OCD remains severe and impairing, consider neurosurgical interventions (Deep Brain Stimulation or ablative procedures).

Criteria for Treatment Refractory OCD
- 3 adequate SRI trials

and
- Add at least two of the following medications for at least 1 month
  - antipsychotic
  - clonazepam
  - lithium
  - buspirone

and
- Adequate CBT with at least 20 hours of EX/RP

FIGURE 12.1 Algorithm for the treatment of obsessive-compulsive disorder. Abbreviations: CBT = cognitive-behavioral therapy; EX/RP = exposure and response prevention; SSRI = selective serotonin reuptake inhibitor; SRI = serotonin reuptake inhibitor (i.e., clomipramine or SSRI).

PSYCHOTHERAPY FOR OCD

Cognitive-Behavioral Therapy

CBT alone or in combination with SRIs is recommended as a first-line treatment for both children and adults with OCD. Historically, CBT has evolved from two traditions: one that relies primarily on behavioral techniques such as EX/RP; and another that focuses primarily on cognitive techniques (CT), such as identifying, challenging, and modifying faulty beliefs. In OCD, the evidence is strongest for EX/RP.

Exposure and response prevention: CBT consisting of exposure and response prevention (called ERP or EX/RP in the literature and EX/RP in this chapter) involves in vivo (i.e., actual) exposures to feared situations, imaginal exposures to feared consequences, and ritual prevention, in which patients refrain from performing compulsions (Foa, Yadin et al. 2012). For example, a patient with harm obsessions and checking rituals would be coached to confront feared situations (e.g., using knives in the kitchen around family members), to imagine feared consequences (e.g., stabbing family members), and to refrain from checking rituals. In EX/RP treatment, the therapist tailors the exposure exercises to the specific fears of the patient.

There are different theories for how EX/RP might work. Recent learning and emotional processing theories posit that fear extinction via repeated exposures to unrealistic fears (as occurs in EX/RP) helps patients disconfirm unrealistic perceptions and beliefs. From this perspective, EX/RP modifies pathological fear structures by first activating the pathological fear associations (via exposures in the absence of rituals) and then incorporating information that is disconfirmatory, such that new learning occurs.

In randomized controlled trials, EX/RP has been shown to be a superior OCD treatment compared to other psychotherapies and control conditions, including pill placebo, anxiety management therapy, self-guided relaxation therapy, therapist-guided progressive muscle relaxation, and wait list control (Koran, Hanna et al. 2007). In a randomized controlled trial, Foa et al. (2005) found that EX/RP with or without clomipramine (CMI) was superior at reducing OCD symptoms to CMI alone and to pill placebo (Figure 12.2). Patients receiving EX/RP with or without CMI also had significantly higher rates of achieving excellent response (Yale-Brown Obsessive Compulsive Scale score ≤ 12; Goodman, Price et al. 1989) than those receiving CMI or placebo alone (58% EX/RP +CMI; 52% EX/RP; 25% CMI; 0% placebo; Simpson, Huppert et al. 2006). When treatment was discontinued, patients receiving EX/RP with or without CMI also had significantly lower relapse rates than those receiving CMI alone (Simpson, Franklin et al. 2005). EX/RP can also augment SRI response.

Different factors can affect EX/RP outcome (Foa, Steketee et al. 1983), including the number and frequency of sessions, the presence of comorbidity (e.g., severe depression), and the patient's degree of insight. Patient adherence to acute treatment is also a robust predictor of both acute and long-term outcome (Simpson, Maher et al. 2011, Simpson, Marcus et al. 2012). After successful treatment, some patients will relapse, but teaching relapse prevention techniques near the end of acute treatment can help patients maintain the gains made in therapy (Hiss, Foa et al. 1994).

Other types of CBT for OCD: Cognitive therapy (CT) has also been studied in OCD. In CT, the patient and therapist identify the patient's distorted patterns of thinking that lead to emotional reactions and then challenge and alter this thinking to change their emotional response. CT has been found to reduce OCD symptoms in several clinical trials (Rosa-Alcázar, Sánchez-Meca et al. 2008), and some of these trials directly compared

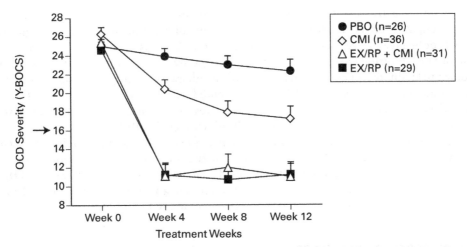

FIGURE 12.2 The effects of clomipramine, exposure and response prevention, and their combination in the treatment of adults with obsessive-compulsive disorder. A 12-week randomized controlled trial compared the effects of clomipramine (CMI), exposure and response prevention (EX/RP), their combination (EX/RP + CMI), and pill placebo (PBO) in adults with obsessive-compulsive disorder. Estimates from linear mixed-effects models of Yale-Brown Obsessive Compulsive Scale (Y-BOCS) mean scores (with standard error bars) over time are shown by treatment group. See text for more details.

CT to EX/RP (e.g., van Balkom, de Haan et al. 1998, Whittal, Robichaud et al. 2008, Olatunji, Rosenfield et al. 2013). Of note, separating these treatments can be procedurally difficult because standard CT includes behavioral experiments that can resemble exposures, and many EX/RP protocols incorporate informal cognitive techniques (e.g., relapse prevention, cognitive processing during exposures). Standard CT that includes behavioral experiments appears similar in efficacy to EX/RP when EX/RP is suboptimally delivered (e.g., 45-minute weekly sessions, self-guided exposure; van Balkom, de Haan et al. 1998). When EX/RP is more optimally delivered (e.g., 120 minute sessions twice-per week, therapist-aided exposure), EX/RP can be superior (Olatunji, Rosenfield et al. 2013). At the same time, a small open trial suggested that CT in the absence of behavioral experiments may help some OCD patients (Wilhelm, Steketee et al. 2009).

Acceptance and commitment therapy (ACT) has recently been tested in OCD. Rather than challenging and restructuring unpleasant thoughts and dysfunctional beliefs, ACT attempts to teach patients to observe and accept these unpleasant thoughts and beliefs without resorting to rituals. One trial found ACT to be superior to relaxation training (Twohig, Hayes et al. 2010).

Since the evidence supporting EX/RP for OCD is stronger than the evidence supporting other psychotherapies, EX/RP remains the recommended first-line psychotherapy for OCD (Koran, Hanna et al. 2007, Koran and Simpson 2013).

Limitations of CBT in the Treatment of OCD

Although EX/RP is a highly effective treatment for OCD, it has important limitations. It is anxiety-provoking for patients, time-consuming for patients and therapists, requires good adherence with treatment procedures for full effects, and is not widely available.

To improve treatment adherence, approaches such as motivational interviewing (Simpson, Zuckoff et al. 2010) and modification of treatment-interfering cognitive beliefs or behaviors have been tried. Another approach stems from animal research: the use of D-cycloserine (a partial agonist at the N-methyl-D-aspartate [NMDA] receptor known to facilitate fear extinction in animals) to enhance learning. Three small randomized trials compared EX/RP to EX/RP augmented with D-cycloserine. In two of these trials, D-cycloserine reduced the time to EX/RP response, but did not result in increased response by the end of the trials (Chasson, Buhlmann et al. 2010).

To increase EX/RP access, technology is being used. For example, web-based platforms can now deliver EX/RP by the Internet, with minimal therapist support provided by email or phone. In a randomized controlled trial, Andersson et al. (2012) found that this online EX/RP therapy was significantly better than an online attention control condition and led to clinically meaningful improvement in OCD symptoms.

PHARMACOTHERAPY FOR OCD

Serotonin Reuptake Inhibitors

Serotonin reuptake inhibitors (SRIs) are the only medications proven effective as a monotherapy for OCD in multi-site randomized controlled trials. SRIs include clomipramine, a tricyclic antidepressant, and the selective SRIs (i.e., fluoxetine, fluvoxamine, sertraline, paroxetine, citalopram, and escitalopram). All but citalopram and escitalopram are approved by the Food and Drug Administration (FDA) for the treatment of OCD. SRIs lead to improvement in 40–60% of patients with OCD, and OCD patients who receive an adequate trial will achieve on average a 20–40% reduction in their symptoms (Koran, Hanna et al. 2007). Thus, SRIs typically lead to amelioration rather than elimination of symptoms. SRIs are thought to reduce OCD symptoms by modulating CSTC circuit function.

Comparative efficacy: SRIs are thought to be equally efficacious, with the possible exception of clomipramine (Koran, Hanna et al. 2007). In meta-analyses, clomipramine, both an SRI and a norepinephrine reuptake inhibitor, had greater effects than the selective SRIs. However, the clomipramine studies were conducted earlier in time and thus were likely to include more treatment-naïve samples. In head-to-head comparisons, clomipramine has not been shown to be clearly superior to selective SRIs. As a result, practice guidelines (Koran, Hanna et al. 2007) recommend that patients first be started on a selective SRI because they have fewer serious side effects than clomipramine. To determine which selective SRI to try first, the clinician should consider prior treatment response, safety and acceptability of particular side effects for the individual patient, and the potential for drug-drug interactions. If there is no response, patients can be switched to another selective SRI. If response is still limited, then a trial of clomipramine is recommended.

Dose: Trials of fluoxetine, paroxetine, and citalopram that randomized patients to different doses of the same medication (i.e., fixed dose studies) found that higher doses produced a higher response rate and/or greater degree of improvement than lower doses; one fixed dose study of sertraline did not find significant differences between the effects of 50 and 200 mg/day (reviewed in Bloch, McGuire et al. 2010). Based on these data, practice guidelines (Koran, Hanna et al. 2007) recommend the following target doses for adults with OCD: fluoxetine 40–60 mg/day, fluvoxamine 200 mg/day, paroxetine 40–60 mg/day, sertraline 200 mg/day, escitalopram 20 mg/day, and clomipramine 100–250 mg/day. The FDA no longer recommends citalopram above 40 mg/day because of dose-dependent QT prolongation. When starting patients on SRIs, it is advised to start patients at a low dose for tolerability (e.g., fluoxetine 10 or 20 mg/day) and to increase the dose every week or two (as tolerated) to doses at least as high as those listed before deciding that a patient will not respond.

When patients do not respond to these doses, doses even higher have been tried in clinical practice (e.g., fluoxetine 120 mg/day, paroxetine 100 mg/day). For example, Ninan et al. (2006) randomized patients who had not responded to 16 weeks of sertraline (titrated from 50 mg/day to 200 mg/day) to continued sertraline (200 mg/day) or to increased sertraline (250–400 mg/day). The high-dose group had significantly more improvement than the lower-dose group, but the clinical difference was modest, and both groups still had clinically significant symptoms. Thus, increasing SRIs to higher than recommended doses may be effective for certain OCD patients, but this strategy is not helpful for all.

Time to response: Many SRI trials for OCD did not show a significant difference between placebo and active medication before 6 weeks. Thus, an adequate trial has been defined as the maximum dose tolerated for a minimum of 6 weeks (Koran, Hanna et al. 2007). Given usual titration schedules, this usually amounts to an 8–12 week trial overall. It is important to explain this time course to patients so that they don't prematurely stop taking their SRI. Based on preclinical studies, it has been hypothesized that this delayed response corresponds to the time course of desensitizing presynaptic serotonin receptors that inhibit serotonin release in the orbito-frontal cortex (El Mansari and Blier 2006).

Side effects: Selective SRIs are generally well-tolerated (Koran, Hanna et al. 2007). Potential side effects include gastrointestinal problems (e.g., nausea or diarrhea), agitation, sleep disturbances (e.g., insomnia, vivid dreams), increased sweating, and sexual side effects (e.g., decrease in libido, trouble ejaculating, delayed orgasm). In addition, weight gain or fatigue can occur. Specific side effects of certain agents have also been reported that are presumed to be due to their unique pharmacological characteristics (e.g., more sedation and constipation due to the mild anticholinergic effects of paroxetine, more anorexia and activation due to the 5HT2C antagonism of fluoxetine). Thus, a patient may tolerate one SRI, but not another. Of note, citalopram can cause dose-dependent QT interval prolongation, which can cause Torsades de Pointes, ventricular tachycardia, and sudden death. Thus citalopram is not recommended in patients with congenital long QT syndrome or who are at risk for QT prolongation (e.g., due to an underlying heart condition or low levels of potassium or magnesium).

Clomipramine not only inhibits serotonin reuptake, it also inhibits norepinephrine reuptake and blocks muscarinic cholinergic receptors, H1 histamine receptors, alpha1 adrenergic receptors, and sodium channels in the heart and brain. Thus, in addition to the SRI side effects described earlier, clomipramine can cause anticholinergic effects (e.g., dry mouth, constipation, delayed urination), antihistamine effects (e.g., sedation, weight gain), antiadrenergic effects (e.g., orthostatic hypotension), and cardiac conduction abnormalities or seizures.

Duration of treatment: Double-blind discontinuation trials that treat patients for a certain period of time and then randomly assign responders to either continue that medication or be switched to pill placebo help determine the risk of relapse if medication is stopped. Several double-blind discontinuation studies in adults with OCD (reviewed in Fineberg, Brown et al. 2012) examined different SRIs, used different designs (e.g., length of follow-up, procedure for placebo substitution), and applied different relapse definitions. The studies came to different conclusions. For example, relapse rates (or discontinuation due to insufficient clinical response) after a double-blind switch to placebo ranged from a high of 89% within 7 weeks for clomipramine, to a low of 24% within 28 weeks for sertraline. Practice guidelines (Koran, Hanna et al. 2007) recommend that an OCD patient who has improved during an adequate SRI trial should stay on that medication for 1–2 years, and that if the medication is discontinued, it should be slowly tapered (e.g., 10–25% every 1–2 months).

If stopped abruptly, SRIs can lead to a drug discontinuation syndrome. This can include flulike symptoms (e.g., dizziness, nausea/vomiting, headache, and lethargy) as well as agitation, insomnia, myoclonic jerks, and paresthesias (Shelton 2006). Drugs with a shorter half-life (e.g., paroxetine) are more likely to cause this than those with a longer half-life and an active metabolite (e.g., fluoxetine).

Venlafaxine and Duloxetine in the Treatment of OCD

Like clomipramine, venlafaxine and duloxetine are both serotonin and norepinephrine reuptake inhibitors. Because they inhibit serotonin reuptake, both are presumed to be effective for the treatment of OCD. However, neither is FDA-approved for OCD. Venlafaxine has been studied more extensively, but the findings conflict (Koran, Hanna et al. 2007). The only randomized placebo-controlled trial in OCD found no significant difference between venlafaxine and placebo. However, the sample was small ($n = 30$), the maximum dose only 225 mg/day, and the trial only 8 weeks long. Other randomized trials compared venlafaxine (or venlafaxine XR) to either paroxetine or clomipramine, using higher doses of venlafaxine (e.g., 225–300 mg/day). In both studies, venlafaxine was as efficacious as the SRI to which it was compared. Finally, in a crossover study of nonresponders, when paroxetine nonresponders were switched to venlafaxine, only 3 of 16 (19%) responded, whereas when venlafaxine nonresponders were switched to paroxetine, 15 of 27 (56%) responded.

Limitations of Serotonin Reuptake Inhibitors

Although SRIs are the only FDA-approved medications for OCD, they have important limitations: only up to 65% of patients will respond to an adequate trial; the typical response is a 20–40% reduction in symptoms; and patients can relapse if the medication is discontinued (Koran, Hanna et al. 2007). Because many patients will have a clinically meaningful but modest reduction in symptoms and some will have no response (e.g., <25% reduction in symptoms), clinicians who treat OCD patients will commonly be faced with both problems.

One strategy is to switch to another SRI and eventually to try clomipramine. Switching to venlafaxine or duloxetine is another option; however, the data for both agents is limited (as reviewed earlier). Switching to mirtazapine, shown in a small double-blind discontinuation study to reduce OCD symptoms, is another option (Koran, Gamel et al. 2005).

A different strategy is to augment SRI response by adding additional treatments. These augmentation strategies have much more empirical support.

Augmentation Strategies

Randomized controlled trials support the addition of EX/RP or antipsychotics to augment SRI response. A recent study (Simpson, Foa et al. 2013) found that EX/RP augmentation was superior to antipsychotic augmentation with risperidone. Many other augmenting agents have also been tried as well and are briefly reviewed.

CBT augmentation: Several randomized controlled trials examined the effects of delivering EX/RP to OCD patients on medications. In the first study, Tenneij and colleagues (2005) compared the effects of continuing medication (paroxetine or venlafaxine) versus adding EX/RP (18, 45-minute sessions over 6 months) in patients with mild OCD symptoms. Adding EX/RP was superior, but the effects were modest. In the second study, Simpson, Foa and colleagues (2008) recruited OCD patients who had received an SRI for at least 12 weeks but who still had clinically significant symptoms. Patients were randomized to EX/RP or to stress management therapy as a control therapy; both treatments included 17, 90-minute sessions delivered over 8 weeks. Patients receiving EX/RP had significantly fewer symptoms at the end of treatment (Figure 12.3A), and significantly more achieved an excellent response (Y-BOCS ≤ 12; 33% versus 4%). These effects were maintained in many patients at a 6 month follow-up (Foa, Simpson et al. 2013). In a third

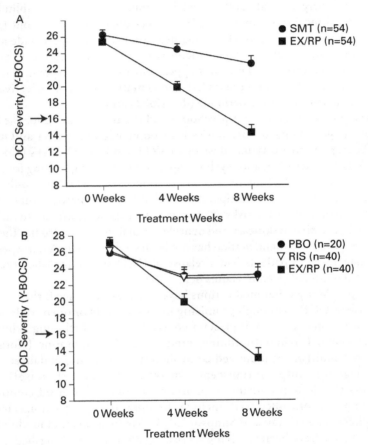

FIGURE 12.3 Augmenting serotonin reuptake inhibitors. (a) The effects of exposure and response prevention versus stress management therapy. An 8-week randomized controlled trial compared the effects of augmenting serotonin reuptake inhibitors (SRIs) with exposure and response prevention (EX/RP) versus stress management therapy (SMT). Estimates from linear mixed-effects models of Yale-Brown Obsessive Compulsive Scale (Y-BOCS) mean scores (with standard error bars) over time are shown by treatment group. See text for more details. (b) The effects of exposure and response prevention versus risperidone. An 8-week randomized controlled trial compared the effects of augmenting serotonin reuptake inhibitors (SRIs) with exposure and response prevention (EX/RP), risperidone (RIS), or pill placebo (PBO). Estimates from linear mixed-effects models of Yale-Brown Obsessive Compulsive Scale (Y-BOCS) mean scores (with standard error bars) over time are shown by treatment group. See text for more details.

study (Simpson, Foa et al. 2013), patients who had received an SRI for at least 12 weeks but who still had clinically significant symptoms were randomized to EX/RP, a low dose of risperidone (up to 4.0 mg/day), or pill placebo. Patients receiving EX/RP had significantly fewer symptoms at the end of treatment (Figure 12.3B), and significantly more achieved an excellent response (Y-BOCS ≤ 12; 43% EX/RP; 13% risperidone; 5% pill placebo). Together, these findings strongly support using EX/RP to augment SRIs in OCD.

Antipsychotic augmentation: Haloperidol, risperidone, quetiapine, olazapine, and aripiprazole have all been shown in randomized controlled trials to augment SRI response. There are also negative studies of these agents (reviewed in Fineberg, Brown et al. 2012, Koran and Simpson 2013). A review of antipsychotic augmentation (Bloch, Landeros-Weisenberger et al. 2006), which combined nine double-blind, randomized controlled clinical trials involving 278 subjects, concluded that about 1/3 of OCD patients will be helped by antipsychotic augmentation. The strongest evidence supports the use of haloperidol or risperidone. Patients with a minimal response to an SRI and/or patients with comorbid Tic Disorders appear most likely to respond. A recent study (Simpson, Foa et al. 2013) found that CBT augmentation was more effective than antipsychotic augmentation with risperidone (described earlier).

Given the potential risks of antipsychotics and the time required for the full effects of SRIs to emerge, adding antipsychotics is recommended only after an OCD patient has failed to respond to a maximal dose of an SRI for at least 12 weeks (Koran, Hanna et al. 2007). Low doses of an antipsychotic appear effective (e.g., <3 mg for risperidone or the equivalent), and the time to response is about 2–4 weeks. Since only a subset of OCD patients will respond, the antipsychotic should be terminated in those who do not clearly benefit to minimize the risks of antipsychotic exposure, which can include metabolic syndrome, tardive dyskinesia, and neuroleptic malignant syndrome. The long-term efficacy of antipsychotic augmentation has not been studied much. A retrospective study suggested that 13 of 15 patients had a relapse of OCD symptoms when their antipsychotic was discontinued (Koran, Hanna et al. 2007).

Other agents: Many other medications have been tested to see if they can enhance SRI response in OCD. Although promising in case reports or open trials, several did not show clear efficacy in small placebo-controlled trials, including lithium, buspirone, clonazepam, L-triiodothyronine, pindolol, and desipramine (Koran, Hanna et al. 2007). A multisite randomized controlled trial of adding ondansetron to SRIs was also negative (http://ir.transcept.com/releasedetail.cfm?ReleaseID=728327). Other agents that look promising in preliminary studies but need confirmation in larger randomized controlled trials include clomipramine, pregabalin, celecoxib, and dextroamphetamine (Koran and Simpson 2013). Medications that modulate the glutamatergic system have been receiving increasing attention, as described next.

Novel Medications that Target Brain Mechanisms

Human genetic studies, imaging studies, and animal models of OCD suggest that glutamatergic abnormalities in cortico-striatal circuits contribute to OCD symptoms (see also chapter 11, Ahmari and Dougherty). Thus, medications that modulate the glutamate system have been tested in OCD (reviewed in Pittenger, Bloch et al. 2011). Various agents, each thought to modulate glutamate in different ways, have shown some promise in case reports, open-label studies, or small controlled trials either as monotherapy or as an adjunct to SRIs. These agents include: *N*-acetylcysteine, memantine, riluzole, lamotrigine, topiramate, and minocycline. In a proof-of-concept small crossover study, a single dose of IV ketamine (an antagonist at the NMDA receptor) led to the rapid resolution of obsessions in unmedicated adults with OCD (Rodriguez, Kegeles et al. 2013). This introduces the exciting possibility that there could be rapidly acting medications for OCD.

TREATMENT OF CHILDREN AND ADOLESCENTS

First-line treatments: CBT alone or in combination with an SRI are first-line treatments for children and adolescents with OCD. This recommendation is supported by the Pediatric OCD Treatment Study (POTS, March, Foa et al. 2004) ($N = 112$, ages 7–17), which compared CBT alone (including cognitive training and EX/RP), SRI alone (sertraline), their combination, and pill placebo. All treatments were superior to placebo, and combination treatment was superior to CBT alone and to SRI alone. Remission rates were 54% for combination treatment, 39% for CBT alone, 21% for SRI alone, and 4% for placebo. The authors concluded that children and adolescents with OCD should begin treatment with CBT alone or in combination with a selective SRI.

A recent meta-analysis of 18 studies of CBT and pharmacological treatments for pediatric OCD concurs with these conclusions (Sánchez-Meca, Rosa-Alcázar et al. 2014). Comparing CBT, pharmacological, and combined treatments in a sample of 1223 patients (656 in the treatment groups and 567 in the control groups), the meta-analysis found that all treatments were efficacious in reducing OCD symptoms (with effect sizes adjusted by the type of control group of $d = 1.203$ for CBT, $d = 0.745$ for pharmacological treatments, and $d = 1.704$ for combination treatments). The specific CBT protocol and hours of treatment influenced the effect size; one of the most effective protocols was the one used in the POTS trial.

In 2004, the FDA placed a "black-box" warning on antidepressant medications, including SRIs, publicizing a two-fold increased risk for suicidal thinking or behavior in children and adolescents taking these medications (2% vs. 4%). On the other hand, a recent analysis of published and unpublished studies (12 adult, 4 geriatric, and 4 youth randomized controlled trials of fluoxetine and venlafaxine) found no evidence of increased suicide risk in youths receiving antidepressant medication. Instead, severity of depression improved with medication and was significantly related to suicide ideation or behavior (Gibbons, Hur et al. 2012). Using SRIs in children and adolescents requires careful balancing of these benefits and costs.

Augmentation strategies: Paralleling findings in adults, the addition of CBT to medication continuation compared to medication continuation alone leads to significantly greater response rates in children and adolescents with OCD (Franklin, Sapyta et al. 2011). Antipsychotics are often used to augment SRI response in clinical practice despite the fact that there are no randomized controlled trials of antipsychotic augmentation in pediatric OCD—only data from retrospective reports, case reports, and open-label studies (Masi, Pfanner et al. 2013). This is concerning given the data from adults that only about 1/3 will benefit from antipsychotic augmentation, and the fact that youth may be particularly vulnerable to the long-term effects of antipsychotics, including weight gain and diabetes.

SURGICAL AND OTHER TREATMENTS FOR OCD

Surgery: A small subset of OCD patients (up to 10%) will not respond to the treatments described earlier. Patients deemed treatment refractory (i.e., failed at least three adequate SRI trials, at least one augmentation trial with clomipramine, an antipsychotic, or clonazepam, and at least one EX/RP trial performed in combination with pharma-cotherapy) are potential candidates for neurosurgical interventions. These interventions include either making lesions in CSTC circuits or altering their activity using deep brain stimulation (DBS). These interventions are reviewed in detail in the companion chapter (chapter 11, Ahmari and Dougherty).

Transcranial magnetic stimulation (TMS): TMS is a noninvasive method for either stimulating or inhibiting neural transmission. Greenberg et al. (1997) found that a single session of stimulation of the right lateral PFC led to a decrease in compulsive urges that lasted for 8 hours. However, meta-analyses of the existing small trials of repetitive TMS (rTMS) studies suggest that rTMS of prefrontal regions (specifically the dorsolateral pre-frontal cortex) may not be effective in OCD, but that low-frequency rTMS targeting the supplemental motor area appears promising (Jaafari, Rachid et al. 2012, Berlim, Neufeld et al. 2013).

Electroconvulsive therapy (ECT): Given the limited data, ECT is not currently recom-mended for patients with OCD unless a patient has a comorbid condition (e.g., severe depression) for which ECT is effective (Koran, Hanna et al. 2007).

CONCLUSION

In summary, OCD is a severe, chronic, and disabling illness. Although all patients have obsessions and compulsions, patients can appear very different from each other because the specific content of obsessions and compulsions varies as does an individual patient's affective response, level of insight, and co-occurring psychiatric disorders. The result is a heterogeneous clinical phenotype. Researchers are working to identify domains of neural dysfunction that underlie the clinical phenotype, and to develop valid and reli-able probes of these domains that could be used in individual patients in clinical prac-tice. Success could ultimately change how we evaluate OCD, enabling clinicians to use not only self-reports of symptoms but also objective measures of brain dysfunction.

Dysfunction in CSTC circuits is implicated in the pathophysiology of OCD. However, what causes an individual to develop CSTC dysfunction and how CSTC dysfunction inter-acts with dysfunction in other circuits (e.g., fear circuitry) to produce the heterogeneous clinical phenotype remains unclear. Whether the obsessions and compulsions that occur in OCD share the same neural correlates as the repetitive thoughts and behaviors that occur in other psychiatric disorders is another question. Answers to these questions can change how we conceptualize OCD, and can help us identify novel targets for treatment development.

CBT consisting of EX/RP, SRIs, or their combination are first-line treatments for OCD, and can help about half of patients achieve minimal symptoms and live high-quality lives. As monotherapy, EX/RP can be more effective than SRIs when delivered expertly to adherent patients. Although FDA-approved for the treatment of OCD, SRIs can take weeks to have their full effects and usually lead to only a partial reduction in symptoms. Evidence-based SRI augmentation strategies include add-ing EX/RP or antipsychotics: recent data strongly support trying EX/RP first. For treatment-refractory patients, neurosurgical interventions are an option.

Faster and more effective treatments for OCD are clearly needed. Ideally, such treat-ments would be tailored to an individual's disease process and would capitalize on emerg-ing knowledge about the genetic vulnerability and neural processes implicated in OCD (e.g., response inhibition, habit formation, fear processing). The ultimate goal would be to preempt the development of OCD and therefore alleviate individual suffering and the public health burden of this disabling illness.

DISCLOSURE STATEMENT

In the last three years, Dr. Simpson has received research funds from the National Institute of Mental Health, the Brain and Behavior Foundation, and the pharmaceutical industry (i.e., Janssen Pharmaceuticals and Transcept Pharmaceuticals); she has also received consulting fees from Quintiles, Inc., and royalties from UpToDate, Inc. and Cambridge University Press. Dr. Foa has received research support from Transcept Pharmaceuticals, Neuropharm Ltd., Pfizer, Solvay, Eli Lilly, SmithKline Beecham, GlaxoSmithKline, Cephalon, Bristol-Myers Squibb, Forest, Ciba-Geigy, Kali-Duphar, and APA. She has been a speaker for Pfizer, GlaxoSmith-Kline, Forest, and APA; and she receives royalties from the sale of two books on obsessive-compulsive disorder from Bantam and Oxford University Press.

REFERENCES

Ahmari, S. E., V. B. Risbrough, M. A. Geyer, and H. B. Simpson (2012). Impaired sensorimotor gating in unmedicated adults with obsessive–compulsive disorder. *Neuropsychopharmacology* 37 (5): 1216–1223.

American Psychiatric Association. (2013). *Diagnostic and Statistical Manual of Mental Disorders, Fifth Edition.* Arlington, VA: American Psychiatric Association.

Ameringen, M., B. Patterson and W. Simpson (2014). DSM-5 obsessive-compulsive and related disorders: Clinical implications of new criteria. *Depress Anxiety* 31 (6): 487–493.

Andersson, E., J. Enander, P. Andren, E. Hedman, B. Ljotsson, T. Hursti, ... C. Ruck (2012). Internet-based cognitive behaviour therapy for obsessive-compulsive disorder: A randomized controlled trial. *Psychol Med* EPUB: 1–11.

Berlim, M. T., N. H. Neufeld, and F. Van den Eynde (2013). Repetitive transcranial magnetic stimulation (rTMS) for obsessive–compulsive disorder (OCD): An exploratory meta-analysis of randomized and sham-controlled trials. *J Psychiatric Res* 47 (8): 999–1006.

Bloch, M. H., A. Landeros-Weisenberger, B. Kelmendi, V. Coric, M. B. Bracken, and J. F. Leckman (2006). A systematic review: antipsychotic augmentation with treatment refractory obsessive-compulsive disorder. *Mole Psychiatry* 11 (7): 622–632.

Bloch, M. H., J. McGuire, A. Landeros-Weisenberger, J. F. Leckman, and C. Pittenger (2010). Meta-analysis of the dose-response relationship of SSRI in obsessive-compulsive disorder. *Mol Psychiatry* 15 (8): 850–855.

Chasson, G. S., U. Buhlmann, D. F. Tolin, S. R. Rao, H. E. Reese, T. Rowley, K. S. Welsh, and S. Wilhelm (2010). Need for speed: evaluating slopes of OCD recovery in behavior therapy enhanced with d-cycloserine. *Behav Res Ther* 48 (7): 675–679.

El Mansari, M., and P. Blier (2006). Mechanisms of action of current and potential pharmacotherapies of obsessive-compulsive disorder. *Prog Neuropsychopharmacol Biol Psychiatry* 30 (3): 362–373.

Fineberg, N. A., A. Brown, S. Reghunandanan, and I. Pampaloni (2012). Evidence-based pharmacotherapy of obsessive-compulsive disorder. *Int J Neuropsychopharmacol* 15 (08): 1173–1191.

Fineberg, N. A., A. Brown, S. Reghunandanan, and I. Pampaloni (2012). Evidence-based pharmacotherapy of obsessive-compulsive disorder. *Int J Neuropsychopharmacol* 15 (8):1173–1191.

Foa, E. B., M. J. Kozak, W. K. Goodman, E. Hollander, M. A. Jenike, and S. A. Rasmussen (1995). DSM-IV field trial: Obsessive-compulsive disorder. *Am J Psychiatry* 152 (1): 90–96.

Foa, E. B., M. R. Liebowitz, M. J. Kozak, S. Davies, R. Campeas, M. E. Franklin, ... X. Tu (2005). "Randomized, placebo-controlled trial of exposure and ritual prevention, clomipramine, and their combination in the treatment of obsessive-compulsive disorder." *Am J Psychiatry* 162 (1): 151–161.

Foa, E. B., H. B. Simpson, M. R. Liebowitz, M. B. Powers, D. Rosenfield, S. P. Cahill, ... M. T. Williams (2013). Six-month follow-up of a randomized controlled trial augmenting serotonin reuptake inhibitor treatment with exposure and ritual prevention for obsessive-compulsive disorder. *J Clin Psychiatry* 74 (5): 464–469.

Foa, E. B., G. Steketee, J. B. Grayson, and H. G. Doppelt (1983). Treatment of obsessive-compulsives: When do we fail? In E. B. Foa and P. M. G. Emmelkamp (Eds.), *Failures in behavior therapy* (10–34). New York, NY: John Wiley & Sons.

Foa, E. B., E. Yadin, and T. K. Lichner (2012). *Exposure and response (ritual) prevention for obsessive-compulsive disorder.* New York, NY: Oxford University Press.

Franklin, M. E., J. Sapyta, J. B. Freeman, M. Khanna, S. Compton, D. Almirall, . . . A. L. Edson (2011). Cognitive behavior therapy augmentation of pharmacotherapy in pediatric obsessive-compulsive disorder: the Pediatric OCD Treatment Study II (POTS II) randomized controlled trial. *J Am Med Assoc* 306 (11): 1224–1232.

Gibbons, R. D., K. Hur, C. H. Brown, J. M. Davis, and J. J. Mann (2012). Benefits from antidepressants: Synthesis of 6-week patient-level outcomes from double-blind placebo-controlled randomized trials of fluoxetine and venlafaxine. *Arch Gen Psychiatry* 69 (6): 572–579.

Gillan, C. M., M. Papmeyer, S. Morein-Zamir, B. J. Sahakian, N. A. Fineberg, T. W. Robbins, and S. de Wit (2011). Disruption in the balance between goal-directed behavior and habit learning in obsessive-compulsive disorder. *Am J Psychiatry* 168 (7): 718–726.

Goodman, W. K., L. H. Price, S. A. Rasmussen, C. Mazure, R. L. Fleischmann, C. L. Hill, G. R. Heninger, and D. S. Charney (1989). The Yale-Brown obsessive compulsive scale: I. Development, use, and reliability. *Arch Gen Psychiatry* 46 (11): 1006–1011.

Greenberg, B. D., M. S. George, J. D. Martin, J. Benjamin, T. E. Schlaepfer, M. Altemus, . . . D. L. Murphy (1997). Effect of prefrontal repetitive transcranial magnetic stimulation in obsessive-compulsive disorder: A preliminary study. *Am J Psychiatry* 154 (6): 867–869.

Hiss, H., E. B. Foa, and M. J. Kozak (1994). Relapse prevention program for treatment of obsessive-compulsive disorder. *J Consult Clin Psychol* 62 (4): 801.

Jaafari, N., F. Rachid, J.-Y. Rotge, M. Polosan, W. El-Hage, D. Belin, N. Vibert, and A. Pelissolo (2012). Safety and efficacy of repetitive transcranial magnetic stimulation in the treatment of obsessive-compulsive disorder: A review. *World J Biol Psychiatry* 13 (3): 164–177.

Koran, L. M., N. N. Gamel, H. W. Choung, E. H. Smith, and E. N. Aboujaoude (2005). Mirtazapine for obsessive-compulsive disorder: An open trial followed by double-blind discontinuation. *J Clin Psychiatry* 66 (4): 515–520.

Koran, L. M., G. L. Hanna, E. Hollander, G. Nestadt, and H. B. Simpson (2007). Practice guideline for the treatment of patients with obsessive-compulsive disorder. *Am J Psychiatry* 164 (7 Suppl): 5–53.

Koran, L. M., and H. B. Simpson (2013). Guideline watch (March 2013): Practice guideline for the treatment of patients with obsessive-compulsive disorder. *APA Prac Guide* 1–22.

Leckman, J. F., D. Denys, H. B. Simpson, D. Mataix-Cols, E. Hollander, S. Saxena, . . . D. J. Stein (2010). Obsessive-compulsive disorder: A review of the diagnostic criteria and possible subtypes and dimensional specifiers for DSM-V. *Depress Anxiety* 27 (6): 507–527.

March, J., E. Foa, P. Gammon, A. Chrisman, J. Curry, D. Fitzgerald, . . . M. Rynn (2004). Cognitive-behavior therapy, sertraline, and their combination for children and adolescents with obsessive-compulsive disorder: The Pediatric OCD Treatment Study (POTS) randomized controlled trial. *J Am Med Assoc* 292 (16): 1969–1976.

Markarian, Y., M. J. Larson, M. A. Aldea, S. A. Baldwin, D. Good, A. Berkeljon, . . . D. McKay (2010). Multiple pathways to functional impairment in obsessive-compulsive disorder. *Clinical Psychol Rev* 30 (1): 78–88.

Masi, G., C. Pfanner, and P. Brovedani (2013). Antipsychotic augmentation of selective serotonin reuptake inhibitors in resistant tic-related obsessive-compulsive disorder in children and adolescents: A naturalistic comparative study. *J Psychiatric Res* 47 (8): 1007–1012.

Milad, M. R., S. C. Furtak, J. L. Greenberg, A. Keshaviah, J. J. Im, . . . S. Wilhelm (2013). Deficits in conditioned fear extinction in obsessive-compulsive disorder and neurobiological changes in the fear circuit. *J Am Med Assoc Psychiatry* 70 (6): 608–618.

Milad, M. R., and S. L. Rauch (2012). Obsessive-compulsive disorder: Beyond segregated cortico-striatal pathways. *Trends Cogn Sci 16* (1): 43–51.

Ninan, P. T., L. M. Koran, A. Kiev, J. R. Davidson, S. A. Rasmussen, J. M. Zajecka, D. G. Robinson, P. Crits-Christoph, F. S. Mandel, and C. Austin (2006). High-dose sertraline strategy for nonresponders to acute treatment for obsessive-compulsive disorder: a multicenter double-blind trial. *J Clin Psychiatry 67* (1): 15–22.

Olatunji, B. O., D. Rosenfield, C. D. Tart, J. Cottraux, M. B. Powers, and J. A. Smits (2013). Behavioral versus cognitive treatment of obsessive-compulsive disorder: An examination of outcome and mediators of change. *J Consult Clin Psychol 81* (3): 415.

Pauls, D. L. (2010). The genetics of obsessive-compulsive disorder: A review. *Dialogues Clin Neurosci 12* (2): 149–163.

Pertusa, A., R. O. Frost, and D. Mataix-Cols (2010). When hoarding is a symptom of OCD: A case series and implications for DSM-V. *Behav Res Ther 48* (10): 1012–1020.

Phillips, K. A., A. Pinto, A. S. Hart, M. E. Coles, J. L. Eisen, W. Menard, and S. A. Rasmussen (2012). A comparison of insight in body dysmorphic disorder and obsessive-compulsive disorder. *J Psychiatric Res 46* (10): 1293–1299.

Pinto, A., J. L. Eisen, M. C. Mancebo, and S. A. Rasmussen (2008). Obsessive-compulsive personality disorder. *Obsessive-compulsive disorder: Subtypes and spectrum conditions.* New York, NY: Elsevier.

Pittenger, C., M. H. Bloch, and K. Williams (2011). Glutamate abnormalities in obsessive compulsive disorder: neurobiology, pathophysiology, and treatment. *Pharmacol Ther 132* (3): 314–332.

Ravizza, L., G. Maina, and F. Bogetto (1997). Episodic and chronic obsessive-compulsive disorder. *Depress Anxiety 6* (4): 154–158.

Rodriguez, C. I., L. S. Kegeles, A. Levinson, T. Feng, S. M. Marcus, D. Vermes, . . . H. B. Simpson (2013). Randomized controlled crossover trial of ketamine in obsessive-compulsive disorder: Proof-of-concept. *Neuropsychopharmacology 38* (12): 2475–2483.

Rosa-Alcázar, A. I., J. Sánchez-Meca, A. Gómez-Conesa, and F. Marín-Martínez (2008). Psychological treatment of obsessive–compulsive disorder: A meta-analysis. *Clin Psychol Rev 28* (8): 1310–1325.

Ruscio, A. M., D. J. Stein, W. T. Chiu, and R. C. Kessler (2010). The epidemiology of obsessive-compulsive disorder in the National Comorbidity Survey Replication. *Mol Psychiatry 15* (1): 53–63.

Sánchez-Meca, J., A. I. Rosa-Alcázar, M. Iniesta-Sepúlveda, and Á. Rosa-Alcázar (2014). Differential efficacy of cognitive-behavioral therapy and pharmacological treatments for pediatric obsessive–compulsive disorder: A meta-analysis. *J Anxiety Disorders 28* (1): 31–44.

Shavitt, R. G., M. A. de Mathis, F. Oki, Y. A. Ferrao, L. Fontenelle, A. R. Torres, . . . M. Q. Hoexter (2014). Phenomenology of OCD: Lessons from a large multicenter study and implications for ICD-11. *J Psychiatric Res 57*: 141–148.

Shelton, R. C. (2006). The nature of the discontinuation syndrome associated with antidepressant drugs. *J Clin Psychiatry 67*: 3–7.

Simpson, H. B., E. B. Foa, M. R. Liebowitz, J. D. Huppert, S. Cahill, M. J. Maher, . . . R. Campeas (2013). Cognitive-behavioral therapy vs risperidone for augmenting serotonin reuptake inhibitors in obsessive-compulsive disorder: A randomized clinical trial. *J Am Med Assoc Psychiatry 70*(11): 1190–1199.

Simpson, H. B., E. B. Foa, M. R. Liebowitz, D. R. Ledley, J. D. Huppert, S. Cahill, . . . E. Petkova (2008). A randomized, controlled trial of cognitive-behavioral therapy for augmenting pharmacotherapy in obsessive-compulsive disorder. *Am J Psychiatry 165* (5): 621–630.

Simpson, H. B., M. E. Franklin, J. Cheng, E. B. Foa, and M. R. Liebowitz (2005). Standard criteria for relapse are needed in obsessive-compulsive disorder. *Depress Anxiety 21* (1): 1–8.

Simpson, H. B., J. D. Huppert, E. Petkova, E. B. Foa, and M. R. Liebowitz (2006). Response versus remission in obsessive-compulsive disorder. *J Clin Psychiatry 67* (2): 269–276.

Simpson, H. B., M. J. Maher, Y. Wang, Y. Bao, E. B. Foa, and M. Franklin (2011). Patient adherence predicts outcome from cognitive behavioral therapy in obsessive-compulsive disorder. *J Consult Clin Psychol 79* (2): 247–252.

Simpson, H. B., S. M. Marcus, A. Zuckoff, M. Franklin and E. B. Foa (2012). "Patient adherence to cognitive-behavioral therapy predicts long-term outcome in obsessive-compulsive disorder." *J Clin Psychiatry* 73(9): 1265–1266.

Simpson, H. B., A. M. Zuckoff, M. J. Maher, J. R. Page, M. E. Franklin, E. B. Foa, . . . Y. Wang (2010). Challenges using motivational interviewing as an adjunct to exposure therapy for obsessive-compulsive disorder. *Behav Res Ther* 48 (10): 941–948.

Skoog, G., and I. Skoog (1999). "A 40-year follow-up of patients with obsessive-compulsive disorder." *Arch Gen Psychiatry* 56 (2): 121–127.

Stewart, S., D. Geller, M. Jenike, D. Pauls, D. Shaw, B. Mullin, and S. Faraone (2004). Long-term outcome of pediatric obsessive–compulsive disorder: A meta-analysis and qualitative review of the literature. *Acta Psychiatrica Scand* 110 (1): 4–13.

Tenneij, N. H., H. J. van Megen, D. A. Denys, and H. G. Westenberg (2005). Behavior therapy augments response of patients with obsessive-compulsive disorder responding to drug treatment. *J Clin Psychiatry* 66 (9): 1169–1175.

Twohig, M. P., S. C. Hayes, J. C. Plumb, L. D. Pruitt, A. B. Collins, H. Hazlett-Stevens, and M. R. Woidneck (2010). A randomized clinical trial of acceptance and commitment therapy versus progressive relaxation training for obsessive-compulsive disorder. *J Consult Clin Psychol* 78 (5): 705.

van Balkom, A. J., E. de Haan, P. van Oppen, P. Spinhoven, K. A. Hoogduin, and R. van Dyck (1998). Cognitive and behavioral therapies alone versus in combination with fluvoxamine in the treatment of obsessive compulsive disorder. *J Nerv Ment Dis* 186 (8): 492–499.

van Velzen, L. S., C. Vriend, S. J. de Wit, and O. A. van den Heuvel (2014). Response inhibition and interference control in obsessive-compulsive spectrum disorders. *Front Human Neurosci* 8: 419.

Whittal, M. L., M. Robichaud, D. S. Thordarson, and P. D. McLean (2008). Group and individual treatment of obsessive-compulsive disorder using cognitive therapy and exposure plus response prevention: A 2-year follow-up of two randomized trials. *J Consult Clin Psychol* 76 (6): 1003–1014.

Wilhelm, S., G. Steketee, J. M. Fama, U. Buhlmann, B. A. Teachman, and E. Golan (2009). Modular cognitive therapy for obsessive-compulsive disorder: A wait-list controlled trial. *J Cog Psychotherapy* 23 (4): 294.

PHOBIAS, FEARS, AND PANIC

13

THE ETIOLOGY OF FEAR AND ANXIETY

The Role of Environmental Exposures

JOHN M. HETTEMA

INTRODUCTION

As expounded upon in prior chapters, there are several aspects of the etiology of fear and anxiety that have been well established:

1. The emotional/behavioral response to threat, as typified by the fight or flight response, is programmed into living organisms to serve one of the most critical instinctual drives: survival.
2. Anxiety disorders (ANX) including generalized anxiety disorder (GAD), panic disorder (PD), agoraphobia (AG), social phobia (SOC), and specific phobias (SP), seem to represent a dysregulation of the normal threat response, in which the response is inappropriate or excessive in regards to the level of potential harm.
3. Since all biological systems are controlled, at various levels, by the genes encoded in DNA, it is not surprising that genetic factors play a substantial role in both the normal expression of fear in animals and humans and its dysregulation as defined by our clinical nosology. Thus, nearly all human traits and disorders, including fear and anxiety disorders, have some inherent genetic basis. This is true even for infectious diseases, in which a clear external pathogen is the direct cause, but the infectious process is influenced by the genetics of the host.

Importantly, risk for disorders of fear and anxiety is also influenced by nongenetic factors, particularly environmental exposures with psychological salience like life experiences. This knowledge comes from two major sources of data: (1) twin studies parse latent (unmeasured) variance into genetic and environmental sources, the former reflected in estimates of heritability. They generally find that all psychiatric disorders have heritability less than 100%, indicating a significant role for environmental effects that varies by disorder. (2) Traditional case-control or cohort studies directly measure the effects of individual putative risk factors on the outcomes of interest. These effects are typically quantified as an odds ratio (OR) or relative risk (RR), depending upon the study design.

Figure 13.1 illustrates the classic twin study design (see Kendler, 2001 for extensive reviews of twin studies of psychiatric phenotypes). The outcome trait is measured in each member of a twin pair (Tw1, Tw2). There are three basic sources (risk domains) of individual differences of any trait: genetic factors (here denoted as A for additive genetic effects, although other types of genetic effects are allowable), familial influences shared by the twins (C, common familial factors), and environmental influences unique to each twin (E, individual specific environmental factors). The fact that these are latent, not measured, influences in this study design is denoted by ovals in the diagram. Double-headed arrows from each risk domain in Twin 1 to the same domain in Twin 2 indicate the average degree of correlation (or resemblance) for each: 1 or ½ for A, depending on whether the pair is monozygotic (MZ) or dizygotic (DZ), respectively; 1 for C, independent of zygosity (equal environment assumption); and no correlation for E (by definition).The strength of A, C, and E factors influencing the trait in each twin is denoted by the path loadings a, c, and e, which can range from 0 to 1 (in standardized notation). The application of twin structural equation modeling to phenotype data allows one to estimate a, c, and e, the proportion of variance of the outcome due to each of these risk domains (See (Neale and Cardon, 1992) for more details.) As reviewed in chapter 4, like many other commonly occurring psychiatric phenotypes (e.g., depression, substance abuse), the influence of genetics in ANX is only moderate (heritability 30–50%), with the remaining variance primarily explained by E in adults (Hettema et al., 2001).

A primary risk study, whether twin pair or traditional single-subject design, first aims to measure the direct (main) effects of genetic and/or environmental factors on the outcome phenotype. However, etiological models also allow the inclusion of a higher-order effect: gene-by-environment interaction (GxE). Psychiatric researchers

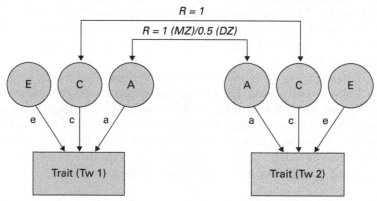

FIGURE 13.1 Classic twin study design in which the outcome trait is measured in each member of a twin pair (Tw1, Tw2). The three basic risk domains are additive genetics (A), familial shared environment (C), and individual specific (nonshared) environment (E). The strengths of A, C, and E factors influencing the trait are denoted by the path loadings a, c, and e. Double-headed arrows from each risk domain in Twin 1 to the same domain in Twin 2 indicate the average degree of correlation, with only A varying by zygosity (MZ = monozygotic pair, DZ = dizygotic pair).

have long postulated that it is the combination of genetic and environmental factors that best explains risk. Thus, genes "prime" the organism to respond to an environmental exposure. When the exposure occurs, different individuals will respond differently based upon their genetic makeup ("genetic sensitivity to the environment"). This is one example of the *stress-diathesis model* (Monroe and Simons, 1991), which asserts that if the combination of the predisposing vulnerability (diathesis) and the environmental stress exceeds a (nonspecified) threshold, the person will develop the disorder.

This is the basic model proposed for the patho-etiology of PTSD, as explained in Section 4: genetic (and other) premorbid factors influence which trauma-exposed individuals are more or less likely to develop PTSD. However, researchers expect a similar mechanism is at work in other disorders. For example, major depressive (MD) episodes more likely occur after stressful events in individuals with a family history of mood disorders. Panic attacks similarly onset or recur during stressful exposures in susceptible individuals.

Note that, in addition to studying the genetics of the observed outcome of interest (i.e., anxiety disorders) as the diathesis, one might examine an inherent trait correlated with it that is intermediate between the direct biological expression of the underlying genes and the diagnostic level outcome. Such "endophenotypes" are generally less complex, often quantitative rather than categorical, and can be reliably measured in unaffected individuals (Gottesman and Gould, 2003). Detection of the endophenotypes in unaffected individuals suggests they represent an unexpressed vulnerability (diathesis). In order to be true endophenotypes and not just biomarkers associated with the illness, the genetic factors underlying their expression must overlap those of the illness ("co-aggregate" in families). Thus, family members might express the vulnerability they carry in their genes via such endophenotypes without ever developing the illness. Some have argued that their relative phenotypic simplicity might translate into a simpler genetic architecture, reducing genetic heterogeneity and increasing power to identify risk variants.

Several psychological, physiological, and brain-based measures have been proposed as potential diatheses for ANX. The most extensively studied category is premorbid anxious temperamental traits, like behavioral inhibition, neuroticism, introversion, and harm avoidance, as reviewed in chapter 4. Other well-studied ANX diatheses include laboratory paradigms of fear-conditioning and extinction (Lissek et al., 2005), startle reflex (Grillon and Baas, 2003), physiologic responsivity to chemical challenges like carbon dioxide (CO_2)-induced panic (Amaral et al., 2013), cognitive or emotional biases to negative stimuli (Armstrong and Olatunji, 2012; Britton et al., 2011), or patterns of neural activation in response to emotional faces (Ball et al., 2012; Britton et al., 2013). While researchers generally consider these as candidate endophenotypes, only neuroticism (Hettema et al., 2006), introversion (Bienvenu et al., 2007), and CO_2 challenge (Battaglia et al., 2008) have been sufficiently examined in genetically informative study designs to establish their genetic overlap with ANX. Of note, many of these are not specific to one or another anxiety disorder, but rather, have variable associations across multiple disorders. This is consistent with, and one of the drivers for, a recent shift in the direction of psychopathological research, as expressed in NIMH's Research Domain Criteria (RDoC) initiative (http://www.nimh.nih.gov/research-priorities/rdoc/index.shtml). RDoC is part of NIMH's strategic plan to "develop new ways of classifying disorders based on dimensions of observable behaviors and brain functions." RDoC aims to serve as a framework for new approaches to research on mental disorders using fundamental dimensions that cut across traditional disorder categories and more closely align with mechanisms that underlie psychopathology at various biological levels from genes to neural circuits to behavioral responses.

Like the main effects of genes and environment, both twin and case-control study designs can detect GxE effects. In principle, the sequence of discovery should follow the same order as that emphasized for testing for main effects of genetic factors: first use a twin design to establish that GxE effects exist for a condition, then search for *which* specific genes account for those effects. However, very few twin studies have directly tested for GxE effects. Most extant GxE studies have focused on symptoms or episodes of depression, generally finding evidence that latent genetic background moderates the depressogenic effect of adverse experiences (Kendler et al., 1995; Wichers et al., 2009). Two juvenile twin studies have thus far reported tentative GxE effects for anxiety symptoms (Lau et al., 2007; Silberg et al., 2001), but no studies have examined this for ANX disorders in children or adults. Chapter 4 of this volume reviews GxE studies conducted with selected candidate genes and environments.

The remainder of this chapter summarizes the extant evidence supporting the role that particular environmental experiences ("exposures") increase and shape the risk of developing ANX. It is meant to be representative rather than exhaustive, focusing on meta-analyses, reviews, or large epidemiological studies. While the focus here is on ANX disorders, there is a much larger research literature addressing the environmental risk factors for depression than for ANX, with PTSD being the obvious exception. Therefore, where relevant and useful, I will compare findings across studies of ANX versus depressive disorders. Environmental exposures have been much less studied for obsessive compulsive and related disorders, so they will not be considered herein. And, given the early and tentative nature of GxE effects for ANX, I restrict the details of this review to environmental main effects.

CHILDHOOD ENVIRONMENT

A range of candidate variables representing key aspects of the family environment experienced by a child during development has been tested for association with ANX. Ones most studied and showing robust effects are early parental loss, parenting style, and childhood abuse. Table 13.1 summarizes the main findings from several large, representative epidemiological studies that assessed these major childhood risk factor domains in relation to various ANX. Strength of association is provided from each study as an OR. For the purposes of this review, effects are roughly summarized across genders when reported separately. Where available, associations between risk domains and MD are provided for comparison.

Early Parental Loss

Early parental loss, via death or separation, has been implicated in adult risk of MD in a fair number of studies, with most finding that disruption of parental care (separation, neglect) is more specifically predictive of adult depression than loss (death) per se (Harris et al., 1986; Veijola et al., 2004). Few large studies have examined the effects of parental loss or separation on ANX. As reported by the two studies included in Table 13.1, parental loss increases risk for most ANX with OR between 1.2 and 2.8. The Virginia Twin Registry (VTR) study separately examined separation and

TABLE 13.1 Association between major domains of childhood adversity and risk for adult anxiety and depressive disorders reported in several large, epidemiologic studies

RISK FACTOR	STUDY (N)	REF	ODDS RATIO (OR)							
			GAD	PD	PHOB	AG	SOC	SP	PTSD	MD
Parental Loss/	EDSP (2427)	Wittchen et al., 2000	2.4	2.3		2.8	2.0	1.2		NS
Separation	VTR[a] (4671)	Kendler et al., 1992; Otowa et al., 2014	1.44	2.06	1.24					1.52
Parenting[a]	NCS (5877)	Enns et al., 2002								
Coldness			1.16	1.08		1.10	1.08	1.08	1.21	1.16
Overprotection			1.06	1.01		1.09	1.06	1.04	1.06	1.04
Parenting[a]	ESSMeD (8232)	Heider et al., 2008								
Coldness			1.40	1.25			1.42	1.15		
Overprotection			1.12	1.23			1.19	1.17		
Parenting[a]	VTR (4671)	Kendler et al., 2000b; Otowa et al., 2013								
Coldness			1.33	1.48	1.26					1.33
Overprotection			1.27	1.24	1.24					1.16
Sexual Abuse[c]	NCS[a] (5877)	Molnar et al., 2001	1.15	1.10		1.05	1.50	1.20	7.75	1.80
	NCS-R (4141)	Cougle et al., 2010	1.28	1.91		0.69 (NS)	1.70	0.85 (NS)	2.38	
	VTR[b] (1411)	Kendler et al., 2000	1.62	1.99						1.72

Blank cells indicate that the disorder was not assessed or not analyzed for association to the risk factor in the referenced study.

[a] OR averaged across genders where reported separately.

[b] Only risk to females was assessed.

[c] Adjusted for other disorders and risk factors.

EDSP = Early Developmental Stages of Psychopathology; VTR = Virginia Twin Registry; NCS = National Comorbidity Study; ESSMeD = European Study of the Epidemiology of Mental Disorders; NCS-R = National Comorbidity Study—Replication; NS = nonsignificant; GAD = generalized anxiety disorder; PD = panic disorder; PHOB = any phobia; AG = agoraphobia; SOC = social phobia; SP = specific phobia; PTSD = posttraumatic stress disorder; MD = major depression.

loss, finding broad effects for the former across all ANX but only phobia predicted by parental death.

Parenting Style

Various psychological theories implicate parenting style in the development of anxiety. Several early, small studies suggested that reduced parental care, characterized by low warmth or neglect, and parental overprotection are associated with risk for many forms of psychopathology, particularly anxiety and depression. A review of the subject of child autonomy and parental overprotection suggests that early experience with diminished control may foster a cognitive style characterized by an increased probability of interpreting or processing subsequent events as out of one's control, which may represent a psychological vulnerability for anxiety (Chorpita and Barlow, 1998). A meta-analysis of 23 observational studies of 1,305 parent-child dyads reported a moderate effect of parental control on child anxiety (Cohen's $d = 0.58$; van der Bruggen et al., 2008). A review and meta-analysis of an array of parental factors potentially influencing the onset of ANX and MD during adolescence concluded that reduced parental warmth, more inter-parental conflict, parental overinvolvement, and aversiveness increased risk for both ANX and depressive disorders (Yap et al., 2014).

Several large studies have simultaneously examined risk for each ANX across multiple parenting dimensions assessed using the Parental Bonding Instrument, which typically produces three correlated factors: warmth (or its inverse, coldness or lack of care), overprotection, and authoritarianism. Results are reported for three such studies in Table 13.1: low parental warmth (coldness) consistently but nonspecifically predicted development of most ANX and MD. On the other hand, the effects of parental overprotection were more variable, with some studies suggesting more specificity for ANX versus depression. Both dimensions of parenting have modest effect sizes on these various outcomes, increasing risk by 50% or less, depending on the study. Interestingly, a pattern emerged in some studies showing that the most consistent associations were seen in children of the same gender as the parent providing the care. Authoritarianism is generally not associated with ANX.

Note that parenting styles likely have complex and bidirectional influences on the child. For example, overprotectiveness might be evoked in parents of anxious or depressed children who are deemed more vulnerable, making this an effect of psychopathology rather than a cause. Anxiety and depression in parents not only can be transmitted genetically to offspring but can directly affect parenting style and adequacy. Furthermore, parenting itself has a genetic component (Kendler, 1996), so no simple model can explain the effects of parenting on psychopathology.

Childhood Abuse

The largest extant systematic review and meta-analysis of the relationship between sexual abuse and lifetime psychopathology was conducted using a total sample size of over 3 million subjects from 37 studies, providing the most accurate and unbiased estimates of this association (Chen et al., 2010). There were statistically significant associations between sexual abuse and Any ANX (OR, 3.09; 95% CI 2.43–3.94), PTSD (OR, 2.34; 95% CI 1.59–3.43), and depression (OR, 2.66; 95% CI 2.14–3.30), among others. The confidence intervals for all of these outcomes overlap, suggesting little overall diagnostic specificity for risk from sexual abuse. Another review examined risk by subtype of abuse, concluding that physical abuse, sexual abuse, and unspecified neglect are generally associated with both mood and ANX disorders (Carr et al., 2013).

The main findings from some of the larger epidemiological studies that examined the effects of childhood sexual abuse (CSA) on individual ANX are shown in Table 1. Kendler and colleagues reported ORs for CSA in females that were comparable between MD, GAD, PD, and alcohol and drug dependence, with stronger effects for more severe forms of abuse (Kendler et al., 2000). These were only mildly attenuated when adjusted for family functioning and parental psychopathology, suggesting that CSA is an independent risk factor for a wide range of psychiatric conditions. Using multivariate analyses in the National Comorbidity Survey (NCS) controlling for parental psychopathology and other forms of abuse, Molnar et al. found modest (OR ~ 1.5) associations between CSA and each ANX and MD in females but no significant associations in males. The exception was PTSD, with strong associations in both female and male CSA survivors (OR = 10.2 and 5.3, respectively; Molnar et al., 2001).

Analyses using the NCS-Replication sample ($N = 4,141$) were conducted to determine the differential impact of physical versus sexual abuse on individual ANX and PTSD. Multivariate analyses found significant associations for physical abuse on PTSD and SP and CSA on PTSD and each ANX except SP, with somewhat smaller effects (OR ranges 1.3–2.4; Cougle et al., 2010). Examining comorbidity, de Graaf and colleagues analyzed the effects of any childhood abuse on prevalence of pure and comorbid ANX and mood disorders in the prior 12 months in the Dutch NEMESIS study (R. de Graaf et al., 2002). After controlling for other adversities, abuse significantly predicted pure any ANX (OR = 1.7), pure any mood disorder (OR = 2.3), and mood plus ANX (OR = 2.7).

These studies were conducted in large samples of adults retrospectively reporting abuse, often decades after it occurred. Fergusson et al. (1996) assessed 1,019 members of a New Zealand birth cohort at age 18 for CSA occurring before age 16 and psychiatric disorders in the prior two years. After adjusting for multiple confounders, their estimated effects of CSA on any ANX and MD were consistent overall with those from the other studies, supporting the validity of those results (Fergusson et al., 1996).

One of the only large epidemiological samples in which the effects of multiple domains of adversity were simultaneously analyzed is the NCS. Kessler et al. (1997) analyzed the effects of 26 specific childhood adversities categorized as interpersonal loss (parental death or divorce), parental psychopathology, interpersonal trauma (e.g., abuse or aggression), and other (e.g., accidents, natural disasters) on adult psychopathology. Most bivariate adversity-diagnosis associations had OR > 1, with 67% significant at $P = 0.05$ level; thus, most adversities were diagnostically nonspecific. The most consistent predictors across diagnoses were parental psychopathologies (93% significant), followed by interpersonal traumas (79% significant). The former result is difficult to interpret, since it could represent the effects of genes and/or parenting or other downstream sequelae of being raised in a household with parental mental illness. The most consistently significant loss event across diagnoses was parental separation or divorce, with death of either parent showing few associations with adult outcomes. Controlling for multiple adversities and prior disorders attenuated most associations; for example, no loss events remained significantly associated with any ANX or MD. The authors caution against overinterpretation of studies analyzing the effects of single adversities on single disorders since they likely have compound, complex effects on child development.

In summary, various aspects of the environment experienced during childhood fairly nonspecifically increase risk for most ANX and depressive disorders. These are, in order of increasing effect size: parental bonding (lack of care/warmth, overprotection/control): OR 1.1–1.5; parental separation/loss: OR 1.5–2; sexual/physical abuse: OR 2–3. While there appear to be specific effects of each type of adversity on risk after controlling for others, often these are experienced in the context of multiple adversities occurring in the same family. It is not surprising that the overall family environment has profound effects on a broad array of developmental outcomes and adult disorders.

STRESSFUL LIFE EVENTS

In this section, I review the role of stressful life events (SLE) occurring after childhood to distinguish their effects from those from childhood adversity. Studying the effects of SLE is difficult to do well. There are many types of SLE, and they can be characterized in multiple ways based upon their hypothesized effects (acute vs. chronic, interpersonal—dependent vs. independent, emotional salience—threat vs. loss, etc.). Because one usually assumes relatively short-term effects, SLEs are often studied in relation to the first onset of a disorder or a recent episode, which makes data on relative timing critical and samples relatively underpowered to detect effects of particular stressors. For this reason, researchers often resort to simply counting the number of recent or lifetime SLE, assuming an additive and cumulative effect, which is crude model for their complex emotional effects in an individual's life.

Several excellent reviews exist that delineate the role for recent SLE in risk of MD (see, for example, Paykel, 1994). Only one such review currently exists for ANX with its focus on PD (Klauke et al., 2010). The reader is referred to their tables listing all studies available at the time of the article's publication. Most are small and heterogeneous in design, producing some variability across them. The authors conclude that the cumulative effects of stress (i.e., count of SLE), as well as specific life events, such as threat, interpersonal and health-related events, impact on the development of PD.

Comparing types of SLE for differential risk of psychiatric outcomes, early studies from Brown and colleagues report that recent SLE involving "loss" were more often related to cases of depression. In comparison, ones involving "danger" (threat of loss) were more often related to anxiety, with comorbid conditions tending to involve both (Finlay-Jones and Brown, 1981).

For ANX, many of the larger studies focus on SLE in GAD in comparison with MD. Newman and Bland compared Life Events Scale scores in 222 subjects with MD and 234 with GAD from 3,070 community survey respondents in Edmonton, Canada (cross-sectional; Newman and Bland, 1994). They observed a significantly increasing trend for total LES scores and certain subscales of events (*entrance, undesirable,* and *marital*): no MD or GAD < GAD only < MD only < both MD and GAD, but no diagnostic specificity for types of events. Pine and colleagues assessed 23 SLE and various internalizing and externalizing disorders in an epidemiologic sample of 760 subjects aged 11–20 years at baseline and again 6 years later (Pine et al., 2002). Significant cross-sectional associations were seen between total number of SLE at baseline and most baseline psychopathology (MD, GAD, phobia, OCD, PD, ADHD, conduct disorder). SLE at baseline was the main predictor variable for psychopathology at follow-up, controlling for age, gender, SES, and diagnosis at baseline.

Kendler et al. examined the effects and specificity of 15 classes of SLE for predicting onsets of MD or a comparable 2-week duration generalized anxiety syndrome (GAS) in the year prior to interview of female subjects from the VTR (Kendler et al., 1998). Thirteen out the 15 were significantly associated with MD risk in the month of occurrence, with OR ranging from 2.5 (personal network illness) to 18 (assault). Similarly, most events were also associated with risk for GAS (OR 2.2 for network illness to 10 for assault). Specificity, as indexed by ratio of OR predicting MD versus GAS, was noted for some events: One event, (network death), was the most specific for MD (ratio 7.6); five events (assault, divorce/separation, and serious financial, housing, or network relationship problems), were modestly specific for MD (ratios 1.3 to 2); three (loss of confidant, and work or legal problems) were modestly specific for GAS (ratios 0.4 to 0.7), and six lacked specificity (ratios 0.8 to 1.2).

Few large studies looked at other individual ANX or ANX as a group. One re-analyzed the lifetime effects of several SLE categories for onset of three phobia types in the NCS, with the following findings: life-threatening accidents, natural disasters, and combat raised risk for AG (OR 2.9, 2.2, 3.5, respectively) but no specific events after childhood significantly increased risk for SOC or SP (Magee, 1999). McLaughlin and colleagues (2010) looked at the effects of past-year SLE on 12-month MD, PTSD, ANX in the very large US National Epidemiological Survey of Alcohol and Related Conditions (NESARC) sample (N = 34,653). Increasing numbers of SLE corresponded to higher prevalence of each outcome. These results were moderated by level of prior childhood adversity, such that greater levels of adversity produced larger effects of SLE. The authors concluded that this supports the stress-sensitization hypothesis, in which individuals exposed to early life adversity become more sensitive to pathogenic effects of SLE as adults (McLaughlin et al., 2010).

In summary, SLE likely increase risk for ANX as they also do for MD, with some suggestion that threat verses loss content of specific domains of SLE are more relevant for ANX. Beyond that, the inherent difficulties in examining the effects of SLE together with insufficient studies of ANX limits the specific inferences one can draw regarding their effects on ANX risk compared to depression.

SOCIAL SUPPORT

Social support has been found to overall reduce the risk of MD in most studies (Paykel, 1994), with little support for the "buffering theory of social support," which postulates that effective social support specifically lessens the depressogenic effects of SLE (Aneshensel and Stone, 1982; Wade and Kendler, 2000). Comparatively little study has been devoted to the effects of social support on risk for ANX. Plaisier and colleagues found evidence for similar levels of protective effects of social support on incidence of both depressive and ANX disorders as a group using longitudinal data from the NEMESIS sample, but they did not analyze effects for specific disorders (Plaisier et al., 2007). In 2065 subjects from Oslo registered in the National Population Register, current perceived social support if ill, among a number of quality of life indicators, was compared for each ANX to: other ANX, other nonanxiety Axis I disorders, and subjects with no Axis I disorder (Cramer et al., 2005). GAD and AG were the only ANX for which significantly lower social support was not seen in any of the comparisons, suggesting that social support has a role in some, but not all, ANX.

CONCLUSIONS

Environmental factors, in general, play a major role in the development of ANX, accounting for 50% or more of individual differences in risk. This likely occurs via both main effects and interactions with prior risk factors, particularly genetics. Several major domains of childhood adversity, including parenting, parental separation/loss, and physical/sexual abuse, each accounts for significantly increased risk that does not vary much across different disorders. The recent or cumulative effects of many types of life events after childhood also contribute to risk of ANX onset during adulthood, although their relevance over and above that of childhood adversity is unclear. Also, insufficient data exists to estimate the importance of gene-by-environment effects in addition their main effects. More research effort needs to be applied to address these outstanding questions.

REFERENCES

Amaral, J. M., Spadaro, P. T., Pereira, V. M., Silva, A. C. and Nardi, A. E. (2013). The carbon dioxide challenge test in panic disorder: A systematic review of preclinical and clinical research. *Rev. Bras. Psiquiatr.* 35, 318–331.

Aneshensel, C. S. and Stone, J. D. (1982). Stress and depression: A test of the buffering model of social support. *Arch. Gen. Psychiatry* 39, 1392–1396.

Armstrong, T. and Olatunji, B. O. (2012). Eye tracking of attention in the affective disorders: A meta-analytic review and synthesis. *Clin. Psychol. Rev.* 32, 704–723.

Ball, T. M., Sullivan, S., Flagan, T., Hitchcock, C. A., Simmons, A., Paulus, M. P. and Stein, M. B. (2012). Selective effects of social anxiety, anxiety sensitivity, and negative affectivity on the neural bases of emotional face processing. *Neuroimage.* 59, 1879–1887.

Battaglia, M., Pesenti-Gritti, P., Spatola, C. A., Ogliari, A. and Tambs, K. (2008). A twin study of the common vulnerability between heightened sensitivity to hypercapnia and panic disorder. *Am. J. Med. Genet. B Neuropsychiatr. Genet.* 147B, 586–593.

Bienvenu, O. J., Hettema, J. M., Neale, M. C., Prescott, C. A. and Kendler, K. S. (2007). Low extraversion and high neuroticism as indices of genetic and environmental risk for social phobia, agoraphobia, and animal phobia. *Am. J. Psychiatry* 164, 1714–1721.

Britton, J. C., Grillon, C., Lissek, S., Norcross, M. A., Szuhany, K. L., Chen, . . . Pine, D. S. (2013). Response to learned threat: An fMRI study in adolescent and adult anxiety. *Am. J. Psychiatry* 170, 1195–1204.

Britton, J. C., Lissek, S., Grillon, C., Norcross, M. A. and Pine, D. S. (2011). Development of anxiety: The role of threat appraisal and fear learning. *Depress. Anxiety.* 28, 5–17.

Carr, C. P., Martins, C. M., Stingel, A. M., Lemgruber, V. B. and Juruena, M. F. (2013). The role of early life stress in adult psychiatric disorders: A systematic review according to childhood trauma subtypes. *J. Nerv. Ment. Dis.* 201, 1007–1020.

Chen, L. P., Murad, M. H., Paras, M. L., Colbenson, K. M., Sattler, A. L., Goranson, E. N., . . . Zirakzadeh, A. (2010). Sexual abuse and lifetime diagnosis of psychiatric disorders: Systematic review and meta-analysis. *Mayo Clin. Proc.* 85, 618–629.

Chorpita, B. F. and Barlow, D. H. (1998). The development of anxiety: The role of control in the early environment. *Psychol. Bull.* 124, 3–21.

Cougle, J. R., Timpano, K. R., Sachs-Ericsson, N., Keough, M. E. and Riccardi, C. J. (2010). Examining the unique relationships between anxiety disorders and childhood physical and sexual abuse in the National Comorbidity Survey-Replication. *Psychiatry Res.* 177, 150–155.

Cramer, V., Torgersen, S. and Kringlen, E. (2005). Quality of life and anxiety disorders: A population study. *J. Nerv. Ment. Dis.* 193, 196–202.

de Graaf R., Bijl, R. V., Smit, F., Vollebergh, W. A. and Spijker, J. (2002). Risk factors for 12-month comorbidity of mood, anxiety, and substance use disorders: Findings from the Netherlands Mental Health Survey and Incidence Study. *Am. J. Psychiatry* 159, 620–629.

Enns, M. W., Cox, B. J., and Clara, I. (2002). Parental bonding and adult psychopathology: results from the US National Comorbidity Survey. *Psychol Med* 32(6), 997–1008.

Fergusson, D. M., Horwood, L. J. and Lynskey, M. T. (1996). Childhood sexual abuse and psychiatric disorder in young adulthood: II. Psychiatric outcomes of childhood sexual abuse. *Am. Acad. Child. Adolesc. Psychiatry* 34, 1365–1374.

Finlay-Jones, R. and Brown, G. W. (1981). types of stressful life event and the onset of anxiety and depressive disorders. *Psychol. Med.* 11, 803–815.

Gottesman, I. I. and Gould, T. D. (2003). The endophenotype concept in psychiatry: Etymology and strategic intentions. *Am. J. Psychiatry* 160, 636–645.

Grillon, C. and Baas, J. (2003). A review of the modulation of the startle reflex by affective states and its application in psychiatry. *Clin. Neurophysiol.* 114, 1557–1579.

Harris, T., Brown, G. W. and Bifulco, A. (1986). Loss of parent in childhood and adult psychiatric disorder: The role of lack of adequate parental care. *Psychol. Med.* 16, 641–659.

Heider, D., Matschinger, H., Bernert, S., Alonso, J., Brugha, T. S., Bruffaerts, R., de G. G., Dietrich, S., and Angermeyer, M. C. (2008). Adverse parenting as a risk factor in the occurrence of anxiety disorders: a study in six European countries. *Soc Psychiatry Psychiatr Epidemiol.* 43(4), 266–272.

Hettema, J. M., Neale, M. C., and Kendler, K. S. (2001). A review and meta-analysis of the genetic epidemiology of anxiety disorders. *Am. J. Psychiatry.* 158, 1568–1578.

Hettema, J. M., Neale, M. C., Myers, J., Prescott, C. A. and Kendler, K. S. (2006). A population-based twin study of the relationship between neuroticism and internalizing disorders. *American. J Psychiatry* 163, 857–864.

Kendler, K. S. (1996). Parenting: A genetic-epidemiologic perspective. *Am. J. Psychiatry* 153, 11–20.

Kendler, K. S. (2001). Twin studies of psychiatric illness: An update. *Arch. Gen. Psychiatry* 58, 1005–1014.

Kendler, K. S., Bulik, C. M., Silberg, J., Hettema, J. M., Myers, J. and Prescott, C. A. (2000). Childhood sexual abuse and adult psychiatric and substance use disorders in women: An epidemiological and cotwin control analysis. *Arch. Gen. Psychiatry* 57, 953–959.

Kendler, K. S., Karkowski, L. M. and Prescott, C. A. (1998). Stressful life events and major depression: Risk period, long-term contextual threat, and diagnostic specificity. *J. Nerv. Ment. Dis.* 186, 661–669.

Kendler, K. S., Kessler, R. C., Walters, E. E., MacLean, C., Neale, M. C., Heath, A. C. and Eaves, L. J. (1995). Stressful life events, genetic liability, and onset of an episode of major depression in women. *Am. J. Psychiatry* 152, 833–842.

Kendler, K. S., Myers, J., and Prescott, C. A. (2000b) Parenting and adult mood, anxiety and substance use disorders in female twins: an epidemiological, multi-informant, retrospective study. *Psychol Med.* 30(2), 281–294.

Kendler, K. S., Neale, M. C., Kessler, R. C., Heath, A. C., and Eaves, L. J. (1992). Childhood parental loss and adult psychopathology in women. A twin study perspective. *Arch Gen Psychiatry.* 49(2), 109–116.

Kessler, R. C., Davis, C. G. and Kendler, K. S. (1997). Childhood adversity and adult psychiatric disorder in the US National Comorbidity Survey. *Psychol. Med.* 27, 1101–1119.

Klauke, B., Deckert, J., Reif, A., Pauli, P. and Domschke, K. (2010). Life events in panic disorder-an update on "candidate stressors." *Depress. Anxiety* 27, 716–730.

Lau, J. Y., Gregory, A. M., Goldwin, M. A., Pine, D. S. and Eley, T. C. (2007). Assessing gene-environment interactions on anxiety symptom subtypes across childhood and adolescence. *Dev. Psychopathol.* 19, 1129–1146.

Lissek, S., Powers, A. S., McClure, E. B., Phelps, E. A., Woldehawariat, G., Grillon, C. and Pine, D. S. (2005). Classical fear conditioning in the anxiety disorders: a meta-analysis. *Behav. Res. Ther.* 43, 1391–1424.

Magee, W. J. (1999). Effects of negative life experiences on phobia onset. *Soc. Psychiatry Psychiatr. Epidemiol.* 34, 343–351.

McLaughlin, K. A., Conron, K. J., Koenen, K. C. and Gilman, S. E. (2010). Childhood adversity, adult stressful life events, and risk of past-year psychiatric disorder: a test of the stress sensitization hypothesis in a population-based sample of adults. *Psychol. Med.* 40, 1647–1658.

Molnar, B. E., Buka, S. L. and Kessler, R. C. (2001). Child sexual abuse and subsequent psychopathology: results from the National Comorbidity Survey. *Am. J. Public Health* 91, 753–760.

Monroe, S. M. and Simons, A. D. (1991). Diathesis-stress theories in the context of life stress research: Implications for the depressive disorders. *Psychol. Bull.* 110, 406–425.

Neale, M. C. and Cardon, L. R. (1992). *Methodology for genetic studies of twins and families*. Dordrecht, The Netherlands: Kluwer Academic Publishers B.V.

Newman, S. C. and Bland, R. C. (1994). Life events and the 1-year prevalence of major depressive episode, generalized anxiety disorder, and panic disorder in a community sample. *Compr. Psychiatry* 35, 76–82.

Otowa, T., Gardner, C. O., Kendler, K. S., and Hettema, J. M. (2013). Parenting and risk for mood, anxiety and substance use disorders: a study in population-based male twins. *Soc Psychiatry Psychiatr Epidemiol.* 48(11), 1841–1849.

Otowa, T., York, T. P., Gardner, C. O., Kendler, K. S., and Hettema, J. M. (2014). The impact of childhood parental loss on risk for mood, anxiety and substance use disorders in a population-based sample of male twins. *Psychiatry Res.* 220(1–2):404–409.

Paykel, E. S. (1994). Life events, social support and depression. *Acta Psychiatr. Scand Suppl* 377, 50–58.

Pine, D. S., Cohen, P., Johnson, J. G. and Brook, J. S. (2002). Adolescent life events as predictors of adult depression. *J. Affect. Disord.* 68, 49–57.

Plaisier, I., de Bruijn, J. G., de Graaf, R., ten Have, M., Beekman, A. T. and Penninx, B. W. (2007). The contribution of working conditions and social support to the onset of depressive and anxiety disorders among male and female employees. *Soc. Sci. Med.* 64, 401–410.

Silberg, J., Rutter, M., Neale, M. and Eaves, L. (2001). Genetic moderation of environmental risk for depression and anxiety in adolescent girls. *Br. J. Psychiatry* 179, 116–121.

van der Bruggen, C. O., Stams, G. J. and Bogels, S. M. (2008). Research review: the relation between child and parent anxiety and parental control: a meta-analytic review. *J. Child Psychol. Psychiatry* 49, 1257–1269.

Veijola, J., Maki, P., Joukamaa, M., Laara, E., Hakko, H. and Isohanni, M. (2004). Parental separation at birth and depression in adulthood: A long-term follow-up of the Finnish Christmas Seal Home Children. *Psychol. Med.* 34, 357–362.

Wade, T. D. and Kendler, K. S. (2000). The relationship between social support and major depression: Cross-sectional, longitudinal, and genetic perspectives. *J. Nerv. Ment. Dis.* 188, 251–258.

Wichers, M., Schrijvers, D., Geschwind, N., Jacobs, N., Myin-Germeys, I., Thiery, E., ... Van, O. J. (2009). Mechanisms of gene-environment interactions in depression: Evidence that genes potentiate multiple sources of adversity. *Psychol. Med.* 39, 1077–1086.

Wittchen, H. U., Kessler, R. C., Pfister, H., and Lieb, M. (2000). Why do people with anxiety disorders become depressed? A prospective- longitudinal community study. *Acta Psychiatr Scand Suppl* 406, 14–23.

Yap, M. B., Pilkington, P. D., Ryan, S. M. and Jorm, A. F. (2014). Parental factors associated with depression and anxiety in young people: A systematic review and meta-analysis. *J. Affect. Disord.* 156, 8–23.

/// 14 /// CLINICAL ASPECTS OF SOCIAL ANXIETY DISORDER AND SPECIFIC PHOBIAS

FRANKLIN SCHNEIER AND ASALA HALAJ

INTRODUCTION

Social anxiety disorder and specific phobia are the two most common anxiety disorders, and they are among the most prevalent of all psychiatric disorders. These diagnostic categories were carved out of the broader category of phobic neuroses in the 1970s. The modern classification of phobias grew out of work by Marks and Gelder (1966) demonstrating different ages of onset for subcategories of phobic disorders. Social anxiety disorder was originally termed "social phobia" in *Diagnostic and Statistical Manual of Mental Disorders,* third edition (DSM-III) and was originally defined by excessive fear of scrutiny in circumscribed situations, such as performance or eating in public. In the 1980s, it was recognized that performance fears often exist on a continuum with broader anxiety about social evaluation in most interpersonal situations (Liebowitz, Gorman, Fyer, and Klein, 1985). These observations led to a broadening of the definition of social phobia to include persons with fears of most social situations, termed the "generalized" subtype, and "social anxiety disorder" was introduced as an alternative term for the disorder. Current DSM-5 nomenclature has retained this broader definition and adopted "social anxiety disorder" (SAD) as the preferred name (see Table 14.1). In recognition of findings that the strongest support for subtyping exists for the more narrowly defined performance-related fears, DSM-5 recognizes a "performance only" subtype (Heimberg et al., 2014).

Specific phobias were previously termed "simple phobias" in DSM-III. In DSM-IV the name was changed to "specific" phobia, and based on findings of significant heterogeneity of gender distribution, age of onset, and other characteristics, five types of specific phobias were identified: blood injection/injury, animal (animals or insects), natural environment (e.g., heights, storms, water), situational (e.g., driving, tunnels, enclosed places, flying), and other (e.g., loud noises, costumed characters, or situations that could lead to choking or vomiting). The specific phobia criteria and subtypes have largely been carried forward in DSM-5 (see Table 14.2) (Lebeau et al., 2010).

TABLE 14.1 Summary of Social Anxiety Disorder Diagnostic Criteria

SOCIAL ANXIETY DISORDER (SOCIAL PHOBIA)

A. Marked fear or anxiety about at least one social situation involving possible scrutiny by others. (In children, anxiety must occur with peers.)

B. Fear of acting in a way or showing anxiety symptoms that will result in negative evaluation (e.g., be humiliating, lead to rejection, or be offensive to others).

C. The feared social situations almost always result in fear or anxiety.

D. The feared social situations are avoided or endured with intense fear or anxiety.

E. The fear is out of proportion to the actual threat.

F. Symptoms last 6 months or more.

G. Symptoms cause clinically significant distress or impairment in functioning.

H./I. Symptoms are not due to a substance or another mental disorder.

J. If a medical condition that draws unwanted attention is present, SAD symptoms are clearly unrelated to it or excessive.

"Performance only" type: fear limited to speaking or performing in public.

TABLE 14.2 Summary of Specific Phobia Diagnostic Criteria

SPECIFIC PHOBIA

A. Marked fear or anxiety about an object or situation (e.g., flying, heights, animals, injection, blood). In children, fear/anxiety may manifest by crying or other distress behaviors.

B. The feared object/situation almost always provokes an immediate fear.

C. The feared object/situation is avoided or endured with intense fear.

D. The fear/anxiety is out of proportion to the object/situation and its context.

E. Symptoms are persistent (e.g., > 6 months).

F. Symptoms cause clinically significant distress or impairment in functioning.

G. Symptoms are not better explained by another mental disorder.

PREVALENCE AND COURSE

The lifetime prevalence of SAD in the community has been estimated at 5–14% in recent surveys, and about one-third of this seems to represent the performance-only subtype (Kessler et al., 1998). About 60% of individuals with SAD in the community are female, but men are overrepresented in treatment-seeking samples (Xu et al., 2012). Onset of SAD may occur as early as age 5, but it is most common in the mid-teens. First onset after age 30 is uncommon. Figure 14.1A, depicts the age-specific cumulative lifetime incidence rates for SAD up to age 33 among females and males as assessed in the 10-year prospective-longitudinal Early Developmental Stages of Psychopathology (EDSP) study (Beesdo et al., 2010). Naturalistic follow-up studies suggest that SAD follows a chronic course in the community, with a mean recovery rate of 40% after 5 years, and recovery rates tend to be lower in clinical samples (e.g., 27% after 5 years) (Steinert, Hofmann, Leichsenring, and Kruse, 2013).

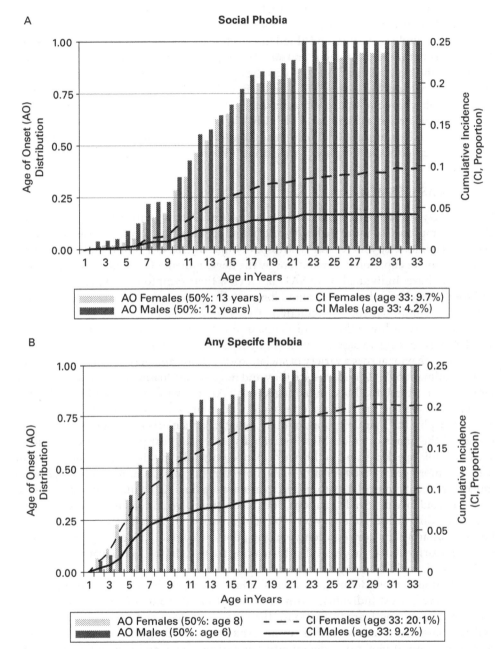

FIGURE 14.1 Cumulative incidence (CI) and age of onset (AO) distribution of A. SAD and B. specific phobias by gender (EDSP; *N* = 3021). Bars show the cumulative age of onset distribution; lines show the age-dependent cumulative lifetime incidence; in phobias impairment was required among subjects aged 18 years or older.

The lifetime prevalence of specific phobias is approximately 12%, with a female-to-male ratio of about 2:1 (Kessler, Petukhova, Sampson, Zaslavsky, and Wittchen, 2012). Prevalence ranges for specific types include 3.3–7% for animal phobias, 8.9–11.6% for natural environment phobias, 5.2–8.4% for situational phobias, and 3.2–4.5% for blood-injury phobias. Animal and blood injury phobia typically have an onset before age 10, whereas natural environment and situational phobias more commonly have an age of onset in the teens. Figure 14.1B depicts the age-specific cumulative lifetime incidence rates for specific phobia in the EDSP study (Beesdo et al., 2010). Most individuals with specific phobia have multiple phobias during their lifetime, and half have three or more lifetime specific phobias (Lebeau et al., 2010). Whereas many specific phobias in childhood prove to be transient or at least tend to improve over time without treatment, in adults most cases of specific phobia are chronic (Silverman and Moreno, 2005).

CLINICAL ASSESSMENT

Social anxiety disorder presentation and clinical features. Persons with SAD typically struggle with symptoms for more than a decade before seeking treatment. Treatment seeking may be precipitated by increasing distress and impairment, as a young adult faces social pressures and occupational demands, or by the development of secondary depression or substance abuse. Individuals with SAD often view their symptoms as a personality flaw and sometimes build their lives around longstanding symptoms, such as by taking a job that requires minimal social interaction. They may tend to underreport the impact of social fear on their life, either out of shame or due to having accommodated to chronic avoidance, so during an assessment it is important to investigate the scope of fear and avoidance behavior across a variety of social, work/school, and performance situations.

The hallmark of SAD is fear of scrutiny and negative evaluation by others in social or performance situations. Most individuals with SAD report fearful cognitions of being judged to be foolish, inarticulate, or anxious, and many are also concerned that others will notice physical manifestations of their anxiety, particularly blushing, sweating, and tremor of the hands or voice. Most individuals with SAD fear performance situations, such as public speaking, and in the performance-only subtype this constitutes the main fear. The more generalized form of SAD, however, is typically more severe and more impairing, and it is more likely to lead to treatment seeking. Avoidance may take the form of overt avoidance of social situations, such as declining invitations to social gatherings or even missing classes, or it may be more subtle, such as by attending a social gathering but not initiating any conversations, making poor eye contact, or cutting conversations short. Impairment may involve difficulty making friends, dating, participating in school, seeking work, and advancing in a career.

In addition to these defining features, a number of other characteristics of SAD have been observed. Most individuals with SAD report marked anticipatory anxiety before important upcoming feared situations. They may lose sleep and play out scenarios of embarrassment and failure in their mind. Anxiety typically peaks upon entering the feared situation. It may reach the intensity of a panic attack and may not decline until the individual leaves the situation. Performance anxiety is particularly associated with autonomic arousal symptoms of tremor and pounding heart (Pull, 2012). After leaving a feared situation, persons with SAD often harshly review their social performance and feel self-loathing and depressed mood. Usually these depressed moods are transitory, but many persons with SAD go on to develop major depressive disorder (see next section on comorbidity). Although persons with SAD may crave social approval, they also often report discomfort with positive evaluation, feeling unworthy, unsure how to respond, and fearing they will be unable to fulfill heightened expectations (Kashdan, Weeks, and Savosyanova, 2011).

Social anxiety disorder comorbidity and differential diagnosis. SAD is most commonly comorbid with other anxiety disorders. In SAD, if panic attacks occur they are limited to the anticipation of (or experience of) being in a social or performance situation, whereas as in panic disorder they occur in a variety of settings and sometimes occur unexpectedly. Generalized anxiety disorder shares symptoms of anticipatory and situational anxiety with SAD, but it encompasses prominent and excessive fears of nonsocial situations as well. Unlike the obsessions in obsessive-compulsive disorder, the fearful ruminations in SAD are experienced as more ego-syntonic than intrusive, and they are accompanied by avoidance rather than by compulsive behaviors.

Depression is a common secondary symptom in SAD, but the social avoidance in SAD is primarily related to fears of negative evaluation, rather than due to the lack of social interest or low energy seen in primary major depressive disorder. The social discomfort of SAD differs from that occurring in psychotic disorders in that individuals with SAD typically can acknowledge their own behavior as the problem, rather than having delusional beliefs that others have singled them out for harm. Body dysmorphic disorder and eating disorders are often accompanied by prominent fears about appearance to others, but these tend to be driven more by extreme internal standards and are less focused on negative evaluation by others. Substance use disorders, particularly alcohol and cannabis dependence, often occur secondary to SAD. Some SAD patients report that these substances initially relieved their SAD symptoms, but that the substances themselves then became problematic (Buckner, Heimberg, Ecker, and Vinci, 2013). Avoidant personality disorder has been shown to greatly overlap the more generalized forms of SAD, and some researchers have argued that these ought to be considered alternative descriptors of the same area of psychopathology. At the other end of the severity spectrum, SAD differs from nonpathological shyness in being more severe, pervasive, and impairing.

Specific phobia presentation, clinical features, and differential diagnosis. The diagnosis of specific phobia is relatively straightforward, given the inherently circumscribed quality of the disorder. The fear in specific phobia must be excessive, persistent, maladaptive, and generally not subject to reason or voluntary control, and it leads to avoidance of the feared stimulus (Silverman and Moreno, 2005). The emotional content of fears in specific phobias is variable. About half of individuals with animal phobia focus on disgust, and about a quarter focus on danger. Most individuals with phobias of the natural environment or situations, however, focus on danger or harm. In blood-injury phobias the focus is usually a physical symptom (e.g., fainting) or disgust (Lebeau et al., 2010). Blood-injury phobias also manifest a distinct physiological response pattern. Whereas response to a feared stimulus in most phobias leads to persistent tachycardia, in blood-injury phobia an initial tachycardia is followed by vasovagal bradycardia and frequently syncope (Marks, 1998).

In addition to comorbid specific phobias, other anxiety disorders and depression are common among individuals with specific phobia. Situational phobias are associated with unexpected panic attacks at a higher rate than other types of specific phobias. Although the circumscribed nature of some specific phobias limits their functional impairment, individuals with specific phobia do evidence impairment in functioning relative to persons with no anxiety disorder (Comer et al., 2011). Blood injury fears can interfere with obtaining medical or dental care, for example, and situational phobias often interfere with travel. Specific phobias are distinguished from normal fears by their severity, persistence, associated impairment, and by not being developmentally age- or stage-specific.

CASE VIGNETTE 1: SOCIAL ANXIETY DISORDER

Mr. A. is a 27-year-old who presented with a chief complaint of social anxiety after being laid off from his job at a media company. He attributed this negative life event to his inability to actively participate in group meetings and his tendency to delay making phone calls, due to fears of negative evaluation. He recalled being a shy child but always had a couple of good friends. He did well in school but tried to avoid speaking up in class unless he was called upon. As a teenager his anxiety around groups of peers intensified, and he began to avoid social gatherings due to fears that he would seem awkward and stumble over his words. He avoided dating until late in college, due to fears of rejection. In his job he did well with written assignments, but worried about making a poor impression in meetings, so he usually remained silent. When he did attempt to speak in meetings, he experienced strong palpitations and sweating, and he was afraid that his anxiety was evident to all his colleagues. He had always hoped he would "grow out" of his social fears, but finally decided he had better get help before it ruined his career prospects.

CASE VIGNETTE 2: SPECIFIC PHOBIA

Ms. B is a 19-year-old woman who has always felt disgusted by the sight of blood. At age 10 she fainted while having blood drawn in her doctor's office. She has been able to comply with doctor's visits at the urging of her family by lying down and looking away when she has had to have blood drawn. She also developed a fear of visiting the dentist, also feeling disgust at seeing small amounts of blood in her saliva after dental work. Since moving away from her family for college, she had stopped going to dental appointments and now has developed severe toothaches requiring multiple extractions. Ms. B also has strong fears of spiders and other small insects, although these are not impairing in her everyday life.

CONCEPTUAL APPROACHES

Social anxiety disorder. A variety of explanatory models have been proposed for SAD. Twin studies suggest that the genetic heritability of SAD is in the range of 20–40% (Kendler, Myers, Prescott, and Neale, 2001), but the role of specific genes remains poorly understood. Developmental models hypothesize that a genetic predisposition and early developmental effects may lead to a behaviorally inhibited temperament, present in 10–15% of toddlers, which in turn is a risk factor for the development of SAD in childhood and adolescence. Parental anxiety and parenting processes such as overprotection and excessive criticism may contribute to the expression of SAD, as may bullying or conditioning events (Ollendick and Benoit, 2012). Often, however, patients report only a gradual onset of fears that they experience as characterologic. Evolutionary models of SAD note its similarities with an excess of submissive behaviors, such as gaze aversion and appeasement behavior in the face of threat, behaviors common to other group-living species (Gilbert, 2001).

Cognitive-behavioral models of SAD incorporate elements of biased attention toward social threats and interpretation of neutral stimuli as threatening. Self-focused attention interferes with social performance and with opportunities to disconfirm fears of negative evaluation. Safety behaviors, such as attempts to conceal anxiety, have the unintended consequences of contributing to the maintenance of social anxiety. Postevent processing is negatively biased and maintains negative self-impressions and future avoidance (Morrison and Heimberg, 2013).

Neurobiological studies have identified abnormalities in multiple neurotransmitter systems, including serotonin, dopamine, and GABA. Dysregulation of the hypothalamic pituitary axis and autonomic arousal has also been noted. As in other anxiety disorders, fMRI studies have implicated hyperactive fear circuitry with impaired cortical regulation of amygdala activity, and dysfunction in medial and parietal regions related to theory of mind and self-consciousness may be more specific to SAD (Brühl et al., 2014). Behaviorally inhibited temperament in early childhood has been shown to be a risk factor for developing pathological social anxiety in humans and nonhuman primates. This temperament is associated with a number of stable neurobiological traits, including increased reactivity of neural circuitry involving the amygdala, hippocampus, prefrontal cortex and insula, decreased connectivity of amygdala with prefrontal cortex, and alterations in gene expression that diminish neuroplasticity of the amygdala (Fox and Kalin, 2014).

Specific phobia. Some specific fears, such as fear of heights, thunderstorms, and animals, have been noted to have innate survival value. This suggests an evolutionary basis for prepared fears, but it does not explain why only some people develop phobias around these situations. Specific phobias have been shown to be highly familial, and rates of genetic heritability vary by type of phobia, with highest rates for animal fear (45%) and blood-injury fears (33%). Animal and situational phobias have also been reported to be strongly influenced by specific environmental factors. Environmental factors that have been shown to play a role in some cases of specific phobia include direct conditioning, vicarious learning (e.g., by observing parental reactions), and instructional learning (Silverman and Moreno, 2005; Van Houtem et al., 2013).

TREATMENT

Social anxiety disorder psychotherapies. Cognitive behavioral therapy (CBT) is the best-established psychotherapy for SAD, supported by randomized, controlled trials and several meta-analyses. In clinical trials, CBT for SAD has typically been administered over 12–16 weekly sessions. One component of CBT treatment is psychoeducation, in which individuals develop an understanding of the onset and examine the causes and triggers of anxiety. The cognitive elements of CBT of SAD feature cognitive restructuring, in which a patient identifies cognitive distortions and learns techniques to utilize helpful thoughts to prevent and manage social fears. The behavioral element of CBT involves systematic exposure to the feared situations with elimination of safety behaviors (Wong, Gordon, and Heimberg, 2012). CBT for SAD often incorporates role-plays to simulate social situations and behavioral experiments to challenge beliefs about feared outcomes. Socratic questioning, logical disputation, relaxation exercises, and social training skills are also commonly used CBT techniques.

Some comparative treatment studies (e.g., Hofmann, 2004) have found that cognitive behavioral therapy is more effective than treatment with exposure alone. In addition, both individual and group formats of CBT have been found to be effective in SAD (Heimberg, Salzman, Holt, and Blendell, 1993; Clark et al., 2003). Group therapy has potential advantages of increased support from other group members and broader opportunities for in vivo exposure, however, group therapy can feel threatening to some individuals with social fears, and scheduling a compatible group of patients can be logistically challenging.

Other psychotherapies have been much less studied. A few studies (e.g., Piet, Hougaard, Hecksher, and Rosenberg, 2010) suggest that mindfulness may not be as effective as CBT. Interpersonal psychotherapy also appeared less effective than CBT in one randomized controlled trial (Strangier, Schramm, Heidenreich, Berger, and Clark, 2011). Psychodynamic therapy is also sometimes used clinically in SAD, and a recent controlled trial found that manualized psychodynamic therapy and CBT did not differ significantly in response rate over 15 weeks of treatment (Leichsenring et al., 2013). In summary, the preponderance of evidence supports CBT as a first line treatment for SAD patients, although recent studies show that other therapies including psychodynamic therapy are possibly efficacious alternatives.

Social anxiety disorder medication therapies. Several classes of medication have been found in randomized clinical trials to have efficacy in treating SAD. The selective serotonin reuptake inhibitors (SSRIs) and the SNRI venlafaxine are the first line medications for SAD, based on more than 20 randomized controlled trials, most with response rates of 50–70% (Ipser, Kariuki, and Stein, 2008). Dosing is similar to that used in depression, such as 20mg/day for paroxetine, but higher doses may be helpful for some patients. Improvement may be noticeable in the first few weeks, but some patients take up to 12 weeks to achieve a response (Stein, Westenberg, Yang, and Barbato, 2003). Improvement sometimes accrues gradually over 6 to 12 months of treatment, and discontinuation of treatment after 3–6 months leads to increased rates of relapse compared to treatment continuation. Paroxetine, sertraline, fluvoxamine, and venlafaxine are approved by the US Food and Drug Administration (FDA) for the indication of SAD.

In respect to other classes of medication, several studies support the efficacy of the benzodiazepine clonazepam administered on a daily schedule. Davidson et al. (1993) examined the efficacy of clonazepam on 75 patients in a 10-week placebo-controlled study, finding a 78% response rate on a mean daily dose of 2.4 mg of clonazepam versus 20% for placebo. Benzodiazepines are a second line treatment for SAD, however, because they are not effective for frequently comorbid depression, and they carry risk of abuse and risk of withdrawal symptoms upon discontinuation. Several controlled trials also support the efficacy of monoamine oxidase inhibitors (MAOIs) in SAD, particularly phenelzine. This class of medications is usually reserved for treatment-refractory patients, however, due to the need for dietary restrictions and risk of hypertensive crisis. Beta-adrenergic antagonists, such as propranolol, are widely used on an as-needed basis for performance anxiety in patients with SAD, although these have been studied only in analogue samples, such as in anxious performers. Typically a 10–20 mg dose of propranolol is administered about an hour before a performance situation. Anecdotal reports suggest that some patients experience a marked diminution in anxiety-related palpitations and tremor, which allows them to focus better on their performance task. Other medications that have shown some evidence for efficacy in small randomized controlled trials or open trials include buspirone, gabapentin, pregabalin, mirtazapine, olanzapine, and quetiapine.

Several studies have attempted to compare the efficacy of CBT and medication treatment for SAD, delivered as monotherapies or in combination. Some of these studies (e.g., Blomhoff et al., 2001; Blanco et al., 2010) suggest that an integration of CBT and medication has been superior to individual modalities of treatment. Several studies have also investigated the efficacy of treatment in SAD with comorbid disorders. In patients with comorbid depression, medications with antidepressant effects, such as SSRIs and SNRIs have advantages over medications like benzodiazepines, which have not been shown effective for depression. SAD symptoms may respond more slowly than depressive symptoms to treatment with an SSRI (Schneier et al.,

2003). In patients with comorbid alcohol abuse, hyperhidrosis, or attention deficit hyperactivity disorder (ADHD), SSRIs have been shown to be safe and effective for SAD symptoms, but additional pharmacological or psychotherapeutic approaches may be needed to fully address the comorbid disorder (Connor, Cook, and Davidson, 2006; Book, Thomas, Randall, and Randall, 2008; Adler et al., 2009).

Specific phobia psychotherapies. CBTs are the best-established approach to treatment of specific phobias. Types of cognitive behavioral interventions that are used in treating specific phobia include exposure treatments, applied relaxation, applied tension, and cognitive restructuring. Exposure treatments are the most common approach for treating specific phobia and appear to be the most beneficial. In exposure treatment, the patient confronts the feared stimulus directly and indirectly. In graduated exposure, a patient with a spider phobia might start with touching a toy spider and gradually increasing proximity to a real one. In vivo exposure is associated with large effect sizes at posttreatment and has been shown to remain effective at follow-ups of 6 months to 1 year.

Immersive computer-generated virtual reality exposure is a form of this therapy that occurs in a virtual environment that can be tightly controlled. Evidence suggests that this form of treatment is associated with positive treatment outcomes and is as effective as in vivo exposure (e.g., Rothbaum et al., 2006). Other specific behavioral approaches include applied muscle tension, which has appeared to be a superior approach for blood injury phobias in some studies (e.g., Ost et al., 1989). Additionally, in some studies a single session of CBT has been beneficial in treating particular specific phobias (spider phobia, blood-injury phobia, injection phobia, claustrophobia, flying phobia, and small animal phobia) and in achieving long-term treatment outcomes (e.g., Hellström, and Fellenius, 1996).

Empirical evidence is limited regarding the effectiveness of cognitive restructuring in treating specific phobia (Choy, Fyer, and Lipsitz, 2007). Thorpe and Salkovskis (1995) suggest that patients with specific phobia can benefit from cognitive restructuring because they tend to experience unreasonable thoughts that contribute to their anxiety symptoms, and cognitive therapy assists them in modifying, constructing, and evaluating these negative thoughts. Several studies suggest that other psychotherapies may be effective for specific phobias, including psychodynamic supportive therapy, (Klein, Zitrin, Woerner, and Ross, 1983), hypnotic therapy (Stanley, Burrows, and Judd, 1990) and eye movement desensitization and reprocessing (EMDR) De Jongh, Ten Broeke, and Renssen, 1999).

Specific phobia medication therapies. Pharmacotherapy of specific phobias has been little studied, with existing research tending to investigate the impact of medication as an adjunct to exposure therapy. For instance, Marks, Viswanathan, Lipsedge, and Gardner (1972) found that a 0.1mg/kg dose of adjunctive diazepam given four hours before exposure treatment was more beneficial than a placebo. Other reports have raised concerns, however, that adjunctive benzodiazepines might interfere with the efficacy of exposure (Marks et al., 1993). Benzodiazepines are also often used clinically on an as-needed basis to treat anxiety related to predictable exposures, such as for flying.

A novel experimental approach to combined treatment has grown out of animal models demonstrating the importance of glutamatergic NMDA-receptor antagonism in extinction learning. The first proof-of-concept of this experimental approach demonstrated that the NMDA-receptor antagonist d-cycloserine, given just prior to exposure sessions, enhanced a brief exposure-based treatment of acrophobia. Further study is needed to determine optimal dosing and to demonstrate whether this combined treatment is superior to a full course of exposure therapy.

CONCLUSIONS

SAD is among the most common psychiatric disorders. Due to its early age of onset, chronicity, and the pervasiveness of social situations, this disorder often significantly interferes with social and work performance. Efficacious pharmacological and psychotherapeutic treatments are available, but a large minority of persons with SAD don't benefit from an initial course of treatment. Future directions of research include better understanding the cause of SAD, in order to predict who might respond best to a specific treatment, and determining the best next-step approaches for those patients who have an inadequate response to a first treatment.

Specific phobias are extremely common, and while they are often transient among children, in adulthood they often represent persistent problems. Although many sufferers do not seek treatment, these conditions can interfere with travel, work, and ability to obtain health care. More research is needed to understand what is unique and what is shared among the various forms of specific phobia. Behavioral therapies are often highly effective, and there is a need to test alternative psychotherapeutic and pharmacological approaches.

DISCLOSURE STATEMENT

Dr. Schneier has received research support from Forest Laboratories. Asala Halaj has no conflicts of interest to report.

REFERENCES

Adler, L. A., Liebowitz, M., Kronenberger, W., Qiao, M., Rubin, R., Hollandbeck, M., and Durell, T. (2009). Atomoxetine treatment in adults with attention-deficit/hyperactivity disorder and comorbid social anxiety. *Depress Anxiety, 26* (3), 212–221.

Beesdo, K., Pine, D. S., Lieb, R., and Wittchen, H. (2010). Incidence and risk patterns of anxiety and depressive disorders and categorization of generalized anxiety disorder. *Arch Gen Psychiatry, 67* (1), 47–57.

Blanco, C., Heimberg, R. G., Schneier, F. R., Fresco, D. M., Chen, H., Turk, C. L., . . . Liebowitz, M. R. (2010). A placebo-controlled trial of phenelzine, cognitive behavioral group therapy, and their combination for social anxiety disorder. *Arch Gen Psychiatry, 67* (3), 286–295.

Blomhoff, S., Haug, T. T., Hellström, K., Holme, I., Humble, M., Madsbu, H. P., and Wold, J. E. (2001). Randomised controlled general practice trial of sertraline, exposure therapy and combined treatment in generalised social phobia. *Br J Psychiatry, 17* 9(1), 23–30.

Book, S. W., Thomas, S. E., Randall, P. K., and Randall, C. L. (2008). Paroxetine reduces social anxiety in individuals with a co-occurring alcohol use disorder. *J Anxiety Disord, 22* (2), 310–318.

Brühl, A.B., Delsignore, A., Komossa, K., Seidt, S. (2014). Neuroimaging in social anxiety disorder: A meta-analytic review resulting in new neurofunctional model. *Neuroscience and Biobehavioral Reviews, 47,* 260–280. http://dx.doi.org/10.1016/j.neubiorev.wo14.08.003.

Buckner, J. D., Heimberg, R. G., Ecker, A. H., and Vinci, C. (2013). A biopsychosocial model of social anxiety and substance use. *Depress Anxiety, 30* (3), 276–284.

Choy, Y., Fyer, A. J., and Lipsitz, J. D. (2007). Treatment of specific phobia in adults. *Clinical Psychology Review, 27* (3), 266–286.

Clark, D. M., Ehlers, A., McManus, F., Hackmann, A., Fennell, M., Campbell, H., . . . Louis, B. (2003). Cognitive therapy versus fluoxetine in generalized social phobia: A randomized placebo-controlled trial. *J Consult Clin Psychol, 71* (6), 1058–1067.

Comer, J. S., Blanco, C., Hasin, D. S., Liu, S. M., Grant, B. F., Turner, J. B., and Olfson, M. (2011). Health-related quality of life across the anxiety disorders. *J Clin Psychiatry, 72* (1), 43–50.

Connor, K. M., Cook, J. L., and Davidson, J. R. (2006). Botulinum toxin treatment of social anxiety disorder with hyperhidrosis: A placebo-controlled double-blind trial. *J Clin Psychiatry, 67* (1), 30–36.

Davidson, J. R., Potts, N., Richichi, E., Krishnan, R., Ford, S. M., Smith, R., and Wilson, W. H. (1993). Treatment of social phobia with clonazepam and placebo. *Journal of Clinical Psychopharmacology, 13*(6), 423–428.

De Jongh, A., Ten Broeke, E., and Renssen, M. R. (1999). Treatment of specific phobias with eye movement desensitization and reprocessing (EMDR): Protocol, empirical status, and conceptual issues. *J Anxiety Disorders, 13* (1), 69–85.

Fox, A. S., and Kalin, N. H. (2014). A translational neuroscience approach to understanding the development of social anxiety disorder and its pathophysiology. *Am J Psychiatry, 171* (11), 1162–1173.

Gilbert, P. (2001). Evolution and social anxiety: The role of attraction, social competition, and social hierarchies. *Psychiatric Clin of North America, 24* (4), 723–751.

Heimberg, R. G., Hofmann, S. G., Liebowitz, M. R., Schneier, F. R., Smits, J. A., Stein, M. B., . . . Craske, M. G. (2014). Social anxiety disorders in DSM-5. *Depress Anxiety, 31* (6), 472–479.

Heimberg, R. G., Salzman, D. G., Holt, C. S., and Blendell, K. A. (1993). Cognitive behavioral group treatment for social phobia: Effectiveness at five-year followup. *Cog Ther Res, 17* (4), 325–339.

Hellström, K., and Fellenius, J. (1996). One versus five sessions of applied tension in the treatment of blood phobia. *Behav Res Ther, 34* (2), 101–112.

Hofmann, S. G. (2004). Cognitive mediation of treatment change in social phobia. *J. Consult Clin Psychol, 72* (3), 392–399.

Ipser, J. C., Kariuki, C. M., and Stein, D. J. (2008). Pharmacotherapy for social anxiety disorder: A systematic review. *Expert RevNeurotheraputics, 8* (2), 235–257.

Kashdan, T. B., Weeks, J. W., and Savostyanova, A. A. (2011). Whether, how, and when social anxiety shapes positive experiences and events: A self-regulatory framework and treatment implications. *Clin Psychol Rev, 31* (5), 786–799.

Kendler, K. S., Myers, J., Prescott, C. A., and Neale, M. C. (2001). The genetic epidemiology of irrational fears and phobias in men. *Archives of General Psychiatry, 58*(3), 257–265.

Kessler, R. C., Petukhova, M., Sampson, N. A., Zaslavsky, A. M., and Wittchen, H. U. (2012). Twelve-month and lifetime prevalence and lifetime morbid risk of anxiety and mood disorders in the United States. *Int J Meth Psychiatric Res, 21* (3), 169–184.

Kessler, R.C., Stein, M.D., and Berglund, P. (1998). Social phobia subtypes in the National Comorbidity Survey. *Am J Psychiatry, 155* (5), 613–619.

Klein, D. F., Zitrin, C. M., Woerner, M. G., and Ross, D. C. (1983). Treatment of phobias: II. Behavior therapy and supportive psychotherapy: Are there any specific ingredients? *Arch Gen Psychiatry, 40* (2), 139–145.

LeBeau, R. T., Glenn, D., Liao, B., Wittchen, H. U., Beesdo-Baum, K., Ollendick, T., and Craske, M. G. (2010). Specific phobia: A review of DSM-IV specific phobia and preliminary recommendations for DSM-V. *Depress Anxiety, 27* (2), 148–167.

Liebowitz, M. R., Gorman, J. M., Fyer, A. J., and Klein, D. F. (1985). Social phobia: Review of a neglected anxiety disorder. *Arch Gen Psychiatry, 42* (7), 729–736.

Leichsenring, F., Salzer, S., Beutel, M. E., Herpertz, S., Hiller, W., Hoyer, J., . . . Leibing, E. (2013). Psychodynamic therapy and cognitive-behavioral therapy in social anxiety disorder: a multicenter randomized controlled trial. *Am J Psychiatry, 170* (7), 759–767.

Marks, I. M., Swinson, R. P., Ba, M., Kuch, K., Noshirvani, H., O'Sullivan, G., . . . Sengun, S. (1993). Alprazolam and exposure alone and combined in panic disorder with agoraphobia. A controlled study in London and Toronto. *Br J Psychiatry, 162* (6), 776–787.

Marks, I. (1988). Blood-injury phobia: A review. *Am J Psychiatry, 145* (10), 1207–1213.

Marks, I. M., Viswanathan, R., Lipsedge, M. S., and Gardner, R. (1972). Enhanced relief of phobias by flooding during waning diazepam effect. *Br J Psychiatry, 121* (564), 493–505.

Marks, I. M., and Gelder, M. G. (1966). Different ages of onset in varieties of phobia. *Am J Psychiatry, 123* (218–221).

Morrison, A. S., and Heimberg, R. G. (2013). Social anxiety and social anxiety disorder. *Annu Rev Clin Psychol, 9,* 249–274.

Ollendick, T. H., and Benoit, K. E. (2012). A parent–child interactional model of social anxiety disorder in youth. *Clin Child Family Psychology Rev, 15* (1), 81–91.

Öst, L. G., Sterner, U., and Fellenius, J. (1989). Applied tension, applied relaxation, and the combination in the treatment of blood phobia. *Behav Res Therapy, 27* (2), 109–121.

Piet, J., Hougaard, E., Hecksher, M. S., and Rosenberg, N. K. (2010). A randomized pilot study of mindfulness-based cognitive therapy and group cognitive-behavioral therapy for young adults with social phobia. *Scand J Psychol, 51* (5), 403–410.

Pull, C. B. (2012). Current status of knowledge on public-speaking anxiety. *Curr Opinion Psychiatry, 25* (1), 32–38.

Rothbaum, B. O., Anderson, P., Zimand, E., Hodges, L., Lang, D., and Wilson, J. (2006). Virtual reality exposure therapy and standard (in vivo) exposure therapy in the treatment of fear of flying. *Behav Ther, 37* (1), 80–90.

Schneier, F. R., Blanco, C., Campeas, R., Lewis-Fernandez, R., Lin, S. H., Marshall, R., . . . Liebowitz, M. R. (2003). Citalopram treatment of social anxiety disorder with comorbid major depression. *Depress Anxiety, 1 7*(4), 191–196.

Silverman, W. K., and Moreno, J. (2005). Specific phobia. *Child Adolesc Psychiatric Clin N Am, 14* (4), 819–843.

Stangier, U., Schramm, E., Heidenreich, T., Berger, M., and Clark, D. M. (2011). Cognitive therapy vs. interpersonal psychotherapy in social anxiety disorder: A randomized controlled trial. *Arch Gen Psychiatry, 68* (7), 692–700.

Stanley, R. O., Burrows, G. D., and Judd, F. K. (1990). Hypnosis in the management of anxiety disorders. *Handb Anxiety, 4,* 537–548.

Stein, D. J., Westenberg, H. G., Yang, H., Li, D., and Barbato, L. M. (2003). Fluvoxamine CR in the long-term treatment of social anxiety disorder: The 12-to 24-week extension phase of a multicentre, randomized, placebo-controlled trial. *Int J Neuropsychopharmacol, 6* (04), 317–323.

Steinert, C., Hofmann, M., Leichsenring, F., and Kruse, J. (2013). What do we know today about the prospective long-term course of social anxiety disorder? A systematic literature review. *Journal of Anxiety Disorders, 27*(7), 692–702.

Thorpe, S. J., and Salkovskis, P. M. (1995). Phobic beliefs: Do cognitive factors play a role in specific phobias? *Behav Res and Therapy, 33* (7), 805–816.

Van Houtem, C. M. H. H., Laine, M. L., Boomsma, D. I., Ligthart, L., Van Wijk, A. J., and De Jongh, A. (2013). A review and meta-analysis of the heritability of specific phobia subtypes and corresponding fears. *J Anxiety Disorders, 27* (4), 379–388.

Xu, Y., Schneier, F., Heimberg, R. G., Princisvalle, K., Liebowitz, M. R., Wang, S., and Blanco, C. (2012). Gender differences in social anxiety disorder: Results from the national epidemiologic sample on alcohol and related conditions. *J Anxiety Disord, 26* (1), 12–19.

Wong, J., Gordon, E. A., and Heimberg, R. G. (2012). Social anxiety disorder. In P. Sturmey and M. Herseen (Eds.), *Handbook of evidence-based practice in clinical psychology* (pp. 621–649). Hoboken, NJ: John Wiley & Sons.

/// 15 /// CLINICAL ASPECTS OF PANIC DISORDER

STEFAN G. HOFMANN

INTRODUCTION

Panic disorder can become a chronic and debilitating psychiatric condition characterized by recurrent unexpected panic attacks. Epidemiological studies report that the lifetime prevalence rate of panic disorder is 7.1% in women and 4.0% in men (McLean, Asnaani, Litz, and Hofmann, 2011); the most common age of onset is between adolescence to early adulthood, with a median age of onset of 24 (Öst, 1987).

This chapter will summarize the clinical aspects of panic disorder. Following a description of the key clinical features and phenotypes, this chapter will review the mechanisms and theories of the disorder, followed by a brief review of the contemporary treatment options. The chapter concludes with some future directions for research.

The most significant change in the diagnostic criteria from DSM-IV (APA, 1994) to the DSM-5 (APA, 2013) is the separation of panic disorder and agoraphobia as two separate diagnostic entities. Prior to the DSM-5, agoraphobia has been described as avoidance of many situations in which having a panic attack could be dangerous or embarrassing or in which it may be difficult to get help. The DSM-IV implied that agoraphobia is typically preceded by spontaneous panic attacks. However, recent longitudinal data show that while a baseline diagnosis of panic disorder is the strongest predictor of the onset of agoraphobia, a baseline diagnosis of agoraphobia without spontaneous panic attacks also predicts the onset of panic disorder (Bienvenu, Onyike, Stein, Chen, Samuels, Nestadt, and Eaton, 2006). Moreover, a study by Kessler et al. (2006) used the NCS-R data (N = 9,282) to compare four mutually exclusive groups: panic attacks only without panic disorder or agoraphobia (22.7% of the sample), panic attacks without panic disorder but with agoraphobia (0.8%), panic disorder without agoraphobia (3.7%), and panic disorder with agoraphobia (1.1%). This study revealed monotonic increases for number of attacks, comorbidity, clinical severity, role impairment, and treatment seeking with lowest values for respondents with panic attacks only, intermediate values for agoraphobia without panic disorder and panic disorder without agoraphobia, and highest values for panic disorder with agoraphobia. The findings suggest that agoraphobia might be a severity marker of panic and confirm the importance of agoraphobia as a separate diagnosis, thus reconsidering the implicitly assumed one-way causal relationship from panic to agoraphobia. The contemporary view assumes that patients with agoraphobia either experience no panic attacks at all or only isolated attacks that do not meet full criteria for panic disorder.

KEY CLINICAL FEATURES/CLINICAL PHENOTYPE

The typical panic attack has a sudden onset, which builds rapidly to a peak and is accompanied by a sense of imminent danger or impending doom and an urge to escape. Ambulatory monitoring of heart rate and blood pressure changes typically show that the average attack is characterized by heart rates of only around 90 bpm, an increase of around 7 bpm compared to control periods 24 hours later, and moderate increases in systolic and diastolic blood pressure (Margraf et al., 1987; White and Baker, 1987).

Panic attacks typically happen during the daytime. A review by Craske and colleagues (2001) suggests that nocturnal panic occurs in 18% to 45% of panic disorder patients who wake up in a state of panic without a period of waking time before panicking and without any obvious trigger (e.g., absence of nightmares as triggers). Panic patients with and without nocturnal panic are equally avoidant and distressed, but individuals with nocturnal panic report daytime panic and general somatic sensations more frequently and were found to be more distressed during a relaxation task (Craske et al., 2001).

Panic disorder is highly comorbid with a number of other disorders. More than half of individuals with panic disorder suffer from comorbid psychiatric conditions (McLean et al., 2011). If left untreated, panic disorder can lead to reduced quality of life with substantial functional impairment (Simon et al., 2002) and excessive health care utilization (Klerman et al., 1991). Patients with panic disorder who had a comorbid medical condition were less likely to be recognized because the symptoms of anxiety were attributed to the physical illness (Roy-Byrne et al., 2000). Referrals to mental health professionals occur typically late in the course of the disorder, and even when the condition is properly diagnosed, patients often do not receive proper treatment or referrals to specialized settings experienced in treating this disorder (Demyttenaere et al., 2004; Roy-Byrne et al., 1999).

It should be noted that panic attacks are not restricted to panic disorder; they also occur in other disorders, such as specific phobia or social anxiety. In these cases, panic attacks have recognizable external triggers (also referred to as cued panic attacks). Many people experiencing panic attacks without meeting criteria of any anxiety disorder (22.7%; Kessler et al., 2006) are not only at risk to develop panic disorder later in life, but also other anxiety disorders or other psychopathologies, especially major depressive disorder, somatoform disorders or alcohol or drug abuse (Kessler et al., 2006).

The panic disorder phenotype is highly heterogeneous in terms of age of onset, familial aggregation, subtypes and severity of panic attacks, comorbidity with agoraphobia and other diagnoses (Bienvenu et al., 2006; Kessler et al., 2006), gender (McLean et al., 2011), ethnicity (Hofmann and Hinton, 2014), and symptom cluster (Meuret, White, Ritz, Roth, Hofmann, and Brown). For example, the latter study found three different subtypes of symptom patterns: cardio-respiratory (palpitations, shortness of breath, choking, chest pain, and numbness); mixed somatic (sweating, trembling, nausea, chills/hot flashes, and dizziness), and cognitive (feeling of unreality, fear of going crazy, and fear of losing control). The cardio-respiratory subtype was a strong predictor of panic severity, frequency of panic attacks, and agoraphobic avoidance, whereas the cognitive subtype primarily predicted worry due to panic. These findings illustrate the heterogeneity of the panic disorder phenotype, even on the symptom level.

MECHANISMS AND THEORIES OF DISORDER

Numerous factors contribute to the development and maintenance of the disorder, including genetic factors, neurobiological factors, and psychosocial factors (for a review, see (Roy-Byrne, Craske, and Stein, 2006)). The most prominent theories to explain the psychopathology and mechanisms leading to panic disorder include biological models, the *cognitive model* (Clark, 1986), the *expectancy theory* (Reiss, 1991), the *interoceptive conditioning model* (Goldstein and Chambless, 1978) and, more recently, the *modern learning perspective* (Bouton, Mineka, and Barlow, 2001; Suárez, Bennett, Goldstein, and Barlow, 2009).

Biological Models

Biological models of panic disorder were founded on the observation that certain pharmacological agents (e.g. sodium lactate, CO2, Yohimbin) trigger panic attacks in panic patients far more often than in healthy volunteers (e.g. Gorman et al., 2004). The original conceptualization of *panic disorder* was partly the result of studies that were aimed at distinguishing two types of anxiety disorder patients based on their pharmacological treatment response, assuming the existence of distinct and mutually exclusive syndromes with an inherently organic etiology and specific treatment indications (Klein, 1964; Klein and Fink, 1962). Specifically, Klein and his colleagues observed that imipramine, a tricyclic antidepressant, was effective for spontaneous anxiety attacks, but not for chronic and anticipatory anxiety. Klein concluded that spontaneous anxiety (panic) and anticipatory anxiety reflect two qualitatively different underlying biological processes.

Klein subsequently developed the suffocation false alarm theory (Klein, 1993), postulating the existence of an evolved physiologic suffocation alarm system that monitors information about potential suffocation. Spontaneous panic attacks are assumed to be caused when the alarm is erroneously triggered. The theory assumes that panic patients who panic in response to CO2 inhalation and lactate infusion show oversensitive chemoreceptors, signaling the potential of asphyxiation and subsequently leading to panic attacks. This model further assumes that separation anxiety and the endogenous opioid system dysfunction is directly linked to the suffocation alarm system (Preter and Klein, 2008). A similar theory was postulated by Levy (1985), which assumes that hyperventilation causes chronic low levels of carbon dioxide partial pressure (pCO2), leading to dyspnea and more hyperventilation, thus establishing a positive feedback loop that may result in panic attacks.

There are several experimental studies that support this association: lowering pCO_2 into the hypocapnic range or increasing pCO_2 into the hypercapnic range often results in panic-like symptoms in PD patients (e.g., Gorman et al., 2004). Furthermore, sustained hypocapnic levels have been observed in patients with panic disorder (e.g., Meuret, Wilhelm, et al., 2008), and a breathing training targeting pCo2 reduced fear of bodily sensations in panic disorder (Meuret, Rosenfield, et al., 2008). The diversity of substances shown to elicit panic in patients with panic disorder suggests that it is not a specific pharmacological effect but rather a common nonspecific effect (e.g., the elicitation of feared physical sensations) that triggers panic attacks. In addition, several studies indicate that the effects of the pharmacological manipulations greatly depend on cognitive factors, e.g. expectation and attribution of symptoms as well as social support (for a review, see Barlow, 2002).

Cognitive Model

According to the cognitive model of panic, first formulated by Clark (1986), panic attacks are viewed as a result of catastrophic misinterpretations of certain bodily sensations, such as palpitations, breathlessness, dizziness, etc. An example of such a catastrophic misinterpretation would be an instance where a healthy individual perceives harmless palpitations as evidence of an impending heart attack. The vicious cycle of the cognitive model suggests that various external (i.e., the feeling of being trapped in a supermarket) or internal stimuli (i.e., body sensations, thought or images) trigger a state of apprehension if these stimuli are perceived as a threat (Figure 15.1). It is assumed that this state is accompanied by fearful bodily sensations, which, if interpreted in a catastrophic fashion, further increase the apprehension and the intensity of bodily sensations (for a critical discussion, see McNally, 1994). Consistent with this model, it has been found that changes in catastrophic cognitions mediate treatment changes during CBT, but not treatment changes during pharmacotherapy (Hofmann et al., 2007).

The model does not rule out biological factors in panic. In contrast, it is assumed that biological variables may contribute to an attack by triggering benign bodily fluctuations or intensifying fearful bodily sensations. For example, the model assumes that pharmacological treatments can be effective if they reduce the frequency of bodily fluctuations, which can trigger panic or if they block the bodily sensations, which accompany anxiety. However, if the patient's tendency to interpret bodily sensations in a catastrophic fashion is not changed, discontinuation of drug treatments should be associated with a high rate of relapse.

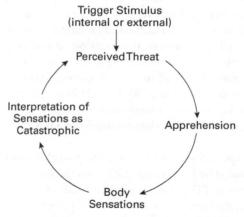

FIGURE 15.1 Cognitive model of panic disorder. Reprinted from "A cognitive approach to panic" by D. M. Clark, 1986, *Behaviour Research and Therapy*, p. 463. Copyright 1986 by Elsevier Publications. Adapted with permission.

Anxiety Sensitivity and Expectancy Theory

Panic patients are characterized by enhanced anxiety sensitivity which refers to fear of anxiety related sensations. This dispositional variable can be assessed with the Anxiety Sensitivity Index (ASI; Reiss et al., 1986). The expectancy model (Reiss, 1991) states that anxiety and avoidance are a function of *expectations* (what one thinks might happen in a situation), and *sensitivities* (why one is afraid of the anticipated event). Especially interesting are prospective studies showing that high ASI scores constitute a risk for panic attacks, panic disorder and avoidance behavior. For example, Schmidt et al. (1997, 1999) observed that about 6% of a cohort of cadets entering the U.S. Air Force Academy experienced panic attacks during the five-week basic training. Most important, ASI scores assessed before training predicted panic even after controlling for several moderating variables.

Reiss (1991) acknowledges that because anxiety sensitivity is defined in terms of irrational beliefs, the concept has similarities to the cognitive model of panic (Clark, 1986), and some individuals with high anxiety sensitivity may misinterpret bodily sensations catastrophically. However, in contrast to the cognitive model, the expectancy model predicts that individuals with high anxiety sensitivity also believe that high arousal itself can lead to harmful consequences without necessarily misinterpreting any specific physical sensations.

Interoceptive Conditioning Model

Goldstein and Chambless (1978) suggested that certain internal bodily sensations become the conditioned stimuli for the conditioned response of a panic attack, which then results in the development of *fear of fear*. This so-called *interoceptive conditioning model* assumes that people become hyper-alert to their sensations and that they interpret feelings of mild to moderate anxiety as signs of upcoming panic attacks and react with such anxiety that the dreaded episode is almost invariably induced after having experienced one or more panic attacks. For a critical discussion, see McNally (1994).

Modern Learning Theory Perspective

A revised learning model of panic disorder is based on the critical distinction between *anxiety*, an anticipatory emotional state that functions to prepare the individual for a threatening event, and *panic*, an emotional state designed to deal with a threatening event that is already in progress (Bouton, Mineka, and Barlow, 2001; Suárez et al., 2009). This model assumes that panic disorder develops as a result of the conditioning of anxiety to exteroceptive and interoceptive cues. The conditioned anxiety then potentiates the next panic attack and anxiety becomes a precursor of panic. This model considers a number of general and specific vulnerability factors that might influence the person's susceptibility to conditioning, such as early experiences with uncontrollable and unpredictable events, and vicarious learning events that focused on certain bodily sensations. This model incorporates supporting data of other theoretical accounts and attempts to correct some of the weaknesses of previous models.

Despite the differences in mechanisms, the various psychological models all share the basic premise that certain bodily symptoms are triggers for panic attacks, leading to a maladaptive fear response. The primary difference between the various models is the principal mechanism through which the stimuli trigger the fear response.

Genetics

Twin and family studies suggest that the heritability of panic disorder is close to 40% (Hettema, Neale, and Kendler, 2011). Although more than 350 candidate genes and 1,000 polymorphisms have been examined, the contribution for most of these genes and single nucleotide polymorphisms (SNPs) remain inconclusive, in part because the majority of the studies have been underpowered (Maron, Hettema, and Shlik, 2010). The most promising SNP is the Val158Met polymorphism of the catechol-O-methyltransferase (COMT) gene, which codes for a methylation enzyme metabolizing the monoamine neurotransmitters (e.g., Domschke, Deckert, O'Donovan, and Glatt, 2007). Moreover, as reviewed by Maron et al. (2010), there is evidence to suggest that genetic variations are differentially associated with different panic disorder phenotypes. For example, Domschke et al. (2007) reported that the association between panic disorder and the COMT 158 Val allele was considerably stronger in Caucasian females.

Developmental Precursors

Panic symptoms wax and wane. For example, the 12-year follow-up study of the Harvard/Brown Anxiety Disorders Program revealed a relatively high cumulative probability of both, recovery (0.82) and relapse (0.56). Similarly, results from the National Epidemiologic Survey on Alcohol and Related Conditions revealed high remission (75%) and recovery rates (12%) of panic disorder over a 3-year interval (Nay, Brown, and Roberson-Nay, 2013).

Despite the fluctuating course of panic disorder, there is some evidence to suggest that there are factors predicting the development of panic disorder. The most consistent predictor of adult panic disorder appears to be childhood separation anxiety disorder, which was proposed by Klein as early as 1964. Consistent with this notion are the results of a 7-year follow-up studies showing that 27.8% of children with separation anxiety disorder but only 14.3% of children with overanxious disorder and 12.3% with social anxiety disorder later developed panic disorder as adults (Aschenbrand et al., 2003). Similarly, a study examining the 5-year trajector of psychiatric disorders in children of patients with or without panic disorder, major depression, or neither disorders suggests that separation anxiety disorder is a major antecendent disorder for the development of panic disorder (Biedermann et al., 2007). Finally, analyses of the Virginia twin study of adolescent behavioral development further showed that childhood separation anxiety disorder (but not overanxious disorder) was uniquely associated with adult onset panic attacks, suggesting that separation anxiety disorder and adult onset panic attacks share a common genetic diathesis (Roberson-Nay, Eaves, Hettema, Kendler, and Silberg, 2012).

TREATMENT

It has been shown that by successfully treating panic disorder, indirect costs associated with this condition can be reduced substantially (Salvador-Carulla et al., 1995). CBT-oriented care has been shown to be strongly associated with the patient's satisfaction with health care (Stein et al., 2011). Moreover, CBT can significantly improve the lives of patients with panic disorder (Hofmann, Wu, and Boettcher, 2014). Similar effects were found for the effects of pharmacotherapy for panic disorder (Hofmann, Wu, Boettcher, and Sturm, 2014). In both meta-analyses, larger symptom reductions were associated with greater improvement in quality of life. These results highlight the importance for correctly diagnosing and delivering appropriate care to panic disorder patients

Medications

Pharmacological agents that have demonstrated efficacy for panic disorder include tricyclic antidepressants (TCAs), monoamine oxidase inhibitors (MAOIs), reversible inhibitors of monoamine oxidase-A (RIMAs), selective serotonin reuptake inhibitors (SSRIs), serotonin-norepinephrine reuptake inhibitors (SNRIs), and other drugs, such as anticonvulsants and atypical antipsychotics (for review, see Ravindran, and Stein, 2010). Due to space limitations, this review will only briefly review the most commonly used drug classes.

The TCAs work by inhibiting both serotonin and norepinephrine reuptake from the synaptic cleft (Feighner, 1999). SSRIs primarily work by inhibiting the reuptake of serotonin at the presynaptic serotonin transporter pump, leading to an increased level of brain 5-HT. Similarly, SNRIs inhibit the reuptake of norepinephrine and serotonin at either end of its dose range. MAOIs work by irreversibly inhibiting monoamine oxidase, an enzyme that is responsible for breaking down monoamines, such as serotonin and norepinephrine, resulting in increased availability of these neurotransmitters in the synaptic cleft.

The oldest class of drugs includes the TCAs and the two most investigated drugs for panic disorder include imipramine and clomipramine. The SSRIs (e.g., paroxetine) and SNRIs (e.g., venlafaxine) are currently the first line medication treatments for panic disorder. Although meta-analytic reviews suggest that these classes of drugs are similarly effective to TCAs (Bakker, van Balkom, and Spinhoven, 2002; Otto, Tuby, Gould, et al., 2001), they showed fewer treatment drop-outs, possibly due to better tolerability (Otto, et al., 2001); in addition, TCAs have more side effects and are more toxic in an overdose than SSRIs or SNRIs. Similarly, MAOIs (e.g., phenelzine) are an older but effective class (Buigues and Vallejo, 1987). However, use of MAOIs requires maintaining a low-tyramine diet because of the risk of a hypertensive crisis.

Psychotherapies

The most efficacious treatment for panic disorder is cognitive-behavior therapy (CBT), which is typically delivered in 12–16 individual hour-long sessions (e.g., Clark, Salkovskis, Hackman, Wells, Ludgate, and Gelder, 1999; Barlow, Gorman, Shear, Woods, 2000). These treatment protocols are based on the same basic treatment rationale but vary in the emphasis on the particular treatment components (such as the amount and type of exposure). One of the most frequently cited CBT protocols is the Panic Control Treatment (PCT) that was employed in the largest comparative treatment study of panic disorder (Barlow et al., 2000). It combines, similar to other CBT protocols, a number of treatment components, including cognitive restructuring, psychoeducation, relaxation, controlled breathing procedures, and exposure techniques. Because the treatment targets panic disorder with no more than mild agoraphobia, the exposure component focuses primarily on internal cues, specifically, frightening bodily sensations (interoceptive exposure). Due to the strong empirical support, some national guidelines recommend CBT as a first-line treatment for panic disorder (e.g., National Institute for Health and Clinical Excellence, 2004; revised 2007). Nevertheless, there is clearly still room for further improvement

(Hofmann and Smits, 2008). One obvious strategy is to combine pharmacotherapy and CBT in order to maximize treatment efficacy.

The largest clinical trial to date compared the efficacy of CBT (PCT) to imipramine, a pill placebo, and combinations of CBT with imipramine or a pill placebo (Barlow et al., 2000). The results showed that imipramine was superior to placebo after acute treatment, 3 months after the beginning of the study, with drug-placebo differences even larger at the end of maintenance treatment 9 months after the beginning of the study. The efficacy of CBT was comparable to imipramine on nearly all measures during treatment, with better maintenance of gains after treatment discontinuation. Combining imipramine and CBT showed limited advantage acutely but more substantial advantage by the end of maintenance than monotherapies. Interestingly, the combination between CBT and imipramine was not more effective than the combination between CBT and placebo, raising important questions about the mechanism of combination treatments. The results of this trial are consistent with other combination studies (Furukawa, Watanabe, and Churchill, 2006).

Other Therapies

CBT and pharmacological treatments are the clearly the treatments of choice. Although still widely used in clinical practices, psychodynamic treatments show very limited support (Milrod et al., 2007) and unsatisfactory results in meta-analytic reviews, even when conducted by psychodynamically oriented authors (Abbass et al., 2014).

FUTURE DIRECTIONS

Although pharmacological and psychological treatments are efficacious, there is clearly room for improvement (Hofmann and Smits, 2008; Ravindran and Stein 2010). The disappointing results of combining conventional therapies highlight the importance of understanding the mechanism though which the treatments work. A more recent approach toward combination therapy is to enhance the mechanism of CBT using pharmacological agents. Some of these approaches are highly promising and support such augmentation strategies to further enhance the efficacy of CBT. Examples of those agents include d-cycloserine, yohimbine, cortisol, oxytocin, propranolol, and various nutritional supplements (Hofmann, Smits, Asnaani, Gutner, and Otto, 2011). Some of these agents, such as d-cycloserine, are especially promising because they appear to act as cognitive enhancers by facilitating extinction learning that is one of the basic mechanisms of CBT (Otto et al., 2010). Future studies also need to focus on the heterogeneity of the panic disorder phenotype. Rather than conducting small-scale studies to examine candidate genes and SNPs that are believed to be implicated in specific pharmacological treatments, the field would benefit more from large-scale and well-powered genome-wide association studies that account for the different panic disorder phenotypes, in combination with neuroimaging and treatment outcome studies.

DISCLOSURE STATEMENT

To my knowledge, all of my possible conflicts of interest, financial or otherwise, including direct or indirect financial or personal relationships, interests, and affiliations, whether or not directly related to the subject of the chapter, are listed here.

I serve on the Advisory Board of Palo Alto Health Sciences and Otsuka America Pharmaceutical, Inc., and receive financial compensation for my participation as an advisor. I receive grant support from NIH/NCCAM (R01AT007257), NIH/NIMH (R01MH099021, R34MH099311, R34MH086668, R21MH102646, R21MH101567, K23MH100259), and the Department of the Army. I also receive royalties from various book publishers and financial compensation for my editorial work from Springer Publications and the American Psychological Association.

REFERENCES

Abbass, A. A., Kisely, S. R., Town, J. M., Leichsenring, F., Driessen, E., DeMaat, S., Gerber, A., Dekker, J., Rabung, S., Rusalovska, S., and Crowe, E. (2014). Short-term psychodynamic psychotherapies for common mental disorders. *Cochrane Database Systematic Rev*, 7, CD004687

American Psychiatric Association (1994). *Diagnostic and statistical manual for mental disorders* (4th ed.). Washington, D.C.: Author.

American Psychiatric Association (2013). *Diagnostic and statistical manual for mental disorders* (5th ed.). Washington, D.C.: Author.

Aschenbrand, S. G., Kendall, P. C., Webb, A., Safford, S. M., Flannery-Schroeder, E. (2003). Is childhood separation anxiety disorder a predictor of adult panic disorder and agoraphobia? A seven-year longitudinal study. *J Am Acad Child Adolesc Psychiatry*, 42, 1478–1485.

Bakker, A., van Balkom, A. J., and Spinhoven, P. (2002). SSRIs vs. TCAs in the treatment of panic disorder: A meta-analysis. *Acta Psychiatr Scand*, 106, 163–167.

Barlow, D. H. (2002). *Anxiety and its disorders*. New York: Guilford Press.

Barlow, D. H., Gorman. J. M., Shear, M. K., Woods, S. W. (2000). Cognitive-behavioral therapy, imipramine, or their combination for panic disorder: A randomized control trial. *J Am Med Assoc*, 283, 2529–2536.

Biedermann, J., Petty, C. R., Hirshfeld-Becker, D. R., et al. (2007). Developmental trajectories of anxiety disorders in offspring at high risk for panic disorder and major depression. *Psychiatric Res*, 153, 245–252.

Bienvenu, O. J., Onyike, C. U., Stein, M. B., Chen, L.-S., Samuels, J., Nestadt, G., and Eaton, W. W. (2006). Agoraphobia in adults: Incidence and longitudinal relationship with panic. *British Journal of Psychiatry*, 188, 432–438.

Bouton, M. E., Mineka, S., and Barlow, D. H. (2001). A modern learning theory perspective on the etiology of panic disorder. *Psychol Rev*, 108, 4–32.

Bruce, S. E., Yonkers, K. A.., Otto, M. W., Eisen, J. L., Weisberg, R. B., Pagano, M., Shea, M., Keller, M. B. (2005). Influence of psychiatric comorbidity on recovery and recurrence in generalized anxiety disorder, social phobia, and panic disorder: A 12-year prospective study. *Am J Psychiatry*, 162, 1179–1187.

Buigues, J., and Vallejo, J. (1987). Therapeutic response to phenelzine in patients with panic disorder and agoraphobia with panic attacks. *J Clin Psychiatry*, 48, 55–59

Clark, D. M. (1986). A cognitive approach to panic. *Behav Res Therapy*, 24, 461–470.

Clark, D. M., Salkovskis, P. M., Hackman, A., Wells, A., Ludgate, J., and Gelder, M. (1999). Brief cognitive therapy for panic disorder: A randomized controlled trial. *J Consult Clin Psychology*, 67, 583–589.

Craske, M. G., Lang, A. J., Tsao, J., Mystkowski, J. L., and Rowe, M. (2001). Reactivity to interoceptive cues in nocturnal panic. *J Behav Therapy Exp Psychiatry*, 32, 173–190.

Demyttenaere, K., Bruffaerts, R., Posada-Villa, J., Gasquet, I., Kovess, V., Lepine, J. P., et al. (2004). Prevalence, severity, and unmet need for treatment of mental disorders in the World Health Organization World Mental Health Surveys. *J Am Med Assoc*, 291, 2581–2590.

Domschke, K., Deckert, J., O'Donovan, M. C., and Glatt, S. J. (2001). Meta-analysis of COMT val158met in panic disorder: Ethnic heterogeneity and gender specificity. *Am J Med Genet B: Neuropsychiatric Genet, 144B,* 667–673.

Feighner, J. P. (1999). Mechanism of action of antidepressant medications. *J Clin Psychiatry, 60 (suppl 4),* 4–11.

Furukawa, T. A., Watanabe, N., and Churchill, R. (2006). Psychotherapy plus antidepressant for panic disorder with or without agoraphobia. *Br J Psychiatry, 188,* 305–312.

Goldstein, A. J., and Chambless, D. L. (1978). A reanalysis of agoraphobia. *Behav Res Ther, 9,* 47–59.

Gorman, J. M, Martinez, J., Coplan, J.D., Kent, J., and Kleber, M. (2004). The effect of successful treatment on the emotional and physiological response to carbon dioxide inhalation in patients with panic disorder. *Biol Psychiatry, 56,* 862–867

Hettema, J. M., Neale, M. C., and Kendler, K. S. (2001). A review and meta-analysis of the genetic epidemiology of anxiety disorders. *Am J Psychiatry, 158,* 1568–1578.

Hofmann, S. G., and Hinton, D. E. (2014). Cross-cultural aspects of anxiety disorders. *Curr Psychiatry Rep, 16*:450.

Hofmann, S. G., Meuret, A. E., Rosenfield, D., Suvak, M. K., Barlow, D. H., Gorman, J. M., Shear, M. K., and Woods, S. W. (2007). Preliminary evidence for cognitive mediation during cognitive behavioral therapy for panic disorder. *J Consult Clin Psychol, 75,* 374–379.

Hofmann, S. G. and Smits, J. A. J. (2008). Cognitive-behavioral therapy for adult anxiety disorders: A meta-analysis of randomized placebo-controlled trials. *J Clin Psychiatry, 69,* 621–632.

Hofmann, S. G., Smits, J. A. J., Asnaani, A., Gutner, C. A., and Otto, M. W. (2011). Cognitive enhancers for anxiety disorders. *Pharmacol Biochem Behav, 99,* 275–284.

Hofmann, S. G., Wu, J. Q., and Boettcher, H. (2014). Effect of cognitive behavioral therapy for anxiety disorders on quality of life: A meta-analysis. *J Consult Clin Psychol, 82,* 375–391.

Hofmann, S. G., Wu, J. Q., Boettcher, H, and Sturm, J. (2014). Effect of pharmacotherapy for anxiety disorders on quality of life: A meta-analysis. *Quality Life Res, 23,* 1141–1153.

Kessler, R. C., Chiu, W. T., Jin, R., Ruscio, A. M., Shear, K., and Walters, E. E. (2006). The epidemiology of panic attacks, panic disorder, and agoraphobia in the National Comorbidity Survey Replication. *Arch Gen Psychiatry, 63,* 415–424.

Klein, D. F. (1964). Delineation of two drug-responsive anxiety syndromes. *Psychopharmacologia, 5,* 397–408.

Klein, D. F. (1993). False suffocation alarms, spontaneous panics, and related conditions. An integrative hypothesis. *Arch Gen Psychiatry, 50,* 306–17.

Klein, D. F., and Fink, M. (1962). Psychiatric reaction patterns to imipramine. *American Journal of Psychiatry, 119,* 432–438.

Klerman, G. L., Weissman, M. M., Ouellette, R., Johnson, J., and Greenwald, S. (1991). Panic attacks in the community. Social morbidity and health care utilization. *J Am Med Assoc, 265,* 742–746.

Ley, R. (1985). Blood, breath and fears: A hyperventilation theory of panic attacks and agoraphobia. *Clin Psychol Rev, 5,* 271–85.

Margraf, J., Taylor, C. B., Ehlers, A., and Roth, W. T. (1987). Panic attacks in the natural environment. *J Nerv Mental Dis, 175,* 558–565.

Maron, E., Hettema, J. M., and Shlik, J. (2010). Advances in molecular genetics of panic disorder. *Mol Psychiatry, 15,* 681–701.

McLean, C. P., Asnaani, A., Litz, B. T., and Hofmann, S. G. (2011). Gender differences in anxiety disorders: Prevalence, course of illness, comorbidity, and burden of illness. *J Psychiatric Res, 45,* 1027–1035.

McNally, R. J. (1994). *Panic disorder. A critical analysis.* New York: Guilford Press.

Meuret, A. E., Rosenfield, D., Hofmann, S. G., Suvak, M. K., and Roth, W. T. (2008). Changes in respiration mediate changes in fear of bodily sensations in panic disorder. *J Psychiatric Res, 43,* 634–641.

Meuret, A. E., White, K. S., Ritz, T., Roth, W. T., Hofmann, S. G. and Brown, T. A. (2006). Panic attack symptom dimensions and their relationship to illness characteristics in panic disorder. *J Psychiatric Res, 40*, 520–527.

Meuret, A. E., Wilhelm, F. H., Ritz T., and Roth, W. T. (2008). Feedback of end-tidal pCO2 as a therapeutic approach for panic disorder. *J Psychiatric Res, 42*, 560–568.

Milrod, B., Leon, A. C., Busch, F., Rudden, M., Schwalberg, M., Clarkin, J., . . . Shear, M. K. (2007). A randomized controlled clinical trial of psychoanalytic psychotherapy for panic disorder. *Am J Psychiatry, 164*, 265–272.

National Institute for Health and Clinical Excellence (NICE). (2004; revised 2007). *Management of anxiety (panic disorder with or without agoraphobia, and generalized anxiety disorder) in adults in primary, secondary and community care.* London: NICE.).

Nay, W., Brown, R., and Roberson-Nay, R. (2013). Longitudinal course of panic disorder with and without agoraphobia using the national epidemiologic survey on alcohol and related conditions (NESARC). *Psychiatric Res, 208*, 54–63.

Öst, L. G. (1987). Age of onset in different phobias. *J Abnormal Psychol, 96*, 223–229.

Otto, M. W., Tolin, D. F., Simon, N. M., Pearlson, G. D., Basden, S., Meunier, S. A., . . . Pollack, M. H. (2010). Efficacy of d-cycloserine for enhancing response to cognitive-behavior therapy for panic disorder. *Biological Psychiatry, 67*, 365–370.

Otto, M. W., Tuby, K. S., Gould, R. A., et al. (2001). An effect size analysis of the relative efficacy tolerability of serotonin selective reuptake inhibitors for panic disorder. *Am J Psychiatry, 158*, 1989–1992.

Preter, M., and Klein, D. F. (2008). Panic, suffocation false alarms, separation anxiety and endogenous opioids. *Progr Neuro-Psychopharmacol Biol Psychiatry, 32*, 603–612.

Ravindran, L. N., and Stein, M. B. (2010). The pharmacologic treatment of anxiety disorders: A review in progress. *J Clin Psychiatry, 71*, 839–854.

Reiss, S. (1991). Expectancy model of fear, anxiety and panic. *Clin Psychol Rev, 11*, 141–153.

Reiss, S., Peterson, R. A., Gursky, D. M., and McNally, R. J. (1986). Anxiety sensitivity, anxiety frequency and the prediction of fearfulness. *Behav Res Therapy, 24*, 1–8.

Roberson-Nay, R., Eaves, L. J., Hettema, J. M., Kendler, K. S., and Silberg, J. L. (2012). Childhood separation anxiety disorder and adult onset panic attacks share a common genetic diathesis. *Depress Anxiety, 29*, 320–327.

Roy-Byrne, P. P., Craske, M. G., and Stein, M. B. (2006). Panic disorder. *Lancet, 368*, 1023–1032.

Roy-Byrne, P. P., Katon, W., Cowley, D. S., Russo, J. E., Cohen, E., Michelson, E., et al. (2000). Panic disorder in primary care: Biopsychosocial differences between recognized and unrecognized patients. *Gen Hosp Psychiatry, 22*, 405–411.

Roy-Byrne, P. P., Stein, M. B., Russo, J., Mercier, E., Thomas, R., McQuaid, J., et al. (1999). Panic disorder in the primary care setting: Comorbidity, disability, service utilization, and treatment. *J Clin Psychiatry, 60*, 492–499.

Salvador-Carulla, L., Segui, J., Fernandez-Cano, P., and Canet, J. (1995). Costs and offset effect in panic disorders. *Br J Psychiatry, 166 (Suppl 27)*, 23–28.

Schmidt, N. B., Lerew, D. R., and Jackson, R. J. (1997). The role of anxiety sensitivity in the pathogenesis of panic: Prospective evaluation of spontaneous panic attacks during acute stress. *J Abnormal Psychol, 106*, 355–364.

Schmidt, N. B., Lerew, D. R., and Jackson, R. J. (1999). Prospective evaluation of anxiety sensitivity in the pathogenesis of panic: Replication and extension. *Journal of Abnormal Psychology, 108*, 532–537.

Simon, N. M., Otto, M. W., Korbly, N. B., Peters, P. M., Nicolaou, D. C., and Pollack, M. H. (2002). Quality of life in social anxiety disorder compared with panic disorder and the general population. *Psychiatric Serv, 53*, 714–8.

Stein, M. B., Roy-Byrne, P. P., Craske, M. G., Campbell-Sills, L., Kang, A. J., Rosen, R. D., Bytritsky, A., Sullivan, G., and Sherbourne, C. D. (2011). Quality of and patient satisfaction with primary health care for anxiety disorders. *J Clin Psychiatry, 72*, 970–976.

Suárez, L., Bennett, S., Goldstein, C., and Barlow, D. H. (2009). Understanding anxiety disorders from a "triple vulnerabilities" framework. In M. M. Antony & M. B. Stein (Eds.), *Oxford handbook of anxiety and related disorders* (pp. 153–172). New York: Oxford.

White, W. B., and Baker, L. H. (1987). Ambulatory blood pressure monitoring in patients with panic disorder. *Arch Internal Med, 147*, 1973–1975.

INTERSECTION OF MEDICAL AND ANXIETY DISORDERS

FEAR, ANXIETY, AVOIDANCE, AND CHRONIC PAIN

GORDON J. G. ASMUNDSON,
HOLLY A. PARKERSON, AND
CHRISTINA A. D'AMBROSIO

INTRODUCTION

It is not uncommon for individuals with psychiatric disorders to present with co-occurring physical and mental health concerns. Over the past few decades, strong associations have been identified between the anxiety disorders and various chronic pain conditions. Individuals with anxiety disorders are two to three times more likely to have chronic pain than the general population (Sareen, Cox, Clara, and Asmundson, 2005). Similarly, individuals with chronic pain are at a two to three fold greater risk for past 12 month (Demyttenaer et al., 2007) and lifetime (McWilliams, Cox, and Enns, 2003) anxiety disorders. While numerous mechanisms have been proposed to account for the co-occurrence of anxiety disorders and chronic pain (for review see Asmundson and Katz, 2009), it is the constructs of fear of pain and pain-related anxiety, as well as related avoidance behaviors, that have provided the theoretical foundation for advances in this area. Whether or not a person with chronic pain has a co-occurring anxiety disorder, pain-related fear and anxiety can be disabling. The purpose of this chapter is fourfold. First, we describe the core characteristics of pain, chronic pain, and related fear and anxiety constructs. Second, we provide a brief overview of state-of-the-art models that have guided research and treatment development for fear of pain and pain-related anxiety. Third, we summarize assessment targets and emerging evidence-based treatments. Finally, we conclude with an agenda that outlines areas in need of additional research.

KEY CLINICAL FEATURES

Pain

Pain has been defined as "an unpleasant sensory and emotional experience associated with actual or potential tissue damage. . ." (International Association for the Study of Pain Subcommittee on Taxonomy, 1994, p. S212). The emotionally aversive nature of pain has adaptive and protective functions; specifically, pain draws attention to potentially dangerous stimuli and motivates action to remove oneself from danger, it facilitates the learning necessary to avoid potentially painful or injurious behaviors and circumstances, and it can prevent a person from engaging in activity that would interrupt the body's natural healing processes or lead to further injury. The adaptive function of pain ceases when it persists beyond the time necessary to facilitate healing.

Chronic Pain

Pain that persists beyond three months from time of onset is typically classified as chronic (International Association for the Study of Pain, 1994). Although not necessarily disabling (i.e., some people function well despite having chronic pain; Asmundson et al., 1997; Turk and Rudy, 1987), chronic pain is one of the most common and costly chronic health conditions in North America (Hardt, Jacobsen, Goldberg, Nickel, and Buchwald, 2008; Reitsma, Tranmer, Buchanan, and Vandenkerkhof, 2012). Health care costs associated with chronic pain have been estimated at over several hundred billion dollars annually in the USA alone (Gaskin and Richard, 2012). Chronic pain is not recognized as a psychiatric disorder in the DSM-5; instead, in cases where a psychiatric diagnosis related to the pain experience is given, people with chronic pain can be diagnosed with somatic symptom disorder with predominant pain or psychological factors that affect other medical conditions. It remains to be determined whether these new diagnostic options will be more useful than the DSM-IV diagnosis of pain disorder, which was controversial and not commonly used by pain practitioners (Collimore, Asmundson, Taylor, and Abramowitz, 2009). Notwithstanding the presence or absence of a psychiatric diagnosis stemming from the pain experience, chronic pain is often associated with fear and anxiety, catastrophizing, hypervigilance to pain and pain-related stimuli, avoidance behavior, and depression, as well as increased risk of developing psychiatric disorders, impaired social and educational/occupational functioning, suicide, and increased medical service utilization in both adults and children (Asmundson and Katz, 2009; Gureje et al., 1998; Kashikar-Zuck et al., 2001; Perquin et al., 2001).

Fear of Pain, Pain-Related Anxiety, and Pain Catastrophizing

Contrary to the traditional medical model, which limited the conceptualization of pain to a sensory experience and nothing more, contemporary models recognize that pain occurs in a context that includes various individual difference factors as well as behavioral and social determinants (Asmundson and Wright, 2004). Amongst the various individual difference factors that influence the pain experience, fear of pain and pain-related anxiety have been shown to play an important role in the complex transition from acute to chronic and disabling pain. Like other presentations of fear and anxiety, fear of pain and pain-related anxiety are distinct constructs (Asmundson. Norton, and Vlaeyen, 2004; Carleton and Asmundson, 2009; McCracken, Gross, Aikens, and Carnrike, 1996). This distinction is potentially useful both theoretically and clinically. Fear of pain is conceptualized as a response to an immediate pain-related threat (e.g., initiating a painful activity), whereas pain-related anxiety is a response that occurs in anticipation of pain-related threat (e.g., expecting an activity to be painful). The focus of fear or anxiety in the context of pain is often on specific activities (e.g., having to lift something or the possibility thereof) or experiences (e.g., noticing muscle tension). The focus can also span to perceptions of self-worth and identity formation (e.g., "I'm not what I once was," Morely and Eccleston,

2004). The related construct of pain catastrophizing refers to a cognitive and emotional schema that results in negative responses to actual or anticipated pain (Sullivan, Thorn, Keefe, Martin, Bradley, and Lefebvre, 2001). Pain catastrophizing is characterized by the tendency to exaggerate the threat value of pain, feelings of helplessness in response to pain, and an inability to suppress or inhibit pain-related thoughts in anticipation of, during, or following pain (Sullivan et al., 2001). Together, fear of pain, pain-related anxiety, and catastrophic interpretations of pain are thought to promote hypervigilance to pain sensations and avoidance of behaviors that, while potentially adaptive in the short-term, often elicit the perpetuation of pain and pain-related disability (Asmundson et al., 2004; Vlaeyen and Linton, 2000).

MODELS AND MECHANISMS

Variants of the fear-avoidance model of chronic musculoskeletal pain (Asmundson, Norton, and Norton, 1999; Vlaeyen and Linton, 2000) have stimulated considerable research on mechanisms and treatment. The fear-avoidance model emerged from a body of literature supporting the role of fear of pain and pain-related anxiety as key factors in the maintenance of disabling musculoskeletal pain (for reviews, see Asmundson et al., 1999; Leeuw et al., 2007; Vlaeyen and Linton, 2000, 2012). The fear-avoidance model, as articulated by Vlaeyen and Linton (2000) and illustrated in Figure 16.1, can be summarized as follows. Pain resulting from an injury or other cause (e.g., disease) is perceived and appraised as either unpleasant, but not catastrophic, or threatening and potentially catastrophic. People who appraise pain as unpleasant engage in appropriate behavioral restrictions (e.g., rest), followed by graduated increases in activity until healing has occurred. People who appraise pain as threatening and potentially catastrophic—a

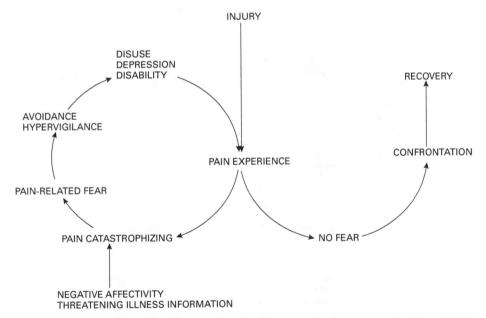

FIGURE 16.1 The fear-avoidance model of chronic musculoskeletal pain from Vlaeyen and Linton (2000). This figure has been reproduced with permission of the International Association for the Study of Pain (IASP). The figure may not be reproduced for any other purpose without permission.

tendency influenced by negative affect and threatening illness information—develop fear of pain which promotes avoidance behavior, hypervigilance to bodily sensations, functional disability, and depression, all of which serve to perpetuate the vicious fear-avoidance cycle.

Although initially developed to explain the maintenance of disabling chronic musculoskeletal pain, evidence indicates that the fear-avoidance model is applicable to many other pain conditions experienced by adults (for review, see Asmundson, Parkerson, Petter, and Noel, 2012a) and children (for review, see Asmundson, Noel, Petter, and Parkerson, 2012b). Researchers and theorists have continued to refine the fear-avoidance model based on emerging data. These data have informed modifications that elaborate on maintenance mechanisms, further delineate putative vulnerability traits and contextual factors that influence threat value attributed to pain experiences, and identify alternate pathways to persistent pain and associated functional disability. For example, Norton and Asmundson (2003) suggested that activation of the sympathetic division of the autonomic nervous system might contribute to protracted muscular tension and other bodily changes that influence avoidance behaviors and contribute to maintenance of pain over time (see Figure 16.2). They also emphasized that anxiety sensitivity (i.e., the fear of anxiety-related bodily sensations based on the belief they may have harmful consequences)—a potential vulnerability factor—warrants consideration as a factor that influences catastrophic appraisals of pain and pain-related fear and anxiety. Hassenbring and Verbunt (2010) suggest that, in addition to the pathways described by Vlaeyen and Linton (2000), pain-related functional disability might arise as a product of physical overuse or overload (i.e., endurance).

The fear-avoidance model and its refinements have been specifically applied to models of co-occurring anxiety disorders and chronic pain. To illustrate, Liedl and Knaevelsrud

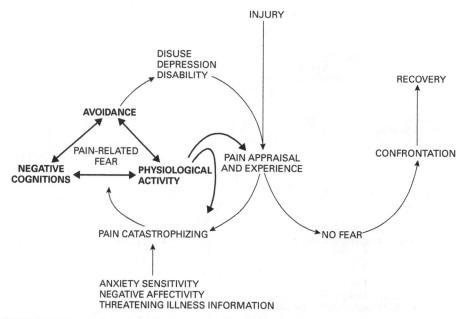

FIGURE 16.2 The amended fear-avoidance model from Norton and Asmundson (2003). This figure has been reproduced with permission of Elsevier Science. The figure may not be reproduced for any other purpose without permission.

(2008) proposed a model incorporating postulates of the cognitive model of posttraumatic stress disorder (PTSD; Ehlers and Clark, 2000) and the Vlaeyen and Linton (2000) formulation of the fear-avoidance model to explain the co-occurrence of PTSD and chronic pain. The essence of this model is that traumatic or painful experiences appraised as threatening (e.g., as a situation that may never resolve) are dealt with in maladaptive ways that perpetuate the fear-avoidance cycle and thereby promote continued emotional distress and functional disability (see Figure 16.3). More detailed consideration of refinements to the fear-avoidance model, as well as specific applications to comorbid presentations of the anxiety disorders and chronic pain, are available elsewhere (Asmundson, 2014; Asmundson and Katz, 2009; Asmundson et al., 2012a).

Despite its heuristic value and considerable influence, as well as the substantive body of empirical support (for reviews, see Asmundson et al., 1999; 2012a, 2012b; Leeuw et al., 2007; Vlaeyen and Linton, 2000), the fear-avoidance model and its various amendments are not without limitations; as such, a number of theorists have recently suggested that further advances in knowledge and treatment effectiveness may require a move away from the simplistic self-perpetuating cyclical relationship described in the fear-avoidance model (see, for example, Wideman et al., 2013). While research stemming from these critiques is emerging, it remains in its infancy and, as such, has not yet influenced the development or provision of evidence-based treatment in a substantive manner.

Acceptance-based approaches, derived from the psychological flexibility model, have emerged as an alternative to the fear-avoidance model and its amendments. The acceptance-based approaches suggest that human suffering, including pain, is a normal part of human existence. These approaches further suggest that attempts to control, suppress, or avoid negative cognitive and emotional states or distressing bodily sensations are counterproductive (Hayes, Strosahl and Wilson, 1999). Psychological acceptance refers to a person's willingness to experience some level of pain (and associated discomfort and distress) in pursuit of greater life goals or values (Dahl, Wilson, and Luciano, 2005). Allowing oneself to experience unwanted or distressing cognitions or

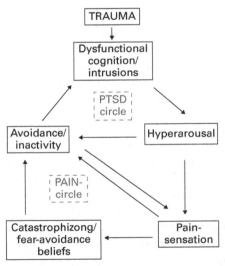

FIGURE 16.3 The perpetual avoidance model from Liedl and Knaevlsrud (2008). This figure has been reproduced with permission of the International Rehabilitation Council of Torture Victims (IRCT). The figure may not be reproduced for any other purpose without permission.

bodily sensations without judgment (or attempts to change or control them) is thought to reduce their emotional impact and increase the capacity for behavior change (Hayes et al., 1999). Acceptance of the uncontrollable aspects of the chronic pain experience (e.g., pain, fatigue, negative thoughts and emotions) is emphasized as a way to modify aspects of the experience that can be changed (e.g., engaging in meaningful activities despite pain). Acceptance-based treatments align with the fear-avoidance model and its refinements, at least in part, as they involve exposure to meaningful life activities that may be painful or anxiety provoking. A substantial body of evidence supports the efficacy of acceptance and commitment therapy (ACT) for improving pain outcomes such as pain intensity, depression, anxiety, and physical well-being (for review, see Veehof, Oskam, Schreurs, and Bohlmeijer, 2011).

ASSESSMENT AND TREATMENT

A variety of treatments for chronic musculoskeletal pain have emerged from the fear-avoidance model and mechanisms it describes. Although a relatively new area of inquiry, with the first report on related treatment published in 2001, a substantive body of research on these new treatment strategies has emerged. These treatment strategies include graded in vivo exposure (GivE), graded activity (GA), ACT, as well as less standardized techniques comprising various aspects of cognitive, behavioral, and other therapies (i.e., mixed therapy). Innovative approaches specifically targeting the co-occurrence of various anxiety disorders (primarily PTSD) and chronic pain are emerging. These treatments are described next. While pharmacotherapy has been shown effective in alleviating chronic pain (for review, see Kroenke, Krebs, and Bair, 2009), there are limited data regarding its application in the context of pain-related fear and anxiety; consequently, we do not discuss pharmacotherapy any further. Since choice of treatment follows from findings of assessment and case conceptualization, we first provide an overview of select assessment targets specific to fear of pain and pain-related anxiety.

Select Assessment Targets

Pain and related emotional responses are not typically targets of assessment for patients presenting with an anxiety disorder; however, given evidence that severe pain negatively impacts treatment outcomes for patients with various anxiety disorders (Teh et al., 2009), it becomes clear that the details of pain experiences are important for comprehensive case conceptualization. It is beyond the scope of this chapter to review the procedures for performing a comprehensive assessment of pain; in brief, this includes consideration of pain severity or intensity, pain location and distribution, attitudes and beliefs about pain and its effects, ways of coping with pain, pain-specific emotional distress (i.e., fear, anxiety, mood changes), and pain-related functional abilities and limitations. Asmundson, McMillan, and Carleton (2011) provide guidelines for conducting a time-efficient yet thorough pain assessment in patients presenting with an anxiety disorder. Here we highlight the core measures pertinent to fear of pain, pain-related anxiety, and pain catastrophizing.

Fear of pain is often measured with the 30-item Fear of Pain Questionnaire-III (FPQ-III; McNeil and Rainwater 1998) and, more recently, the 20-item Fear of Pain Questionnaire-Short Form (FPQ-SF; Asmundson, Bovell, Carleton, and McWilliams,

2008b). Items on both scales are rated using a 5-point Likert scale ranging from 1 (not at all) to 5 (extreme). The short-form resulted from a factor analytic finding suggesting removal of unstable items and revision of the three-factor structure of the FPQ-III (i.e., minor pain, severe pain, medical pain) into a more robust four-factor structure. The factorially distinct subscales of the FPQ-SF are each related to a specific type of pain, including minor pain (e.g., biting your tongue while eating), severe pain (e.g., having someone slam a heavy car door on your hand), injection pain (e.g., having a blood sample drawn with a hypodermic needle), and dental pain (e.g., having one of your teeth drilled). While both measures have sound psychometric properties (Asmundson et al., 2008; McNeil and Rainwater, 1998), the brevity of the FPQ-SF has made it an increasingly appealing option in experimental and treatment applications.

Pain-related anxiety is most commonly measured with either the original 40-item Pain Anxiety Symptoms Scale (McCracken, Zayfet, and Gross, 1992) or the 20-item Pain Anxiety Symptoms Scale-20 (PASS-20; McCracken and Dhingra, 2002). Items on both scales are rated using a 6-point Likert scale anchored from 0 (never) to 5 (always). Both measures consist of four factorially distinct components of pain-related anxiety including cognitive anxiety (e.g., I can't think straight when in pain), pain-related fear (e.g., Pain sensations are terrifying), escape and avoidance (e.g., I try to avoid activities that cause pain), and physiological anxiety (e.g., Pain makes me nauseous). Both measures have sound psychometric properties (McCracken and Dhingra, 2002; McCracken et al., 1992); as such, they are frequently used to assess pain-related anxiety in clinical and nonclinical samples.

Pain catastrophizing is commonly assessed with the Pain Catastrophizing Scale (PCS; Sullivan, Bishop, and Pivik, 1995). The PCS is a 13-item self-report measure designed to assess the extent to which people experience catastrophic thoughts and feelings when in pain. The measure is comprised of three factorially distinct subscales, including rumination (e.g., I can't seem to keep it out of my mind), magnification (e.g., I become afraid that the pain will get worse), and helplessness (e.g., It's awful and I feel that it overwhelms me). Items are rated on a 5-point Likert scale ranging from 0 (not at all) to 4 (all the time). The PCS has demonstrated strong internal reliability as well as discriminant, concurrent, and criterion-related validity (Osman, Barrios, Gutierrez, Kopper, and Grittmann, 2000). The measure has also been validated for use in many languages and across age groups (Parkerson et al., 2013).

Graded in vivo Exposure

GivE is a cognitive behavioral method that was developed by Vlaeyen and colleagues (2001) to target fear of pain and pain-related anxiety. The basic premise of GivE is that fear of pain, pain-related anxiety, and associated disability can be reduced by deliberately exposing patients to movements and tasks that have been avoided because of fear of pain or pain-related anxiety. GivE begins with psychoeducation about the fear-avoidance model, followed by a series of interactive therapy sessions involving graded exposure techniques and behavioral experiments. Patients and therapists collaborate to create an individualized hierarchy of feared activities (e.g., bending over to pick up an object). In subsequent sessions, patients are gradually exposed to the activities in their hierarchy, providing ratings of fear and pain expectation before and following each activity exposure. Therapists encourage patients to practice exposing themselves to the activities in their hierarchy as homework assignments between treatment sessions. It remains to be determined whether therapists need to model behaviors in a biomechanically appropriate fashion. It has been suggested that focusing on proper biomechanics may be counter-intuitive to patients who fear pain (Vlaeyen et al., 2001); indeed, fearful patients may misinterpret this information to mean that catastrophe will occur if they do not perform activities exactly as demonstrated by the therapist.

Graded Activity

GA, like GivE, is an active therapy used for treating chronic musculoskeletal pain. It works by using positive reinforcement of predefined activity quotas to shape healthy behaviors (Fordyce, 1976; Vlaeyen, de Jong, Sieben, and Crombez, 2002). Patients first identify specific functional activities that have been suspended as a result of chronic musculoskeletal pain (e.g., playing with children, driving). Patients are asked to describe their tolerance level for performing each of the suspended activities and treatment goals are formulated around these initial tolerances. For example, a patient might avoid bending at the waist while being able to tolerate bending halfway (45 degrees) for a maximum of 10 minutes. The avoided activities and associated tolerances form a time-contingent treatment schedule, not unlike a fear hierarchy. Patients begin engaging in the activities at 70 to 80% of their baseline tolerance levels (e.g., bending over to 35 degrees for 8 minutes) and gradually increase the activity engagement over time.

Despite their similarities, GA and GivE differ in an important way. GA is based on operant conditioning principles, whereas GivE uses principles from both classical and operant conditioning. More specifically, GA takes advantage of a progressive positive reinforcement schedule to modify behaviors while GivE works by first modifying behavior and, thereafter, applying positive and negative reinforcement schedules in order to change behavioral activity patterns. Although it was previously thought that exposure worked by abolishing pairings between conditioned and unconditioned stimuli, more recent evidence suggests that inhibitory learning occurs during exposure (Craske et al., 2008; Craske, this volume; Crombez et al., 2002).

Acceptance and Commitment Therapy

ACT is based on concepts of mindfulness, acceptance, and values-based action (Hayes and Duckworth, 2006; Hofmann and Asmundson, 2008). This approach has garnered considerable recent attention as a means of treating chronic musculoskeletal pain (Vowles and McCracken, 2008) and is based on the premise that patients with chronic pain need to shift the focus of their life away from the pain and onto things of greater interest, value, or importance. Acceptance occurs when one is willing to experience pain without attempting to control it—patients are taught to acknowledge their pain, observe it as a sensation, and then accept it as part of present reality without judgment. Through this process, individuals learn to accept pain as part of life rather than attempting to use coping strategies to manage it. Values based action occurs when values are clarified and actions are performed in line with those values; that is, patients are encouraged to consciously choose to engage in satisfying and rewarding activities despite their pain. The shift reduces or ameliorates the catastrophic cognitions and avoidance behaviors associated with debilitating chronic musculoskeletal pain, while also serving to diminish pain intensity (Vowles, McCracken, and Eccleston, 2008). It is noteworthy that, like GivE and GA, the effects of ACT on fear of pain may result from exposure (e.g., engaging in a pain-provoking experience and working to accept the pain sensation; Dahl et al., 2004), at least in part.

Other Mixed and Innovative Protocols

There are several other protocols that combine a variety of cognitive and behavioral techniques to treat fear, anxiety, and avoidance associated with chronic musculoskeletal pain (e.g., Linton and Ryberg, 2001). These alternatives may target the same fear of pain and pain-related anxiety beliefs as GA, GivE, and ACT; however, they utilize less detailed protocols. To illustrate, protocols have included problem-solving, cognitive re-appraisal, goal-setting, coping skills training, relaxation training, and assertiveness training. Since positive treatment outcomes are reduced for patients presenting with a co-occurring anxiety disorder and chronic pain (Teh et al., 2009), several innovative approaches to treating the co-occurrence have also been developed. These treatments, described in detail by Asmundson and colleagues (Asmundson, 2014; Asmundson, Gomez-Perez, and Fetzner, 2014), have focused primarily on early intervention, integrated treatment, and targeting shared vulnerabilities (or risk factors) in the co-occurrence of PTSD and chronic pain. For example, early interventions that combine brief CBT to relieve acute trauma symptoms while simultaneously promoting gradual increases in physical activity (i.e., GA) to reinstate pre-injury functioning may serve to prevent the onset of comorbid PTSD and chronic pain. Similar effects may be obtained through administration of opioid analgesics, which have been shown to diminish acute pain experiences and also reduce the risk of developing PTSD (Holbrook, Galarneau, Dye, Quinn, and Dougherty, 2010; Morgan, Krystal, and Southwick, 2003). Integrated treatments that include psychoeducation, cognitive restructuring, emotion regulation strategies, activity planning, and prolonged exposure and GivE may reduce both post-trauma and pain-relevant indices in patients with comorbid PTSD and chronic pain. Likewise, emerging treatment strategies that target the putative shared maintenance and vulnerability mechanisms of anxiety sensitivity and selective attentional bias—interoceptive exposure and attention modification programming—may serve to simultaneously reduce the symptoms of both conditions and, depending on when administered in the transition from acute to chronic, may prevent chronicity or curtail its maintenance.

Evidence

Each of the treatments for fear of pain and pain-related anxiety associated with chronic musculoskeletal pain described (i.e., GivE, GA, ACT, and the mixed CBT protocols) has received varying levels of empirical support. It is beyond the scope of this chapter to comprehensively review the evidence; however, a recent review of 17 treatment studies conducted by Bailey and colleagues (2010) suggests that GivE and ACT, but not mixed CBT protocols, produce superior outcomes with respect to fear of pain, avoidance, pain severity and associated disability when compared against GA and wait-list. GivE was generally more successful than GA and wait-list in reducing fear of pain, pain-related catastrophizing, and disability and marginally more successful than GA and wait-list in reducing pain severity. ACT was effective in reducing pain severity and disability and showed potential for reducing fear of pain; however, results from the ACT studies need to be interpreted with caution given that few of the available studies assessed the effectiveness of ACT relative to comparison groups. The available data on number of hours required for treatment and dropout rates for each of GiveE and ACT suggest that the former requires fewer hours (17 versus 50, on average) whereas the latter has a lower dropout rate (29% versus 39%, on average). Given that innovative approaches specifically targeting the co-occurrence of various anxiety disorders and chronic pain are just emerging, sufficient evidence on which to judge their effectiveness or efficacy has not yet accumulated; however, preliminary finding are encouraging (for review, see Asmundson, 2014).

SUMMARY AND FUTURE DIRECTIONS

People with disabling chronic pain often experience significant pain-related fear and anxiety. It has been well documented that fear and anxiety play an important role in the transition from acute to chronic pain. The fear-avoidance model and its variants have guided considerable research on mechanisms and treatment; indeed, a number of relevant assessment targets (e.g., pain-related anxiety, fear of pain, pain catastrophizing) have been identified and several empirically supported treatments (e.g., GivE, GA, ACT) have been developed to reduce pain-related fear and anxiety and associated disability. More recently, observations that many people with an anxiety disorder experience co-occurring chronic pain and that pain negatively impacts anxiety treatment outcomes have prompted efforts to explain the co-occurrence and develop effective means of treatment. The models and treatments resulting from these efforts have been derived, in large part, from postulates of the fear-avoidance model and its variants.

Though existing work on the associations between fear, anxiety, and chronic pain is rapidly growing and already clinically meaningful, further research is needed. First, models guiding research and treatment require continued refinement. For example, the fear-avoidance model and its refinements have been criticized for focusing exclusively on factors that predict maladaptive responses to chronic pain (Wideman et al., 2013). Many individuals with chronic pain are well-adjusted and their pain is not associated with disability. Theorists have suggested that advances in knowledge and treatment may require a greater focus on resilience factors that predict successful adaptation to chronic pain (Wideman et al., 2013) as well as patterns of successful recovery and rehabilitation (Pincus and McCracken, 2013). A clearer understanding of how resilience factors interact with patterns of pain-related fear, anxiety, and avoidance would also help guide future adaptations of existing models.

Second, theorists have suggested a need for continued refinement in the conceptualization and measurement of fear of pain, which currently shares characteristics with phobic disorders (Turk and Wilson, 2010; Wideman et al., 2013). Treatments that utilize graded exposure techniques align with a phobic conceptualization of fear of pain. There is evidence to suggest that fear of pain may not be well represented as a phobic disorder, as individuals with chronic pain do not often see their fear as excessive or unreasonable (Williams and McCracken, 2004) and their brain activation patterns are not consistent with those exposed to feared stimuli (Barke, Baudewig, Schmidt-Samoa, Dechent, and Kröner-Herwig, 2012). Likewise, fear of pain measures do not follow as closely to this conceptualization, as they often assess only expectancies and beliefs while overlooking other components of phobic disorders (e.g., negative affect, distress-related behaviors). There are also no objective measures of avoidance that reliably and validly assess pain-related avoidance behaviors (Vlaeyen and Linton, 2012). Development of such assessment tools may provide clearer behavioral targets for treatment and, thereby, increase the effectiveness of treatment. Future research is necessary to develop consistency between conceptualization, measurement, and treatment of fear of pain.

Finally, treatment of co-occurring anxiety disorders and chronic pain is still in its infancy and requires continued development and testing of new and innovative treatment approaches. Established treatment approaches for anxiety (e.g., problem-solving, cognitive re-appraisal, goal-setting, coping skills training, relaxation training, assertiveness training) could be combined with components of GA, GivE, and ACT protocols in an effort to maximize the effectiveness of interventions for co-occurring anxiety disorders and chronic pain. Increasing activity via regular and vigorous participation in various forms of exercise (e.g., resistance training, aerobic training, hatha yoga) may also prove beneficial for those with co-occurring anxiety disorders and chronic pain. Some progress has already been made in efforts to treat co-occurring PTSD and chronic pain; however, these treatments are in the early stages of development and evaluation of effectiveness (Asmundson, 2014) and extension to other anxiety disorders is warranted.

DISCLOSURE STATEMENT

Preparation of this paper was supported, in part, by the University of Regina President's Chair for Academic Excellence in Adult Mental Health Research awarded to G.J.G.A. and a Canadian Institutes of Health Research (CIHR) Regional Partnership Program Doctoral Award to H.A.P. The authors have nothing further to disclose.

REFERENCES

Asmundson, G. J. G. (2014). The emotional and physical pains of trauma: Contemporary and innovative approaches for treating co-occurring PTSD and chronic pain. *Depress Anxiety, 31*, 717–720.

Asmundson, G. J. G., Bovell, C. V., Carleton, N. R., and McWilliams, L. A. (2008). The fear of pain questionnaire-short form: Factorial validity and psychometric properties. *Pain, 134*, 51–58.

Asmundson, G. J. G., Gomez-Perez, L., and Fetzner, M. (2014). Chronic pain and posttraumatic stress disorder and. In N. Feeny and L. Zoellner (Eds.), *Facilitating resilience and recovery following trauma* (pp. 265–290). New York: Guilford.

Asmundson, G. J. G., and Katz, J. (2009). Understanding the co-occurrence of anxiety disorders and chronic musculoskeletal pain: The state-of-the-art. *Depress Anxiety, 26*, 888–901.

Asmundson, G. J. G., McMillan, K. A., and Carleton, R. N. (2011). Understanding and managing clinically significant pain in patients with an anxiety disorder. *Focus: J Lifelong Learning Psychiatry, 9*, 264–272.

Asmundson, G. J. G., Noel, M., Petter, M., and Parkerson, H. A. (2012b). Pediatric fear-avoidance model of chronic pain: Foundation, application, and future directions. *Pain Res Manage, 17*, 397–405.

Asmundson, G. J. G., Norton, G. R., and Allerdings, M. D. (1997). Fear and avoidance in dysfunctional chronic back pain patients. *Pain, 69*, 231–236.

Asmundson, G. J. G., Norton, P. J., and Norton, G. R. (1999). Beyond pain: The role of fear and avoidance in chronicity, *Clin Psychol Rev, 19*, 97–119.

Asmundson, G. J. G., Norton, P. J., and Vlaeyen, J. W. S. (2004). Fear-avoidance models of chronic pain: An overview. In G. J. G. Asmundson, J.W.S. Vlaeyen, and G. Crombez (Eds.), *Understanding and treating fear of pain* (pp. 3–24). Oxford, England: Oxford University Press.

Asmundson, G. J. G., Parkerson, H. A., Petter, M., and Noel, M. (2012a). What is the role of fear and escape/avoidance in chronic pain? Models, structural analysis, and future directions. *Pain Manage, 2*, 295–303.

Asmundson, G.J.G., and Wright, K.D. (2004). The biopsychosocial model of pain. In T. Hadjistavropoulos, and K. D. Craig (Eds.), *Pain: Psychological perspectives* (pp. 35–57). Hillsborough, NJ: Lawrence Erlbaum.

Bailey, K. M., Carleton, R. N., Vlaeyen, J. W., and Asmundson, G. J. G. (2010). Treatments addressing pain-related fear and anxiety in patients with chronic musculoskeletal pain: A preliminary review. *Cog Behav Ther, 39*, 46–63.

Barke, A., Baudewig, J., Schmidt-Samoa, C., Dechent, P., Kröner-Herwig, B. (2012). Neural correlates of fear of movement in high and low fear-avoidant chronic low back pain patients: an event-related fMRI study. *Pain, 153*, 540–552.

Carleton, N. R., and Asmundson, G. J. G. (2009). The multidimensionality of fear of pain: Construct independent for the fear of pain questionnaire-short form and the pain anxiety symptoms scale-20. *J Pain, 10*, 29–37.

Collimore, K. C., Asmundson, G. J. G., Taylor, S., and Abramowitz, J. S. (2009). Classification of hypochondriasis and other somatoform disorders. In D. McKay, J. S. Abramowitz, S. Taylor, and G. J. G. Asmundson. (Eds.), *Current perspectives on the anxiety disorders: Implications for DSM-V and Beyond* (pp.431–447). New York, NY: Springer.

Craske, M. G., Kircanski, K., Zelikowsky, M., Mystkowski, J., Chowdhury, N., and Baker, A. (2008). Optimizing inhibitory learning during exposure therapy. *Behav Res Ther, 46*, 5–27.

Crombez, G., Eccleston, C., Vlaeyen, J. W., Vansteenwegen, D., Lysens, R., and Eelen, P. (2002). Exposure to physical movements in low back pain patients: Restricted effects of generalization. *Health Psychol, 21*, 573–578.

Dahl, J., Wilson, K. G., and Luciano, C. (2005). *Acceptance and commitment therapy for chronic pain.* Reno: Context Press, 2005.

Demyttenaer, K., Bruffaerts, R., Lee, S., Posasa-Villa, J., Kovess, V., Angermeyer, M. C., . . . Von Korff, M. (2007). Mental disorders among persons with chronic back or neck pain: Results from the World Mental Health Surveys. *Pain, 129*, 332–342.

Ehlers, A., and Clark, D. M. (2000). A cognitive model of posttraumatic stress disorder. *Behav Res Ther, 38*, 319–345.

Fordyce, W. E. (1976). *Behavioral Methods for Chronic Pain and Illness.* St. Louis, MO: C. V. Moseby Company.

Gaskin, D. J., and Richard, P. (2012). The economic costs of pain in the Unites States. *J Pain, 13*, 715–724.

Gureje, O., Von Korff, M., Simon, G. E., and Gater, R. (1998). Persistent pain and well-being: A world health organization study in primary care. *J Am Med Assoc, 280*, 147–151.

Hardt, J., Jacobsen, C., Goldberg, J., Nickel, R., and Buchwald, D. (2008). Prevalence of chronic pain in a representative sample in the United States. *Pain Med, 9*, 803–812.

Hasenbring, M. I., and Verbunt, J. A. (2010). Fear-avoidance and endurance-related responses to pain: New models of behavior and their consequences for clinical practice. *Clin J Pain, 26*, 747–753.

Hayes, S. C., and Duckworth, M. P. (2006). Acceptance and commitment therapy and traditional cognitive behavior therapy approaches to pain. *Cogn Behav Pract, 13*, 185–187.

Hayes, S. C., Strosahl, K. D., and Wilson, K. G. (1999). *Acceptance and commitment therapy: An Experiential approach to behavior change.* New York, NY: The Guilford Press.

Hofmann, S. G., and Asmundson, G. J. (2008). Acceptance and mindfulness-based therapy: New wave or old hat? *Clin Psychol Rev, 28*, 1–16.

Holbrook, T. L., Galarneau, M. R., Dye, J. L., Quinn, K., and Dougherty, A. L. (2010). Morphine use after combat injury in Iraq and post-traumatic stress disorder. *N Engl J Med, 362*, 110–117.

International Association for the Study of Pain Subcommittee on Taxonomy. (1994). Classification of chronic pain: Descriptions of chronic pain syndromes and definitions of pain terms. *Pain Suppl* 3:S1–S226.

Kashikar-Zuck, S., Goldschneider, K. R., Powers, S. W., Vaught, M. H., and Hershey, A. D. (2001). Depression and functional disability in chronic pediatric pain. *Clin J Pain, 17* (4), 341–349.

Kroenke, K., Krebs, E. E., and Bair, M. J. (2009). Pharmacotherapy of chronic pain: A synthesis of recommendations from systematic reviews. *Gen Hosp Psychiatry, 31*, 206–219.

Leeuw, M., Goossens, M. E., Linton, S. J., Crombez, G., Boersma, K., and Vlaeyen, J. W. S. (2007). The fear-avoidance model of musculoskeletal pain: Current state of scientific evidence. *J Behav Med, 30*, 77–94.

Liedl, A., and Knaevelsrud, C. (2008). Chronic pain and PTSD: The perpetual avoidance model and its treatment implications. *Torture, 18*, 69–76.

Linton, S. J., and Ryberg, M. (2001). A cognitive behavioral group intervention as prevention for persistent neck and back pain in a non-patient population: A randomized controlled trial. *Pain, 90*, 83–90.

McCracken, L. M., and Dhingra, L. (2002). A short version of the pain anxiety symptoms scale (PASS—20): Preliminary development and validity. *Pain Res Manage, 7*, 45–50.

McCracken, L. M., Gross, R. T., Aikens, J., and Carnrike, C. L. M. Jr. (1996). The assessment of anxiety and fear in persons with chronic pain: A comparison of instruments. *Behav Res Ther, 34*, 927–933.

McCracken, L. M., Zayfert, C., and Gross, R. T. (1992). The pain anxiety symptoms scale: Development and validation of a scale to measure fear of pain. *Pain, 50*, 67–73.

McNeil, D. W., and Rainwater, A. J. (1998). Development of the Fear of Pain Questionnaire-III. *J Behav Med, 21*, 389–410.

McWilliams, L. A., Cox, B. J., and Enns, M.W. (2003). Mood and anxiety disorders associated with chronic pain: An examination in a nationally representative sample. *Pain, 106*, 127–133.

Morgan, C. A. III, Krystal, J. H., and Southwick, S. M. (2003). Toward early pharmacological post-traumatic stress intervention. *Biol Psychiatry, 53*, 834–843.

Morley, S., and Eccleston, C. (2004). The object of fear in chronic pain. In G. J. G. Asmundson, J. W. S. Vlaeyen, and G. Crombez (Eds.), *Understanding and treating fear of pain.* (pp. 163–188). Oxford, England: Oxford University Press.

Norton, P. J., and Asmundson, G. J. G. (2003). Amending the fear-avoidance model of chronic pain: What is the role of physiological arousal? *Behav Therapy, 34*, 17–30.

Osman, A., Barrios, F. X., Gutierrez, P. M., Kopper, B. A., Merrifield, T., and Grittmann, L. (2000). The pain catastrophizing scale: Further psychometric evaluation with adult samples. *J Behav Med, 23*, 351–365.

Parkerson, H. A., Noel, M., Pagé, M. G., Fuss, S., Katz, J., and Asmundson, G. J. G. (2013). Factorial validity of the English-language version of the pain catastrophizing scale-child version. *J Pain, 14*, 1383–1389.

Perquin, C. W., Hunfeld, J. A. M., Hazebroek-Kampschreur A. A. J. M., van Suijlekom-Smit, L. W. A., Passchier, J., Koes, B. W., and van der Wouden, J. C. (2001). Insights in the use of health care services in chronic benign pain in childhood and adolescence. *Pain, 94*, 205–213.

Pincus, T., and McCracken, L. M. (2013). Psychological factors and treatment opportunities in low back pain. *Best Pract Res Clin Rheumatol, 27*, 625–635.

Reitsma, M. L., Tranmer, J. E., Buchanan, D. M., and VanDenKerkhof, E. G. (2012). The epidemiology of chronic pain in Canadian men and women between 1994 and 2007: Results from the longitudinal component of the National Population Health Survey. *Pain Res and Manage J Canadian Pain Soc, 17*, 166–172.

Sareen, J., Cox, B. J., Clara, I., and Asmundson, G. J. G. (2005). The relationship between anxiety disorders and physical disorders in the US National Comorbidity Survey. *Depress Anxiety, 21*, 193–202.

Sullivan, M. J., Bishop, S. R., Pivik, J. (1995). The pain catastrophising scale: Development and validation. *Psychol Assess, 7*, 524–532.

Sullivan, M. J. L., Thorn, B., Haythornthwaite, J. A., Keefe, F., Martin, M., Bradley, L. A., and Lefebvre, J. C. (2001). Theoretical perspectives on the relation between catastrophizing and pain. *Clin J Pain, 17*, 52–64.

Teh, C. F., Morone, N. E., Karp, J. F., Belnap, B. H., Zhu, F., Weiner, D. K., and Rollman, B. L. (2009). Pain interference impacts responses to treatment for anxiety disorders. *Depress Anxiety, 26*, 222–228.

Turk, D. C., and Rudy, T. E. (1987). Towards a comprehensive assessment of chronic pain patients. *Behav Res Ther, 25*, 237–249.

Turk, D. C., & Wilson, H. D. (2010). Fear of pain as a prognostic factor in chronic pain: Conceptual models, assessment, and treatment implications. *Curr Pain Headache Rep, 14*, 88–95.

Veehof, M. M., Oskam M., Schreurs, K. M. G., and Bohlmeijer, E. T. (2011). Acceptance-based interventions for the treatment of chronic pain: A systematic review and meta-analysis. *Pain, 15*, 533–542.

Vlaeyen, J. W., de Jong, J., Geilen, M., Heuts, P. H., & van Breukelen, G. (2001). Graded exposure in vivo in the treatment of pain-related fear: A replicated single-case experimental design in four patients with chronic low back pain. *Behav Res Ther, 39*, 151–166.

Vlaeyen, J. W., de Jong, J., Sieben, J., Crombez, G. (2002). Graded exposure in vivo for pain-related fear. In D. C. Turk and R.J. Gatchel (Eds.), *Psychological approaches to pain management* (2nd ed.), (pp. 210–233). New York, NY: Guilford Press.

Vlaeyen, J. W., and Linton, S. J. (2000). Fear-avoidance and its consequences in chronic musculoskeletal pain: A state of the art. *Pain, 85*, 317–332.

Vlaeyen, J. W., and Linton, S. J. (2012). Fear-avoidance model of chronic musculoskeletal pain: 12 years on. *Pain, 153*, 1144–1147.

Vowles, K. E., and McCracken, L. M. (2008). Acceptance and values-based action in chronic pain: A study of treatment effectiveness and process. *J Consult Clin Psychol, 76*, 397–407.

Vowles, K. E., McCracken, L. M., and Eccleston, C. (2008). Patient functioning and catastrophizing in chronic pain: The mediating effects of acceptance. *Health Psychology, 27* (Suppl.), S136–S143.

Wideman, T. H., Asmundson, G. J. G., Smeets, R. J. E. M., Zautra, A. J., Simmonds, M. J., Sullivan, M. J. L., . . . Edwards, R. R. (2013). Rethinking the fear avoidance model: Toward a multidimensional framework of pain-related disability. *Pain, 154*, 2262–2265.

Williams, A. C. de C., and McCracken, L. (2004). Cognitive-behavioral therapy for chronic pain: An overview with specific reference to fear and avoidance. In G. J. G. Asmundson, J. Vlaeyen, and G. Crombez (Eds.), *Understanding and treating fear of pain* (pp. 293–312). Oxford, England: Oxford University Press.

/// 17 /// DETECTION AND TREATMENT OF ANXIETY DISORDERS IN PRIMARY CARE SETTINGS

CARA H. FUCHS AND RISA B. WEISBERG

INTRODUCTION

It is well established that the majority of mental health treatment in the United States is delivered in primary care settings (Wang et al., 2005, 2006). As a result, interest in integrating mental and behavioral health services into primary care has been rapidly growing. Fortunately, with the passage of the Affordable Care Act, support for integration is also growing. Anxiety is the most common mental health condition in the United States and significantly contributes to disability, functional impairment, and rising health care costs. In this chapter, we present: (1) a rationale for addressing anxiety disorders in primary care, (2) a brief overview of primary care behavioral health and health care reform efforts, (3) an overview of anxiety screening and treatment research in primary care, (4) the challenges to implementation, and (5) future directions with respect to detecting and treating anxiety disorders within a primary care behavioral health model.

WHY SCREEN FOR AND TREAT ANXIETY IN PRIMARY CARE?

Anxiety disorders are highly prevalent in the US, with lifetime prevalence estimates as a high as 15.6% for specific phobias and 10.7% for social phobia (Kessler, Petukhova, Sampson, Zaslavsky, and Wittchen, 2014). Overall, 28.8% of the general US population is estimated to have at least one anxiety disorder during their lifetime (Kessler et al., 2005). Further, the estimated current prevalence of an anxiety disorder among primary care patients is as high as 19.5% (Kroenke, Spitzer, Williams, Monahan, and Lowe, 2007) and more than half of patients with an anxiety disorder receive their treatment from a primary care provider (Harman, Rollman, Hanusa, Lenze, and Shear, 2002; Wang et al, 2006). In 2007, almost half of all prescriptions for antidepressants and anxiolytics were written in primary care settings (Schappert and Rechsteiner, 2011).

Primary care patients with anxiety disorders tend to experience considerable disability, functional impairments, and health care needs. They are high health care utilizers, with utilization rates as high as patients with chronic physical health conditions (Stein et al., 2005).

Comorbidities with other mental health disorders are particularly high in this population. Rodriguez et al. (2004) found that among primary care patients with anxiety disorders, 80% reported a lifetime history of at least one additional axis I disorder. At the time of assessment, 60% had more than one current anxiety disorder and 40% were currently experiencing at least one anxiety disorder and a major depressive episode These comorbidity rates are particularly notable given that primary care patients are not necessarily seeking treatment for anxiety. This challenges the notion that treatment-seeking populations are more impaired than individuals with mental health disorders who are not seeking treatment.

Primary care patients with anxiety disorders are likely to have comorbid physical health conditions. A study of primary care patients with chronic musculoskeletal pain found that almost half (45%) met criteria for one or more anxiety disorders and these patients reported worse health-related quality of life compared to patients without an anxiety disorder (Kroenke, et al., 2013). Gastrointestinal (GI) problems are common among primary care patients (Thompson, Heaton, Smyth, and Smyth, 2000). Data from the patient health questionnaire (PHQ) anxiety study revealed that primary care patients who reported GI symptoms were at elevated risk for anxiety disorders (Mussell et al., 2008). More specifically, complaints of constipation, loose bowels, or diarrhea were associated with a more than two-fold risk of having Generalized anxiety disorder (GAD), panic disorder (PD), or social anxiety disorder (SAD). Primary care patients with anxiety disorders are more likely to have medically unexplained symptoms like chest pain and rapid heart rate that often lead to costly, nonurgent emergency department visits (Stein et al., 2005). It is estimated that 30–50% of patients who visit the emergency department for "nonspecific chest pain" have an anxiety disorder (Demiryoguran, et al., 2006; Gibler et al., 1995; Kontos, 2001).

Identifying primary care patients with anxiety symptoms and intervening early has the potential of lowering health care costs and possibly preventing the development of anxiety disorders. Primary care is also a natural fit for addressing the ways in which anxiety disorders affect physical health problems and interfere with effective health maintenance. However, detecting and treating anxiety disorders in primary are not without challenges, as we will discuss in later sections of this chapter. First, we will present an overview of integrated primary care and a model of integrating behavioral health services into primary care. A brief discussion of the health care reform efforts that have affected integrated primary care will also be presented.

INTEGRATED PRIMARY CARE AND ANXIETY DISORDERS

Given the prevalence and associated impairment of anxiety and other mental health problems in primary care patients and the fact that most patients with these problems seek care in general medical settings rather than specialty mental health settings, the past decade has brought increased focus on models of better integrating behavioral health care into the primary care setting. Integrated primary care may be thought of as a continuum, ranging from coordinated to integrated care (Blount, 2003). Coordinated care refers to behavioral health and medical care provided in different settings but in which there is a mechanism in place to allow for communication and coordination between providers. Co-located care, residing between coordinated and integrated care, is when behavioral health and medical care is provided separately but in the same location with shared resources. Integrated care is defined by one comprehensive treatment plan that acknowledges the intersections between mental and physical health. Many primary care practices contain elements of coordination and co-location, however full integration requires resources and practice support that is currently less common.

The Primary Care Behavioral Health (PCBH) Model

One of the most commonly used methods of delivering behavioral health services in primary care settings is that of the primary care behavioral health (PCBH) model (Robinson and Reiter, 2007). In this model, a behavioral health consultant (BHC), often within the disciplines of psychology, social work, or nursing, serves as a member of the primary care team providing consultation to physicians and direct service to patients. The BHC can provide (1) assessment of behavioral health issues, (2) consultation to the primary care providers on how they can help their patients better manage behavioral health issues, (3) brief treatment to primary care patients, often using cognitive behavioral-based treatment principles, and (4) guidance regarding triage to specialty mental health or other related services. Like physicians, BHCs can also consult intermittently throughout a patient's lifespan as needed.

Table 17.1 outlines some of the key differences between the roles of a mental health provider in specialty mental health versus primary care. Visits with a BHC tend to be brief (15–30 minutes) and focused. To be useful in primary care, the BHC needs to be easily accessible and able to work at the fast pace of primary care. BHCs can be called upon by patients during an office visit with their physician (warm hand-off) or a walk-in visit (open access). Therefore, the BHC needs to be ready at all times. Unless the referral question is a diagnostic one (e.g., differentiating between unipolar and bipolar depression), assessments are typically focused on functioning rather than diagnosis. Interventions often target discrete lifestyle changes (i.e. increasing physical activity, enhancing medication adherence) or coping strategies (i.e. mindfulness practices, assertiveness skills). In integrated practices, behavioral health notes are included in the shared medical record and used to communicate information to physicians and coordinate care. Like primary care physicians, BHCs need to be able to function as generalists. Holistic approaches to care are critical. BHCs need to be skilled at identifying the role that mental health issues like anxiety play in causing, exacerbating, and maintaining physical health conditions.

TABLE 17.1 The Roles of a Mental Health Provider

	SPECIALTY MENTAL HEALTH	PRIMARY CARE BEHAVIORAL HEALTH
Length of session	45–60 minutes	15–30 minutes
Session schedule	Fixed	Flexible, open access
Assessments	Diagnostic	Functional
Interventions	In-depth, disorder-specific	Targeted, focused on lifestyle changes and/or coping strategies
Chart notes	Private, written for treating clinician	Shared, written for referring physician
Clinician orientation	Specialist	Generalist

Content from Robinson and Reiter, 2007.

It should be clear at this point that the role of a BHC is dramatically different from a specialty mental health provider. Further, it is difficult to disseminate and implement traditional treatments for anxiety disorders, which often require at least 12–16 weekly sessions of in-depth, disorder-specific treatment, in this setting. In later sections of this chapter, we will review the research on behavioral treatments for anxiety disorders in primary care and discuss how anxiety might be best addressed in a PCBH model.

Health Care Reform and Patient-Centered Medical Home

Alongside the integration movement has been the advent of the patient-centered medical home (PCMH) model. PCMH is a way of organizing service delivery in a coordinated manner. The core components of the PCMH include (1) patient-centered care, where care is approached as an active partnership between patients and providers, (2) comprehensive, coordinated, team-based care in which there is a focus on the whole person and the physician consults with a team of specialists and community providers, (3) continuous access to care, where patients can access care when they need it and utilize multiple methods of communication to do so, and (4) population-based approaches to quality and safety, such that important health metrics are monitored in the entire patient population to allow for proactive intervention with high risk patients and tracking of health outcomes. Behavioral health issues like anxiety are often interwoven with physical health problems and are best addressed in a coordinated treatment plan. Therefore, integrated primary care behavioral health dovetails nicely within the PCMH mission to provide comprehensive, team-based care.

The passage of the Affordable Care Act in 2010 brought further momentum to the integrated care movement as it expanded access to mental health and substance abuse treatment. Measures embedded within the Affordable Care Act reward practices for attending to primary prevention and including care management, thus creating an incentive for having integrated behavioral health services.

This movement in medical care creates both opportunities and challenges for the treatment of anxiety disorders. As medical sites vie to attain certification as PCMHs and eventually as accountable care organizations (ACOs) there will be increased need to place behavioral health expertise in the primary care sites. With clear tools for anxiety screening and tested methods of treatment, this presents the opportunity for greatly improved public health. However, new more capitated care payment models for ACOs can potentially lead healthcare sites to look for the least costly methods of addressing mental and behavioral health problems, and, as anxiety disorders can be difficult to diagnose accurately and may require specialized treatments, there is a risk that less than adequate care may continue to be provided.

DETECTION OF ANXIETY DISORDERS IN PRIMARY CARE

Accurate detection of anxiety disorders in primary care is critical to providing appropriate and timely treatment. Despite the high prevalence of anxiety disorders in primary care populations, the detection and treatment of anxiety disorders in primary care has historically taken a back seat to depression. In this section, we will review the challenges in detecting and screening for anxiety disorders in primary care and lessons learned from depression screening that might inform anxiety-screening efforts.

Challenges of Screening for Anxiety Disorders in Primary Care

It is estimated that only 10–30% of primary care patients with anxiety disorders are recognized as having anxiety (Karlsson, Joukamaa, and Lehtinen, 2000; Wittchen et al., 2002). Further, when anxiety is recognized in primary care, a differential DSM diagnosis is not likely to be applied. The majority of recorded anxiety diagnoses by physicians are "anxiety state, unspecified" (Harman, Rollman, Hanusa, Lenze, and Shear, 2002).

Accurate diagnosis of anxiety disorders in primary care is complicated by several factors. In contrast to depression, there are many anxiety disorders each with greatly overlapping symptoms. Thus, to make a particular DSM anxiety disorder diagnosis, a primary care provider would first need to be well versed in the diagnostic criteria and clinical presentations of each individual anxiety disorder. In addition to this pre-requisite knowledge, the provider would then have the difficult and often time-consuming task of making a differential diagnosis. This task can be more challenging in primary care settings, as it is often accomplished only via careful questioning of patients with regard to the particular source of their fear and situations that they avoid. Primary care patients may have less insight than mental health specialty patients about their mental health symptoms or language to describe them and thus have more difficulty reporting. Further complicating anxiety disorder diagnosis in primary care is the task of differentiating between anxiety and somatic symptoms related to medical conditions. Primary care patients are much more likely to present with somatic complaints than with emotional concerns. There is considerable overlap between the symptoms of anxiety, depression, and somatization disorders and, as a result, they have shared effects on functioning and quality of life (Lowe et al., 2008). In fact, when primary care patients present with a physical or somatic complaint, the correct psychiatric diagnosis is only made 50% of the time (Kroenke and Mangelsdorff, 1989). This underscores the importance of having useful screening measures to assist primary physicians with population-based screening of anxiety disorders.

Depression Screening in Primary Care

The importance of managing depression in primary care is well established. The patient health questionnaire (PHQ-9) was the first depression screening measure developed for use in primary care (Kroenke, Spitzer, and Williams, 2001) and has been demonstrated to be a valid tool for monitoring clinically meaningful symptom changes over time (Lowe et al., 2004). When the PHQ-9 is routinely used to screen and monitor depression symptoms severity, it is predictive of physician-initiated treatment changes (Moore, et al., 2012).

The PHQ-2 was developed as an even shorter depression screening measure, including just two items of the PHQ-9 assessing depressed mood and anhedonia. The PHQ-2 has demonstrated strong validity (Kroenke, Spitzer, and Williams, 2003) and high sensitivity for detecting major depression in primary care (Arroll, et al., 2010). The PHQ-2 can be used as a first-step in the screening process, to be followed by the more comprehensive PHQ-9 if the PHQ-2 is positive to determine depression severity, inform treatment decisions, and monitor progress over time (Whooley, Avins, Miranda, and Browner, 1997). However, the extent to which this process is implemented in practice and how physicians use information from the PHQ-2 and PHQ-9 to guide treatment decisions is not known.

The perception of some physicians is that targeted screening of at-risk populations is more feasible and useful than screening the entire population and question the utility of structured assessments like the PHQ-9, as they are seen as impersonal and generally less reliable than clinical judgment (Henke, et al., 2008). A national survey of physicians found that physicians tend to selectively use depression screening measures to confirm a diagnosis in patients they believe are likely to be diagnosed with a mood disorder (Mojtabai, 2011).

Applying Lessons Learned from Depression Screening in Primary Care to Anxiety Disorders

The US Preventative Services Task Force recommends routine depression screening of all adults in clinical practices in which depression treatment and follow-up is available. However, what we have learned from depression screening in practice is that it needs to be one part of a larger process in which positive screens lead to further evaluation, which lead to changes in care. Time constraints, staffing limitations, and physicians' preference to use their clinical judgment often preclude follow-up on positive depression screens. Therefore, in order for population-based anxiety screening to become a part of usual care, practice support and a follow-up treatment plan are crucial.

Many primary care physicians are more comfortable with treatment of depression than anxiety. While selective serotonin reuptake inhibitors (SSRIs) and serotonin–norepinephrine reuptake inhibitors (SNRIs) are front-line recommended pharmacotherapies for both depression and anxiety, these medications are classified and commonly referred to as "antidepressants." "Anxiolytics" is used mostly to refer to benzodiazpines, a class of medications that many primary care providers are very reluctant to prescribe, given side effects and abuse potential. This naming of medication class by disorder may contribute to a lack of confidence among primary care providers in how to best treat patients with anxiety disorders. Additionally, many primary care physicians are familiar with the behavioral activation approach to treating depression and will naturally encourage increased activation in conjunction with a psychopharmacological approach. However, physicians may be less comfortable encouraging behavioral interventions for treating anxiety disorders such as repeated exposure to feared situations, as they seem less straightforward to treat. Therefore, increased education for physicians about *common mechanisms* underlying anxiety disorders (i.e., experiential avoidance, attention bias, interpretation bias, and intolerance of uncertainty) and how cognitive behavioral treatment components address these mechanisms might improve physician-initiated treatment of anxiety disorders.

TREATMENT RATES AMONG PRIMARY CARE PATIENTS WITH ANXIETY DISORDERS

Despite the relatively low detection rates, the majority of mental health treatment of anxiety continues to occur in primary care (Harman, Rollman, Hanusa, Lenze, and Shear, 2002; Wang et al, 2006). Relatively few US adults with anxiety disorders receive mental health treatment from a mental health specialist. In this section, we will review the research on the rates of treatment for anxiety disorders among primary care patients and the adequacy of these treatments.

The Primary Care Anxiety Project (PCAP) was the first longitudinal study of primary care patients with anxiety disorders and provided a naturalistic view of anxiety treatment in 15 primary care practices in New England (Weisberg, Bruce, Machan, et al., 2002). Results from this study revealed that 53% of primary care patients with anxiety disorders were receiving any treatment for psychiatric problems at baseline, 25% were receiving both psychopharmacological treatment and psychotherapy, 21% were receiving medication only, and 7% were receiving psychotherapy only (Weisberg, Dyck, Culpepper, and Keller, 2007). A similar study of primary care patients with anxiety disorders revealed that 13% of patients were receiving both psychopharmacological treatment and psychotherapy, 42% of patients were receiving medication only, 4% were receiving psychotherapy only, and 41% were not receiving any form of treatment (Kroenke, Spitzer, Williams, Monahan, and Lowe, 2007).

Further, *adequate* treatment of anxiety disorders in primary care patients, both pharmacotherapy and psychotherapy, is variable. Cross-sectional data from PCAP revealed that very few primary care patients were receiving adequate doses of psychiatric medication (20%), psychotherapy (14%), or both (5%) (Weisberg, Beard, Moitra, Dyck, and Keller, 2013). However, these rates increased over the course of the 5-year follow-up period, with almost two-thirds of the patients eventually receiving adequate treatment for anxiety. Two other US-based, cross-sectional studies examining the quality of care that primary care patients with anxiety disorders received found similar rates with 31 to 41% of patients receiving appropriate care for anxiety (Stein et al., 2004; Stein et al., 2011).

In summary, there is considerable variability in the extent to which anxiety disorders are effectively recognized and treated in primary care. Failure to screen systematically for anxiety disorders, challenges in differentiating anxiety disorders from somatic symptoms related to physical health problems, and limited outpatient referral options may contribute to the low treatment rates. Despite the fact that efficacious psychological treatments for anxiety disorders exist, a very large proportion of primary care patients with anxiety disorders are not being treated adequately, or at all. In the next section, we describe a screening measure, much like the PHQ-9, that is easy to administer and interpret, and has the potential to improve population-based detection and treatment of anxiety disorders among primary care patients.

AN ANXIETY SCREENING MEASURE IN PRIMARY CARE

The GAD-7 is the most well-known and validated anxiety screening measure in primary care. It was developed by Spitzer, Kroenke, Williams, and Lowe (2006) to identify probable cases of GAD but has since been recognized as a useful screening measure for other anxiety disorders as well. Scores on the GAD-7 range from 0 to 21 with scores of 5, 10, and 15 representing mild, moderate, and severe anxiety symptoms, respectively. The first two items of the GAD-7 assess the two core diagnostic criteria for GAD: (1) nervousness, anxious, or on edge feelings and (2) difficulty controlling worry. In a study of primary care patients, the GAD-7 had high sensitivity and good specificity for detecting GAD, panic disorder, social anxiety disorder, and posttraumatic stress disorder (Kroenke, Spitzer, Williams, Monahan, and Lowe, 2007). Specifically, at a cutpoint of ≥ 10, sensitivity and specificity was greater than .80. The GAD-2 consists of the first two items of the GAD-7 and scores range from 0 to 6. A cutpoint of ≥ 3 denotes clinically significant anxiety and should prompt the completion of the full GAD-7 and/or clinical interview (Kroenke, Spitzer, Williams, Monahan, and Lowe, 2007). The GAD-7 has been found to be associated with degree of disability as measured by the WHO-DAS II (Ruiz et al., 2010), the MOS SF-20 (Spitzer, Kroenke, Williams, and Lowe, 2006; Kroenke, Spitzer, Williams, Monahan, and Lowe, 2007), and the SF-36 (Ramsawh, Stein, Belik, Jacobi, and Sareen, 2009).

While the GAD-7 is a useful screening measure in primary care as it is brief and easy to administer, it is not without limitations. The GAD-7 is a measure of anxiety severity and "anxiety disorder caseness." It should not be used as a diagnostic measure as it does not include items related to fear, avoidance, or panic symptoms, all of which are central constructs in most anxiety disorders. Therefore, additional diagnostic clarification is needed for a diagnosis. However, in terms of population-based screening of anxiety disorders, the GAD-7 is quite useful, as it can alert physicians to patients at risk for having an anxiety disorder. Additionally, the GAD-7 can be used to monitor treatment response when documented along with other health metrics in the medical record.

TREATMENT OF ANXIETY IN PRIMARY CARE

As discussed earlier, the utility of depression screening in primary care has hinged upon practice support, appropriate follow-up, and access to treatment. While the GAD-7 may be a useful method of screening for anxiety disorders across primary care populations, low treatment rates suggest that improvements in access to treatment are also needed. Efforts have been made to investigate the effectiveness of treatments for anxiety disorders with primary care patients. In this section, we provide an overview of these treatment studies and the challenges to implementing these treatments in practice.

Computer-assisted CBT

One method of making evidence-based treatments for anxiety disorders more accessible to primary care patients is through guided computer- or Internet-based CBT. Perhaps the most well-known computer-based CBT program in primary care is the Coordinated Anxiety Learning and Management program (CALM; Sullivan et al., 2007). CALM is a computer-assisted CBT program that contains disorder-specific packages that address panic disorder, generalized anxiety disorder, social anxiety disorder, and posttraumatic stress disorder. There are five generic modules (education, self-monitoring, hierarchy development, breathing training, and relapse prevention) as a well as three disorder-specific modules (cognitive restructuring, exposure to internal and external stimuli). An anxiety clinical specialist (ACS), a role similar to that of a behavioral health consultant, assists patients in navigating the computer program which uses a web-based system to track patient outcomes. CALM was examined in 17 primary care clinics across the country and compared to usual care. In this randomized clinical trial, patients randomized to CALM were offered CBT, pharmacotherapy, or both, in accordance to their preference. If patients met criteria for more than one anxiety disorder, they were asked to choose the most disabling one on which to focus treatment. CALM was acceptable and effective at reducing anxiety disorder symptoms and improving functioning among primary care patients (Roy-Byrne et al., 2010). However, as we will discuss in the next section, the feasibility of implementing treatments like CALM is not without barriers.

Cognitive behavioral therapy (CBT) is an evidence-based treatment approach that targets the relationships between cognitions, emotions, and behaviors that are maintaining psychopathology. A recent review of CBT for depressive and anxiety disorders delivered in primary care revealed that Internet- or computer-based CBT delivered in primary care was more effective for treating mild to moderate depression and anxiety compared to usual care (Høifødt et al., 2011). The same review found that clinician-delivered CBT did not outperform usual care, but noted that variability in CBT training and adherence to treatment may partially account for that finding. Computer-based treatments have an advantage in primary care of reducing the effects of such variability in behavioral health provider knowledge and experience with CBT.

Collaborative Care

Collaborative care (CC) is a team-based model of care delivery that typically involves a care manager, physician, and a mental health provider (often an off-site psychiatrist) working together to help patients manage chronic illnesses. The care manager has the most regular contact with patients and serves to coordinate care between the patient and other providers. The care manager can meet with patients in the clinic, by phone, in the community, and at patients' homes. In many CC models, the care manager offers the patient a combination of (1) self-help resources, (2) psychopharmacological treatment, and/or (3) referral to specialty mental health. The care manager monitors the patient's progress and communicates with the primary care physician via the electronic medical record. A recent Cochrane review of 79 RCTs comparing collaborative care for depression and anxiety to usual care showed significant improvements in anxiety outcomes at 6, 12, and 24 months (Archer et al., 2012). Collaborative care was associated with higher rates of pharmacotherapy for anxiety at 12 months and better mental health-related quality of life at 6, 12, and 24 months compared to usual care.

One example of collaborative care for the treatment of an anxiety disorder is the reengineering systems of primary care treatment of depression and PTSD in the military (RESPECT-Mil; Engel et al., 2008) program. RESPECT-Mil is a collaborative care approach to recognizing and treating depression and PTSD in primary care, modeled from the RESPECT-D collaborative depression care program. It uses the Three Component Model (3CM) of collaborative care, which involves (1) education and screening tools, (2) care management, and (3) support from a psychiatrist who serves as a supervisor to the care managers, a consultant to the primary care physician, and a facilitator of mental health referrals. RESPECT-Mil was initially demonstrated to be feasible and associated with pre–post changes in depression and PTSD symptoms during an open trial conducted with active duty patients at an army troop medical clinic primary care site.

Difficulties with Implementation of Treatment for Anxiety Disorders in Primary Care

While the evidence for the efficacy of computer-based CBT and CC for anxiety disorders among primary care patients is promising, financial and organizational barriers present considerable challenges to implementing these interventions in a way that allows them to be sustainable after the research structure and funding ends. A recent qualitative study by Curran et al. (2012) identified some of the major barriers to implementing CALM in practice. Variable buy-in from key stakeholders (i.e. physicians, nurses) was a significant barrier to implementation. They found that while some physicians referred patients to CALM frequently, others failed to refer at all. High numbers of part-time physicians at the practice sites may have been partly to blame for this, though this is not very uncommon in general practice. Additionally, many nurses reported feeling like they were often kept out of the loop, and as a result, were less enthusiastic about the program. Providers identified that the most significant barrier to sustainability was the inability to pay for the services of the anxiety clinical specialist (ACS) after the study funding was complete. The implementation and sustainability of collaborative care interventions are also affected by inconsistent reimbursement for the services of the care manager (Bachman et al., 2006).

In addition to the financial and organization barriers that hinder implementation efforts, anxiety disorders appear to present some unique implementation challenges.

For example, while RESPECT-Mil was demonstrated to be feasible and showed promise at reducing PTSD symptoms in soldiers during an open trial study, a recent RCT comparing usual care to RESPECT-PTSD (similar to RESPECT-Mil except implemented in Veterans Administration medical centers and focused more specifically on PTSD), found marginal improvements in PTSD symptoms in both groups, with no significant between-group differences in patient outcomes (Schnurr et al., 2013). Limited knowledge about and confidence in treating PTSD among primary care providers was one explanation for the results. The authors also suggested that models that incorporate co-located behavioral health consultants might be required to more adequately manage severe PTSD in primary care.

Finally, none of these treatments directly address the co-morbid health problems that are present in many primary care patients with anxiety disorders. In the CALM study, ACSs noted that the presence of chronic diseases, psychosocial stressors, and low socio-economic status contributed to lower treatment adherence (Curran et al., 2012). Chronic diseases that can contribute to and exacerbate anxiety disorders may be the most significant concern for some primary care patients. Therefore, failing to attend to comorbid chronic diseases when treating anxiety may prevent patient engagement in treatment. One of the benefits of integrating behavioral health services into primary care is that attention to the "whole person" is more feasible, with providers from multiple disciplines working together under one roof. In the next section, we will discuss how anxiety disorders might be treated within a PCBH model.

TREATING ANXIETY DISORDERS WITHIN A PCBH MODEL

Now that we have discussed the challenges in disseminating evidence-based treatments for anxiety disorders in primary care, we would like to offer suggestions for how these challenges might be addressed. As stated earlier, the PCBH model is dramatically different from specialty mental health. Managing health issues at the population level is emphasized in PCBH, whereas providing an in-depth course of treatment that meets the unique needs of each individual client is the focus of specialty mental health. Population-based care involves recording and monitoring health metrics that are relevant to the population often through the use of the electronic medical record (EMR) and proactively intervening with patients at high risk for health problems. One of the goals of population-based care is to provide cost-effective services to the entire patient population rather than intensive services to a select number of patients (Robinson and Reiter, 2007). Patients who require a higher level of care are recommended to be managed by the team of providers and specialists, with the physician and patient serving as the co-leaders of that team.

In order to create a sustainable approach to detecting and treating anxiety disorders within a PCBH model, a population-based approach is essential. This would start with population-based screening for anxiety disorders. As stated earlier in this chapter, acquiring practice support for such an initiative is necessary. Use of the GAD-7 is standard in some practices and is the most likely fit for such an initiative, though other measures may be used instead. Integrating the administration of a universal screener with all primary care patients involves determining (1) who in the practice will administer the measure (e.g., medical assistants, front desk staff, nurses, physicians), (2) how/where the measure will be recorded, (3) who will discuss the results of the measure with the patient, (4) who will follow-up on elevated scores, (5) what types of treatment will be offered, and (6) how progress will be monitored over time. Creating registries of patients in the practice based on important health metrics can help identify high-risk patients. Treatment options can be offered in a stepped-care fashion based on anxiety screener severity scores. Treatments might include psychoeducation, "watchful waiting," psychopharmacology, consultation with a BHC, and referral to outpatient psychotherapy.

With respect to treatment, there remains little research examining the effectiveness of a PCBH model of care for treating anxiety disorders, including meetings with a BHC. Further, though much has been written about the structure of the BHC role, less guidance and research exists on the content of the brief sessions between a BHC and patients. Such research is greatly needed in order to guide the field as staffing and financial decisions are made across practices and in the forming of Accountable Care Organizations.

Case Example

We conclude this chapter with a case example that illustrates a PCBH approach to treatment of anxiety. A primary care physician in one of our practices consulted with us about a 65-year-old male with a history of heart disease, recent heart attack and bypass surgery, and suspected panic disorder. Since his surgery six months prior, the patient had been to the emergency department (ED) five times for chest pain that was determined to be noncardiac. The patient and physician both agreed that his frequent ED visits were problematic and potentially avoidable. Prior to the referral to behavioral health, the physician had introduced brief psychoeducation about panic disorder and prescribed a short course of a benzodiazepine. The referral to behavioral health requested help confirming the diagnosis of panic disorder and treatment for panic disorder in an effort to avoid future unnecessary ED visits.

The initial visit with the BHC focused on assessment of panic symptoms, a discussion about the ways that panic symptoms were interfering with his life, and a brief history of his heart disease. The BHC and the patient agreed that he was likely misinterpreting panic symptoms as signs of a heart attack, which was leading him to seek medical attention in the ED. They discussed how difficult it was for the patient to notice the chest discomfort without assuming that it was another heart attack and how his visits to the ED were preventing him from learning to tolerate the uncertainty associated with chest discomfort. The patient's partner would often encourage the ED visits, as he was also concerned that the patient was having a heart attack. The BHC and patient agreed to meet biweekly for 4-5 sessions and then re-evaluate the need for additional treatment or referral to a specialist. Treatment focused on cognitive behavioral strategies for managing panic attacks with a focus on understanding normal chest discomfort related to his prior surgery. For example, psychoeducation about the nature of anxiety, the fear response, and the roles of avoidance and reassurance seeking in maintaining and exacerbating anxiety was provided. The patient was encouraged to monitor his physical symptoms and the thoughts, feelings, and behaviors that they triggered. Mindful diaphragmatic breathing was introduced and the patient was encouraged to notice and gently challenge worries that he had about his physical symptoms. The BHC consulted with the physician about what to expect after bypass surgery and the warning signs of a heart attack so that she could best advise the patient on how to differentiate these experiences. The physician and the patient agreed that the patient would gradually taper off of the benzodiazepine, as it was serving as a form of avoidance. The BHC and the patient developed a list of strategies for responding to chest pain/discomfort and a plan for what he would do if the pain increased in intensity. They involved the patient's partner in the plan so that he could encourage effective coping and discourage unnecessary ED visits. The BHC and the patient met for eight 20–30 minute visits over the course of 5 months, during which time the patient did not make any trips to the ED. The patient reported improved quality of life and decreases in the number and intensity of panic attacks. The BHC documented the coping strategies that the patient was utilizing in the EMR and encouraged the patient's physician to reinforce the use of these strategies. The BHC and the patient continued to meet monthly for 4 months to ensure that the he maintained his progress.

This case example illustrates a number of key factors about treatment of anxiety in primary care. First, in this instance, the BHC was sought out by recommendation of the primary care provider, not because the patient was seeking psychotherapy. One of the main factors generating this referral was the patient's overutilization of costly emergency department services. Thus, it was a population-based, public health concern guiding the referral request, in addition to concern about individual patient symptoms and functioning. Second, this patient was seen for a total of 12 visits, each 20-30 minutes long, spaced over the course of nine months, thus allowing for the BHC to also serve many other patients during this time frame. Such recurrent visits are feasible within a PCBH model when they are brief and spaced out over time. Third, the BHC sessions flexibly applied evidence-based principles of CBT for anxiety disorders with careful attention to co-morbid physical health problems. Lastly, the treatment plan involved the patient, the BHC, and the physician all working collaboratively. This was crucial, as in this case, as is common, specific medical input about the patient's cardiac health was needed, and the plan called for a change in medication use.

Disclosure Statement: No conflicts to disclose (RW and CF).

ACKNOWLEDGMENT

The authors thank Haran Mennillo for his assistance with the literature review for this chapter.

REFERENCES

Archer, J., Bower, P. Gilbody, S., Lovell, K., Richards, D., Gask, L., Dickens, C., and Coventry, P. (2012). Collaborative care for depression and anxiety problems. *Cochrane Database Systematic Rev*, *10*: CD006525.

Arroll, B., Goodyear-Smith, F., Crengle, S., Gunn, J., Kerse, N., Fishman, T., Falloon, K. and Hatcher, S. (2010). Validation of the PHQ-2 and PHQ-9 to screen for major depression in the primary care population. *Ann Fam Med*, *8*(4), 348–353.

Bachman, J., Pincus, H. A., Houtsinger, J. K., and Unützer J. (2006). Funding mechanisms for depression care management: Opportunities and challenges. *Gen Hosp Psychiatry*, *28*(4), 278–288.

Blount, A. (2003). Integrated primary care: Organizing the evidence. *Families, Systems Health*, *21*, 121–134.

Curran, G. M., Sullivan, G., Mendel, P., Craske, M. G., Sherbourne, C. D., Stein, M. B., McDaniel, A., and Roy-Byrne, P. (2012). Implementation of the CALM intervention for anxiety disorders: A qualitative study. *Implementation Science*, *7*, 1–11.

Demiryoguran, N. S., Karcioglu, O., Topacoglu, H., Kivan, S., Ozbav, D., Onur, E., Korkmaz, T., and Demir, O. F. (2006). Anxiety disorder in patients with non-specific chest pain in the emergency setting. *Emergency Med J*, *23*(2), 99–102.

Engel, C. C., Oxman, T., Yamamoto, C., Gould, D., Barry, S., Steward, P., Kroenke, K., Williams, J. W., and Dietrich, A. J. (2008). RESPECT-Mil: Feasibility of a systems-level collaborative care approach to depression and post-traumatic stress disorder in military primary care. *Military Med*, *173* (10), 935–940.

Gibler, W. B., Runyon, J. P., Levy, R. C., Sayre, M. R., Kacich, R., Hattemer, C. R., Hamilton, C., Gerlach, J. W., and Walsh, R. A. (1995). A rapid diagnostic and treatment center for patients with chest pain in the emergency department. *Ann Emergency Med*, 25, 1–8.

Harman, J. S., Rollman, B. L., Hanusa, B. H., Lenze, E. J., and Shear, M. K. (2002). Physician office visits of adults for anxiety disorders in the United States, 1985–1998. *J G Int Med*, 17 (3), 165–172.

Henke, R. M., Chou, A. F., Chanin, J. C., Zides, A. B., and Hudson Scholle, S. (2008). Physician attitude toward depression care interventions: Implications for implementation of quality improvements. *Implement Sci 3* (40), 1–10.

Høifødt, R. S., Strøm, C., Kolstrup, N., Eisemann, M., and Waterloo, K. (2011). Effectiveness of cognitive behavioural therapy in primary health care: A review. *Fam Pract*, 28 (5), 489–504.

Karlsson, H., Joukamaa, M., and Lehtinen, V. (2000). Differences between patients with identified and not identified psychiatric disorders in primary care. *Acta Psychiatrica Scandinavica*, 102 (5), 354–358.

Kessler, R. C., Berglund, P., Demler, O., Jin, R., Merikangas, K. R., and Walters, E. E. (2005). Lifetime prevalence and age-of-onset distributions of DSM-IV disorders in the National Comorbidity Survey Replication. *Arch Gen Psychiatry*, 62 (6), 593–602.

Kessler, R. C., Petukhova, M., Sampson, N. A., Zaslavsky, A. M., and Wittchen, H. U. (2012). Twelve-month and lifetime prevalence and lifetime morbid risk of anxiety and mood disorders in the United States. *Int J Meth Psychiatric Res*, 21 (3), 169–184.

Kontos, M. C. (2001). Evaluation of the emergency department chest pain patient. *Cardiol Rev*, 9, 266–75.

Kroenke K. and Mangelsdorff A. D. (1989). Common symptoms in ambulatory care: Incidence, evaluation, therapy, and outcome. *Am J Med*, 86, 262–266.

Kroenke, K., Outcalt, S., Krebs, E., Bair, M. J., Wu, J., Chumbler, N., and Yu, Z. (2013). Association between anxiety, health-related quality of life and functional impairment in primary care patients with chronic pain. *Gen Hosp Psychiatry*, 35 (4), 359–365.

Kroenke, K., Spitzer, R. L., and Williams, J. B. (2001). The PHQ-9: validity of a brief depression severity measure. *J Gen Internal Med*, 16 (9), 606–613.

Kroenke, K., Spitzer, R. L., and Williams, J. B. (2003). The Patient Health Questionnaire-2: Validity of a two-item depression screener. *Med Care*, 41 (11), 1284–1292.

Kroenke K., Spitzer R. L., Williams J. B., Monahan P. O., and Löwe B. (2007). Anxiety disorders in primary care: Prevalence, impairment, comorbidity, and detection. *Ann Int Med*, 146 (5), 317–325.

Löwe, B., Kroenke, K., Herzog, W., and Gräfe, K. (2004). Measuring depression outcome with a brief self-report instrument: sensitivity to change of the Patient Health Questionnaire (PHQ-9). *J Affect Disorders*, 81 (1), 61–66.

Löwe, B., Spitzer, R. L., Williams, J. B., Mussell, M., Schellberg, D., and Kroenke, K. (2008). Depression, anxiety and somatization in primary care: Syndrome overlap and functional impairment. *Gen Hosp Psychiatry*, 30 (3), 191–199.

Mojtabai, R. (2011). Does depression screening have an effect on the diagnosis and treatment of mood disorders in general medical settings? An instrumental variable analysis of the national ambulatory medical care survey. *Med Care Res Rev*, 68 (4), 462–489.

Moore, M., Ali, S. Stuart, B., Leydon, G. M., Ovens, J., Goodall, C., and Kendrick, T. (2012). Depression management in primary care: an observational study of management changes related to PHQ-9 score for depression monitoring. *British Journal of General Practice*, 62(599), e451–e457.

Mussell, M., Kroenke, K., Spitzer, R. L., Williams, J. B., Herzog, W., & Löwe B. (2008). Gastrointestinal symptoms in primary care: Prevalence and association with depression and anxiety. *J Psychosomatic Res*, 64 (6), 605–612.

Rawsawh, H. J., Stein, M. B., Belik, S. L., Jacobi, F., and Sareen, J. (2009). Relationship of anxiety disorders, sleep quality, and functional impairment in a community sample. *J Psychiatric Res*, 43 (**10**), 926–933.

Robinson, P. J. and Reiter, J. T. (2007). *Behavioral consultation and primary care: A guide to integrating services.* New York: Springer Science-Media.

Rodriguez, B. F., Weisberg, R. B., Pagano, M. E., Machan, J. T., Culpepper, L., and Keller, M. B. (2004). Frequency and patterns of psychiatric comorbidity in a sample of primary care patients with anxiety disorders. *Comp Psychiatry, 45* (2), 129–137.

Schappert, S. M. and Rechtsteiner, E. A. (2007). Ambulatory medical care utilization estimates for 2007. *Vital Health Stat, 13* (169), 1–38.

Schnurr, P. P., Friedman, M. J., Oxman, T. E., Dietrich, A. J., Smith, M. W., Shiner, B., . . . Thurston, V. (2013). RESPECT-PTSD: Re-engineering systems for the primary care treatment for PTSD, a randomized controlled trial. *J Gen Int Med, 28* (1), 32–40.

Spitzer, R. L., Kroenke, K., Williams, J. B., and Löwe, B. (2006). A brief measure for assessing generalized anxiety disorder: The GAD-7. *Arch Int Med, 166* (10), 1092–1097.

Stein M. B., Roy-Byrne P. P., Craske M. G., Bystritsky, A., Sullivan, G., Pyne, J. M., Katon, W., and Sherbourne, C. D. (2005). Functional impact and health utility of anxiety disorders in primary care outpatients. *Med Care, 43*, 1164–1170.

Stein, M. B., Roy-Byrne, P. P., Craske, M. G., Campbell-Sills, L., Lang, A. J., Golinelli, D., Rose, R. D., Bystritsky, A., Sullivan, G., and Sherbourne, C. D. (2011). Quality of and patient satisfaction with primary health care for anxiety disorders. *Journal of Clinical Psychiatry. 72(7),* 970–976.

Stein, M. B., Sherbourne, C. D., Craske, M. G., Means-Christensen, A., Bystritsky, A., Katon, W., Sullivan, G., and Roy-Byrne, P. P. (2004). Quality of care for primary care patients with anxiety disorders. *Am J Psychiatry, 161*, 2230–2237.

Sullivan, G., Craske, M. G., Sherbourne, C., Edlund, M. J., Rose, R. D., Golinelli, D., . . . Roy-Byrne, P. P. (2007). Design of the coordinated anxiety learning and management (CALM) study: Innovations in collaborative care for anxiety disorders. *Gen Hosp Psychiatry, 29*, 379–387.

Thompson, W. G., Heaton, K. W., Smyth, G. T., and Smyth, C. Irritable bowel syndrome in general practice: Prevalence, characteristics, and referral. *Gut, 46*, 78–82.

Wang, P. S., Demler, O., Olfson, M., Pincus, H. A., Wells, K. B., and Kessler, R. C. (2006). Changing profile of service sectors used for mental health care in the U.S. *Am J Psychiatry, 163* (7), 1187–1198.

Wang, P. S., Lane, M., Olfson, M., Pincus, H. A., Wells, K. B., and Kessler, R. C. (2005). Twelve-month service use of mental health services in the United States. *Arch Gen Psychiatry, 62*, 629–640.

Weisberg, R. B., Beard, C., Moitra, E., Dyck, I., and Keller, M. B. (2014). Adequacy of treatment received by primary care patients with anxiety disorders. *Depress Anxiety, 31* (5), 443–450.

Weisberg, R. B., Bruce, S. E., Machan, J. T., Kessler, R. C., Culpepper. L., and Keller, M. B. (2002). Nonpsychiatric illness among primary care patients with trauma histories and post-traumatic stress disorder. *Psychiatric Serv, 53* (7), 848–854.

Weisberg, R. B., Dyck, I., Culpepper, L., and Keller, M. B. (2007). Psychiatric treatment in primary care patients with anxiety disorders: A comparison of care received from primary care providers and psychiatrists. *Am J Psychiatry, 164* (2), 276–282.

Whooley, M. A., Avins, A. L., Miranda, J., and Browner, W. S. (1997). Case-finding instruments for depression. Two questions are as good as many. *J Gen Int Medi, 12* (7), 439–445.

Wittchen, H. U., Kessler, R. C., Beesdo, K., Krause, P., Höfler, M., and Hoyer, J. (2002). Generalized anxiety and depression in primary care: Prevalence, recognition, and management. *J Clin Psychiatry, 63* (8), 24–34.

/// 18 /// GASTROINTESTINAL DISORDERS, IRRITABLE BOWEL SYNDROME, AND ANXIETY

R. BRUCE LYDIARD

INTRODUCTION

The close association of gastrointestinal (GI) sensations with emotional experience is evidenced by common expressions such as "a lump in my throat', "gut-wrenching experience," "hating his guts," or "butterflies in my stomach" that are used to describe intense emotions. Various emotional states are accompanied by changes in GI blood flow, secretions and motility; more recent research suggests that that gut-to-brain signals can affect our emotions (Mayer, 2013). Using IBS as a model for functional GI disorders, this chapter highlights evidence linking GI distress and anxiety with particular emphasis on panic disorder (PD). In addition, recent emerging information is presented on how the microbial content of the GI system affects brain-gut communication.

IRRITABLE BOWEL SYNDROME

Irritable bowel syndrome (IBS) is a common, potentially disabling functional GI disorder, which affects an estimated 8–17% of the general population (D. A. Drossman et al., 1994). The key features of IBS include continuous or recurrent abdominal pain or discomfort, associated with a change in bowel frequency or consistency with typical relief with defecation. It is classified as a functional disorder because there are no consistent physical or laboratory abnormalities indicative of an organic etiology. Psychosocial factors such as acute and chronic stress, poor coping skills, psychiatric diagnosis, and prior physical or sexual abuse history can play a crucial role in the clinical course of functional gastrointestinal disorders (FGID).

In both clinical and population-based IBS samples, women are twice as frequently affected as men. IBS most often appears during the second or third decades but can occur in earlier or later life. The typical course of IBS is chronic, generally worsening during stressful periods. Symptom severity varies within and between individuals, ranging from mild to incapacitating. Most individuals who seek treatment for their

IBS symptoms exhibit significant emotional distress and functional impairment. IBS has been estimated to rank second only to the common cold as a cause for work absenteeism (Whitehead, Schuster, 1985). The published diagnostic criteria for IBS varied widely until 1994 when a committee of international experts established consensus criteria for the 20 FGIDs, including IBS (D. A. Drossman et al., 1994). IBS frequently co-exists with other FGIDs and 'extra-intestinal' functional conditions (fibromyalgia, chronic fatigue, others) suggesting some shared vulnerability (Goddard, Barth, & Lydiard, 2007).

OVERLAP OF IBS AND PSYCHIATRIC DISORDERS

For many years, it was believed that less than half of individuals with IBS sought treatment for it (D. A. Drossman, Sandler, McKee, & Lovitz, 1982) and that those who did had high levels of neuroticism, more illness behavior, utilized ineffective coping styles, and consumed more health services. Drossman et al. (1990) first reported that women with FGIDs including IBS had an increased likelihood of prior sexual and physical abuse, a finding which has been reported by other groups (Irwin et al., 1996).

Among individuals diagnosed with IBS, a significant percentage have concomitant anxiety and/or mood disorders (Table 18.1) (Blanchard, Scharff, Schwarz, Suls, & Barlow, 1990; Blewett et al., 1996; Irwin et al., 1996; R. B. Lydiard, Fossey, Marsh, & Ballenger, 1993; Walker, Roy-Byrne, & Katon, 1990; Singh et al., 2012). Conversely, individuals with anxiety or mood disorders have unexpectedly high rates of IBS (17%–60%) (R. B. Lydiard, & Falsetti, 1999). A recent meta-analysis (Fond et al., 2014) included 10 recent studies that employed validated diagnostic criteria for IBS and psychometric assessments for anxiety. This study indicated that there were higher levels of symptomatic anxiety in IBS patients ($n = 885$) compared with healthy controls ($n = 1384$).

Community studies (R. B. Lydiard et al., 1994; Walker, Katon, Jemelka, & Roy-Bryne, 1992) suggest that the high rates of anxiety and mood disorders in IBS are not necessarily related to treatment-seeking behavior. One community study

TABLE 18.1 Percentage of Treatment-seeking IBS Patients with Comorbid Psychiatric Disorders*

STUDY DISORDER	MDE	DYSTHYMIA	PANIC DISORDER	GAD	SOCIAL PHOBIA	SOMATOFORM
Blewett et al., 1996 ($n = 63$)	17	5	16	5	n/a	n/a
Irwin et al., 1996 ($n = 50$)*	18	n/a	18	4	10	n/a
Walker et al., 1993 ($n = 71$)	15	39	28	58	n/a	17
Lydiard et al., 1993 ($n = 36$)	23	9	26	26	26	12
Walker et al., 1990 ($n = 19$)	21	n/a	7	11	11	32**
Blanchard et al., 1990 ($n = 44$)	6	4	0	88	7	1
Singh et al., 2013 ($n = 184$)	47	17	44	NA	NA	NA

n/a = not available; GI = gastrointestinal; Sx = symptoms; * = total percentage may exceed 100% since some patients have >1 disorder; ** = Lifetime, not current.

(R. B. Lydiard et al., 1994) found that PD (n = 194) had a significant association with medically unexplained GI symptoms that resemble IBS (unexplained abdominal pain, diarrhea or constipation, bloating). After controlling for gender, age, marital status, race, socioeconomic status, concomitant psychiatric disorder, and survey site, individuals with PD were several times more likely (OR 4.6) to endorse the combination of IBS-like symptoms compared with the combined group of other anxiety disorders, other psychiatric disorders, and no psychiatric disorder. Of note, unexplained nausea without vomiting in the PD group was the symptom with the highest OR (4.7) compared to the other groups combined.

This study also found a significant temporal association between PD/panic attacks and IBS-like GI symptoms. A subsample of 143 respondents who endorsed PD and IBS-like symptoms at the initial interview were subsequently re-interviewed two years later. Those who continued to have PD/panic attacks (n = 88) continued to endorse IBS-like symptoms while those who no longer endorsed PD/panic attacks (n = 58) were significantly less likely to report IBS-like symptoms. These findings suggested that the association between PD and IBS–like symptoms may represent a more fundamental relationship between PD and IBS, and raised the question of shared pathophysiology between them.

PANIC DISORDER: ASSOCIATION WITH OTHER FGIDS

Evolving diagnostic systems for both the psychiatric disorders and for the FGIDs hampered efforts to assess the potential relationship between FGIDs and psychiatric disorders until relatively recently. The development of internationally accepted diagnostic criteria for the FGIDs and corresponding diagnostic interview questions provided the opportunity to estimate the prevalence of all 20 of the FGIDs in both clinical and community samples.

To assess whether PD was associated with FGIDs other than IBS, we surveyed a group of individuals with DSM-IV PD utilizing a validated survey for FGIDs (R. B. Lydiard, 2005). Due to the substantial methodological differences used in obtaining the data

TABLE 18.2 Psychiatric Diagnosis and IBS Treatment-Seeking History (%)

DSM-IV AXIS I DISORDER	IBS SOUGHT TREATMENT (N = 60)	IBS NEVER SOUGHT TREATMENT (N = 27)	CONTROLS (N = 121)	P
Depression—Current	38.3	37.0	8.3*	.0000
Depression—Lifetime	60.0	63.0	21.5*	.0000
Panic Dis.—Current	3.3	0	0*	.08
Panic Dis.—Lifetime	10.0	3.7	1.7*	.03
Panic Attacks Lifetime	33.3	25.9	9.9*	.0004
PTSD—Current	11.7	11.1	.8*	.003
PTSD—Lifetime	20.0	18.5	5.0*	.004
Generalized Social Phobia—Current	18.3	18.5	3.3*	.001

*Significant differences were between the IBS groups and the control groups only

(R. B. Lydiard, 2011).

from our PD sample (direct interview of treatment-seeking PD patients) and those in the U.S. Householder Survey sample (self-report response to mailed questionnaire), only descriptive comparisons are presented (D. A. Drossman et al., 1993). As can be seen in Table 18.2, individuals with PD had higher rates of IBS (about 25%) than did the US Householders survey sample. Both women and men with PD met diagnostic criteria for an average of ~4 FGIDs and nearly equal prevalence (about 25%) of IBS in both genders, in contrast to the usual finding of a preponderance of women as was found in the US Householder survey.

PANIC DISORDER AND IBS: DOES TREATMENT-SEEKING BEHAVIOR MATTER?

Much of the literature prior to the 1990s suggested that IBS sufferers who sought treatment for it reported more psychosocial stress and exhibited more illness behavior than those with IBS that had not sought treatment for it. It was widely believed that the frequently comorbid psychiatric disorders in IBS consulters were the cause for illness behavior and excessive healthcare-seeking. The availability of standardized interviews for both FGIDs (D. A. Drossman et al., 1994) and psychiatric disorders (APA, 1994), made it possible to conduct a US population survey (R. B. Lydiard, 2005) (R. B. Lydiard, 2011). This 1996 US population survey employed a validated random digit-dialing telephone method prior to the widespread use of cell phones. Samples selected included respondents with current IBS who had sought treatment in the past 6 months (IBS consulters), respondents who met criteria for IBS but had never sought treatment for it (IBS nonconsulters), and respondents with no history of IBS or other GI illnesses (healthy controls). Results are shown in Table 18.3.

In this survey psychiatric disorders (PD, generalized social anxiety, PTSD and major depression) and a victimization history were quite prevalent and were similar in frequency in both the IBS consulters and nonconsulter groups while the rates of psychiatric disorder and victimization were approximately at the level of the US population values in the healthy no-IBS group. Psychiatric disorders, physical and sexual abuse, and IBS appeared to be strongly linked with each other in both IBS consulters and nonconsulters but not in healthy controls. Between-groups comparisons may have been affected by the small sample size in the IBS nonconsulters group ($n = 27$).

IBS, STRESS AND ANXIETY

Stress meaningfully contributes to the development and persistence of anxiety and mood disorders (McEwen, 2003). Likewise, it may play a similar role in IBS symptoms (Chang, 2011; D. A. Drossman et al., 1988; Mayer, Craske, and Naliboff, 2001). In vulnerable individuals, sustained stress can alter brain circuitry function in a manner which promotes the development of anxiety, depression and/or additional functional somatic disorders which often coexist with IBS (fibromyalgia, chronic fatigue, and other somatic disorders) (Chang, 2011; Goddard et al., 2007). This pathophysiologic stress model for IBS broadly accounts for the stress reactivity, frequent comorbidity with anxiety and mood disorders, frequently reported history of physical, sexual or emotional abuse, persistent low-level gut inflammation, altered GI motility and disrupted visceral perception in IBS. In particular, early adverse events appear to contribute to persistent dysfunction of the stress system and the development of stress-related conditions (Mayer, 2013; Chang, 2011).

TABLE 18.3 Prevalence of Functional Gastrointestinal Disorders in DSM-IV Panic Disorder and the US Householder Survey

	PANIC DISORDER	USHS
Size (n)	73	5430
Age (SD)	33 (10.3)	49.1 (15.9)
% Women	67.1	51.0
FGID Diagnosis	(%)	(%)
Functional Esophageal		
Globus	33.0	12.5
Rumination	12.3	10.9
Functional Chest Pain	58.9	13.6
Functional Heartburn	58.1	32.6
Functional Dysphagia	14.1	7.5
Functional Gastroduodenal		
Functional Dyspepsia	25.3	2.9
Ulcer-like Dyspepsia	35.6	0.3
Dysmotility-like Dyspepsia	12.3	1.1
Aerophagia	26.3	23.4
Functional Bowel		
Irritable Bowel Syndrome	26.3	11.6
Functional Bloating	12.3	30.7
Functional Constipation	13.7	3.6
Functional Diarrhea	0.0	1.8
Functional Abdominal Pain	0.0	2.2
Functional Biliary Pain		
Sphincter of Oddi Dysfunction	1.3	1.5
Functional Anorectal		
Functional Incontinence	6.9	7.8
Functional Anorectal Pain	10.9	11.6
Proctalgia Fugax	11.0	8.0

THE BRAIN-GUT AXIS: A BIDIRECTIONAL COMMUNICATION SYSTEM

The term "brain-gut axis" is used to identify the pathway by which the brain and gut communicate. An important component is enteric nervous system (ENS), a neuronal network which is diffusely embedded in the gut wall. The ENS contains between 200 and 600 million neurons (approximately the same number as the spinal cord). The ENS is actually a third division of the autonomic nervous system (ANS) in addition to sympathetic and parasympathetic divisions. It has been called 'the 'second brain' (Mayer, 2013) because of its size, complexity, and relative functional autonomy. Most neurotransmitters found in the brain are found in the ENS including serotonin, norepinephrine, acetylcholine, cytokines, peptide neurotransmitters such as CRF and other signaling molecules (O'Malley, Quigley, Dinan, and Cryan, 2011). There are at least 20 hormones secreted by thousands of entero-endocrine cells. The gut-associated immune system contains two-thirds of the immune cells in the body. Sensory information is communicated to the brain via several types of afferent cells (mostly vagal), including primary afferent cells, immune cells and entero-endocrine cells (O'Malley et al., 2011; Mayer, 2013).

The brain-gut axis includes the brain, spinal cord, ANS, the ENS, the neuroendocrine system, and the immune system, which function as one unit under normal circumstances. Brain–to-gut communication occurs via the, ANS (both sympathetic and parasympathetic divisions), the ENS, the hypothalamic–pituitary–adrenal axis (HPA axis), sympatho-adrenal axis (which also modulates the GI immune system), and via descending spinal monoaminergic pathways which modulate spinal reflexes and dorsal horn excitability (Mayer, 2013). This rich and complex brain-gut interface is necessary for maintaining homeostasis. Two critical brain structures generate the outputs from brain to gut: the hypothalamus and the amygdala. These outputs are integrated in the periaquductal grey nucleus (motor), brainstem structures (serotonergic raphe nuclei, the locus coeruleus complex, dorsal vagal complex and motor nucleus of the vagus), all of which are in turn modulated by a variety of hormonal and humoral factors (Mayer, 2013; O'Malley et al., 2011). These same structures are also known to play a crucial role in modulating stress, anxiety and depression (Beurel and Nemeroff, 2014).

Corticotropin-releasing factor (CRF) is a neuropeptide which initiates the stress response in the HPA axis. In conjunction with other stress mediators, CRF elicits autonomic, metabolic and behavioral responses to stress. CRF plays an important role in mediating fear and arousal, anxiety, depression, pain, and other functional disorders which overlap with IBS. Experimental administration of CRF to healthy individuals or to patients with IBS causes aversive GI responses. These include abdominal discomfort and altered motility symptoms which can be prevented by pretreatment with CRF antagonists (Labus et al., 2013; Taché, Kiank, and Stengel, 2009; Beurel and Nemeroff, 2014). The pontine locus ceruleus is a CRF-responsive nucleus containing high concentrations of norepinephrine and is known to mediate symptoms of fear and arousal and also to regulate GI motility in health and under stressful conditions (Taché et al., 2009; Beurel and Nemeroff, 2014). CRF and related peptides also occur within the gastrointestinal system modulating enteric, endocrine, and immune cells and colonic manifestations of IBS, especially during stress (Beurel and Nemeroff, 2014; O'Malley et al., 2011). Type 1 and Type II CRF receptors are present in both in brain and in the GI system and appear to play different, sometimes opposing roles (Taché et al., 2009; Goddard et al., 2007) in the GI response to stress.

Other work implicates shared neurobiology of anxiety and GI function. For example, psychotherapeutic agents effective in anxiety and mood disorders, including tricyclic antidepressants, serotonin selective-reuptake inhibitors and benzodiazepines, also effectively reduce IBS symptoms. Moreover, each drug class noted has been shown to reduce or antagonize CRF function in the brain (Camilleri et al., 2006).

THE BRAIN–GUT–INTESTINAL MICROBIOME AXIS AND IBS

Disrupted bidirectional brain-gut interactions are thought to influence pathophysiology of IBS and other FGIDs (Chang, 2011; Rhee, Pothoulakis, and Mayer, 2009; Mayer, 2013; Dinan and Cryan, 2013; Cryan and Dinan, 2012). Evidence derived from preclinical models and limited human data suggest an important 'bottom-up' influence on CNS function modulated by the large population of microbes in the GI system. The term microbiome refers to the total population of microbes present in the gut (the gastrointestinal microbiome).

A novel concept of a 'microbiome–gut–brain axis' has evolved over the past five years (Rhee et al., 2009). The microbiome interacts with the brain via neural, immune and endocrine pathways (Cryan and Dinan, 2012). In health, the human GI tract is colonized by over 100 trillion bacteria and other microbes (over 10 times the number of human cells in the body and 150 times as many genes as the human genome) (Cryan and Dinan, 2012). There are an estimated 1000 species and 7000 strains of microbes in the gut microbiome, primarily bacteria but also smaller numbers of fungi, protozoa, and other microbes (Mayer, Savidge, and Shulman, 2014). Recent preclinical research suggests that gastrointestinal microbiome plays an important role in postnatal development of CNS programming and signaling, and development of the HPA axis, immune and endocrine systems, (Desbonnet et al., 2010; Borre, Moloney, Clarke, Dinan, and Cryan, 2014).

The 'normal' gut microbiome is required for health homeostasis. It modulates the integrity of the gut mucosal barrier, promotes metabolism and absorption of certain necessary nutrients for the host organism, secretes various neuroactive molecules including norepinephrine, serotonin, dynorphin, cytokines and others (Mayer et al., 2014; Cryan and Dinan, 2012; Dinan and Cryan, 2013; R. D. Moloney, Desbonnet, Clarke, Dinan, and Cryan, 2014; R. D. Moloney, Desbonnet, Dinan, and Cryan, 2015; Montiel-Castro, González-Cervantes, Bravo-Ruiseco, and Pacheco-López, 2013; K. A. Neufeld, N. Kang, J. Bienenstock, and J. A. Foster, 2011).

Alteration of normal gut microbiome function has recently been proposed as a plausible mechanism contributing to the development IBS and other FGIDs as well as anxiety and mood disorders which often co-exist with FGIDs. Stress (either physical or psychological) increases permeability of the gut mucosal membrane, exposing the normally protected ENS to gut contents, activates the gut mucosal immune system, ENS and HPA axis, alters pain perception and gut motility via release of cytokines and other stress mediators (Mayer et al., 2014).

Preclinical research suggests that alteration of the brain-gut- microbiome axis may be implicated in the stress-related disorders such as IBS, anxiety, and depression (K. M. Neufeld, N. Kang, J. Bienenstock, and J. A. Foster, 2011; O'Mahony et al., 2014; Mayer et al., 2014; see Figure 18.1 and Box 18.1). Rodents raised in a germ-free environment were shown as adults to exhibit excessive HPA reactivity and impaired immune system development. These abnormalities were attenuated by transfer of fecal matter from control animals early in development (Cryan and Dinan, 2012; K. A. Neufeld et al., 2011). Other preclinical studies have reported that early stress is associated with abnormal concentrations of neurotransmitters in relevant brain nuclei (serotonin and norepinephrine) in adult rodents raised in germ-free conditions or exposed to early maternal separation (R. D. Moloney et al., 2014; Montiel-Castro et al., 2013; K. A. Neufeld et al., 2011; K. M. Neufeld et al., 2011).

Findings from this exciting new area of investigation raise the possibility that probiotics, antibiotics or other interventions that affect the brain-gut-microbiome axis could eventually play a role in ameliorating human stress reactivity and possibly anxiety and depression via gut-brain signaling (Bravo et al., 2012). There is limited evidence for benefits of probiotics in IBS. In normal human volunteers, probiotics have recently been reported to reduce anxiety symptoms and alter brain activity (Messaoudi et al., 2011; Tillisch et al., 2013). At this time, there is more evidence supporting a brain effect on the gut microbiome via 'top

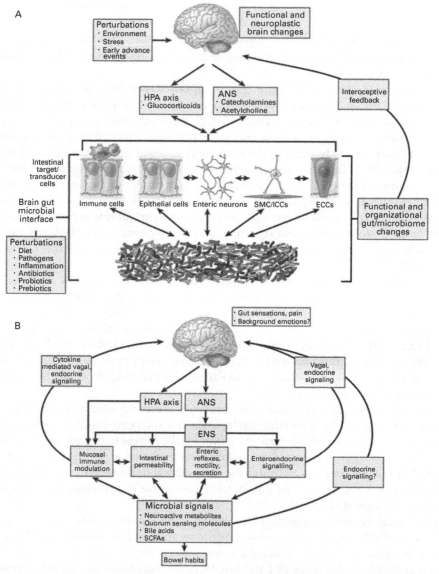

FIGURE 18.1 The brain-gut-microbiome axis.* **A**. Components of the brain-gut-microbiome axis During physical or emotional stress, the brain signals the gut via the ANS, its ENS subdivision, and HPA axis. Specialized cells located in the gut contribute to this bidirectional communication (ECC = enterochromaffin cells; SMC = smooth muscle cells; ICC =interstitial cells) between the brain, gut, and microbiome. In contrast to transient stress, sustained stress may contribute to alterations in the gut microbiome. Persistent perturbations of the gut microbiome may lead to altered gut-brain communication via multiple signaling pathways, potentially changes causing neuroplastic changes in the brain. **B**. Functional and symptom-related consequences of brain gut microbial interactions. IBS symptoms are modulated both by the brain via the ANS/ENS and via signals from the gut microbiome. Molecules released by the microbiome communicate with the brain via activation of vagal and/or spinal afferents via release of cytokines and neurotransmitters from enteric immune or entero-endocrine cells or directly via endocrine-type circulation to the brain. Microbiome-derived molecules (neuroactive metabolites, bile acids), short-chain fatty acids (SCFA) and others may contribute to gut-brain signaling via alteration of abdominal pain perception and enteric reflexes that may contribute to symptoms of IBS. (Modified with permission from Mayer et al., 2014.)

BOX 18.1

REPORTED EFFECTS OF THE GUT MICROBIOME ALTERATIONS ON BRAIN DEVELOPMENT AND BEHAVIOR IN RODENTS*

Altered HPA reactivity
Increased anxiety-like behavior
Altered brain architecture
Altered pain perception
Abnormal emotional behavior
Changes is postnatal brain neurotransmitters concentrations

*Adapted from Mayer et al., 2014.

down' modulation via the ANS and HPA axis (Mayer et al., 2014). As our knowledge base grows, the development of new therapies targeting the gut microbiome may prove useful for the treatment of anxiety, depression, and other stress-related disorders.

CONCLUSIONS

The close association between anxiety disorders and functional gastrointestinal disorders, especially IBS, has been described. Increased rates of anxiety disorders are present in individuals with IBS, and increased rates of functional GI disorders are associated with anxiety disorders—in particular PD. There is evidence for shared neurobiology between IBS, anxiety, depression and other functional disorders which often overlap with them. The most studied is the association between PD and IBS. New evidence for an important role of the intestinal microbiome in the development of the brain, immune, and endocrine systems as well as in health homeostasis. Experimental manipulation of the microbiome resulting in altered anxiety-like behavior suggests an area of potential for future development of novel therapeutic approaches to functional GI disorders, anxiety, depression, and related conditions.

REFERENCES

American Psychiatric Association (APA). (1994). *Diagnostic and Statistical Manual for Mental Disorders* (4th ed.). Washington, D.C.: American Psychiatric Press, Inc.

Beurel, E., and Nemeroff, C. B. (2014). Interaction of Stress, Corticotropin-Releasing Factor, Arginine Vasopressin and Behaviour. *Curr Top Behav Neurosci. 18*, 67–80. doi: 10.1007/7854_2014_306

Blanchard, E. B., Scharff, L., Schwarz, S. P., Suls, J. M., and Barlow, D. H. (1990). The role of anxiety and depression in the irritable bowel syndrome. *Behav Res Ther, 28* (5), 401–405.

Blewett, A., Allison, M., Calcraft, B., Moore, R., Jenkins, P., and Sullivan, G. (1996). Psychiatric disorder and outcome in irritable bowel syndrome. *Psychosomatics, 37*(2), 155–160. doi: 10.1016/S0033-3182(96)71582-7

Borre, Y. E., Moloney, R. D., Clarke, G., Dinan, T. G., and Cryan, J. F. (2014). The impact of microbiota on brain and behavior: mechanisms and therapeutic potential. *Adv Exp Med Biol, 817*, 373–403. doi: 10.1007/978-1-4939-0897-4_17

Bravo, J. A., Julio-Pieper, M., Forsythe, P., Kunze, W., Dinan, T. G., Bienenstock, J., and Cryan, J. F. (2012). Communication between gastrointestinal bacteria and the nervous system. *Curr Opin Pharmacol, 12* (6), 667–672. doi: 10.1016/j.coph.2012.09.010

Camilleri, M., Bueno, L., de Ponti, F., Fioramonti, J., Lydiard, R. B., and Tack, J. (2006). Pharmacological and pharmacokinetic aspects of functional gastrointestinal disorders. *Gastroenterology, 130* (5), 1421–1434.

Chang, L. (2011). The role of stress on physiologic responses and clinical symptoms in irritable bowel syndrome. *Gastroenterology, 140,* 761–763.

Cryan, J. F., and Dinan, T. G. (2012). Mind-altering microorganisms: The impact of the gut microbiota on brain and behaviour. *Nat Rev Neurosci, 13* (10), 701–712. doi: 10.1038/nrn3346

Desbonnet, L., Garrett, L., Clarke, G., Kiely, B., Cryan, J. F., and Dinan, T. G. (2010). Effects of the probiotic Bifidobacterium infantis in the maternal separation model of depression. *Neuroscience, 170* (4), 1179–1188. doi: 10.1016/j.neuroscience.2010.08.005

Dinan, T. G., and Cryan, J. F. (2013). Melancholic microbes: a link between gut microbiota and depression? *Neurogastroenterol Motil, 25* (9), 713–719. doi: 10.1111/nmo.12198

Drossman, D. A., Li, Z., Andruzzi, E., Temple, R. D., Talley, N. J., Thompson, W. G., . . . et al. (1993). U.S. householder survey of functional gastrointestinal disorders. Prevalence, sociodemography, and health impact. *Digest Dis Sci, 38* (9), 1569–1580.

Drossman, D. A., McKee, D. C., Sandler, R. S., Mitchell, C. M., Cramer, E. M., Lowman, B. C., . . . (1988). Psychosocial factors in the irritable bowel syndrome. A multivariate study of patients and nonpatients with irritable bowel syndrome. *Gastroenterology, 95,* 701–708.

Drossman, D. A., Richter, J. E., Talley, N. J., Thompson, W. G., Corazziari, E., and Whitehead, W. E. (1994). *The functional gastrointestinal disorders. diagnosis, pathophysiology and treatment: A multinational consensus.* New York, NY: Little, Brown and Company.

Drossman, D. A., Sandler, R. S., McKee, D. C., and Lovitz, A. J. (1982). Bowel patterns among subjects not seeking health care. Use of a questionnaire to identify a population with bowel dysfunction. *Gastroenterology, 83,* 529–534.

Fond, G., Loundou, A., Hamdani, N., Boukouaci, W., Dargel, A., Oliveira, J., . . . Boyer, L. (2014). Anxiety and depression comorbidities in irritable bowel syndrome (IBS): a systematic review and meta-analysis. *Eur Arch Psychiatry Clin Neurosci.* doi: 10.1007/s00406-014-0502-z

Goddard, E., Barth, K., and Lydiard, R. B. (2007). Disorders which frequently overlap with irritable bowel syndrome: Can shared neurobiology explain their frequent association? *Primary Psychiatry, 14*(4), 69–73.

Irwin, C., Falsetti, S. A., Lydiard, R. B., Ballenger, J. C., Brock, C. D., and Brener, W. (1996). Comorbidity of posttraumatic stress disorder and irritable bowel syndrome. *J Clin Psychiatry, 57*(12), 576–578.

Labus, J. S., Hubbard, C. S., Bueller, J., Ebrat, B., Tillisch, K., Chen, M., . . . Mayer, E. A. (2013). Impaired emotional learning and involvement of the corticotropin-releasing factor signaling system in patients with irritable bowel syndrome. *Gastroenterology, 145* (6), 1253–1261. doi: 10.1053/j.gastro.2013.08.016

Lydiard, R. B. (2005). Increased Prevalence of Functional Gastrointestinal Disorders in Panic Disorder: Clinical and Theoretical Implications. *CNS Spectrums, 10* (11), 899–908.

Lydiard, R. B. (2011). *Pain, PTSD, psychiatric disorders and irritable bowel syndrome.* Paper presented at the Collaborating with CTSAS to Advance Pain Research., National Institutes of Health, Bethesda, MD.

Lydiard, R. B., and Falsetti, S. A. (1999). Experience with anxiety and depression treatment studies: implications for designing irritable bowel syndrome clinical trials. *Am J Med., 107,* 65S–73S.

Lydiard, R. B., Fossey, M. D., Marsh, W., and Ballenger, J. C. (1993). Prevalence of psychiatric disorders in patients with irritable bowel syndrome. *Psychosomatics, 34* (3), 229–234. doi: 10.1016/S0033-3182(93)71884-8

Lydiard, R. B., Greenwald, S., Weissman, M. M., Johnson, J., Drossman, D. A., and Ballenger, J. C. (1994). Panic disorder and gastrointestinal symptoms: findings from the NIMH Epidemiologic catchment area project. *Am J Psychiatry*, *151* (1), 64–70.

Mayer, E. A. (2013). Gut sensations—not so gut specific after all? *Pain*, *154* (5), 627–628. doi: 10.1016/j.pain.2013.02.014

Mayer, E. A., Craske, M., and Naliboff, B. D. (2001). Depression, anxiety, and the gastrointestinal system. *J Clin Psychiatry*, *62 Suppl 8*, 28–36; discussion 37.

Mayer, E. A., Savidge, T., and Shulman, R. J. (2014). Brain-gut microbiome interactions and functional bowel disorders. *Gastroenterology*, *146* (6), 1500–1512. doi: 10.1053/j.gastro.2014.02.037

McEwen, B. S. (2003). Mood disorders and allostatic load. *Biol Psychiatry*, *54* 200–207.

Messaoudi, M., Violle, N., Bisson, J. F., Desor, D., Javelot, H., and Rougeot, C. (2011). Beneficial psychological effects of a probiotic formulation (Lactobacillus helveticus R0052 and Bifidobacterium longum R0175) in healthy human volunteers. *Gut Microbes*, *2* (4), 256–261. doi: 10.4161/gmic.2.4.16108

Moloney, R. D., Desbonnet, L., Clarke, G., Dinan, T. G., and Cryan, J. F. (2014). The microbiome: Stress, health and disease. *Mamm Genome*, *25* (1–2), 49–74. doi: 10.1007/s00335-013-9488-5

Moloney, R. D., Desbonnet, L., Dinan, T. G., and Cryan, C. F. (2015). Serotonin, tryptophan metabolism and the brain-gut-microbiome axis. *Behav Brain Res*, *277C*, 32–48. doi: 10.1016/j.bbr.2014.07.027.

Montiel-Castro, A. J., González-Cervantes, R. M., Bravo-Ruiseco, G., and Pacheco-López, G. (2013). The microbiota–gut–brain axis:neurobehavioral correlates, health and sociality. *Fron Integ Neuroscience*, *7*, 1–15.

Neufeld, K. A., Kang, N., Bienenstock, J., and Foster, J. A. (2011). Effects of intestinal microbiota on anxiety-like behavior. *Commun Integr Biol*, *4* (4), 492–494. doi: 10.4161/cib.4.4.15702

Neufeld, K. M., Kang, N., Bienenstock, J., and Foster, J. A. (2011). Reduced anxiety-like behavior and central neurochemical change in germ-free mice. *Neurogastroenterol Motil*, *23* (3), 255–264, e119. doi: 10.1111/j.1365-2982.2010.01620.x

O'Mahony, S. M., Felice, V. D., Nally, K., Savignac, H. M., Claesson, M. J., Scully, P., . . . Cryan, J. F. (2014). Disturbance of the gut microbiota in early-life selectively affects visceral pain in adulthood without impacting cognitive or anxiety-related behaviors in male rats. *Neuroscience* (Aug 1 Epub ahead of print).

O'Malley, D., Quigley, E. M., Dinan, T. G., and Cryan, J. F. (2011). Do interactions between stress and immune responses lead to symptom exacerbations in irritable bowel syndrome? *Brain Behav Immun*, *25* (7), 1333–1341. doi: 10.1016/j.bbi.2011.04.009

Rhee, S. H., Pothoulakis, C., and Mayer, E. A. (2009). Principles and clinical implications of the brain-gut-enteric microbiota axis. *Nat Rev Gastroenterol Hepatol*, *6* (5), 306–314. doi: 10.1038/nrgastro.2009.35

Singh, P., Agnihotri, A., Pathak, M. K., Shirazi, A., Tiwari, R. P., Sreenivas, V., . . . Makharia, G. K. (2012). Psychiatric, somatic and other functional gastrointestinal disorders in patients with irritable bowel syndrome at a tertiary care center. *J Neurogastroenterol Motil*, *18* (3), 324–331. doi: 10.5056/jnm.2012.18.3.324

Taché, Y., Kiank, C., and Stengel. (2009). A Role for Corticotropin-releasing Factor in Functional Gastrointestinal Disorders. *Current Gastroenterology Reports*, *11*, 270–277.

Tillisch, K., Labus, J., Kilpatrick, L., Jiang, Z., Stains, J., Ebrat, B., . . . Mayer, E. A. (2013). Consumption of fermented milk product with probiotic modulates brain activity. *Gastroenterology*, *144* (7), 1394–1401, 1401 e1391–e1394. doi: 10.1053/j.gastro.2013.02.043

Walker, E. A., Katon, W. J., Jemelka, R. P., and Roy-Byrne, P. P. (1992). Comorbidity of gastrointestinal complaints, depression, and anxiety in the epidemiologic catchment area (ECA) study. *Am J Med*, *92* (1A), 26S–30S.

Walker, E. A., Roy-Byrne, P. P., and Katon, W. J. (1990). Irritable bowel syndrome and psychiatric illness. *Am J Psychiatry*, *147* (5), 565–572.

Walker, E. A., Roy-Byrne, P. P., Katon, W. J., Li, L., Amos, D., and Jiranek, G. (1990). Psychiatric illness and irritable bowel syndrome: A comparison with inflammatory bowel disease. *Am J Psychiatry, 147* (12), 1656–1661.

Whitehead, W. E., Schuster, M. M., (Eds.). (1985). *Gastrointestinal disorders. Behavioral and physiological basis for treatment.* New York, NY: Academic Press.

/// 19 /// ANXIETY DISORDERS AND CARDIOVASCULAR ILLNESS

MICHAEL J. ZVOLENSKY, JAFAR BAKHSHAIE, AND CHARLES BRANDT

INTRODUCTION

Despite the long-standing, colloquial view that anxious states (e.g., worry, fear, panic) derive from the heart (e.g., "My heart aches," "I have an anxious heart"), only in the past 50 years have scientists sought to systemically explore the associations between the heart and mind. This work arguably began with the now classic work of Friedman and Rosenman's on Type A behavior and personality style (Friedman and Rosenman, 1974). Presently, there is a clear recognition, across diverse disciplines, that the heart (cardiovascular system) and mind are closely interconnected. Yet, the bi-directional relations between anxiety and cardiac pathology are only beginning to be understood.

In this chapter, we explore the linkages between anxiety and its disorders with cardiovascular disease, and we orient the discussion on coronary heart disease (CHD). CHD is a leading cause of death and disability in the United States and in other regions of the world, especially among western nations.[1] Indeed, cardiovascular disease has been the leading cause of death in the United States for over a century, and rates proportionately continue to grow (See Figure 19.1). There is now widespread recognition that psychological processes (e.g., stress, anger, depression, isolation), including in more recent years emotional states such as anxiety and fear, can contribute to the presentation and course of CHD and related conditions. For instance, some research suggests that sudden, strong emotional reactions such as panic attacks are one of the most common precipitating events experienced prior to sudden cardiac death (Lampert et al., 2005).

There are a range of definitions that can be used to describe anxiety and its associated sensations. However, in the current chapter, we refer to anxiety in the context of all anxiety disorders as outlined in the DSM-5 (APA, 2013). The DSM-5 categorizes

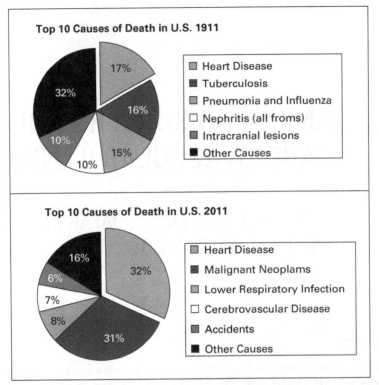

FIGURE 19.1 Top 10 causes of death in the United States by percentage; 1911 and 2011.

individual anxiety disorders (e.g. Specific Phobia, Panic Disorder, and Generalized Anxiety Disorder), while simultaneously recognizing that all anxiety disorders share certain commonalities. Specifically, anxiety disorders share features of excessive fear (the emotional response to real or perceived threat) and anxiety (anticipation of a future threat; APA, 2013). These features often lead to behavioral disturbances, including "life interfering" avoidance of feared stimuli.

There is recent empirical recognition that heart-related sensations contribute to the presentation and course of anxiety states and disorders. For example, at least 3 million patients across the United States who annually visit emergency departments suffer from some forms of chest pain in the presence of angiographically normal coronary arteries and no significant heart disease (Marchand et al., 2012). Although many of these patients are satisfied with negative medical examination results, others will worry about the possibility of suffering from a yet undiagnosed physical disease. These persons are worried about chest pain and/or other heart-related sensations because of their potential negative consequences (e.g., pain, death), and continue to seek help for these symptoms; a phenomenon often referred to as "heart-focused anxiety" (Eifert, Zvolensky, and Lejuez, 2001).

Together, the purpose of the present chapter is to provide an overview of the linkages and interplay between anxiety and its disorders and cardiovascular illness. First, we discuss the clinical significance of chest pain, and we make distinctions between cardiac chest pain and noncardiac chest pain (NCCP) and their relevance to anxiety and its disorders. Second, we briefly present epidemiologic data pertaining to the co-occurrence of anxiety and cardiovascular illness and NCCP. Third, we summarize studies that detail the relations between anxiety and cardiovascular illness. Fourth, we address the role of anxiety and its disorders in the nature of noncardiac chest pain. Fifth, we then provide an overview of some possible biobehavioral processes that may undergird the interplay between anxiety disorders and cardiovascular illnesses. We conclude with a discussion of treatment considerations for these comorbid conditions.

CHEST PAIN AND HEART DISEASE

Chest pain. Persons experiencing chest pain present with a wide variety of cardiorespiratory symptoms including sensations of chest tightening, heart palpitations, pain in limbs/extremities, dyspnea, choking/suffocation sensations, sweating, and numbness. These recurrent symptoms typically occur in an abrupt and intense manner, and frequently in response to stressful life events. Because these physical symptoms mimic cardiac problems, many individuals believe that they are experiencing angina or a heart attack. Physical sensations also may be accompanied by fears and thoughts of dying and/ or other catastrophic thoughts.

The pooled prevalence of chest pain in community samples of healthy persons has been estimated around 13% (Ford, Suares, and Talley, 2011). Additionally, of those individuals who seek help in an emergency room, approximately 7%–10% present with a primary complaint of chest pain. In fact, with a 10% three-year incidence rate, chest pain is the single most common somatic symptom reported for general medical visits, with a physical cause found in only one of every ten patients.

It is perhaps not surprising that many persons who experience chest pain seek immediate medical attention, prompting physicians and other medical specialists to search for "biological causes" of the complaints. This search typically begins with a medical examination and blood tests followed by various types of electrocardiograph tests, and in persistent cases, more costly procedures such as cardiac catheterization. Estimates suggest that these medical evaluations lead to millions of hospitalizations annually; costing more than $8 billion per year (Amsterdam et al., 2010). An important factor contributing to these high costs is that many patients seeking professional consultation for cardiac-related chest pain do so on more than one occasion and for extended periods of time.

As chest pain manifests with symptoms that are associated with both medical and psychological (anxiety) conditions (see Table 19.1), accurate assessment and diagnosis of both types of conditions is a difficult task, particularly in busy medical settings. Several studies have attempted to identify criteria to differentiate cardiac from NCCP. At a descriptive level, it is useful to note that cardiac chest pain typically is described by patients in straightforward terms as a tight, gripping, central chest pain that often occurs during or soon after exercise. It is most often substernal or symmetrical, and is rapidly relieved by rest or nitroglycerine. Patients with NCCP, by contrast, often describe pain in complex metaphorical terms as occurring spontaneously, usually away from the midline of the chest. It is typically felt unilaterally in the vicinity of the cardiac apex, and is associated with local or diffuse tenderness over the anterior chest wall. NCCP can last for several hours, rarely occurs with physical exertion, and is not relieved by rest or nitroglycerine.

Heart disease. Heart disease is a general label for a number of syndromes that are a function of ischemia—an imbalance between supply/demand of the heart for oxygenated blood. Given that most instances of myocardial ischemia are caused by coronary artery obstruction due to arteriosclerosis, myocardial ischemia is frequently referred to as CHD. Depending on the rate and severity at which arterial narrowing occurs, distinct

TABLE 19.1 Common Symptoms of Cardiac Chest Pain and Anxiety

CARDIOVASCULAR SYMPTOMS	ANXIETY SYMPTOMS	SHARED SYMPTOMS
• Pain in extremities	• Fear of death	• Chest tightening
	• Out-of-body experience	• Chest pain
		• Heart palpitations
		• Dyspnea
		• Choking Sensations
		• Sweating
		• Numbness
		• Dizziness

cardiac syndromes may develop (e.g., angina pectoris, chronic coronary artery disease, myocardial infarction, and sudden cardiac death). Even when obstruction of the main coronary arteries can be ruled out as a cause of chest pain, such pain may be accounted for by other cardiac problems (e.g., Prinzmetal's angina and microvascular angina). Although there is a unique type of pathogenesis for each of the aforementioned cardiac conditions, all are characterized, to a greater or lesser extent, by chest pain or discomfort. Here, it should, again, be noted that chest pain can also be caused by noncardiac medical problems, most commonly esophageal reflux.

EPIDEMIOLOGY

When addressing the co-occurrence of anxiety and cardiovascular illness, it is first important to recognize at least two key issues. First, prevalence rates will vary as a function of the referenced population. For example, prevalence rates will differ depending on whether one is examining lifetime prevalence rates of anxiety disorders among individuals with CHD or lifetime prevalence rates of CHD among persons with anxiety disorders. Thus, it is necessary to explicate the target population when discussing prevalence rates for two conditions and understand their rate of co-occurrence within this context. Second, a number of studies have examined anxiety-cardiovascular illness comorbidity, but have focused on anxiety disorders in general rather than specific anxiety disorders. In particular, researchers have often not divided anxiety disorder diagnoses into specific anxiety conditions. Given the marked structural and functional differences in the nature of various anxiety conditions and anxiety-related emotional states, these studies, although useful in providing a general context for understanding anxiety disorder-CHD associations may inflate or deflate base rate estimates for particular conditions.

Anxiety and CHD. There is broad-based evidence that anxiety symptoms and disorders are associated with increased co-occurrence of CHD. For example, estimates across studies suggest that anxiety disorders are associated with a 26% increased risk of CHD and a 48% increased risk of cardiac death (Roest, Martens, de Jonge, and Denollet, 2010). Within the range of anxiety disorders, panic-spectrum problems (panic attacks, panic disorder) appear to show the strongest relationship with CHD. Consistent with this perspective, Katerndahl (2008), in a comprehensive review of individuals visiting emergency wards, found a 1.2 relative risk for CVD patients meeting DSM-IV diagnostic criteria for panic disorder. In one classic study, Fleet and colleagues (1998) investigated the presence of panic disorder in 250 consecutive walk-in patients seeking emergency room care for chest pain. The results of this study indicated that of the 74 (30%) persons who had coronary artery disease, 25 (34%) met criteria for panic disorder, as indexed by a structured clinical interview for anxiety disorders. In a recent study among 763 cases of cerebrovascular disease, after adjusting for conventional risk factors of CVD, 12-month prevalence of panic disorder and phobia (assessed through the Composite International Diagnostic Interview) were associated with increased odds of CVD (Tully, and Baune, 2014). Other studies have produced similar findings and highlight that other anxiety disorders also may be evident among CHD populations. Indeed, generalized anxiety disorder has been reported at an increased rate in CHD patients (Tully, and Cosh, 2013). For example, in a recent review, three studies have reported that generalized anxiety disorder, independent of depression, is associated with poorer prognosis in CHD patients (Tully, Cosh, and Baune, 2013). Notably, cardiac patients with co-occurring anxiety tend to have poorer prognosis and disease progression. For instance, anxiety symptoms, such as panic and worry, are related to poor cardiac functioning, adverse cardiac events, compliance problems with medical treatment, and mortality (Fleet et al., 2005).

Anxiety and NCCP. Notably NCCP, also referred to in the literature as atypical chest pain, nonorganic chest pain, or syndrome X, is defined as chest pain or discomfort in the absence of coronary artery disease or other medical conditions such as esophageal reflux. Research indicates that around 30% of patients presenting to emergency rooms with chest pain are ultimately found to have no detectable cardiac-basis for their cardiac concerns (Tavella, and Eslick, 2013). With recent advances in imaging technology like utilization of CT angiography instead of traditional catheterization methods these rates are even increasing (Cury, Budoff, and Taylor, 2013). In the large majority of NCCP cases, individuals are offered no other treatment beyond feedback that there is "nothing physically wrong with them." Further, even when psychological conditions are present, few of these patients actually receive a psychological diagnosis and referral (White, 2010). As a result, these individuals remain "active" in the health care system for many years. Indeed, NCCP patients demonstrate similar levels of medical utilization, functional (life) impairment, and fear of pain and autonomic sensations as coronary artery disease patients (Eslick, 2008). Yet, the incidence of death as a function of myocardial infarction or another cardiac problem in this population is not significantly higher than in the general population (Eslick and Talley, 2008).

ANXIETY SYMPTOMS AND DISORDERS RELATION TO CARDIOVASCULAR ILLNESS

Despite the close interconnection between the heart and mind, there has historically been less scientific attention focused on anxiety, relative to other negative emotions, in regard to cardiovascular pathology. Notably, the vast majority of research has also employed measurement tactics that tap what is often referred to as "phobic anxiety," which has no clear role in the present diagnostic system. It is likely that phobic anxiety actually reflects numerous anxiety symptoms and conditions.

There have been a variety of relatively recent large-scale community-based prospective studies on anxiety and cardiac pathology among initially healthy samples (i.e., no CHD at baseline). These studies have indicated, across populations, that there is a consistent and clinically significant "signal" between anxiety and subsequent death due to cardiac pathology (Roest et al., 2010). One recent population-based cohort study of 24,128 participants across 7 years indicated that both somatic and psychological symptoms of anxiety were associated with development of acute cardiac events (Nabi et al., 2010). After controlling for sociodemographic characteristics, biobehavioral risk factors, and clinically significant symptoms of depression, these associations were completely attenuated for men but not for women. Other investigations have found similar results among other populations, including health professionals with no history of cardiac problems at baseline (e.g., Kawachi et al., 1994). A study has suggested that anxiety symptoms may be unique explanatory factors, relative to negative emotional distress in general, in regard to the future development of CHD (Kubzansky, Cole, Kawachi, Vokonas, and Sparrow, 2006). Such findings are clinically important, as they suggest that anxiety plays a pivotal, clinically significant role in cardiac disease that is not better accounted for by other negative mood states (e.g., anger, depression).

There have been more recent movements, albeit limited, to index specific anxiety and related disorders rather than "phobic anxiety" in CHD relations. For instance, one study explored the association between posttraumatic stress disorder (PTSD) symptoms and CHD among 1,059 women participating in an Epidemiologic Catchment Area study. Results indicated that women with 5 or more symptoms were at over three times the risk of incident CHD and this effect was evident even after adjusting for depression and trait anxiety (Kubzansky, Koenen, Jones, and Eaton, 2009).

Other prospective studies have sought to probe the role of anxiety among persons with existing histories of CHD. This corpus of work has produced mixed results. Some studies have found significant relationships between anxiety and CHD whereas other have not (see Suls and Bunde, 2005, for a review). It is presently unclear why the discrepancies exist across work, but methodological differences across them are apt to play a role. One recent study has explored over 3522 patients with confirmed CHD. They found that symptoms of persistent anxiety were related to the occurrence of new cardiac events such as recurrent fatal and nonfatal myocardial infarction (Moser, et al., 2011). Moreover, the anxiety effect was not better explained by depression or other cardiac risk factors. Similar results employing different methodologies have been reported (e.g., Grace, Abbey, Irvine, Shnek, and Stewart, 2004). Although these studies exemplify the "positive effect" for anxiety in terms of cardiac pathology, other have reported null results. For example, there was no effect for anxiety among 500 patients following myocardial infarction and arrhythmia in terms of future cardiac events (Mayou et al., 2000). Another study among 470 patients referred for percutaneous coronary interventions found a reduction in both mortality and major adverse cardiovascular events over 7 years in anxious (compared to nonanxious) patients (Meyer, Hussein, Lange, and Herrmann-Linge, 2015). One possible explanation for this discrepancy could be the interactive effect of anxiety and severity of heart problems. In fact, the heart function may moderate—i.e., exacerbate in this case—the prognostic effects of anxiety (Perk et al., 2012).

Overall, extant prospective studies suggest anxiety may play a role among healthy samples in terms of future CHD risk, but evidence among persons with existing cardiac pathology history are less clear. There are many methodological challenges to this body of work as a whole, including lack of comparison groups, poor or limited measurement of anxiety via multidimensional, evidenced-based scales, adjustment for health behavior (e.g., eating, exercise, smoking), and limited scope in terms of sampling approach (e.g., nonrepresentative survey tactics). There also is relative little study of the role of clinical anxiety per se, as indexed by an anxiety disorder diagnosis, in relation to CHD onset/maintenance. Indeed, there is a striking paucity of empirical work that has sought to examine the role of CHD in the onset and maintenance of anxiety and its disorders. Thus, while there is widespread evidence of a "co-occurrence of CHD-anxiety," and some evidence of anxiety contributing to CHD and related cardiac problems, far lesser is known about the specific role of CHD prospectively contributing to anxiety psychopathology. This is an area of work in need of further empirical scrutiny and potential clinical attention.

RELATIONSHIP BETWEEN ANXIETY SYMPTOMS AND DISORDERS TO NONCARDIAC CHEST PAIN

Although linkages between anxiety and cardiovascular illness is clearly important, possibly equally important is the association between anxiety and NCCP. Estimates suggest, for example, that 1.8 billion dollars is spent annually to care for patients who are admitted with suspected ischemic symptoms but who do not sustain acute myocardial infarction (Leise et al., 2010). Individuals with NCCP differ from patients with coronary artery disease and normal controls at the psychological level of analysis, including reporting (1) a greater hypersensitivity to cardiac-related stimuli, disease conviction, and cardioprotective behavior relative to coronary artery disease patients; (2) reporting significantly elevated levels of cardiac-related distress; and (3) NCCP patients report significantly greater levels of catastrophic thinking and emotional distress focused on cardiac cues relative to persons with a cardiac problem as well as nonclinical controls (Zvolensky, Feldner, Eifert, Vujanovic, and Solomon, 2008). Collectively, these findings suggest that NCCP patients may have a history that promotes a "hypervigilance" for cardiac sensations and events. This psychological process often can also be found in anxiety disorders such as panic disorder. Thus, NCCP is apt to involve interplay between physical symptoms (e.g., pain) and psychological vulnerabilities (e.g., heart-focused anxiety). Consistent broadly with this type of perspective, many studies have found that more than 50% of patients with normal or near-normal coronary arteries have predominantly psychiatric rather than cardiac disorders (e.g., Fleet et al., 1996). Yet there is relatively little known about the prospective interplay between anxiety states and disorders and NCCP beyond studies that document their co-occurrence. This is a fecund area for further pursuit.

Together, there is consistent empirical evidence that NCCP co-occurs with anxiety symptoms and disorders, most notably panic-spectrum problems. There also is evidence that NCCP is characterized by psychological vulnerabilities for threat stimuli focused on the cardiac region. However, there has thus far been little study of the relation between anxiety states and disorders and NCCP over time or in controlled settings. Thus, major gaps in knowledge exist in regard to how these problems interplay with one another. This body of work also is limited by a lack of comparison groups, adjustment for health behavior and other physical illnesses, and generalizability to the population as a whole.

POTENTIAL MECHANISMS

There are a variety of biobehavioral processes that might play a mechanistic role in anxiety-CHD as well as NCCP relations. This work is situated in the larger tradition of studying psychological processes as risk processes for physical illness and vice versa. As applied to anxiety and CHD and related cardiac illness, much of this work is in its infancy. Nonetheless, some promising mechanisms are starting to emerge.

Physiology: Adverse cardiac-related physiologic changes and stress responses. Anxiety-CHD relations may be affected by physiologic changes, including physical disease and stress responses. For example, some work has linked atherosclerosis to anxiety-CHD comorbidity (Seldenrijk et al., 2013). Other work has found anxiety is associated with hypertension (Player and Peterson, 2011). Anxiety states also may trigger cardiac changes via hyperreactivity of nervous system response, including altered cardiac autonomic tone. For instance, amplified sympathetic stimulation as well as impaired vagal control are each associated CHD and anxiety psychopathology (Olafiranye, Jean-Louis, Zizi, Nunes, and Vincent, 2011). Although the precise process by which this may unfold is not fully clear, broadly, decreased heart rate variability may be one possible mechanism (Chalmers, Quintana, Maree, Abbott, and Kemp, 2014). Some scholars also have suggested ventricular arrhythmias (i.e., abnormal rhythms of the heart) also may link anxiety and CHD, although extant work has thus far been mixed in support of this matter. Others have theorized that anxiety may contribute to excessive activation of the HPA axis and sympathetic nervous system, producing inflammation, plasma catecholamines that may damage the vascular endothelium, and the release of fatty acids. Anxiety is also hypothesized to increase cardiovascular reactivity to stress leading to greater strain on the heart as a result of increased resting heart rate, baroreflex dysfunction and variability in ventricular repolarization.

Behavior: health behavior. There is recognition that anxiety-CHD as well as NCCP may be interconnected via maladaptive health behavior. These health behaviors can include sleep, diet, exercise, substance use (e.g., tobacco, alcohol), as well as possible medication adherence processes. There are large literatures linking anxiety and CHD, and to a lesser extent NCCP, with unhealthy behavior patterns (Zvolensky and Smits, 2008). For example, smoking (tobacco) is related to the increased risk and onset of anxiety psychopathology, particularly panic attacks as well as CHD. Similar effects are apparent for other health behaviors such as obesity and physical activity. Thus, it is possible such behaviors may serve to regulate, in part, aversive internal experiences such as negative mood states, stress, or physical sensations in the short-term, but such behaviors promote increased risk of anxiety psychopathology and CHD and related cardiac illnesses in the longer-term.

Cognition: threat biases for cardiac events. Specific fears of cardiac-related stimuli may also play a figurative role in anxiety-CHD and NCCP relations. For example, persons who fear the consequences of anxiety-related sensations, including cardiac events and symptoms, are significantly more likely to avoid activities that produce such interoceptive activity (e.g., exercise, caffeine intake). In addition to loss of physical capabilities and vigor, this individual actually increases the chance of experiencing anxiety and chest pain through negative reinforcement. Cardioprotective behavior is apt to result in the temporary, but immediate postponement (i.e., avoidance) or reduction (escape) of pain and distress. Over time, reduced levels of cardiac-related activity, particularly physical exercise, is likely to result in a further loss of physical endurance and strength. As an extension, when heart-focused anxiety contributes to persistent avoidance, an individual may fail to learn that cardiac activity due to physical exertion does not indicate danger, thereby perpetuating what may be a "vicious cycle" of emotional distress and greater long-term risk for CHD and related cardiac problems.

Affective processes: negative affect. As noted in earlier sections of this chapter, acute episodes of negative affect such as fear/panic attacks can trigger cardiac events, including myocardial infarction. These findings are broadly in line with the literature on mental stress and its effect on a wide range of behavior and physical states. For example, among individuals without CHD, severe and sudden emotional distress is related to stress cardiomyopathy (Wittstein et al., 2005). These types of findings suggest that discrete, abrupt fear states such as panic attacks may also trigger cardiac dysfunction. It also is possible that such anxiety states can contribute to more chronic negative affect or greater emotional reactivity to stressors. In one important study in this domain, Fleet and colleagues (2005) found that panic attacks were related to provoked myocardial perfusion defects in CAD patients with panic disorder compared to those without panic disorder. Other work has suggested that psychological stress may be related to hypertension, although direct studies on anxiety states per se have not been conducted.

TREATMENT CONSIDERATIONS

The most popular and wide spread approach to cardiac intervention is cardiac rehabilitation; a multicomponent program often involving health education, exercise, and assistance with cardiac risk factor modification. More recent efforts in cardiac rehabilitation have included psychosocial components to help with adherence, and less commonly, stress management that is focused on cultivating specific skills (e.g., relaxation techniques, problem-solving skills, coping strategies). There is a large literature on cardiac rehabilitation programs. As applied to the present topic of anxiety-CHD, perhaps the most notably finding is that these programs produce small to moderate changes in mood states like anxiety (e.g., Whalley et al., 2011). Yet, these programs often do not reduce relative risk for cardiac problems (Whalley et al., 2011).

Although this corpus of work documents the feasibility of integrating psychosocial or combined (pharmacological and psychosocial) programming for CHD and related problems, it has not included many of the evidenced-based change tactics (e.g., exposure) involved in traditional anxiety disorder treatment. Moreover, the literature as applied to anxiety and its disorders and CHD is highly limited in general. Notably, this work is in line with studies focused on depression management among CHD patients via pharmacological and psychological interventions that have shown some promise (e.g., Swenson et al., 2003). These data may suggest that there is merit to exploring the role of the early recognition and treatment of anxiety in patients with CHD and related problems (e.g., NCCP).

In terms of NCCP (including psychiatric causes of chest pain), besides pharmacotherapy (e.g. anxiolytics), several types of psychological interventions are used (see Table 19.2) including: cognitive behavior therapies, relaxation therapies, hyperventilation control therapies, and hypnotherapies (Kisely, Campbell, Skerritt, and Yelland, 2010). In general, these interventions have been reported to provide modest to moderate reduction in reports of chest pain in the first three months following the intervention and increase in the total number of "chest pain free" days. Interventions using a cognitive-behavioral or hypnotherapy framework and prolonged interventions seem to be more beneficial (Kisely et al., 2010).

In efforts aimed at early detection/intervention, it is likely that a greater level of attention to *heart-focused anxiety* will help raise awareness of this specific and common psychological concern that is apparent across various clinical populations. This is important because research suggests elevated heart-focused anxiety increases the probability that individuals, regardless of their specific condition, will become upset and worried about chest pain and/or other heart-related sensations (e.g., heart palpitations). As a result, individuals tend to anxiously monitor their heart and pulse, avoid activities believed to bring on symptoms, and in an attempt to reduce anxiety, repeatedly seek reassurance from health care professionals. Thus, in persons without physical disease, heart-focused anxiety frequently results in costly cycles of reassurance seeking (unnecessary doctor visits, medical examinations) followed by renewed anxiety and worry. In patients with CHD, heart-focused anxiety can provoke and exacerbate the severity

TABLE 19.2 Behavioral Therapy Modalities for NCCP

TYPE OF THERAPY	THEORIZED MECHANISMS OF CHANGE
Cognitive behavioral therapy (CBT)	Changing of maladaptive negative thoughts, and safe exposure to feared physical sensations
Relaxation therapy	Tightening and relaxation of muscles to reduce long-term tension and reduce physical symptoms of anxiety
Hyperventilation control	Quick breathing to stimulate symptoms of cardiac anxiety in a safe, controlled manner; similar to exposure (CBT)
Hypnotherapy	Eye closure followed by guided progressive muscle relaxation and deep breathing to reduce anxiety
Other behavioral therapies	Psychoeducation; health education; diet and exercise changes

and frequency of angina attacks and increase the probability of cardiovascular death (Walters, Rait, Petersen, Williams, and Nazareth, 2008). It is likely that early recognition could facilitate appropriate referrals and treatment of such patients, regardless of their medical status. For instance, a more accurate and timely diagnosis and treatment of heart-focused anxiety could decrease patients' levels of functional impairment, increase their quality of life, and reduce health care costs. Thus, identifying heart-focused anxiety in patients *with* CHD may help in their rehabilitation and minimize their functional impairment just as it helps heart-anxious persons *without* heart disease to break the cycle of heart-focused anxiety, increased attention and worry, reassurance-seeking, and renewed anxiety.

CONCLUSIONS

Together, there is clear empirical evidence that anxiety and its disorders co-occurs with CHD and related cardiac problems as well as NCCP. This co-occurrence is highly clinically significant due to its impact on the individual and society from economic and personal points of reference. Yet, there is presently little systematic work on anxiety and cardiac pathology that helps us uncover the enigmas of their relations, although some work is suggesting anxiety can impart a negative impact on certain cardiac events. Future theory-driven, translational research is needed to better understand these relations and the mechanisms that underlie them. With such knowledge, tailored therapeutic approaches can likely be developed to address the specific and complex needs of this difficult-to-treat population.

DISCLOSURE STATEMENT

All authors have no conflict of interest to disclose. All authors have contributed to and approved the final manuscript.

NOTE

1. Coronary artery disease (CAD) and CHD are often used synonymously and are used in this manner in the current chapter.

REFERENCES

Amsterdam, E. A., Kirk, J. D., Bluemke, D. A., Diercks, D., Farkouh, M. E., Garvey, J. L., . . . Thompson, P. D. (2010). testing of low-risk patients presenting to the emergency department with chest pain: A scientific statement from the American Heart Association. *Circulation, 122,* 1756–1776. doi: 10.1161/CIR.0b013e3181ec61df.

American Psychiatric Association (APA) (2013). Diagnostic and statistical manual for mental disorders (5th ed.). Washington, D.C.: Author.

Chalmers, J. A., Quintana, D. S., Maree, J., Abbott, A., and Kemp, A. H. (2014). Anxiety disorders are associated with reduced heart rate variability: A meta-analysis. *Front Psychiatry, 5,* 80. doi: 10.3389/fpsyt.2014.00080

Cury, R. C., Budoff, M., and Taylor, A. J. (2013). Coronary CT angiography versus standard of care for assessment of chest pain in the emergency department. *J Cardio Comput Tomogr, 7,* 79–82. doi: 10.1016/j.jcct.2013.01.009

Eifert, G. H., Zvolensky, M. J., and Lejuez, C. W. (2001). Heart-focused anxiety in medical and anxiety-related psychological conditions. In G. J. G. Asmundson, S. Taylor, and B. Cox (Eds.). *Health anxiety: Clincial research perspectives on hypochondriasis and related disorders* (pp. 277–297). New York: Wiley.

Eslick, G. D. (2008). Health care seeking behaviors, psychological factors, and quality of life of noncardiac chest pain. *Disease-a-Month, 13,* 604–612. doi:10.1016/j.disamonth.2008.06.004

Eslick, G. D., and Talley, N. J. (2008). Natural history and predictors of outcome for non-cardiac chest pain: a prospective 4-year cohort study. *Neurogastroenterol Motil, 20,* 989–997. doi: 10.1111/j.1365-2982.2008.01133.x

Fleet, R. P., Dupuis, G., Marchand, A., Burelle, D., Arsenault, A. and Beitman, B. D. (1996). Panic disorder in emergency department chest pain patients: Prevalence, comorbidity, suicidal ideation, and physician recognition. *Am J Med, 101,* 371–380. doi:10.1016/S0002-9343(96)00224-0

Fleet, R. P., Dupuis, G., Marchand, A., Kaczorowski, J., Burelle, D., Arsenault, A., and Beitman, B. D. (1998). Panic disorder in coronary artery disease patients with noncardiac chest pain. *J Psychosom Res, 44* (1), 81–90. PMID: 9483466

Fleet, R. P., Lesperance, F., Arsenault, A., Gregoire, J., Lavoie, K., Laurin, C., . . . Frasure-Smith, N. (2005). Myocardial perfusion study of panic attacks in patients with coronary artery disease. *Am J Cardiol, 96,* 1064–1068. doi: 10.1016/j.amjcard.2005.06.035

Ford, A. C., Suares, N. C., and Talley, N. J. (2011). Meta-analysis: The epidemiology of noncardiac chest pain in the community. *Aliment Pharmacol Therapeut, 34,* 172–180. doi: 10.1111/j.1365-2036.2011.04702.x

Friedman, M., and Rosenman, R. H. (1974).*Type A behavior and your heart.* New York, NY: Knopf.

Grace, S. L., Abbey, S. E., Irvine, J., Shnek, Z. M., and Stewart, D. E. (2004). Prospective examination of anxiety persistence and its relationship to cardiac symptoms and recurrent cardiac events. *Psychother Psychosom, 73,* 344–352. doi:10.1159/000080387

Katerndahl, D. A. (2008). The association between panic disorder and coronary artery disease among primary care patients presenting with chest pain: An updated literature review. *Primary Care Comp J Clin Psychiatry, 10,* 276–285. doi:10.4088/PCC.v10n0402

Kawachi, I., Colditz, G. A., Ascherio, A., Rimm, E. B., Giovannucci, E., Stampfer, M. J., and Willett, W. C. (1994). Prospective study of phobic anxiety and risk of coronary heart disease in men. *Circulation, 89,* 1992–1997.

Kisely, S. R., Campbell, L. A., Skerritt, P., and Yelland, M. J. (2010). Psychological interventions for symptomatic management of non-specific chest pain in patients with normal coronary anatomy. *Cochrane Database System Rev, 20,* CD004101. doi:10.1002/14651858.CD004101.pub3.

Kubzansky, L. D., Cole, S. R., Kawachi, I., Vokonas, P., and Sparrow, D. (2006). Shared and unique contributions of anger, anxiety, and depression to coronary heart disease: A prospective study in the normative aging study. *Ann Behav Med, 31,* 21–29. doi:10.1207/s15324796abm3101_5

Kubzansky, L. D., Koenen, K. C., Jones, C., and Eaton, W. W. (2009). A prospective study of post-traumatic stress disorder symptoms and coronary heart disease in women. *Health Psychology, 28*, 125–130. doi: 10.1037/0278-6133.28.1.125.

Lampert, R., Shusterman, V., Burg, M. M., Lee, F. A., Earley, C., Goldberg, A., . . . Soufer, R. (2005). Effects of psychologic stress on repolarization and relationship to autonomic and hemodynamic factors. *J Cardiovasc Electrophysiol, 16*, 372–377.

Leise, M. D., Locke, G. R., Dierkhising, R. A., Zinsmeister, A. R., Reeder, G. S., and Talley, N. J. (2010). Patients dismissed from the hospital with a diagnosis of noncardiac chest pain: Cardiac outcomes and health care utilization. *Mayo Clinic Proc, 85*, 323–330. doi:10.4065/mcp.2009.0428

Marchand, A., Belleville, G., Fleet, R., Dupuis, G., Bacon, S. L., Poitras, J., . . . and Lavoie, K. L. (2012). Treatment of panic in chest pain patients from emergency departments: Efficacy of different interventions focusing on panic management. *Gen Hosp Psychiatry, 34*, 671–680. doi: 10.1016/j.genhosppsych.2012.06.011.

Mayou, R., Gill, D., Thompson, D., Hicks, N., Volmink, J., and Heil, A. (2000). Depression and anxiety as predictors of outcome after myocardial infarction. *Psychosom Med, 62*, 212–219. doi:10.1097/00006842-200003000-00011

Meyer, T., Hussein, S., Lange, H. W., and Herrmann-Lingen, C. (2015). Anxiety is associated with a reduction in both mortality and major adverse cardiovascular events five years after coronary stenting. *Eur J Prev Cardiol, 22* (1), 75–82. doi:10.1177/2047487313505244

Moser, D. K., McKinley, S., Riegel, B., Doering, L. V., Meischke, H., Pelter, M., . . . Dracup, K. (2011). Relationship of persistent symptoms of anxiety to morbidity and mortality outcomes in patients with coronary heart disease. *Psychosom Med, 73*, 803–809. doi: 10.1097/PSY.0b013e3182364992

Nabi, H., Hall, M., Koskenvuo, M., Singh-Manoux, A., Oksanen, T., Suominen, S., . . . Vahtera, J. (2010). Psychological and somatic symptoms of anxiety and risk of coronary heart disease: The health and social support prospective cohort study. *Biol Psychiatry, 67*, 378–385. doi: 10.1016/j.biopsych.2009.07.040

Olafiranye, O., Jean-Louis, G., Zizi, F., Nunes, J., and Vincent, M. T. (2011). Anxiety and cardiovascular risk: Review of epidemiological and clinical evidence. *Mind and brain: The journal of psychiatry, 2*, 32–37. PMCID: PMC3150179

Perk, J., De Backer, G., Gohlke, H., Graham, I., Reiner, Ž., Verschuren, M., . . . Baigent, C. (2012). European guidelines on cardiovascular disease prevention in clinical practice (version 2012). The Fifth Joint Task Force of the European Society of Cardiology and Other Societies on Cardiovascular Disease Prevention in Clinical Practice (constituted by representatives of nine societies and by invited experts). *Eur Heart J, 33*, 1635–1701. doi: 10.1093/eurheartj/ehs092

Player, M. S., and Peterson, L. E. (2011). Anxiety disorders, hypertension, and cardiovascular risk: A review. *International J Psychiatry Med, 41*, 365–377. doi:10.2190/PM.41.4.f

Roest, A. M., Martens, E. J., de Jonge, P., and Denollet, J. (2010). Anxiety and risk of incident coronary heart disease: A meta-analysis. *J Am Coll Cardiol, 56*, 38–46. doi: 10.1016/j.jacc.2010.03.034

Seldenrijk, A., van Hout, H. P., van Marwijk, H. W., de Groot, E., Gort, J., Rustemeijer, C., . . . Penninx, B. W. (2013). Sensitivity to depression or anxiety and subclinical cardiovascular disease. *J Affect Disord, 146*, 126–131. doi: 10.1016/j.jad.2012.06.026

Suls, J., and Bunde, J. (2005). Anger, anxiety, and depression as risk factors for cardiovascular disease: The problems and implications of overlapping affective dispositions. *Psychol Bull, 131*, 260–300.

Swenson, J. R., O'Connor, C. M., Barton, D., Van Zyl, L. T., Swedberg, K., Forman, L. M., . . . Glassman, A. H. (2003). Influence of depression and effect of treatment with sertraline on quality of life after hospitalization for acute coronary syndrome. Sertraline Antidepressant Heart Attack Randomized Trial (SADHART) Group. *Am J Cardiol, 92*, 1271–1276.

Tavella, R., and Eslick, G. D. (2013). Epidemiology of Cardiac Syndrome X and Microvascular Angina. In J. C. Kaski, G. D. Eslick, and C. N. Bairey Merz (Eds.) *Chest pain with normal coronary arteries* (pp. 37–47). London: Springer.

Tully, P. J., and Baune, B. T. (2014). Comorbid anxiety disorders alter the association between cardiovascular diseases and depression: The German National Health Interview and Examination Survey. *Soc Psychiatry Psychiatric Epidemiol, 49*, 683–691. doi: 10.1007/s00127-013-0784-x

Tully, P. J., and Cosh, S. M. (2013). Generalized anxiety disorder prevalence and comorbidity with depression in coronary heart disease: A meta-analysis. *J Health Psychol, 18*, 1601–1616. doi: 10.1177/1359105312467390

Tully, P. J., Cosh, S. M., and Baune, B. T. (2013). A review of the effects of worry and generalized anxiety disorder upon cardiovascular health and coronary heart disease. *Psychol Health Med, 18*, 627–644. doi: 10.1080/13548506.2012.749355

Walters, K., Rait, G., Petersen, I., Williams, R., and Nazareth, I. (2008). Panic disorder and risk of new onset coronary heart disease, acute myocardial infarction, and cardiac mortality: Cohort study using the general practice research database. *Eur Heart J, 29*, 2981–2988. doi: 10.1093/eurheartj/ehn477

Whalley, B., Rees, K., Davies, P., Bennett, P., Ebrahim, S., Liu, Z., . . . Taylor, R. S. (2011). Psychological interventions for coronary heart disease. *Cochrane Database Syst Rev, 10*, CD002902. doi: 10.1002/14651858.CD002902.pub3.

White, K. S. (2010). Assessment and treatment of psychological causes of chest pain. *Med Clin N Am, 94*, 291–318. doi: 10.1016/j.mcna.2010.01.005

Wittstein, I. S., Thiemann, D. R., Lima, J. A., Baughman, K. L., Schulman, S. P., Gerstenblith, G., . . . Champion, H. C. (2005). Neurohumoral features of myocardial stunning due to sudden emotional stress. *N Engl J Med, 352*, 539–548.

Zvolensky, M. J., Feldner, M. T., Eifert, G. H., Vujanovic, A. A., and Solomon, S. E. (2008). Cardiophobia: A critical analysis. *Transcult Psychiatry, 45*, 230–252. doi: 10.1177/1363461508089766

Zvolensky, M. J., and Smits, J. A. (Eds.) (2008). *Anxiety in health behaviors and physical illness: Contemporary theory and research.* New York, NY: Springer.

INTERSECTION OF ANXIETY WITH MOOD AND SUBSTANCE DISORDERS

SUBSTANCE ABUSE AND COMORBIDITY WITH ANXIETY

JENNA L. MCCAULEY, SUDIE E. BACK, AND KATHLEEN T. BRADY

INTRODUCTION

Prevalence of Comorbidity

As highlighted in previous chapters, anxiety disorders (AD) are the most prevalent class of mental health disorders in the United States. Substance use disorder (SUD) diagnoses in DSM-5 combine the previous DSM-IV categories of substance abuse and substance dependence into a single disorder assessed on a severity continuum from mild (2–3 symptoms in a year) to severe (6 or more symptoms in a year). Diagnostic criteria include: (1) use resulting in failure to fulfill major role obligations; (2) use in situations that are physically hazardous; (3) continued use despite recurrent social or interpersonal problems; (4) tolerance; (5) withdrawal; (6) use of larger amounts or over longer periods than intended; (7) persistent desire or repeated efforts to cut down on use; (8) great deal of time dedicated to use or recovery from use; (9) reduction of functional activities due to use; (10) use despite knowledge of physical and psychological problems caused or exacerbated by substances; and (11) craving to use the substance.

The National Comorbidity Survey Replication (NCS-R; Kessler et al., 2005) estimated 14.6% lifetime prevalence for any SUD, with the prevalence for specific DSM-IV diagnoses ranging from 13.2% (alcohol abuse) to 3.0% (drug dependence). Comorbidity estimates from the National Epidemiological Survey on Alcohol and Related Conditions (NESARC; Hasin, Stinson, Ogburn, and Grant, 2007) indicated that among individuals with SUD, 17.7% met criteria for an AD. Conversely, among individuals with an AD, 15% reported past year SUD. AD diagnosis conferred significant risk for past year alcohol use disorder (Odds Ratio [OR] = 1.7) and past year drug use disorder (OR = 2.8). Overall, patterns of comorbidity tend to be similar for men and women, but the magnitude (OR) of associations between AD and SUD tended to be greater among women.

Etiology

Three major theories exist to explain the etiology of AD/SUD comorbidity (see Table 20.1). The *common factors theory* posits that shared mechanisms underpin the AD/SUD association. Mechanisms receiving empirical attention have included personality (e.g., anxiety sensitivity), neurobiological mechanisms (e.g., corticotrophin releasing factor, endogenous opioids, noradrenergic), and genetic factors (Stewart and Conrod, 2008). The *substance-induced anxiety* model posits that the biopsychosocial impact of chronic substance use initiates or exacerbates anxiety symptoms (for review see, Smith and Randall, 2012). Finally, the predominant etiologic model is the *self-medication hypothesis,* which posits that the SUD develops as result of attempts to dampen symptoms of a pre-existing AD; due to the temporary alleviation of anxiety, substance use is negatively reinforced and, over time, develops into disordered use (Robinson, Sareen, Cox, and Bolton, 2009). Empirical support exists for each of these models, highlighting the importance of assessing the specific association and order of onset between AD and SUD for each presenting patient. Once developed, evidence suggests that symptoms of AD and SUD sustain one another, forming a positive feedback loop (Stewart and Conrod, 2008). As reviewed in detail by Smith and Randall (2012), this mutual maintenance model underpins findings that ADs can heighten the severity, duration, and worsen the treatment response of comorbid SUD. Conversely, SUD can enhance the severity, duration and worsen the treatment response of comorbid ADs.

General Diagnostic Considerations

Differential diagnosis of AD/SUD can be challenging. The main diagnostic difficulty is differentiating between independent versus substance-induced anxiety symptoms. Anxiety symptoms are common during both acute intoxication and withdrawal from most substances of abuse. For this reason, observation and assessment of AD symptoms should ideally take place during a period of prolonged abstinence. The specific duration of abstinence required varies dependent on the specific AD in question and the half-life of the substance of abuse. If assessment of symptoms during prolonged abstinence is not possible, documented onset of AD prior to initiation of substance use, family history of AD, or collateral reports of sustained anxiety during previous periods of prolonged abstinence are often indicative of an independent AD, as opposed to a substance-induced AD.

TABLE 20.1 Empirically Supported Etiologic Models for Comorbid Anxiety and Substance Use Disorders

ETIOLOGIC MODEL	DESCRIPTION
Common factors theory	Shared mechanisms (e.g., genetic, environment, anxiety sensitivity) contribute to the development of both the anxiety disorder and the substance use disorder.
Substance-induced anxiety model	The biopsychosocial impact of chronic substance use results in the initiation or exacerbation of anxiety symptoms and disorders.
Self-medication hypothesis	Substances are used to try and mitigate symptoms of anxiety. The substance use may provide short-term relief from anxiety symptoms and is, therefore, negatively reinforcing.

Early diagnosis and treatment for AD/SUD has been associated with improved clinical outcomes. For this reason, screening for comorbidities should ideally take place at the outset of treatment in both mental health and substance abuse treatment facilities, as well as in primary health care settings. Of note, few diagnostic tools have been updated to reflect fully the recent DSM-5 criteria; however, the National Institutes of Health have promoted the use of the NIDA ASSIST (National Institute on Drug Abuse, 2012) for SUD assessment across a range of health care settings. In addition to assessing for abuse of alcohol and illicit substances, it is important to assess for use of certain over-the-counter agents (e.g., pseudoephedrine, diet pills) and caffeine, which can also elicit or increase symptoms of anxiety. Reducing the use of these agents can often help reduce overall anxiety.

General Treatment Considerations

The presentation of comorbid AD/SUD brings with it an array of treatment considerations beyond those for treatment of either disorder in isolation. Comorbid presentation is associated with worse overall treatment prognosis and therefore requires attention throughout the treatment process. Individuals with AD/SUD may be more likely than their singly diagnosed counterparts to have unmet treatment needs. For those SUD patients who do receive treatment, the presence of an AD is likely associated with increased ambivalence toward participation in SUD treatment. Conversely, presence of an SUD may introduce additional issues with respect to compliance and effectiveness of anxiety treatment. Whereas specific considerations for unique permutations of AD/SUD will be discussed in detail throughout the remainder of this chapter, several concepts and principles apply broadly to the treatment of comorbid AD/SUD.

Currently, three main models for treatment of comorbid AD/SUD exist—sequential, parallel, and integrated approaches (see Table 20.2). In the *sequential approach,* one disorder (usually the SUD) is treated prior to initiation of treatment for the comorbid disorder. The sequential model may be appropriate in cases where patient motivation is only present for treatment of one disorder at the outset. However, careful attention should be given during this initial phase of treatment to highlight connections between SUD and anxiety symptoms, as well as educate the patient regarding the benefits of addressing both disorders to prevent relapse of symptoms. The *parallel model* consists of the patient receiving treatment for the SUD and the AD during the same timeframe, but provided in disparate settings by different treatment providers. This parallel approach is theoretically preferred to the sequential approach as it addresses both disorders; however, coordination between treatment providers and patient time and resources often become challenges to successful implementation of this approach. Finally, with the *integrated approach* a patient receives treatment from a single provider that addresses the SUD and the AD simultaneously. Integrated approaches highlight connections between symptoms and promote discussion of the mechanisms through which the mutual maintenance model may sustain active symptom presentation and promote relapse. To date, the majority of research regarding psychotherapeutic and pharmacologic treatments address SUD and anxiety in sequential or parallel fashion. In fact, most randomized clinical trials exclude participants with comorbidity and thereby limit the extant information regarding the comparative effectiveness of treatment combinations. However, recent empirical attention and growing support has been given to integrated treatment approaches. Integrated treatments are discussed in more detail in the section on *Posttraumatic Stress Disorder.*

TABLE 20.2 Common Approaches to the Treatment of Comorbid Anxiety and Substance Use Disorders

APPROACH	DESCRIPTION	ADVANTAGES	DISADVANTAGES
Sequential treatment	The substance use disorder is generally treated first. Treatment of the anxiety disorder is delayed until the substance use disorder has been resolved.	• Consistent with structure of majority of treatment facilities • Majority of evidence-based treatments target diagnoses in isolation • Consistent with predominant disorder-specific training models for treatment providers	• Costly for patients (time and money) • Patient attrition • Untreated symptoms of anxiety often promote relapse to substances of abuse
Parallel treatment	The substance use disorder and the anxiety disorder are treated simultaneously, by different health care providers.	• Addresses both disorders at the same time • May enhance treatment outcomes and reduce risk of relapse promoted by anxiety disorder symptoms • Treating one disorder is consistent with structure of majority of treatment facilities • Majority of evidence-based treatments target diagnoses in isolation • Consistent with predominant disorder-specific training models for treatment providers	• Costly for patients (time and money) • Need for coordination efforts between treatment care providers • May not adequately promote patient understanding of connections between comorbid anxiety and substance use disorder symptoms
Integrated treatment	The anxiety disorder and the substance use disorder are treated simultaneously, by a single health care provider.	• Addresses both disorders at the same time • Increasing array of evidence-based integrated treatment options available • Reduces cost to patients (time and money) • Promotes patient understanding of connections between comorbid symptoms • Reduces burden of provider coordination (compared to parallel approach)	• Fewer evidence-based treatment approaches available • Fewer providers trained in delivery of integrated treatments

Psychotherapeutic Treatments

Maximizing non-pharmacologic methods of symptom management (e.g., self-regulation, alternative coping strategies) is an important goal of psychotherapy, whether it is used as an adjunct to medication or in isolation. Cognitive-behavioral therapy (CBT) approaches have garnered the most empirical support for the treatment of both AD and SUD (Hofmann and Smits, 2008). Evidence-based strategies often found in AD treatment packages include exposure and response prevention, cognitive restructuring, and anxiety self-management skills (e.g., relaxation, coping strategies). With respect to treatment of SUD, abstinence-oriented treatments (e.g., 12-Step, Alcoholics/Narcotics Anonymous), motivational interviewing, harm reduction approaches, relapse prevention, and community reinforcement approaches each have empirical support (Smith and Randall, 2012).

Although integrated treatments are gaining traction, particularly in the arena of SUD/PTSD comorbidity, clinicians wishing to integrate treatment for comorbid patients are often left to do so guided by their conceptualization of the patient's presenting symptoms and ongoing assessment of changes elicited over the course of treatment. Two specific considerations are warranted when integrating CBT approaches for AD/SUD patients. First, exposure-based protocols may include temporary escalation of anxious arousal. Equipping patients with SUD relapse prevention skills and opting for exposure methods that allow for greater control of the dosing effect (e.g., imaginal or graded exposure) is advised. Second, CBT for SUD promotes the avoidance of people, places, and situations that are "triggers" and place the individual at high-risk for relapse to substances (e.g., bars, former using friends). It is important, therefore to address the distinction between avoiding high-risk "triggers" for SUD and not avoiding safe but anxiogenic situations (see, Smith and Randall, 2012).

Pharmacological Treatments

Use of pharmacotherapy for AD symptoms is often discouraged among SUD populations. However, in scenarios where benefits outweigh the risks, pharmacotherapy can be effective, particularly among individuals who may not have the time or financial resources to invest in weekly psychotherapy. As discussed in other chapters, selective serotonin reuptake inhibitors (SSRI), serotonin-norepinephrine reuptake inhibitors (SNRI), tricyclic antidepressants (TCA), and monoamine oxidase inhibitors (MAO-I) have empirical support for their effectiveness in treating AD. Due to potential interactions with some substances of abuse (e.g., alcohol), TCAs and MAO-Is should generally be avoided in comorbid populations. SSRIs and SNRIs present safer and equally effective options for management of anxiety symptoms among AD/SUD patients. Whereas benzodiazepines are regularly considered as adjunctive medication during the early treatment phase when activation or latency of onset of the therapeutic effect of antidepressants is an issue, a special caution is warranted with regard to their use among SUD populations (Smith and Randall, 2012). If benzodiazepines are prescribed to patients in SUD remission, close monitoring and limiting prescribed doses is recommended. A helpful guide to treatment decisions relevant to use of benzodiazepines with comorbid patients is provided by Sattar and Bathia (2003). In general, use of benzodiazepines should be avoided in patients with a current SUD, approached with caution among patients with a history of SUD, and a last resort option for management of chronic anxiety symptoms.

Fewer effective pharmacological options exist for the treatment of SUD. Disulfiram for alcohol use disorders works by interfering with the metabolism of ethanol and induces an aversive reaction to alcohol consumption. For this reason, disulfiram is most useful when a patient's goal is abstinence; however, problems with medication compliance are common with disulfiram. Acamprosate works by counteracting the effects of alcohol on GABA and has evidence suggesting that compliant use promotes abstinence. Naltrexone has shown promise in reducing use of both alcohol and opioids; however, use of naltrexone requires monitoring of liver functioning and may be less effective than alternatives for individuals with opioid use disorders. Medical treatment for opioid use disorders has received increased attention due to the epic rise in abuse of prescription opioids. Although methadone is a well-established, effective pharmacological treatment for opioid use disorders, buprenorphine offers the advantages of being available in medical office-based settings (for approved providers), as well as a lower abuse liability.

Overall, a handful of treatment options exist for patients with comorbid AD/SUD. Limited empirical work has been conducted to examine the differential effects of combined pharmacotherapy/psychotherapy treatment versus monotherapy, and some evidence suggests that adding CBT to SSRI/SNRI may promote better long-term outcomes and prevent relapse (Fatseas et al., 2010). Whether used alone or as part of a combined approach, any patient concerns regarding the use of pharmacotherapy (e.g., thoughts of being defective, failure, etc.) should be addressed with patients at the outset of treatment and as needed throughout treatment. Special attention should be given to address and monitor potential interactions between prescribed medications, illicit drugs of abuse, or alcohol. Options with the lowest abuse potential should be used whenever possible with SUD populations.

ADVANCES AND CONSIDERATIONS BY ANXIETY DISORDER

The subsequent sections discuss advances in epidemiology, etiology, diagnostic, and treatment considerations specific to each AD diagnosis. For most AD diagnoses, the preponderance of literature focuses on comorbid alcohol use disorders. However, literature specific to other substances of abuse will be highlighted when available.

Posttraumatic Stress Disorder (PTSD)

PTSD is one of the most frequently co-occurring stressor-related disorders among individuals in with SUD. Data from the 2010 National Epidemiologic Survey on Alcohol and Related Conditions (NESARC; N = 34,653) reported that among individuals with lifetime PTSD, nearly half (46.4%) met criteria for an SUD (Pietrzak et al., 2011). Rates of SUD treatment-seeking individuals as well as Veteran populations evidence particularly high rates of PTSD and trauma.

Treatment

Over the past decade, several integrated treatments for comorbid PTSD/SUD have been developed and tested. These studies show promise and, contrary to early concerns that trauma work would worsen SUD symptoms, demonstrate that the inclusion of trauma work among PTSD/SUD patients results in significant decreases in both PTSD and SUD (Torchalla et al., 2012; van Dam et al., 2012).

The most studied integrated treatment to date is Seeking Safety (SS), a present-focused, 24-session manualized CBT emphasizing coping skills and psychoeducation (Najavits, 2002). In a study of SS compared to relapse prevention among women, Hien and colleagues (2004) found that both treatments resulted in improved substance use and PTSD, however no significant between group differences in PTSD or SUD symptoms were observed. In a larger national multisite community study, SS was compared to a women's health education (WHE) group (Hien et al., 2009). Both SS and WHE resulted in significantly improved PTSD symptoms, however neither group resulted in a significant reduction in abstinence rates over time. Najavits and colleagues recently developed a 17-session treatment called Creating Change (CC). A pilot study of 7 individuals treated individually with CC found reductions in PTSD and SUD symptoms over time (Najavits and Johnson, 2014). Although CC allows for discussion of the past and emotions related to the trauma, it does not include exposure-based components. Further controlled trials are warranted.

Another integrated treatment for PTSD/SUD is called COPE (Concurrent Treatment of PTSD and Substance Use Disorders using Prolonged Exposure; Back et al., 2014). COPE is a 12-session exposure-based, manualized CBT treatment that integrates relapse prevention for SUD with Prolonged Exposure (PE) for PTSD. COPE is the only integrated treatment developed to date that includes both in vivo and imaginal exposure techniques. COPE was initially tested as a 16-session intervention in an uncontrolled study among patients with comorbid PTSD and cocaine dependence (Brady et al., 2001). In this study, no signs of increased substance use were observed with the inclusion of PE. Treatment resulted in significant improvements in PTSD symptoms and cocaine use that were maintained at 6-month follow-up. Mills and colleagues (2012) completed a randomized control trial of COPE plus treatment as usual (TAU) vs. TAU alone among 103 participants. From baseline to 9-month follow-up, significant reductions in PTSD symptoms were found for both groups; however, the COPE group demonstrated a significantly greater reduction in PTSD symptom severity. No significant between-group differences in rates of abstinence, number of SUD dependence criteria met or retention were found. The findings from these studies indicate that integrated PTSD/SUD treatments employing PE techniques can be used safely and lead to sustained improvements. COPE has been modified to a 12-session treatment and several ongoing randomized controlled trials among civilians and veterans are underway and show promise (Back et al., 2012). In addition, several other studies have explored the use of integrated psychosocial treatments in preliminary or uncontrolled studies with generally positive results (see Torchalla et al., 2012 and van Dam et al., 2012 for comprehensive reviews).

There has been little investigation of the pharmacologic treatment of co-occurring PTSD/SUD and the few studies that have been conducted suggest only a modest response (Batki et al., 2014; Brady et al., 2005; Foa et al., 2013; Petrakis et al., 2012; Sofuoglu et al., 2014). In a double-blind, placebo-controlled, 12-week trial, Brady and colleagues (2005) investigated the use of sertraline in individuals with PTSD and alcohol dependence. Cluster analysis revealed that patients with early onset PTSD and less severe SUD (i.e., primary PTSD) demonstrated improvement in alcohol use severity with sertraline treatment ($p < .001$), while patients with secondary PTSD evidenced more favorable alcohol use outcomes when treated with placebo. Secondary analysis of the temporal course of improvement revealed that improvements in PTSD symptoms had a much greater impact on improvement in SUD symptoms than the reciprocal relationship (Back et al., 2006), highlighting the importance of assessing and treating the comorbid anxiety disorder in SUD patients with PTSD.

Among 254 outpatients with alcohol dependence and comorbid psychiatric disorders (42.9% met DSM-IV criteria for comorbid PTSD), Petrakis and colleagues (2005) investigated the benefits of disulfiram alone, naltrexone alone, or their combination in a 12-week randomized trial. Treatment with naltrexone or disulfiram, as compared to placebo, resulted in more consecutive weeks of abstinence and fewer drinking days per week. Disulfiram-treated participants reported less craving from pre- to posttreatment than naltrexone-treated participants. While specific comorbid psychiatric disorders were not investigated, participants treated with active medication evidenced greater overall symptom improvement (e.g., less anxiety). No clear advantage of combining disulfiram and naltrexone was observed.

Foa and colleagues (2013) compared (1) PE plus naltrexone, (2) PE plus placebo, (3) supportive counseling plus naltrexone, and (4) supportive counseling plus placebo in individuals with PTSD and comorbid alcohol use disorders. All four groups evidenced significant reductions in PTSD severity and frequency of drinking, with the naltrexone-treated groups showing the greatest reductions in alcohol use frequency. At 6-month follow-up, a higher percentage of participants in the PE plus naltrexone group had low levels of PTSD (i.e., $a \geq 10$ point reduction on the Posttraumatic Symptom Severity Interview scale) compared to the other groups ($p \leq .02$). More recently, Batki and colleagues (2014) conducted a 12-week, double-blind study to examine the preliminary efficacy and safety of topiramate among 30 veterans with PTSD and alcohol dependence. Preliminary results were promising and indicate that topiramate resulted in significant reductions in frequency and amount of alcohol use, craving, as well as PTSD symptoms. Further testing in larger studies is warranted.

Social Anxiety Disorder

High rates of comorbid SUD and social anxiety disorder (SAD) have been documented in the general population as well as treatment-seeking samples. SAD increases the risk of illicit drug use, with odds ratios from community samples ranging from 1.6 to 2.3 (Sareen, Chartier, Paulus, and Stein, 2006). Consistent with the self-medication model, the onset of SAD generally precedes the development of SUD (Sareen, Chartier, Kjernisted, and Stein, 2001). Individuals with SAD frequently endorse consuming substances to help reduce fear of criticism or embarrassment, cope with negative emotions, or conform to social situations (Bolton, Cox, Clara, and Sareen, 2006; Carrigan and Randall, 2003).

Diagnostic Considerations
Because the average onset of SAD is before adolescence, symptoms of SAD are often present before the initiation of alcohol or drug use (Sareen et al., 2001). Also, the cardinal symptom of SAD, fear of public scrutiny, is fairly specific to the anxiety disorder and not mimicked by substance use, intoxication or withdrawal. SAD symptoms that arise only in the context of acute intoxication or withdrawal are insufficient to meet criteria for a diagnosis of SAD.

Treatment
Using data from the NESARC, Iza and colleagues (2014) showed that only half of individuals with SAD ever seek treatment, and among those who do the median time from onset of symptoms to first treatment contact is16 years. There have been several studies examining psychosocial and pharmacologic treatment for co-occurring SAD/SUD and the findings are mixed. Randall and colleagues (2001a) compared a 12-week, manual-based

CBT for alcohol dependence to an integrated CBT for SAD/SUD. Contrary to hypothesis, patients who received the SUD treatment evidenced better outcomes than patients who received the integrated intervention. Schade and colleagues (2004) randomly assigned individuals with alcohol dependence and comorbid SAD and/or agoraphobia to receive relapse prevention (RP), or integrated RP plus CBT for SAD. The majority (93%) of the sample was diagnosed with SAD. Both groups were offered concomitant SSRI pharmacotherapy (fluvoxamine), but 53% refused medication. Individuals who received the integrated psychosocial treatment evidenced significantly greater improvement in anxiety symptoms than those who received treatment addressing alcohol dependence only. No significant differences between groups in alcohol use severity were observed. Fluvoxamine treatment was not associated with improved outcome for anxiety or alcohol use severity.

Few medication trials have been conducted targeting SAD/SUD. Randall and colleagues (2001b) conducted an 8-week pilot study to examine the efficacy of paroxetine in 15 individuals with alcohol dependence and SAD. The paroxetine-treated group had significantly lower SAD symptoms at the end of treatment, as compared to placebo, but no significant differences in alcohol use frequency or quantify was revealed. Gabapentin is an anticonvulsant agent with demonstrated efficacy in the treatment of SAD (Pande et al., 1999) and alcohol withdrawal (Voris, Smith, Rao, Thorne, and Flowers, 2003). Unlike benzodiazepines, gabapentin has no abuse potential. No controlled trials among comorbid SAD/SUD patients have been conducted.

Panic Disorder

Early estimates of the prevalence of panic disorder (PD) and SUD provided by the Epidemiologic Catchment Area study conducted in the early 1980s indicate that, among the 1.5% of the general population with a lifetime history of PD, 36% endorsed comorbid SUD (Regier et al., 1990). Although the preponderance of research has focused on comorbid alcohol use disorder and PD, recent estimates from the NCS-R document associations between PD and alcohol abuse (OR = 3.50), alcohol dependence (OR = 4.29), drug abuse (OR = 3.39), and drug dependence (OR = 4.07) indicative of a notable link between PD and SUD (Marmorstein, 2012). Further, NESARC data indicate that the presence of PD with agoraphobia approximately doubles the rates of comorbid SUD (Robinson et al., 2009).

Diagnostic Considerations

Alcohol dependence typically develops subsequent to the onset of PD. Age of SUD onset occurs significantly earlier among individuals with pre-existing PD and, conversely, the age of PD onset occurs earlier among individuals with pre-existing SUD. Self-medication is often posited as a mechanism for initial onset of PD, followed by subsequent development of SUD. However, use of and withdrawal from certain substances may actually induce panic attacks and promote the development of PD. For example, data from the NSDUH indicate a greater than three-fold increase in reported panic attacks among adults using cocaine (O'Brien, Wu, and Anthony, 2005). Stimulants—like cocaine, amphetamines, and phencyclidine—act on the noradrenergic system, potentially accounting for their ability to induce panic attacks. Panic attacks may also develop within the context of marijuana use, as well as sedative hypnotic and alcohol withdrawal (Crippa et al., 2009). The existing research in this area suggests that most panic attack symptoms elicited by withdrawal will remit following protracted abstinence; only PD symptoms persisting during abstinence should be considered for independent diagnosis.

Treatment

Generally, pharmacological treatment options mimic those presented in the general overview: SSRIs, TCAs, MAO-Is, and benzodiazepines. As previously discussed, use of benzodiazepines for management of PD symptoms can be effective, but should be approached with caution and monitoring among comorbid SUD populations. MAO-Is and TCAs are generally avoided as initial treatment options due to dietary restrictions necessary to prevent potential hypertensive crisis to which individuals with comorbid SUD/PD may have difficulty consistently adhering. SSRIs often present the safest option for initial pharmacological treatment of PD/SUD and some evidence suggests that SSRIs may be particularly effective in reducing symptoms of PD as well as alcohol use (Pettinati et al., 2000). PD/SUD patients should be educated and closely monitored for a potential increase in panic symptoms during the initial weeks of their treatment with SSRIs; however, the risk of side effects can be lessened by starting with a lower dosage and will often remit within 2–6 weeks when the medication reaches peak effectiveness. Finally, for special consideration among individuals with comorbid PD and cocaine use, limited preliminary evidence suggests that carbamazepine may be helpful in reducing limbic excitability produced by cocaine use that has been purported to underlie the association between cocaine use and panic (Brady et al., 2002). Research on psychotherapeutic treatments specifically addressing comorbid PD/SUD is sparse. CBTs that often employ exposure, cognitive restructuring, and relaxation training techniques have the most empirical support in the treatment of PD. Non-pharmacological treatment for PD/SUD may afford individuals opportunities to learn and implement new coping skills (instead of substance use) and practice anxiety management strategies.

Generalized Anxiety Disorder

In the NESARC study, approximately 90% of individuals with generalized anxiety disorder (GAD) had at least one other co-occurring disorder and GAD was strongly associated with SUD (Grant et al., 2005). In adolescents, the presence of GAD is associated with a more rapid progression from age of first drink to alcohol dependence (Sartor et al., 2007). GAD follows a chronic course with low rates of remission and frequent relapses/recurrences. Comorbid SUD decreases the likelihood of recovery from GAD and increases the risk of exacerbation.

Differential Diagnosis

GAD symptoms have considerable overlap with acute intoxication from stimulants and withdrawal from alcohol, opiates, sedative, and hypnotic drugs. Because of this, distinguishing substance-induced anxiety symptoms from GAD can be challenging. The DSM-V diagnostic criteria of GAD require a 6 month duration of symptoms not directly related to the physiological effects of a substance; however many substance abusers will have difficulty maintaining abstinence for 6 months, so earlier diagnosis could be important to successful recovery. Careful history taking can establish the timing of GAD relative to the SUD. Both SUD and GAD can result in significant occupational, social, and health problems, so it can be challenging to discern if the impairments are related to the SUD, GAD, or both. As patients engage in recovery, on-going assessment of anxiety symptoms will provide valuable information regarding diagnosis and need for continued treatment.

Treatment

Benzodiazepines have been very effective in the treatment of GAD, however, as previously discussed, their abuse liability limits their utility in individuals with SUD. Buspirone is a non-benzodiazepine anxiolytic with no abuse potential which has shown efficacy in a double-blind, placebo-controlled trial of anxious alcoholics in decreasing alcohol consumption and symptoms of anxiety (Krantzler et al., 1994). However, other studies of buspirone have had mixed results. In a placebo-controlled trial, McRae et al., (2004) explored the use of buspirone in a group of methadone-maintained patients with high anxiety ratings and found decreased anxiety in the medication-treated group. Because of the low abuse potential and reports of success in well-controlled studies, buspirone may be a good choice in individuals with comorbid GAD/SUD.

First-line medications for the treatment of GAD include paroxetine, escitalopram, sertraline, and venlafaxine XR. Second line agents include alprazolam, lorazepam, diazepam, buspirone, imipramine, pregabalin, and buproprion XL. Third line medications to be considered are mirtazapine, citalopram, trazodone, hydroxyzine and adjunctive olanzapine or risperidone. While SSRIs have not been specifically studied in individuals with co-occurring GAD/SUD, they are efficacious in the treatment of uncomplicated GAD and relatively safe to use in individuals with SUD, so would be a reasonable choice in individuals with co-occurring disorders. Buproprion should be avoided or used with caution in individuals at risk for seizures such as alcoholics with a history of withdrawal seizures. While effective for some individuals, controlled trials do not support the use of beta-blockers. Paroxetine, escitalopram, and venlafaxine have demonstrated long-term efficacy with increasing response rates over 6 months. Because approximately 20–40% of patients with GAD relapse within 6–12 months after the discontinuation of pharmacotherapy, long-term treatment may be needed (McKeehan et al., 2002). Psychosocial treatments are efficacious in the treatment of GAD. Cognitive behavioral therapy (CBT) has been most often used in combination with SUD treatment with goals of managing anxious states without substances (McKeehan et al., 2002).

Obsessive-Compulsive Disorder

The association of obsessive-compulsive disorder (OCD) and SUD is less robust than for other anxiety disorders. In the NCS-R study, OCD was negatively correlated with SUD (Kessler et al, 2005). Studies in treatment-seeking samples also suggest a non-significant relationship.

Differential Diagnosis

Diagnosing OCD in substance users is less problematic than with other anxiety disorders, as the characteristic symptoms of OCD are fairly unique. Craving in SUD has been compared to the intrusive recurrent thoughts that drive behavior in OCD, but thoughts and compulsions in individuals with SUD are restricted to substances and easily distinguished from OCD.

Treatment

Fals-Stewart and colleagues (1993) randomly assigned 60 individuals with OCD/SUD in a drug-free therapeutic community to a) combined OCD and SUD treatment, b) SUD treatment alone, or c) SUD treatment plus progressive muscle relaxation. At 12 months, the group receiving combined treatment had higher abstinence, longer duration in treatment, and a greater reduction in OCD symptoms.

There are no controlled studies of pharmacological treatment of co-occurring OCD/SUD. First-line medications for OCD are clomipramine, fluoxetine, fluvoxamine, paroxetine, and sertraline. In individuals with SUD, SSRIs are preferable to clomipramine because of more favorable side effect profiles. The use of psychotherapeutic techniques in combination with pharmacotherapy is particularly important in the treatment of OCD. CBT treatments including exposure and response prevention have reliably been shown to be effective in the treatment of OCD (van Oppen and Arntz, 1994).

CONCLUSIONS

Over the past two decades, evidence regarding the prevalence and negative impact of comorbid AD/SUD has become increasingly clear. Treatment of both disorders is encouraged in order to improve long-term therapeutic outcomes. Specific considerations in choosing a pharmacologic agent for use in patients with SUD include safety, toxicity and abuse liability. Although recent developments in the area of comorbid AD/SUD provide cause for considerable optimism, much work remains to be done. As the legal use of marijuana for medical purposes increases in the US, it will be important to better understanding the impact on pre-existing or new AD symptoms.

REFERENCES

Back, S. E., Brady, K. T., Sonne, S. C., and Verduin, M. L. (2006). Symptom improvement in co-occurring PTSD and alcohol dependence. *J Nerv Ment Dis, 194* (9), 690–696.

Back, S. E., Killeen, T., Foa, E. B., Santa Ana, E. J., Gros, D. F., and Brady, K. T. (2012). Use of an integrated therapy with prolonged exposure to treat PTSD and comorbid alcohol dependence in an Iraq veteran. *Am J Psychiatry, 169* (7), 688–691.

Back, S. E., Killeen, T. K., Teer, A. P., Hartwell, E. E., Federline, A., Beylotte, F., and Cox, E. (2014). Substance use disorders and PTSD: an exploratory study of treatment preferences among military veterans. *Addict Behav, 39* (2), 369–373.

Batki, S. L., Pennington, D. L., Lasher, B., Neylan, T. C., Metzler, T., Waldrop, A.,. . . Herbst, E. (2014). Topiramate treatment of alcohol use disorder in veterans with posttraumatic stress disorder: A randomized controlled pilot trial. *Alcohol Clin Exp Res, 38* (8), 2169–2177.

Bolton, J., Cox, B., Clara, I., and Sareen, J. (2006). Use of alcohol and drugs to self-medicate anxiety disorders in a nationally representative sample. *J Nerv Ment Dis, 194* (11), 818–825.

Brady, K. T., Dansky, B. S., Back, S. E., Foa, E. B., and Carroll, K. M. (2001). Exposure therapy in the treatment of PTSD among cocaine-dependent individuals: Preliminary findings. *J Subst Abuse Treat, 21* (1), 47–54.

Brady, K. T., Sonne, S., Anton, R. F., Randall, C. L., Back, S. E., and Simpson, K. (2005). Sertraline in the treatment of co-occurring alcohol dependence and posttraumatic stress disorder. *Alcohol Clin Exp Res, 29* (3), 395–401.

Brady, K. T., Sonne, S. C., Malcolm, R. J., Randall, C. L., Dansky, B. S., Simpson, K., . . . Brondino, M. (2002). Carbamazepine in the treatment of cocaine dependence: Subtyping by affective disorder. *Exp Clin Psychopharmacol, 10* (3), 276–285.

Carrigan, M. H., and Randall, C. L. (2003). Self-medication in social phobia: A review of the alcohol literature. *Addict Behav, 28* (2), 269–284.

Crippa, J. A., Zuardi, A. W., Martin-Santos, R., Bhattacharyya, S., Atakan, Z., McGuire, P., and Fusar-Poli, P. (2009). Cannabis and anxiety: A critical review of the evidence. *Hum Psychopharmacol, 24* (7), 515–523.

Fals-Stewart, W., Marks, A. P., and Schafer, J. (1993). A comparison of behavioral group therapy and individual behavior therapy in treating obsessive-compulsive disorder. *J Nerv Ment Dis, 181* (3), 189–193.

Fatseas, M., Denis, C., Lavie, E., and Auriacombe, M. (2010). Relationship between anxiety disorders and opiate dependence—a systematic review of the literature: Implications for diagnosis and treatment. *J Subst Abuse Treat, 38* (3), 220–230.

Foa, E. B., Yusko, D. A., McLean, C. P., Suvak, M. K., Bux, D. A. Jr., Oslin, D.,. . . Volpicelli, J (2013). Concurrent naltrexone and prolonged exposure therapy for patients with comorbid alcohol dependence and PTSD: A randomized clinical trial. *J Am Med Assoc, 310,* 488–495.

Grant, B. F., Hasin, D. S., Stinson, F. S., Dawson, D. A., June Ruan, W., Goldstein, R. B., . . . Huang, B. (2005). Prevalence, correlates, co-morbidity, and comparative disability of DSM-IV generalized anxiety disorder in the USA: Results from the National Epidemiologic Survey on Alcohol and Related Conditions. *Psychol Med, 35* (12), 1747–1759.

Hasin, D. S., Stinson, F. S., Ogburn, E., and Grant, B. F. (2007). Prevalence, correlates, disability, and comorbidity of DSM-IV alcohol abuse and dependence in the United States: Results from the National Epidemiologic Survey on Alcohol and Related Conditions. *Arch Gen Psychiatry, 64* (7), 830–842.

Hien, D. A., Cohen, L. R., Miele, G. M., Litt, L. C., and Capstick, C. (2004). Promising treatments for women with comorbid PTSD and substance use disorders. *Am J Psychiatry, 161* (8), 1426–1432.

Hien, D. A., Wells, E. A., Jiang, H., Suarez-Morales, L., Campbell, A. N. C., Cohen, L. R., . . . Nunes, E. V. (2009). Multi-site randomized trial of behavioral interventions for women with co-occurring PTSD and substance use disorders. *J Consult Clin Psychol, 77,* 607–619.

Hofmann, S. G., and Smits, J. A. (2008). Cognitive-behavioral therapy for adult anxiety disorders: A meta-analysis of randomized placebo-controlled trials. *J Clin Psychiatry, 69* (4), 621–632.

Iza, M., Wall, M. M., Heimberg, R. G., Rodebaugh, T. L., Schneier, F. R., Liu, S. M., and Blanco, C. (2014). Latent structure of social fears and social anxiety disorders. *Psychol Med, 44* (2), 361–370.

Kessler, R. C., Chiu, W. T., Demler, O., Merikangas, K. R., and Walters, E. E. (2005). Prevalence, severity, and comorbidity of 12-month DSM-IV disorders in the National Comorbidity Survey Replication. *Arch Gen Psychiatry, 62* (6), 617–627.

Kranzler, H. R., Burleson, J. A., Del Boca, F. K., Babor, T. F., Korner, P., Brown, J., and Bohn, M. J. (1994). Buspirone treatment of anxious alcoholics. A placebo-controlled trial. *Arch Gen Psychiatry, 51* (9), 720–731.

McKeehan, M. B. and Martin, D., (2002). Assessment and treatment of anxiety disorders and co-morbid alcohol/other drug dependency. *Alcoholism Treatment Quarterly, 20* (1), 45–59.

McRae, A. L., Sonne, S. C., Brady, K. T., Durkalski, V., and Palesch, Y. (2004). A randomized, placebo-controlled trial of buspirone for the treatment of anxiety in opioid-dependent individuals. *Am J Addict, 13* (1), 53–63.

Mills, K. L., Teesson, M., Back, S. E., Brady, K. T., Baker, A. L., Hopwood, S., . . . Ewer, P. L. (2012). Integrated exposure-based therapy for co-occurring posttraumatic stress disorder and substance dependence: A randomized controlled trial. *J Am Med Assoc, 308* (7), 690–699.

Najavits, L. M. (2002). *Seeking safety: A treatment manual for PTSD and substance abuse.* New York, NY: Guilford Press.

Najavits, L. M., and Johnson, K. M. (2014). Pilot study of Creating Change, a new past-focused model for PTSD and substance abuse. *Am J Addict, 23* (5), 415–422. National Institute on Drug Abuse (2012). The NIDA Quick Screen. In *Resource Guide: Screening for Drug Use in General Medical Settings.* Retrieved from http://www.drugabuse.gov/publications/resource-guide-screening-drug-use-in-general-medical-settings/nida-quick-screen on September 18, 2014

O'Brien, M. S., Wu, L. T., and Anthony, J. C. (2005). Cocaine use and the occurrence of panic attacks in the community: a case-crossover approach. *Subst Use Misuse, 40* (3), 285–297.

Pande, A. C., Davidson, J. R., Jefferson, J. W., Janney, C. A., Katzelnick, D. J., Weisler, R. H., . . . Sutherland, S. M. (1999). Treatment of social phobia with gabapentin: a placebo-controlled study. *J Clin Psychopharmacol, 19* (4), 341–348.

Pettinati, H. M., Volpicelli, J. R., Kranzler, H. R., Luck, G., Rukstalis, M. R., and Cnaan, A. (2000). Sertraline treatment for alcohol dependence: Interactive effects of medication and alcoholic subtype. *Alcohol Clin Exp Res, 24* (7), 1041–1049.

Petrakis, I. L., Poling, J., Levinson, C., Nich, C., Carroll, K., and Rounsaville, B. (2005). Naltrexone and disulfiram in patients with alcohol dependence and comorbid psychiatric disorders. *Biol Psychiatry, 57* (10), 1128–1137.

Petrakis, I. L., Ralevski, E., Desai, N., Trevisan, L., Gueorguieva, R., Rounsaville, B., and Krystal, J. H. (2012). Noradrenergic vs. serotonergic antidepressant with or without naltrexone for veterans with PTSD and comorbid alcohol dependence. *Neuropsychopharmacology, 37,* 996–1004.

Pietrzak, R. H., Goldstein, R. B., Southwick, S. M., and Grant, B. F. (2011). Prevalence and Axis I comorbidity of full and partial posttraumatic stress disorder in the United States: Results from Wave 2 of the National Epidemiologic Survey on Alcohol and Related Conditions. *J Anxiety Disord, 25* (3), 456–465.

Randall, C. L., Johnson, M. R., Thevos, A. K., Sonne, S. C., Thomas, S. E., Willard, S. L., et al. (2001b). Paroxetine for social anxiety and alcohol use in dual-diagnosed patients. *Depress Anxiety, 14* (4): 255–262.

Randall, C. L., Thomas, S., and Thevos, A. K. (2001a). Concurrent alcoholism and social anxiety disorder: A first step toward developing effective treatments. *Alcohol Clin Exp Res, 25* (2), 210–220.

Regier, D. A., Farmer, M. E., Rae, D. S., Locke, B. Z., Keith, S. J., Judd, L. L., and Goodwin, F. K. (1990). Comorbidity of mental disorders with alcohol and other drug abuse. Results from the Epidemiologic Catchment Area (ECA) Study. *J Am Med Assoc, 264* (19), 2511–2518.

Robinson, J., Sareen, J., Cox, B. J., and Bolton, J. (2009). Self-medication of anxiety disorders with alcohol and drugs: Results from a nationally representative sample. *J Anxiety Disord, 23* (1), 38–45. doi: 10.1016/j.janxdis.2008.03.013

Sareen, J., Chartier, M., Kjernisted, K. D., and Stein, M. B. (2001). Comorbidity of phobic disorders with alcoholism in a Canadian community sample. *Can J Psychiatry, 46* (8), 733–740.

Sareen, J., Chartier, M., Paulus, M. P., and Stein, M. B. (2006). Illicit drug use and anxiety disorders: Findings from two community surveys. *Psychiatry Res, 142* (1), 11–17.

Sartor, C. E., Lynskey, M. T., Heath, A. C., Jacob, T., and True, W. (2007). The role of childhood risk factors in initiation of alcohol use and progression to alcohol dependence. *Addiction, 102* (2), 216–225.

Sattar, S. P., and Bhatia, S. (2003). Benzodiazepines for substance abusers: Yes or no? *Current Psychiatry, 2,* 943–955.

Schade, A., Marquenie, L. A., Van Balkom, A. J., Koeter, M. W., De Beurs, E., Van Den Brink, W., and Van Dyck, R. (2004). Alcohol-dependent patients with comorbid phobic disorders: a comparison between comorbid patients, pure alcohol-dependent and pure phobic patients. *Alcohol Alcohol, 39* (3), 241–246.

Smith, J. P., and Randall, C. L. (2012). Anxiety and alcohol use disorders: Comorbidity and treatment considerations. *Alcohol Res, 34* (4), 414–431.

Sofuoglu, M, Rosenheck, R, and Petrakis, I (2014). Pharmacological treatment of comorbid PTSD and substance use disorder: Recent progress. *Addict Behav, 39,* 428–433.

Stewart, S. H., and Conrod, P. J. (2008). Anxiety disorder and substance use disorder co-morbidity: Common themes and future directions. In S. H. Stewart and P. J. Conrod (Eds.), *Anxiety and Substance Use Disorders: The Vicious Cycle of Comorbidity* (pp. 239–257). New York, NY: Springer.

Torchalla, I., Nosen, L., Rostam, H., and Allen, P. (2012). Integrated treatment programs for individuals with concurrent substance use disorders and trauma experiences: a systematic review and meta-analysis. *J Subst Abuse Treat, 42* (1), 65–77.

van Dam, D., Vedel, E., Ehring, T., and Emmelkamp, P. M. (2012). Psychological treatments for concurrent posttraumatic stress disorder and substance use disorder: a systematic review. *Clin Psychol Rev,* 32 (3), 202–214.

van Oppen, P., and Arntz, A. (1994). Cognitive therapy for obsessive-compulsive disorder. *Behav Res Ther,* 32 (1), 79–87.

Voris, J., Smith, N. L., Rao, S. M., Thorne, D. L., and Flowers, Q. J. (2003). Gabapentin for the treatment of ethanol withdrawal. *Subst Abus,* 24 (2), 129–132.

/// 21 /// COMORBIDITY OF ANXIETY AND DEPRESSION

AMANDA W. CALKINS, ANDREW H. ROGERS,
ALLISON A. CAMPBELL, AND
NAOMI M. SIMON

INTRODUCTION

Comorbidity of psychiatric disorders is quite common—in a 12-month period, almost 50% of adults in the United States with any psychiatric disorder had two or more disorders (Kessler et al., 2006). Notably, the prevalence of comorbid anxiety disorders and major depressive disorder (MDD) is very frequent—as high as 60% (Kessler et al., 2006). Individuals affected by both anxiety and depressive disorders concurrently have generally shown greater functional impairment, reduced quality of life, and poorer treatment outcomes compared with individuals with only one psychiatric disorder (depression or anxiety disorder). In this chapter, we will discuss the epidemiology, etiology and impact of comorbid anxiety and depression as well as methods for treating these commonly co-occurring conditions. Finally, we will touch on some of these issues for individuals with co-occurring anxiety disorders and bipolar disorder.

Currently, the formal diagnosis of comorbid anxiety and depression is based on the presence of meeting *DSM-5* criteria for more than one of the individual disorders (APA 2013). There is, however, a syndrome—mixed anxiety and depression—which includes symptoms of anxiety and depression that do not surpass the threshold required by DSM-5 criteria for individual diagnoses of an anxiety or depressive disorder. This newly defined syndrome may prove to be clinically useful, but requires further research at this time.

Clinicians are well aware that many patients with an anxiety or depression diagnosis have variable subthreshold mood or anxiety symptoms—even beyond those that may overlap across diagnoses—that can add to distress and impairment, and benefit from clinical attention. In this chapter, however, we will focus on the impact of comorbid depression on the *DSM-5* anxiety disorder diagnoses: panic disorder (PD), social anxiety disorder (SAD) and generalized anxiety disorder (GAD).

EPIDEMIOLOGY AND IMPACT

Panic Disorder and Depression

Comorbidity in PD is common; the National Comorbidity Study (NCS-R) revealed that 83% of the PD-only group and 100% of the PD with agoraphobia group met criteria for one or more lifetime comorbid conditions (Kessler et al., 2006). Additionally, having a diagnosis of PD both with or without agoraphobia was commonly associated with the mood disorders, including major depressive disorder (MDD) (35% and 39%, respectively), bipolar disorders (14% and 33%, respectively), and dysthymia (10% and 15%, respectively; Kessler et al., 2006).

The presence of co-occurring PD and depression bodes poorly for a variety of psychological, functional, and treatment outcomes. For example, increased rates of suicide and suicide attempts have been associated with PD with comorbid depression (Goodwin and Roy-Byrne., 2006), with some research suggesting that rates of lifetime suicide attempts in patients with PD and MDD is more than double that of the two disorders independently (Goodwin et al, 2001). Additionally, both medical and psychiatric comorbidities significantly impact quality of life in individuals with PD (Davidoff et al., 2012). Kaplan and colleagues (2006) also found that compared to controls or individuals with PD alone, those with comorbid PD and MDD demonstrated negative attentional bias and visual discrimination along with working memory deficits. Across the anxiety disorders (PD, Agoraphobia, SAD, and GAD), having a comorbid depressive disorder was predictive of a chronic course in a large prospective study (Batelaan, Rhebergen, Spinhoven, van Balkom, and Penninx, 2014).

Social Anxiety Disorder and Depression

SAD has also been shown to be highly co-morbid with depression. In the NCS, MDD was present in 37% of those with SAD (Kessler et al., 2006) and lifetime rates of co-morbid MDD in clinical samples have been reported near 60% (Merikangas and Angst, 1995). SAD typically pre-dates the onset of MDD by many years, and thus individuals presenting with SAD alone may still be at significant risk for the later development of depression (Kessler, DuPont, Berglund, and Wittchen, 1999). In a longitudinal study, participants with SAD and depression in adolescence or early adulthood were found to be at greatest risk for subsequent depression as well as substance abuse and suicide (Stein et al., 2001). Individuals with comorbid SAD also experienced longer episodes of depression (Stein et al., 2001). Research also demonstrates that individuals with SAD and depression are at increased risk of suicidal ideation and suicide attempts (Davidson et al., 1993) as well as experience greater impairment in social and occupational function (Magee et al., 1996). Furthermore, the presence of comorbid MDD also adversely impacts response to SAD treatment (Magee et al., 1996).

Generalized Anxiety Disorder and Depression

Considerable research attention has been paid to the relationship between GAD and depression (Brown and Barlow, 2005). According to data from the NCS and NCS-R follow-up studies, depression and GAD were strongly comorbid; the odds-ratios of having GAD were 6.6–7.5 in individuals with lifetime MDD (Kessler et al., 1994; 2008). Additionally, 62% of individuals with GAD also met criteria for MDD (Kessler et al., 1994; 2008). Similar or higher comorbidity rates of depressive disorders have been reported in clinical samples. For instance, in the Harvard/Brown Anxiety Disorders Research Program study, 54% of patients with GAD had either current MDD or dysthymia (Massion et al., 1993). Other work has demonstrated that between 35%–50% of patients with current MDD also meet criteria for GAD (Roy-Byrne and Katon, 1997).

In general, when MDD occurs comorbidly with GAD, there is a poorer prognosis in terms of impairment, course of illness, and treatment response (Kessler et al., 1999). For example, the NCS-R demonstrated that people with co-morbid GAD and a mood disorder reported greater interference with life activities, and more interpersonal problems (Kessler et al., 2005). Similarly, Wittchen and colleagues (2002) found that patients with GAD and MDD were slightly more impaired than patients with GAD without depression or MDD without GAD. In other work, greater social disability was reported by patients in a primary care setting meeting criteria for both GAD and another psychiatric disorder (46%) compared to patients with GAD alone (25%), as well as medical disorders without a psychiatric diagnosis (20%; (Maier and Falkai, 1999)). Treatment response may also be complicated by comorbid GAD and MDD. In one study the initial treatment response to CBT was equivalent for individuals with GAD with or without MDD; however, those with MDD did not maintain treatment gains upon two year follow-up (Newman et al., 2010). In another study, Treatment response to nortriptyline or interpersonal therapy was delayed in individuals with comborbid GAD and MDD (Brown, Schulberg, Madonia, Shear, and Houck, 1996)

Anxiety Comorbidity with Bipolar Disorder

Anxiety disorders have also been found to occur at elevated rates in individuals with bipolar disorder, with 51% of bipolar I or II patients having at least 1 type of lifetime anxiety disorder (Simon, 2009). Comorbid anxiety disorders in bipolar disorder have been reported at rates of 10.6–62.5% for PD, 7.8–47.2% for SAD, and 7–32% for GAD (Simon et al., 2004). Additionally, anxiety comorbidity in bipolar disorder has been associated with greater symptom severity and dysfunction (Simon et al., 2004, Simon, 2009). Comorbid anxiety in bipolar disorder has been associated with younger age of bipolar onset, poorer role functioning, decreased quality of life, greater suicidality, increased substance abuse, lower lithium responsivity and less time spent euthymic (Keller, 2006; Simon, 2009).

KEY CLINICAL FEATURES AND CLINICAL PHENOTYPE

Complicating the understanding of anxiety and mood disorder comorbidity is that some symptoms are characteristic of both disorders, while others are specific to just one disorder. This has been most closely studied in GAD and depression (Van Ameringen, Stein and Hermann, 2013). For example, symptoms believed to be specific to depression include: sadness, loss of interest, weight change/poor appetite, psychomotor retardation, feelings of guilt or worthlessness, thoughts of death. Symptoms believed to be specific to anxiety include: excessive worry, autonomic hyperactivity, increased startle response and muscle tension. Symptoms common to anxiety and depression include: irritability, restlessness, difficulty concentrating, trouble sleeping, and fatigue (see Figure 21.1 for diagram of overlapping and distinct symptoms of anxiety and depression; Van Ameringen, Stein and Hermann, 2013). In actual practice however even greater overlap may be present: for example, symptoms of nausea and gastrointestinal distress present

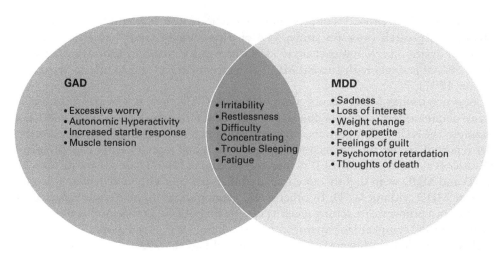

FIGURE 21.1 Overlapping and distinct symptoms of GAD and MDD.

in some patients with severe anxiety related to GAD may result in reduced appetite and weight loss. There are similar overlapping symptoms for GAD and bipolar disorder as well (see Figure 21.2 for diagram of overlapping and distinct symptoms of anxiety and bipolar disorder).

In terms of age of onset, the median age of onset has been reported as 11 years for anxiety disorders (early childhood in SAD and adolescence/early adulthood in GAD, and PD) and 30 years of age for mood disorders (Kessler et al., 2005). When anxiety and depression occur comorbidly, the age of onset has been reported to vary depending on which disorder was classified as the primary or the pre-dating disorder. In a pre-dating/primary anxiety disorder with comorbid depression, age of onset for the comorbid conditions closely followed that of an anxiety disorder alone. In a pre-dating/primary depressive disorder with comorbid anxiety disorder the age of onset more closely followed that of a depressive disorder alone (Kessler et al., 2005).

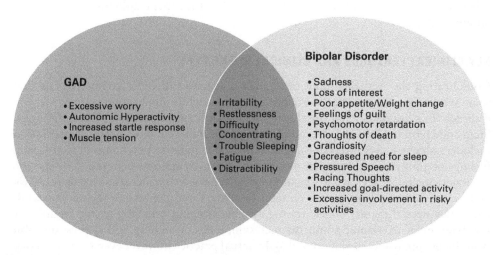

FIGURE 21.2 Overlapping and distinct symptoms of GAD and bipolar disorder.

Some differences within the anxiety disorders in terms of comorbid depression include that SAD and GAD more often predate depression onset, while PD has been reported to postdate depression onset in some research (Fava et al., 2000). Differences are also evident in life course with the recovery rate being substantially higher for MDD than the anxiety disorders (with the exception of panic disorder without agoraphobia; Bruce et al., 2005).

Overall, the presence of anxiety with comorbid depression is associated with significantly lower odds of recovery, greater time to therapeutic onset for pharmacotherapy (Kessler et al., 2005), and a more chronic course than when either anxiety or depression occurs alone (Kessler et al., 2008). Depression is generally episodic in nature with moderate rates of recovery, and high rates of relapse, while anxiety disorders tend to be chronic and unremitting but with a waxing and waning course, with low levels of recovery and moderate levels of relapse (Bruce et al., 2005; Kessler et al., 2008).

In the NCS-R, individuals with a GAD diagnosis had an increased likelihood of having a major depressive episode (MDE) as well as increased persistence of MDD compared to those who had no past or current GAD diagnosis (Kessler et al., 2008). By comparison, individuals who were ever diagnosed with an MDE had increased likelihood of having an onset of GAD but no increased persistence of GAD episode, which may be due to GAD's chronic nature (Kessler et al., 2008). In a longitudinal study of patients with GAD or PD, those with comorbid major depression were half as likely to recover, compared with either GAD or PD alone (Grant et al., 2005). This study also found that those with GAD and comorbid MDD were significantly more impaired in perceived mental health quality and social functioning, compared with those with GAD alone (Grant et al., 2005).

MECHANISMS AND THEORIES OF DISORDER

Family and Genetics

Research suggests there are shared genetic factors associated with risk across depression and anxiety. This genetic link may contribute to the high susceptibility to comorbidity among these disorders (Demirkan et al., 2011). As previously mentioned, the NCS-R found that of individuals diagnosed with MDD, 60% were also diagnosed with an anxiety disorder in their lifetime (Kessler et al., 2006). However, genes do not set a specific code for the symptoms of depression or anxiety; rather genes may add to the vulnerability of individuals to develop these symptoms (Kendler, Heath, Martin, and Eaves, 1987). Twin studies and some family studies have supported this notion of genetic vulnerability, while others suggest the comorbidity of anxiety or depression as an epiphenomenon of the other disorder (Middeldorp, Cath, Van Dyck, and Boomsma, 2005). See chapter 4 of this text for additional information on genetics of anxiety disorders.

Overall, twin studies conducted to date have provided moderate to strong support for shared genetic risk factors between MDD and anxiety disorders. The strength of these genetic associations depends upon the specific anxiety disorder: GAD is most closely related genetically to MDD, followed by panic disorder and then the specific phobias (Hettema, 2008). One twin study of 1128 individuals found that variations in glutamate decarboxylase 1 gene (GAD1), the gene that encodes one of the several forms of the enzyme glutamic acid decarboxylase (synthesizes GABA from glutamate), may contribute to individual differences in trait neuroticism and play a role in susceptibility across anxiety disorders (GAD, PD, agoraphobia and SAD) and major depressive disorder (Hettema et al., 2006). Genetic association studies have looked at the 5-HTTLPR polymorphism (serotonin-transporter linked polymorphic region) as well as the functional Val158Met polymorphism of catechol-O-methyltransferase (COMT), with a significant number of positive and negative findings published to date and no consistent conclusions across studies so far.

Heritability for shared risk between nuclear family members is estimated at 0.25 (95% CI = .22–.27), with a significant correlation on the symptom checklist (SCL-90) assessing symptoms of anxiety and depression (Czajkowski, Roysamb, Reichborn-Kjennerud, and Tambs, 2010). Research suggests that parental psychopathology is associated with the development of comorbid depression and anxiety in offspring. Biedel and Turner (1997) found that children of anxious parents were more vulnerable to develop only an anxiety disorder. Additional findings suggested the children of comorbid anxious and depressed parents were more likely to develop a more varied scope of disorders and more likely to have comorbid diagnoses. Meta-analyses of heritability studies estimate the heritability to be between 30–40% for comorbid anxiety and depression development, with environmental factors playing a role in the remaining variance (Hettema, Neale, and Kendler, 2001). As more is understood about the interplay of genetics, stress and environmental risk, as well as the genetics associated with core neurobiological features of mood and anxiety symptoms, it is likely that even more of the overlap between depression and anxiety will be elucidated.

Environmental Risk

Environmental risk is a key factor in the development of anxiety and depression, and can present itself in various ways. First, Kendler et al. (1992) found that depression and generalized anxiety disorder (GAD) may exist comorbidly due to exposure to non-familial environmental factors. In other words, if one family member experiences a stressful life event, that individual is now more susceptible to developing depression and GAD. Environmental factors in early childhood including parenting style/separation also may be associated with developing comorbid anxiety and depression. Research has emphasized early-life stressors/adversities and their influence on long term psychological health via biological embedding and interaction with genetic risk (Shonkoff, Boyce. and McEwen, 2009). With the development of psychopathology in children, comes an increased risk of continued psychopathology into adulthood. Children who develop an anxiety disorder have a two to three fold increased risk for anxiety and MDD in adulthood (Britton, Lissek, Grillon, Norcross, and Pine, 2011), often with a more severe and chronic course, and greater risk for additional mood and anxiety related psychopathology after exposure to major stressors such as trauma and loss.

Biomarkers

Brain mechanisms are another important factor contributing to the development of comorbid depression and anxiety. The field of neuroimaging has established a vast number of studies supporting that the pre-frontal cortex and the amygdala play a significant role in anxiety and depression. The amygdala has been recognized as crucial for emotion regulation and processing, due in part to its role in emotional memory formation and memory retrieval (Ressler and Mayberg, 2007). Specifically, individuals with anxiety disorders have shown a stronger brain activation response in the amygdala when displaying negative emotional responses (Etkin and Wager, 2007). Frodl, Moller and Meisenzahl (2008) suggest that this increased activation in the amygdala may also contribute to the susceptibility to developing depression.

The prefrontal cortex has also been examined heavily in relation to anxiety and depression. Research suggests the prefrontal cortex is involved in emotional experience and processing, with neural connections to and modulation of the amygdala (Ressler and Mayberg, 2007). Neuroimaging has also clearly demonstrated abnormalities in the prefrontal cortex of individuals with anxiety disorders (Berkowitz, Coplan, Reddy, and Gorman, 2007). Meta-analytic studies examining the neural correlates of anxiety and depression have also found abnormal modulation of prefrontal brain activity in both a resting state and during emotional-cognitive tasks (Messina, Sambin, Palmieri, and Viviani, 2013).

A number of other potential biomarkers have been studied and may add to the predictive validity of anxiety and depression. For example, Nelson. et al (2013) found heightened sensitivity to threat and reduced sensitivity to reward as displayed via abnormal EEG asymmetry, suggesting threat/reward sensitivity may serve as a biomarker for MDD and panic disorder. Initial work has also identified brain-derived neurotrophic factor (BDNF) as a biomarker related to both anxiety and depression. BDNF is the protein encoded in humans by the BDNF gene, and affects the survival and function of neurons in the central nervous system by encouraging the outgrowth of dendrites. BDNF plays an active role in facilitating plasticity particularly in the hippocampus, cortex, and basal forebrain, which are areas critical to the learning process (Gatt et al., 2009). Though this work is still in its early stages, early life stress in combination with the BDNF Met allele and alterations in serotonergic activity may increase the risk of depression and anxiety in human and rodent studies (Gatt et al., 2009).

Cognitive and Personality Correlates

In addition to biological underpinnings, individual personality traits can add to the susceptibility to developing both depression and anxiety, which also may contribute to their high rate of comorbidity. In particular, neuroticism is a specific construct that has been linked to these disorders. Neuroticism is defined as a disposition to emotional instability, anxiety, and self-consciousness or the tendency to stay in negative mood states (Enns and Cox, 1997). Multiple studies have shown that those who are high on neuroticism scales are more vulnerable to develop depression (Kendler, Gardner, and Prescott, 2002; Kendler, Kuhn, and Prescott, 2004) and anxiety (Hettema, Prescott, and Kendler, 2004). For example, Jylha and Isometsa (2006) found that neuroticism scores were strongly associated with anxiety and depressive symptoms, with high neuroticism best explained by these symptoms, even after adjusting for other variables such as age, gender, and education. Further, high levels of neuroticism have been shown to interact with stressful life events to heighten the risk on new onset depression (Kendler et al., 2004).

Anxiety sensitivity, a cognitive vulnerability factor, has received significant research attention and is also believed to play a role in developing and maintaining both anxiety and depression. Anxiety sensitivity is the level of fear associated with anxiety-related bodily sensations, and the interpretation that these sensations are harmful (Taylor, Koch, Woody, and McLean, 1996). The fear can be broken into three components: fear of publicly observable symptoms, fear of loss of cognitive control, and fear of bodily sensations. The first and third factors have been shown to correlate with anxiety, and the fear of loss of cognitive control is correlated with depression (Taylor et al., 1996). Overall, anxiety sensitivity serves as another vulnerability factor for developing psychopathology (Schmidt et al., 2007) and could contribute to the high overlap of the conditions.

Another personality correlate which may be related to comorbid depression and anxiety is behavioral inhibition. Behavioral inhibition is characterized by a shy and fearful temperament, with the individual often quiet and withdrawn in unfamiliar situations (Hirshfeld et al., 1992). Behavioral inhibition is another vulnerability factor for developing anxiety disorders; children and adolescents who have high behavioral inhibition also display greater psychopathological symptoms than their peers who have low or moderate behavioral inhibition (Hirshfeld et al., 1992). Muris et al. (2001) conducted a study which tested hypothetical models examining the role of behavioral inhibition in child anxiety and depression; the best fitting model suggested that behavioral inhibition leads to anxiety, which in turn leads to depression.

Together the cognitive and personality based factors in this section are all at work in contributing to the larger biopsychosocial model of comorbid anxiety and depression. As discussed, genetics and heritability contribute to the likelihood of comorbid anxiety and depression being passed from parent to offspring; however, parenting styles and stressful life events also contribute to psychopathological development. Neurobiological factors including functioning of the amygdala, the prefrontal cortex (PFC) and related neurocircuitry additionally may play a role in comorbid anxiety and depression development and maintenance. However, much more is understood about the direct role of this neurocircuitry in fear and avoidance based conditions such as posttraumatic stress, social anxiety and panic disorder than in depression comorbidity. In brief, research has found hyperactivation of the fear circuit (amygdala, insula, anterior cingulate and PFC) as well as hyperactivation of medial parietal and occipital regions (posterior cingulate, precuneus, cuneus) and a reduction in connectivity between parietal, limbic and prefrontal networks to be implicated in comorbid depression and anxiety (see chapter 3 on the neurobiology of anxiety disorders in this edition for more information; Bruhl et al., 2014). Finally, personality/cognitive correlates including neuroticism, anxiety sensitivity, and behavioral inhibition contribute as additional vulnerability factors that likely interact with a range of biological and environmental risk factors that together contribute to the etiology of comorbid anxiety and depression.

TREATMENT

Medication

A number of medications have demonstrated efficacy for individuals suffering from anxiety or depression, but medication management may be more complicated with comorbid anxiety and depression. Antidepressants, such as selective serotonin reuptake inhibitors (SSRIs) and serotonin norepinephrine reuptake inhibitors (SNRIs) are the first line treatments for comorbid anxiety and depression, with tricyclic antidepressants (TCAs) or monoamine oxidase inhibitors (MAOIs) as potent agents which are less commonly used due to their side effect profiles (Wittchen et al., 2002). Both SSRIs, such as fluoxetine, and SNRIs, such as venlafaxine, have been shown to be effective treatments for both anxiety and depression; however, some but not all research has suggested that dual action drugs, such as the SNRIs, might be superior to SSRIs for treating the two disorders (Baldwin, 2006). In the setting of comorbid anxiety and depression, antidepressants should be started at half the indicated dose for depression because patients experiencing anxiety (and especially those with high levels of anxiety sensitivity or panic) tend to be more sensitive to some of the early anxiogenic side effects of antidepressant medication; however, after initiation-related side effects resolve, medication doses should be titrated up to achieve optimal effect (Simon and Rosenbaum, 2003).

While SSRIs and SNRIs are the first line recommended medications for comorbid anxiety and depression, for some patients with comorbid panic disorder and depression or obsessive-compulsive disorder and depression, TCAs or other agents may be more beneficial (Aina and Susman, 2006; Wittchen et al., 2002). Regardless of the comorbidity, antidepressants are preferred for the treatment of comorbid anxiety and depression over other medications, such as benzodiazepines, which alone do not treat depression and carry the potential for abuse and dependence (Barclay and Barclay, 2014). Benzodiazepines are, however, useful anxiolytic agents with well-established safety and efficacy for the anxiety disorders and for acute anxiolysis. This class of drugs is particularly useful in the early stages of pharmacological treatment of comorbid anxiety and depression, and may enable some patients to better tolerate up titration of antidepressants, but they might not be necessary beyond the first few weeks of treatment when used with an antidepressant (Simon and Rosenbaum, 2003). Combining an SSRI (fluoxetine) with a benzodiazepine has been shown to result in much quicker improvement in anxiety and depression symptoms compared to an SSRI alone (Pollack, 2005). Overall, the presence of anxiety disorders or symptoms with depression have been demonstrated to predict poorer response to initial and next step pharmacotherapy, but anxiety did not predict differential response to switching from a first SSRI to a second SSRI, an SNRI, or bupropion for non-responders in a large randomized depression trial (Fava et al., 2008).

While antidepressants and benzodiazepines are the most common pharmacological treatments for comorbid anxiety and depression, other drugs exist as both first line pharmacological treatments and adjuncts to existing and effective treatments. For example, buspirone, generally used to treat anxiety, acts on serotonin and dopamine and might have anti-depressant effects at higher doses (Pollack, 2005). Buspirone alone has shown modest reductions of anxiety and depressive symptoms in comorbid anxiety and mild depression, but may be more effective when used as an adjunct to other pharmacological treatments (Simon and Rosenbaum, 2003). Finally, for those refractory to or unable to tolerate other agents, some atypical antipsychotics have demonstrated efficacy alone or as adjuncts for both depression and anxiety, though antipsychotics may carry risks of metabolic syndrome and/or tardive dyskinesia, depending on the type. Finally, some anticonvulsants such as gabapentin can also be useful adjuncts to antidepressant treatment for refractory anxiety in the context of depression. See Box 21.1 for treatment considerations relating to comorbid anxiety in mood disorders and chapters 10, 16, and 24 for additional information about medications and treatment for PD, SAD, and GAD.

Therapy

Individuals suffering from comorbid anxiety and depression often seek psychotherapy rather than, or in conjunction with, pharmacological therapy to address symptoms (Malhi et al., 2014). Cognitive-behavioral therapy (CBT) is a well-documented, effective treatment for both anxiety and depression; adults with comorbid anxiety and depression have been shown to have significant decreases in both anxiety and depressive symptoms with group CBT compared to a waitlist group (Wuthrich and Rapee, 2013). CBT works by altering thoughts and behaviors that lead to or maintain distressing emotions; CBT aims to help patients develop a set of skills to be more aware of their thoughts and emotions and how the thoughts and behaviors influence how they feel. These skills along with homework assignments and the structured, brief nature of the therapy, set CBT apart from traditional talk therapy; see section 9 of this text for a greater explanation of CBT and its therapeutic mechanisms (Cully and Teten, 2008).

BOX 21.1

TREATMENT CONSIDERATIONS FOR ANXIETY DISORDERS IN THE SETTING OF COMORBID DEPRESSION OR BIPOLAR DISORDER

- Consider adding behavioral activation to CBT in the context of depression
- In terms of psychotherapy approaches, lead with anxiety disorder specific evidenced based treatments (CBT, Unified Protocol, MBSR, etc.) and consider enhancing engagement of depressed patients with the use of motivational interviewing
- In GAD with comorbid depression, differentiate worry from rumination in psychotherapy; although similar cognitive strategies can be utilized for both, worry exposure may not be effective for rumination
- In PD and SAD differentiate avoidance and amotivation/anhedonia and use appropriate therapeutic strategies for each (e.g., exposure vs. motivational interviewing/behavioral activation)
- Consider starting antidepressants at half the usual dose to limit initiation side effects with anxiety and depression comorbidity, but titrate to full efficacy
- Use caution when prescribing SSRI's for anxiety in bipolar disorder due to risk of inducing a manic episode
- Avoid prescribing benzodiazepines alone with mood disorder comorbidity as they do not address mood symptoms
- Enhance clinical monitoring of suicidality and substance use in the context of comorbid mood and anxiety
- Consider atypical antipsychotics with demonstrated efficacy for anxiety and bipolar depression in context bipolar comorbidity, as they can result in dual efficacy without inducing manic episode
- Place extra emphasis on maintaining regular daily and nightly routines, possibly including sleep, social and interpersonal activity when bipolar is present

---

While CBT is an effective strategy to treat comorbid anxiety and depression, there exists some debate on how to most effectively treat both disorders concurrently. In a research study examining people with comorbid social anxiety disorder and depression receiving CBT, there were significant improvements for both anxiety and depressive symptoms when CBT directly targeted the social anxiety (Fracalanza, McCabe, Taylor, and Antony, 2014). However, contradictory research exists that showed that targeting one disorder in CBT for treating comorbid anxiety and depression will not be as effective (Pollack, 2005). Additionally, patients presenting with anxiety and severe, untreated depression might have less success with CBT, as the depression can interfere with both the treatment of the anxiety and the depression. In that case, it would be important to focus on motivational interventions, cognitive work, depressive symptoms, and the low motivation that accompanies the severe depression.

An example of CBT used to treat comorbid anxiety and depression is the Unified Protocol for the Treatment of Emotional Disorders (Kaufman and Baucom, 2014). In this treatment approach, emotions are accessed and provoked using various exposure techniques, such as in vivo, introceptive, and imaginal. The therapy is divided up into three fundamental components that are identified to be generally relevant in treating emotional disorders: reducing negative thoughts, diminishing avoidance of emotions, and reducing safe behaviors aimed at ameliorating anxiety. While the structure of the therapy is the same for each patient, the exercises and situations used differ from person to person. This treatment may represent a more efficient and effective strategy for treating comorbid anxiety and depression (Barlow, Allen, and Choate, 2004).

Mindfulness based treatments are also used to treat comorbid anxiety and depression, as they are thought to help clients confront aversive behaviors brought on by thoughts and memories (Kaufman and Baucom, 2014). An example of a commonly used, mindfulness based treatment is acceptance and commitment therapy (ACT). ACT focuses on the ways in which clients understand their difficulties through language. Additionally, this therapy focuses on how clients avoid their own uncomfortable thoughts and emotions, which is thought to be the cause of the pathology. The goal of the therapy is to teach clients how to control or eliminate the uncomfortable thoughts and emotions by accepting and embracing them (Hayes, Strosahl, and Wilson, 1999).

Novel Strategies for Treatment

There are many different novel treatments that have been tried for treating anxiety and depression, including psychological and pharmacological therapy; however more research needs to be done solidify the strategies as effective strategies for treating comorbid anxiety and depression.

One such novel strategy focuses on changes in attention. Evidence has shown that attention as a treatment target for both anxiety and depression might be effective in reducing symptoms. Attention Bias Modification (ABM), used in the treatment of anxiety, targets threat-related biases that are prevalent in anxiety and not targeted in CBT. ABM helped to reduce anxiety in a clinical population (Hakamata et al., 2010). Research has yet to prove, however, if ABM is superior to CBT or medications for the treatment of anxiety, but might be an important step in managing anxiety over time. Additionally, attentional control training has been used in the treatment of depression to help prevent relapse; integrating cognitive therapy and attentional control training to manage depression over time might be an effective, long lasting treatment strategy (Teasdale, Segal, and Williams, 1995).

Cognitive control might be another target for novel treatments for comorbid anxiety and depression, as significant neuropsychiatric impairment often goes along with depression and anxiety (Lyche, Jonassen, Stiles, Ulleberg, and Landro, 2010). Additionally, youth experiencing comorbid anxiety and depression showed that they were able to improve their cognitive control under incentive conditions, identifying cognitive control as a potential target for treatment (Hardin, Schroth, Pine, and Ernst, 2007). In fact, in one study, cognitive control training (CCT) was effective in reducing both depressive symptoms as well as physiological arousal associated with depression (Siegle, Ghinassi, and Thase, 2007). Little research has been done on the effects of CCT on comorbid anxiety and depression, but past research suggests that it might be a good strategy for treatment.

FUTURE DIRECTIONS

In our current diagnostic system (DSM-5) diagnosing co-occurring anxiety and depression, and similarly anxiety and bipolar disorder, relies upon meeting criteria for at least two individual disorders which are diagnosed by presenting signs and symptoms, with the result that these diagnoses my not accurately reflect relevant underlying neurobiological and behavioral systems. The National Institute of Mental Health's research domain criteria (RDoC) initiative (see chapter 2 for more information) asserts that this impedes research on etiology, pathophysiology and treatment development. This project was started in 2009 to create a new classification system for mental disorders based upon dimensions of neurobiology and observable behavior. RDoC examines biobehavioral dimensions that cut across current DSM-5 diagnoses. This is very relevant for comorbid anxiety and depression which are both heterogeneous categories with significant overlap in symptoms and risk factors. RDoC research may provide new psychiatric nosologies better routed in research which can better account for the co-occurrence of anxiety and depression (Cuthbert and Insel, 2013).

RDoC represents a significant paradigm shift, by considering psychiatric disorders from a translational science perspective. This initiative begins by conducting an inventory of the fundamental, behavioral functions that the brain conducts, and to specify the neural circuits responsible for implementing these functions. The next step is to consider/diagnose psychopathology in terms of dysfunction of various kinds and degrees in particular systems, as studied from an integrative, multi-systems point of view. Although still in the early stages of research development with limited application to the clinic, RDoC ultimately may provide an improved system for diagnosing anxiety and comorbid depression, and open new avenues to treatment in the future. Until then, identification of individuals who carry the dual burden of comorbid diagnoses of depression and anxiety disorders is important in clinical practice to optimize treatment interventions and outcomes.

Disclosure Statement: Dr. Simon has research support from the American Cancer Society, the American Foundation for Suicide Prevention, the Department of Defense, the Highland Street Foundation and the National Institutes of Health.

REFERENCES

Aina, Yemi, and Susman, Jeffrey L. (2006). Understanding comorbidity with depression and anxiety disorders. *J Am Osteopathic Assoc*, 106 (5 suppl 2), S9–S14.

American Psychiatric Association. (2013). *Diagnostic and statistical manual of mental disorders* (5th ed.). Arlington, VA: American Psychiatric Publishing.

Baldwin, D. S. (2006). Serotonin noradrenaline reuptake inhibitors: A new generation of treatment for anxiety disorders. *Int J Psychiatry Clin Pract*, 10 Suppl 2, 12–15. doi: 10.1080/13651500600637056

Barclay, T. H., and Barclay, R. D. (2014). A clinical trial of cranial electrotherapy stimulation for anxiety and comorbid depression. *J Affect Disord*, 164, 171–177. doi: 10.1016/j.jad.2014.04.029

Barlow, David H., Allen, Laura B., and Choate, Molly L. (2004). Toward a unified treatment for emotional disorders. *Behavior Therapy*, 35 (2), 205–230.

Batelaan, N. M., Rhebergen, D., Spinhoven, P., van Balkom, A. J., and Penninx, B. W. (2014). Two-year course trajectories of anxiety disorders: do DSM classifications matter? *J Clin Psychiatry.* doi: 10.4088/JCP.13m08837

Beidel, D. C., and Turner, S. M. (1997). At risk for anxiety: I. Psychopathology in the offspring of anxious parents. *J Am Acad Child Adolesc Psychiatry*, 36 (7), 918–924. doi: 10.1097/00004583-199707000-00013

Berkowitz, R. L., Coplan, J. D., Reddy, D. P., and Gorman, J. M. (2007). The human dimension: How the prefrontal cortex modulates the subcortical fear response. *Rev Neurosci*, 18 (3–4), 191–207.

Britton, J. C., Lissek, S., Grillon, C., Norcross, M. A., and Pine, D. S. (2011). Development of anxiety: The role of threat appraisal and fear learning. *Depress Anxiety*, 28 (1), 5–17. doi: 10.1002/da.20733

Brown, T. A., and Barlow, D. H. (2005). Dimensional versus categorical classification of mental disorders in the fifth edition of the Diagnostic and Statistical Manual of Mental Disorders and beyond: comment on the special section. *J Abnorm Psychol*, *114* (4), 551–556. doi: 10.1037/0021-8 43x.114.4.551

Brown, C., Schulberg, H. C., Madonia, M. J., Shear, M. K., and Houck, P. R. (1996). Treatment outcomes for primary care patients with major depression and lifetime anxiety disorders. *Am J Psychiatry*, *153* (10), 1293–1300.

Bruce, S. E., Yonkers, K. A., Otto, M. W., Eisen, J. L., Weisberg, R. B., Pagano, M., . . . Keller, M. B. (2005). Influence of psychiatric comorbidity on recovery and recurrence in generalized anxiety disorder, social phobia, and panic disorder: A 12-year prospective study. *Am J Psychiatry*, *162* (6), 1179–1187. doi: 10.1176/appi.ajp.162.6.1179

Bruhl, A. B., Delsignore, A., Komossa, K., and Weidt, S. (2014). Neuroimaging in social anxiety disorder: A meta-analytic review resulting in a new neurofunctional model. *Neurosci Biobehav Rev*, *47*, 260–280.

Cully, J. A., and Teten, A. L. (2008). *A Therapist's Guide to Brief Cognitive Behavioral Therapy*. Houston: Department of Veterans Affairs South Central MIRECC.

Cuthbert, B. N., and Insel, T. R. (2013). Toward the future of psychiatric diagnosis: The seven pillars of RDoC. *BMC Med*, *11*, 126. doi: 10.1186/1741-7015-11-126

Czajkowski, N., Roysamb, E., Reichborn-Kjennerud, T., and Tambs, K. (2010). A population based family study of symptoms of anxiety and depression: the HUNT study. *J Affect Disord*, *125* (1–3), 355–360. doi: 10.1016/j.jad.2010.01.006

Davidoff, J., Christensen, S., Khalili, D. N., Nguyen, J., and Ishak, W. W. (2012). Quality of life in panic disorder: Looking beyond symptom remission. *Qual Life Res*, *21*, 945–959.

Davidson, J. R., Hughes, D. L., George, L. K., and Blazer, D. G. (1993). The epidemiology of social phobia: Findings from the Duke Epidemiological Catchment Area Study. *Psychol Med*, *23*, 709–718.

Demirkan, A., Penninx, B. W., Hek, K., Wray, N. R., Amin, N., Aulchenko, Y. S., . . . Middeldorp, C. M. (2011). Genetic risk profiles for depression and anxiety in adult and elderly cohorts. *Mol Psychiatry*, *16* (7), 773–783. doi: 10.1038/mp.2010.65

Enns, M. W., and Cox, B. J. (1997). Personality dimensions and depression: review and commentary. *Can J Psychiatry*, *42* (3), 274–284.

Etkin, A., and Wager, T. D. (2007). Functional neuroimaging of anxiety: A meta-analysis of emotional processing in PTSD, social anxiety disorder, and specific phobia. *Am J Psychiatry*, *164* (10), 1476–1488. doi: 10.1176/appi.ajp.2007.07030504

Fava, M., Rankin, M. A., Wright, E. C., Alpert, J. E., Nierenberg, A. A., Pava, J., and Rosenbaum, J. F. (2000). Anxiety disorders in major depression. *Compr Psychiatry*, *41* (2), 97–102.

Fava, M., et al. (2008). Difference in treatment outcome in outpatients with anxious and nonanxious depression: A STAR*D report. *Am J Psychiatry*, *165*, 342–351.

Fracalanza, K., McCabe, R. E., Taylor, V. H., and Antony, M. M. (2014). The effect of comorbid major depressive disorder or bipolar disorder on cognitive behavioral therapy for social anxiety disorder. *J Affect Disord*, *162*, 61–66. doi: 10.1016/j.jad.2014.03.015

Frodl, T., Moller, H. J., and Meisenzahl, E. (2008). Neuroimaging genetics: New perspectives in research on major depression? *Acta Psychiatr Scand*, *118* (5), 363–372. doi: 10.1111/j.1600-0447. 2008.01225.x

Gatt, J. M., Nemeroff, C. B., Dobson-Stone, C., Paul, R. H., Bryant, R. A., . . . Williams, L. M. (2009). Interactions between BDNF Val66Met polymorphism and early life stress predict brain and arousal pathways to syndromal depression and anxiety. *Mol Psychiatry*, *14* (7), 681–695. doi: 10.1038/ mp.2008.143

Goodwin, R. D., Ofson, M., Feder, A., Fuentes, M., Pilowsky, D. J., and Weissman, M. M. (2001). Panic and suicidal ideation in primary care. *Depress Anxiety*, *14*, 244–246.

Goodwin, R. D., and Roy-Byrne, P. (2006). Panic and suicidal ideation and suicide attempts: Results from the National Comorbidity Survey. *Depression and Anxiety*, *23*, 124–132. doi: 10.1002/da.20151

Grant, B. F., Hasin, D. S., Stinson, F. S., Dawson, D. A., June Ruan, W., Goldstein, R. B., . . . Huang, B. (2005). Prevalence, correlates, co-morbidity, and comparative disability of DSM-IV generalized anxiety disorder in the USA: Results from the National Epidemiologic Survey on Alcohol and Related Conditions. *Psychol Med*, 35 (12), 1747–1759. doi: 10.1017/s0033291705006069

Hakamata, Yuko, Lissek, Shmuel, Bar-Haim, Yair, Britton, Jennifer C., Fox, Nathan A., Leibenluft, Ellen, . . . Pine, Daniel S. (2010). Attention bias modification treatment: A meta-analysis toward the establishment of novel treatment for anxiety. *Biological Psychiatry*, 68 (11), 982–990. doi: 10.1016/j. biopsych.2010.07.021

Hardin, M. G., Schroth, E., Pine, D. S., and Ernst, M. (2007). Incentive-related modulation of cognitive control in healthy, anxious, and depressed adolescents: development and psychopathology related differences. *J Child Psychol Psychiatry*, 48 (5), 446–454. doi: 10.1111/j.1469-7610.2006.01722.x

Hayes, Steven C, Strosahl, Kirk D, and Wilson, Kelly G. (1999). *Acceptance and commitment therapy: An experiential approach to behavior change*: Guilford Press.

Hettema, J. M., Neale, M. C., and Kendler, K. S. (2001). A review and meta-analysis of the genetic epidemiology of anxiety disorders. *Am J Psychiatry*, 158 (10), 1568–1578.

Hettema, J. M., Prescott, C. A., and Kendler, K. S. (2004). Genetic and environmental sources of covariation between generalized anxiety disorder and neuroticism. *Am J Psychiatry*, 161 (9), 1581–1587. doi: 10.1176/appi.ajp.161.9.1581

Hettema, J. M. (2008). The nosologic relationship between generalized anxiety disorder and major depression. *Depress Anxiety*, 25, 300–316. doi: 10.1002/da.20491

Hettema, J. M., An, S. S., Neale, M. C., Bukszar, J., van den Oord, E. J., . . . Chen, X. (2006). Association between acid decarboxylase genes and anxiety disorders, major depression, and neuroticism. *Mol Psychiatry*, 11 (8), 752–762.

Hirshfeld, D. R., Rosenbaum, J. F., Biederman, J., Bolduc, E. A., Faraone, S. V., Snidman, N., . . . Kagan, J. (1992). Stable behavioral inhibition and its association with anxiety disorder. *J Am Acad Child Adolesc Psychiatry*, 31 (1), 103–111. doi: 10.1097/00004583-199201000-00016

Jylha, P., and Isometsa, E. (2006). The relationship of neuroticism and extraversion to symptoms of anxiety and depression in the general population. *Depress Anxiety*, 23 (5), 281–289. doi: 10.1002/da.20167

Kaplan, J. S., Erickson, K., Luckenbaugh, D. A., Weiland-Fiedler, P., Geraci, M., Sahakian, B. J., . . . Neumeister, A. (2006). Differential performance on tasks of affective processing and decision-making in patients with Panic Disorder and Panic Disorder with comorbid Major Depressive Disorder. *J Affect Disord*, 95 (1–3), 165–171. doi: 10.1016/j.jad.2006.04.016

Kaufman, Erin A., and Baucom, Katherine J. W. (2014). Treating comorbid social anxiety and major depression: The challenge of diagnostic overshadowing. *Clinical Case Studies*, 13 (3), 265–281.

Keller, M. B. (2006). Prevalence and impact of comorbid anxiety and bipolar disorder. *J Clin Psychiatry*, 67, 5–7.

Kendler, K. S., Gardner, C. O., and Prescott, C. A. (2002). Toward a comprehensive developmental model for major depression in women. *Am J Psychiatry*, 159 (7), 1133–1145.

Kendler, K. S., Heath, A. C., Martin, N. G., and Eaves, L. J. (1987). Symptoms of anxiety and symptoms of depression. Same genes, different environments? *Arch Gen Psychiatry*, 44 (5), 451–457.

Kendler, K. S., Kuhn, J., and Prescott, C. A. (2004). The interrelationship of neuroticism, sex, and stressful life events in the prediction of episodes of major depression. *Am J Psychiatry*, 161 (4), 631–636.

Kendler, K. S., Neale, M. C., Kessler, R. C., Heath, A. C., and Eaves, L. J. (1992). Major depression and generalized anxiety disorder. Same genes, (partly) different environments? *Arch Gen Psychiatry*, 49 (9), 716–722.

Kessler, R. C., Berglund, P., Demler, O., Jin, R., Merikangas, K. R., and Walters, E. E. (2005). Lifetime prevalence and age-of-onset distributions of DSM-IV disorders in the National Comorbidity Survey Replication. *Arch Gen Psychiatry*, 62 (6), 593–602. doi: 10.1001/archpsyc.62.6.593

Kessler, R. C., Chiu, W. T., Jin, R., Ruscio, A. M., Shear, K., and Walters, E. E. (2006). The epidemiology of panic attacks, panic disorder, and agoraphobia in the National Comorbidity Survey Replication. *Arch Gen Psychiatry*, 63, 415–424.

Kessler, R. C., DuPont, R. L., Berglund, P., and Wittchen, H. U. (1999). Impairment in pure and comorbid generalized anxiety disorder and major depression at 12 months in two national surveys. *Am J Psychiatry, 156* (12), 1915–1923.

Kessler, R. C., Gruber, M., Hettema, J. M., Hwang, I., Sampson, N., and Yonkers, K. A. (2008). Co-morbid major depression and generalized anxiety disorders in the National Comorbidity Survey follow-up. *Psychol Med, 38* (3), 365–374. doi: 10.1017/s0033291707002012

Lyche, P., Jonassen, R., Stiles, T. C., Ulleberg, P., and Landro, N. I. (2010). Cognitive control functions in unipolar major depression with and without co-morbid anxiety disorder. *Front Psychiatry, 1*, 149. doi: 10.3389/fpsyt.2010.00149

Magee, W. J., Eaton, W. W., Wittchen, H. U., McGonagle, K. A., and Kessler, R. C. (1996). Agoraphobia, simple phobia, and social phobia in the National Comorbidity Survey. *Arch Gen Psychiatry, 53*, 159–168.

Maier, W., and Falkai, P. (1999). The epidemiology of comorbidity between depression, anxiety disorders and somatic diseases. *Int Clin Psychopharmacol, 14 Suppl 2*, S1–S6.

Malhi, G. S., Fritz, K., Coulston, C. M., Lampe, L., Bargh, D. M., Ablett, M., . . . Hopwood, M. (2014). Severity alone should no longer determine therapeutic choice in the management of depression in primary care: Findings from a survey of general practitioners. *J Affect Disord, 152–154*, 375–380. doi: 10.1016/j.jad.2013.09.040

Massion, A. O., Warshaw, M. G. and Keller, M. B. (1993). Quality of life and psychiatric morbidity in panic disorder and generalized anxiety disorder. *Am J Psychiatry, 150* (4):600–607.

Merikangas, Kathleen Ries, and Angst, Jules. (1995). Comorbidity and social phobia: evidence from clinical, epidemiologic, and genetic studies. *Eur Arch Psychiatry Clin Neurosci, 244* (6), 297–303.

Messina, I., Sambin, M., Palmieri, A., and Viviani, R. (2013). Neural correlates of psychotherapy in anxiety and depression: a meta-analysis. *PLoS One, 8* (9), e74657. doi: 10.1371/journal.pone.0074657

Middeldorp, C. M., Cath, D. C., Van Dyck, R., and Boomsma, D. I. (2005). The co-morbidity of anxiety and depression in the perspective of genetic epidemiology. A review of twin and family studies. *Psychol Med, 35* (5), 611–624.

Muris, P., Merckelbach, H., Schmidt, H., Gadet, B. B., and Bogie, N. (2001). Anxiety and depression as correlates of self-reported behavioural inhibition in normal adolescents. *Behav Res Ther, 39* (9), 1051–1061.

Nelson, B. D., McGowan, S. K., Sarapas, C., Robison-Andrew, E. J., Altman, S. E., Campbell, M. L., . . . Shankman, S. A. (2013). Biomarkers of threat and reward sensitivity demonstrate unique associations with risk for psychopathology. *J Abnorm Psychol, 122* (3), 662–671. doi: 10.1037/a0033982

Newman, M. G., Przeworski, A., Fisher, A. J., and Borkovec, T. D. (2010). Diagnostic comorbidity in adults with generalized anxiety disorder: Impact of comorbidity on psychotherapy outcome and impact of psychotherapy on comorbid diagnosis. *Behavior Therapy, 41*, 59–72.

Pollack, M. H. (2005). Comorbid anxiety and depression. *J Clin Psychiatry, 66 Suppl 8*, 22–29.

Pollack, M. H., Otto, M. W., Roy-Byrne, P. P., Coplan, J. D., Rothbaum, B. O., Simon, N. M., and Gorman, J. M. (2008). Novel treatment approaches for refractory anxiety disorders. *Depress Anxiety, 25* (6), 467–476. doi: 10.1002/da.20329

Ressler, K. J., and Mayberg, H. S. (2007). Targeting abnormal neural circuits in mood and anxiety disorders: from the laboratory to the clinic. *Nat Neurosci, 10* (9), 1116–1124. doi: 10.1038/nn1944

Roy-Byrne, P. P., and Katon, W. (1997). Generalized anxiety disorder in primary care: the precursor/modifier pathway to increased health care utilization. *J Clin Psychiatry, 58*, 34–38.

Schmidt, N. B., Eggleston, A. M., Woolaway-Bickel, K., Fitzpatrick, K. K., Vasey, M. W., and Richey, J. A. (2007). Anxiety Sensitivity Amelioration Training (ASAT): A longitudinal primary prevention program targeting cognitive vulnerability. *J Anxiety Disord, 21* (3), 302–319. doi: 10.1016/j.janxdis.2006.06.002

Shonkoff, J. P., Boyce, W. T., and McEwen, B. S. (2009). Neuroscience, molecular biology, and the childhood roots of health disparities: Building a new framework for health promotion and disease prevention. *JAMA, 301* (21), 2252–2259. doi: 10.1001/jama.2009.754

Siegle, Greg J., Ghinassi, Frank, and Thase, Michael E. (2007). Neurobehavioral therapies in the 21st century: Summary of an emerging field and an extended example of cognitive control training for depression. *Cogn Ther Res, 31* (2), 235–262.

Simon, N. M., Otto, M. W., Wisniewski, S. R., Fossey, M., Sagduyu, K., . . . Pollack, M. H. (2004). Anxiety disorder comorbidity in bipolar disorder patients: Data from the first 500 participants in the systematic treatment enhancement program for bipolar disorder (STEP-BD). *Am J Psychiatry, 161,* 2222–2229.

Simon, N. M. (2009). Generalized anxiety disorder and psychiatric comorbidities such as depression, bipolar disorder and substance abuse. *J Clin Psychiatry, 70,* 10–14.

Simon, N. M., and Rosenbaum, J. F. (2003). Anxiety and depression comorbidity: implications and intervention. Retrieved 7/25/14, from http://www.medscape.com/viewarticle/451325_print

Stein, M. B., et al. (2001). Social anxiety disorder and the risk of depression: A prospective community study of adolescents and young adults. *J Am Med Assoc Psychiatry, 58,* 251–256.

Taylor, S., Koch, W. J., Woody, S., and McLean, P. (1996). Anxiety sensitivity and depression: how are they related? *J Abnorm Psychol, 105* (3), 474–479.

Teasdale, J. D., Segal, Z., and Williams, J. M. (1995). How does cognitive therapy prevent depressive relapse and why should attentional control (mindfulness) training help? *Behav Res Ther, 33*(1), 25–39.

Van Ameringen, M., N. M., Stein, M. B. and Hermann, R. (2013). Comorbid anxiety and depression: Epidemiology, clinical manifestations, and diagnosis. Retrieved 7/25/14, from http://www.uptodate.com/contents/comorbid-anxiety-and-depression-epidemiology-clinical-manifestations-and-diagnosis

Wittchen, H. U., Kessler, R. C., Beesdo, K., Krause, P., Hofler, M., and Hoyer, J. (2002). Generalized anxiety and depression in primary care: prevalence, recognition, and management. *J Clin Psychiatry, 63 Suppl 8,* 24–34.

Wuthrich, V. M., and Rapee, R. M. (2013). Randomised controlled trial of group cognitive behavioural therapy for comorbid anxiety and depression in older adults. *Behav Res Ther, 51* (12), 779–786. doi: 10.1016/j.brat.2013.09.002

/// 22 /// GENERALIZED ANXIETY DISORDER

EMMANUEL GARCIA, MEGAN E. RENNA, AND DOUGLAS S. MENNIN

INTRODUCTION

> Living with GAD is like being on an endless rollercoaster ride. Some days I feel like a "normal" person, or at least what I imagine a "normal" person feels like. Other days I feel like the day is a weight that is too heavy for me to carry. All I want to do is put the weight down and crawl into my bed to escape the immense worry that I am feeling. And during major moments of anxiety, nothing matters but what I am worried about. Not receiving a call or text back from someone I care about can throw my mind into a state of terror; imagining all the horrible things that could have happened when in fact, they just didn't hear their phone ring or they are busy with something else. If I had to describe GAD in one word, I would say it is *paralyzing*.
>
> Janine

It is safe to assume that the experience of anxiety is familiar to most people, reflecting the capacity of our brains to imagine, anticipate, adapt, and plan for future goals and events (Mennin and Fresco, 2014). In this sense, anxiety is advantageous (Barlow, 2000). On a very different end of the anxiety spectrum are people like Janine, who live with *generalized anxiety disorder* (GAD). GAD can be a chronic, treatment resistant psychological disorder, characterized by heightened and persistent levels of worry and distressing physical symptoms (e.g. restlessness, irritability). If our ability to experience anxiety is a defining characteristic of being human, then people living with GAD may at times feel cursed as *too human*.

Despite the associated impairment, GAD is sometimes viewed as a mild problem of the "worried well" (Newman, Llera, Erickson, Przeworski, and Castonguay, 2013). As a result, research on GAD lags behind that of other disorders (Covin, Ouimet, Seeds, and Dozois, 2008; Newman et al., 2013). Nevertheless, the last 30 years has spawned a compelling body of research on GAD (e.g. Behar, DiMarco, Hekler, Mohlman, and Staples, 2009).

This chapter highlights the current state of GAD nosology, theory, and treatment. Specifically, the chapter reviews (1) how GAD is currently defined and classified both categorically and dimensionally, (2) advances in conceptual models, (3) advances in treatment, and (4) future research directions.

WHAT IS GENERALIZED ANXIETY DISORDER?

Diagnostic Criteria

Two categorical classification systems exist that treat GAD as a unique diagnostic category: the International Classification of Diseases (ICD-10; World Health Organization, 1992), and the Diagnostic and Statistical Manual of Mental Disorders (DSM-5; American Psychiatric Association, 2013). As concordance between the two systems is only fair, and the DSM-5 focus on excessive anxiety and worry is more closely aligned with contemporary empirical research, this chapter highlights the DSM-5.

Pathological versus Nonpathological Anxiety and Worry

The defining feature of GAD is chronic and excessive worry (Huppert and Sanderson, 2002). Research advances stem from a fine-grained understanding of "the nature and functions of worry" (Borkovec, Alcaine, and Behar, 2004). The DSM-5 outlines some important distinctions between the anxiety and worry individuals with GAD experience, in contrast to non-pathological anxiety and worry. First, for people with GAD, anxiety and worry is *excessive*, or out of proportion with both the likelihood and potential impact of the apprehensively anticipated event. Unlike the day-to-day worries of the general population, for people with GAD, worries are distressing, arresting, and debilitating—contributing to marked disturbances in functioning. Second, for people with GAD, anxiety and worry are *pervasive*, in terms of frequency, duration, and range of worry topics. People with GAD worry more often, much longer, and about many more things than the general population; and often worries arise with no clear precipitants. Third, for people with GAD, worry and anxiety are accompanied by discomforting and disruptive *physical symptoms* (e.g. restlessness, difficulty concentrating, sleep disturbances), which also are distressing and impairing.

GENERALIZED ANXIETY DISORDER AND THE RESEARCH DOMAIN CRITERIA

The DSM manuals have provided useful heuristics. However, a classification system based solely on signs and symptoms is limited, and the nosological history of GAD in the DSM has been historically problematic. Limitations have led to questions about the suitability of diagnostic categories for isolating and elucidating the fundamental mechanisms underlying GAD and other mental disorders. For example, worry is featured in the DSM, but not in a way that captures its putative dimensional and transdiagnostic features (Brown and Barlow, 2009). In addition, neural, genetic, and other biological substrates of biopsychosocial constructs central to clinical research and practice, cannot be easily integrated into the DSM categorical framework—hindering progress in research and treatment (Hyman, 2007; Insel et al., 2010).

Recognition of these limitations prompted the National Institute of Mental Health (NIMH) Research Domain Criteria (RDoC) project, an effort "to create a framework for research on pathophysiology . . . which ultimately will inform future classification schemes (Insel et al., 2010, p. 748)." This RDoC framework is presented as a matrix of constructs and variables that represent fundamental units of analysis meant to serve as a starting point for engendering clinical research and input from the field.[1] The RDoC initiative encourages researchers and clinicians to incorporate insights from clinical science and genetics as they engage in an ongoing constructive dialogue aimed at better aligning research findings with clinical judgments (Insel et al., 2010). It is expected that data from these combined efforts will enhance conceptual and treatment models of GAD by expanding clinical evaluation of the disorder (e.g. by elucidating underlying mechanisms such as apprehension in the negative valence domain of RDoC).

Reasons You Should Worry about GAD

GAD is one of the most common anxiety disorders (Fisher, 2007). Results from the National Comorbidity Study Lifetime prevalence estimates (NCS-R) indicate that the 12-month prevalence of GAD is 3.1% (Kessler et al., 2005b) and the lifetime prevalence is 5.7% (Kessler, et al., 2005a). However, these statistics are based on retrospective assessments, which may underestimate the prevalence of psychopathology. In a recent prospective study the 12-month prevalence of GAD was 4.2% and the lifetime prevalence was 14.2% (Moffitt et al., 2010). Women are twice as likely to be diagnosed with GAD as men (with lifetime prevalence rates of 5.3% versus 2.8% for men; Newman et al., 2013). GAD symptoms start to appear in childhood and both incidence and prevalence continue into late adulthood (Kessler, Walters, and Wittchen, 2004). GAD is possibly the most common anxiety disorder among people aged 55–85 years (Beekman et al., 1998). Caucasian and Native American individuals have higher 12-month prevalence rates of GAD than Black, Asian, and Latina/o individuals (Newman et al., 2013).

GAD is the most frequently seen anxiety disorder in primary care settings both in the U.S. (Barrett, Barrett, Oxman, and Gerber, 1988) and throughout the world (Kessler et al., 2004). As a result, GAD is associated with significantly increased health care utilization and costs, decreased productivity, and significant role impairment (e.g., Greenberg et al., 1999; Newman et al., 2013; Wittchen, Krause, Hoyer, Beesdo, Jacobi, Hofler, and Winter, 2001). Further, Whisman and colleagues (2000) found GAD to have the highest rate of marital dissatisfaction among psychiatric disorders in the Ontario Health Survey Mental Health Supplement (i.e., OHS). Several studies indicate that the degree of impairment experienced by persons with GAD is similar to that experienced by persons with major depression (e.g., Kessler and Wittchen, 1999; Wittchen et al., 2001) and panic disorder (e.g., Hunt, Slade, and Andrews, 2004). GAD characteristically follows a chronic course (Tyrer and Baldwin, 2006) and the rate of spontaneous remission over a five-year period is low (Yonkers, Dyck, Warshaw, and Keller, 2000). Most people diagnosed with GAD still suffer with the disorder six to twelve years after the initial diagnosis (Tyrer and Baldwin, 2006).

Finally, GAD is highly comorbid with other disorders (Kessler and Wittchen, 1999). Although "pure" presentations may be higher in primary care settings than are typically reported in psychiatric settings (Wittchen et al., 2001), non-comorbid GAD is rare when evaluated longitudinally (Bruce, Machan, Dyck, and Keller, 2001). Approximately three out of every five people with GAD are also diagnosed with comorbid depression (Fisher,

2007; Tyrer and Baldwin, 2006; Newman et al., 2013). Around four out of every five individuals with lifetime GAD suffer from a mood disorder at some point (Judd et al., 1998). Even in countries with wide access to treatment, the high comorbidity of GAD with other disorders makes treatment of both of GAD and comorbid disorders less efficacious and more costly, and recovery less predictable and stable. GAD is the least successfully treated anxiety disorder (Newman et al., 2013), and people with comorbid GAD and depression may engage more in negative self-referential thought—making them especially treatment refractory (Mennin and Fresco, 2013).

CONCEPTUAL ADVANCES OF GENERALIZED ANXIETY DISORDER

Over the past several decades, important advances have been made in the conceptualization of generalized anxiety disorder (GAD) and its core features. Contemporary conceptual models of GAD share common origins, but contain important "evidence based" theoretical differences that impact treatment approaches and contribute to heterogeneity (Behar et al., 2009; Newman et al., 2013). Progress towards the integration of these models may be possible by considering each perspective as a contributing chapter to a larger volume of evolving best-practice GAD research and treatment. At the heart of each perspective are several basic shared tenets that converge on the central roles of avoidance and worry in the development and maintenance of GAD.

Barlow (2000) set the stage for such integration; he defines anxiety as *anxious apprehension* and describes it as a state of preparation that draws on our cognitive and emotional faculties to anticipate, minimize, and cope with future threat(s). Anxious apprehension is generically modeled as a process that involves: (1) preexisting biopsychosocial vulnerabilities; (2) conscious or unconscious cues or triggers that evoke anxiety; (3) overwhelming negative affect accompanied by central and peripheral nervous system arousal that is experienced as aversive and uncontrollable; (4) a shift to self-focused attention; (5) cognitive distortions driven by biases and hypervigilance to threat; and (6) behavioral avoidance and worry as coping mechanisms.

In the cognitive avoidance model of worry and GAD, Borkovec and colleagues (2004) expand conceptually on anxious apprehension in GAD by first demonstrating that people with GAD are predisposed to detect threat cues "that exist solely in the mind [and] refer to possible bad events in the future which do not actually exist in the present moment (p. 16)." Catastrophic mental images trigger the anxiety process, which is intensified by the additional threat of subsequent overwhelming aversive emotional and physiological distress. Worry is conceptualized as a functional verbal linguistic process ("talking to oneself in anxious ways") and a self-focused cognitive avoidance strategy. People with GAD worry as an attempt to simultaneously (a) shift attention away from, or mute by interrupting, aversive mental images and emotional/ physiological arousal, and (b) solve the anxiously anticipated problem of perceived threat. Worry fails as a coping mechanism by preventing exposure to a full range of experiences that could lead to extinction. Instead, worry is reinforced when it provides relief from aversive internal images and hyperarousal, perhaps by making the world feel more predictable and controllable (Huppert and Sanderson, 2002). Positive beliefs about worry as an effective means to avoid or prevent perceived threats are generated and/or reinforced—which paradoxically produces and maintains GAD pathology.

Subsequent conceptual models of GAD differentially combine and expand on aspects of this earlier work. Each model maintains a core emphasis on avoidance of overwhelming threatening and aversive internal experiences, and features excessive worry (Behar et al., 2009; Fisher, 2007; Llera and Newman, 2014). Models of GAD diverge when (1) emphasizing *what* exactly people are predisposed to experience as most threatening and aversive—prompting avoidance and (2) explaining *how* worry contributes to the maladaptive processes that produce and maintain GAD. These models emphasize cognitive (i.e., intolerance of uncertainty: Robichaud and Dugas, 2006; meta-worry: Wells and King, 2006), interpersonal (Newman and Erickson, 2010), and emotional (i.e., non-acceptance: Roemer, Orsillo, and Salters-Pedneault, 2008; dysregulation: Mennin and Fresco, 2014; contrast avoidance; Llera and Newman, 2014) processes in GAD. The Contrast Avoidance Model extends the functional perspective of GAD by clarifying that worry becomes reinforced by increasing the predictability of negative emotional experiences, often at the cost of experiencing positive and rewarding states (i.e., diminishing emotional contrasts; Llera and Newman, 2014). However, Newman and colleagues emphasize negative emotional contrasts, rather than aversive emotional/physiological arousal, as the main focus of anxious apprehension, and suggest that people with GAD cope by using worry to "recruit, rather than to avoid" negative emotional arousal (Llera and Newman, 2014).

The burgeoning field of affect science may provide a comprehensive yet empirically sound framework for integrating these findings and theorizations, particularly in relation to compensatory functions of worry and other destructive forms of self-referential mentation that are common in GAD and related disorders. Mennin and Fresco (2014) have posited that dysfunction in GAD can best be understood as follows:

1. *Motivational mechanisms.* People with GAD experience elevated subjective emotional intensity/distress, reflecting greater temperamental negative affect and the activation of underlying motivational systems. For people with GAD greater temperamental affect creates bias to prioritize obtaining safety (from perceived threat) over attaining reward.

2. *Regulatory mechanisms.* People with GAD may respond poorly to the motivational conflicts resulting from prioritizing safety over reward (e.g. conflicts with valued goals and actions), demonstrating deficits in both lesser (i.e., attentional) and more elaborative (i.e., meta-cognitive) forms of emotion regulation. To compensate for their inability to manage distressing emotions and motivational conflicts, people with GAD may then resort to perseverative strategies (e.g., worry, rumination, and self-criticism) for relief.

3. *Contextual learning consequences.* The net result of these regulatory failures is a paradoxical maintenance of the very negative states that people with GAD seek to avoid (Newman et al., 2013)—along with reduced clarity in understanding and optimally responding to these negative states. Indeed, worry results in increased ability to be conditioned to threat, greater stimulus generalization, and diminished ability to discriminate stimuli and learning contingencies, and GAD is associated with restrictions in valued actions and goals. Further, rumination, often found in GAD especially when comorbid with MDD, is associated with decreases in the likelihood of new reward-based learning, weakens instrumental action, and engagement of potentially rewarding social networks (see Figure 22.1 for a summary of normative and GAD-related deficits in these components; for a more detailed description of this model, see Mennin and Fresco, 2014). Further research is necessary to support this affect science conceptualization and whether it provides a useful framework for the extant approaches to GAD.

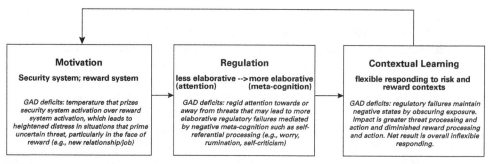

FIGURE 22.1 Affect-science-based integrative model of GAD.

TREATMENT ADVANCES FOR GENERALIZED ANXIETY DISORDER

Treatment Approaches

Well studied treatments include: cognitive behavioral therapies (CBTs) and other psychotherapies; non-psychotherapeutic interventions (e.g. attention-bias modification); hybrid approaches; and existing/new biologically based treatments (e.g. pharmacotherapy; repetitive transcranial magnetic stimulation).

Cognitive behavioral therapies (CBTs). The American Psychological Association (APA) Division 12 (Clinical Psychology) Task Force on Psychological Interventions currently lists cognitive and behavioral therapies as having a "strong research support" status,[2,3] and similar support comes from The National Institute for Clinical Excellence in the United Kingdom, International Consensus Group on Anxiety and Depression, and Dutch guidelines for treatment of anxiety (see Huppert and Sanderson, 2002 for a review). Average effect sizes range from moderately large (ES = 0.73) to large (ES = –1.15 for the reduction of worry; see Covin et al., 2008), but vary based on comparison group(s) and method of outcome assessment (see Cuijpers, Sijbrandij, Koole, Huibers, Berking, and Andersson, 2014). CBT is well-received by clients, and has one of the lowest dropout rates among all types of therapies (Borkovec, Newman, Pincus, and Lytle, 2002).

CBT comes in different flavors, or packages, which have been referred to collectively as the "family of CBTs" (Mennin, Ellard, Fresco, and Gross, 2013). CBTs differ from one another mainly by what is emphasized during treatment based on conceptual perspectives. For example, key components of CBT guided by the cognitive avoidance model of worry and GAD (Borkovec et al., 2004) have included: self-monitoring, relaxation techniques, self-control desensitization, gradual stimulus control, cognitive restructuring, worry outcome monitoring, present-moment focus, and expectancy free living. CBT components aimed at increasing tolerance for and acceptance of uncertainty (e.g. intolerance of uncertainty education, evaluating worry beliefs, etc.; Robichaud and Dugas, 2006), and altering a client's beliefs and coping strategies related to worry (case formation; discussing uncontrollability, danger, and positive beliefs about worry, etc.; Wells and King, 2006) have been featured in CBTs focused on cognitive processes in GAD.

CBTs focused on intolerance of uncertainty in GAD have included: psycho-education about CBT and GAD; worry awareness training; coping with uncertainty; re-evaluating beliefs about the usefulness of worry; improving problem orientation and problem-solving ability; (6) processing core fears through imaginal exposure; and relapse prevention (Robichaud and Dugas, 2006). Integrated approaches have focused both on correcting maladaptive interpersonal problems and understanding the relationship of emotions to the clients' interpersonal needs (e.g. Newman, Jacobson, and Castonguay, 2014). Mindfulness and acceptance based CBTs have emphasized the therapeutic relationship, client self-monitoring, mindfulness practices, values articulation, and behavioral change strategies, with the goal of helping clients relate to their internal emotional experiences differently—thus reducing avoidance behaviors (e.g. Hayes-Skelton, Orsillo, and Roemer, 2013). Further, congruent with an affect science framework, Mennin and Fresco (2014) have developed Emotion Regulation Therapy (ERT), which draws from traditional and contemporary CBT, as well as experiential therapy, in order to form an integrated, mechanism-targeted, CBT. Specifically, ERT was designed to improve acute and enduring treatment efficacy for GAD, especially when comorbid with MDD. ERT clients focus on increasing motivational awareness, developing a range of regulatory capacities (from less to more elaborate), and engaging novel contexts to generate new learning repertoires (Mennin and Fresco, 2014).

Pharmacological treatments. When considering safety, tolerability, and effectiveness, the current consensus is that selective serotonin re-uptake inhibitor (SSRI; e.g. escitalopram, paroxetine, sertraline) and serotonin-norepinephrine re-uptake inhibitor (SNRI; e.g. venlafaxine, duloxetine) antidepressants are the best both acute and longer-term pharmacological treatments for GAD, followed by benzodiazepines for acute symptom management (Baldwin and Polkinghorn, 2005). A detailed account of the advantages and disadvantages of pharmacological treatments, including a more extensive list of available options, is beyond the scope of this chapter—and readers are encouraged to consult extant reviews and standards (e.g. Anderson and Palm, 2006; Baldwin and Polkinghorn, 2005).

CBTs verses Pharmacological treatments. CBT is widely considered to be a preferred first-line treatment for GAD, while others emphasize pharmacological therapy as a first-line treatment. The reality is that there is not enough evidence to support either view, or whether it is advantageous to combine CBT with pharmacological therapy (Cuijpers et al., 2014; Durham, 2007; Newman et al., 2013). There is some preliminary evidence, however, that CBT is more effective than pharmacotherapy for long-term treatment gains (Durham, 2007).

In addition, many studies have shown that psychotherapies (CBTs in particular) are as effective as pharmacological treatments for GAD (Cuijpers et al., 2014). In the long-term, CBTs may even be more effective than pharmacotherapy (Hunt, 2000), as CBTs feature psychoeducation and training (e.g., coping skills) that may lead to increases in feelings of control and mastery in clients, translating to more durable GAD remission (Behar et al., 2009). A recent meta-analysis on CBTs for GAD reports a large overall effect size for treatment effects on depression ($g = 0.71$) in addition to GAD ($g = 0.90$; Cuijpers et al., 2014). Finally, potentially adverse side effects of medications and evidence that pharmacotherapy may not significantly impact worry (Anderson and Palm, 2006) may dissuade some from favoring pharmacological treatments for GAD.

However, many people with GAD are unwilling or unable to avail themselves of psychotherapy (Kazdin and Blase, 2011), so may prefer or have no alternatives to pharmacotherapy (Durham, 2007). About 80% of people with GAD seek treatment in primary care settings, where advances in GAD research and clinical practice remain poorly understood and recognized, leading to non-specific treatment that may or may not include a referral to high-quality psychotherapy (Crits-Christoph et al., 2011). Antidepressants are the most commonly used type of pharmaceutical to treat GAD and may also alleviate both symptoms of GAD and comorbid depression, making them a potentially attractive option to people with GAD and comorbid depressive disorders.

Nontherapeutic interventions. Some limitations of first-line therapeutic and pharmacological interventions for GAD have led to the development of non-therapeutic interventions, which may augment existing treatments or eventually serve as stand-alone treatments. CBT and pharmacotherapy have about a 50% success rate in GAD remission (Durham, 2007) leaving substantial room for improvement. There are also practical barriers (e.g. cost, stigma, limited time) that prevent people from receiving first-line treatment for GAD (Greenberg et al., 1999). Also, extant treatments were largely formulated based on the categorical diagnostic criteria of the DSM manuals, which does not suitably incorporate insights from clinical science and genetics that may lead to better interventions (Insel et al., 2010; Mennin and Fresco, 2013). Two examples of non-therapeutic interventions for GAD are attention bias modification (ABM) and repetitive transcranial magnetic stimulation (rTMS).

Attention bias modification. ABM was developed based on cognitive and behavioral accounts identifying attentional bias (termed the "threat bias") as an important mechanism underlying the onset, etiology, and maintenance of anxiety disorders (Bar-Haim, 2010). ABM protocols for GAD are designed to both measure and manipulate early, automatic, unconscious biases to threatening stimuli by systematically training attention away from threat and towards neutral or pleasant stimuli. The idea is that by creating attentional competition (i.e., threatening vs. neutral stimuli) and repeatedly directing people's attention to the neutral stimuli, threat bias is reduced (see Bar-Haim, 2010 for a review). There is evidence from a recent meta-analysis that ABM is effective in reducing threat bias with a large effect size ($d = 1.16$) that is maintained at between one and six month follow-ups (Hakamata et al., 2010). Two studies have reported success in remission of GAD symptoms after ABM training, however more studies are needed to determine the optimal use of ABM in GAD treatment specifically (Bar-Haim, 2010). ABM is user friendly and circumvents many of the barriers inherent to first-line treatments (Amir and Taylor, 2012). Continuing research on a recently released gamified mobile version of ABM has captured the attention of both researchers and the general public (Dennis and O'Toole, 2014), which is a strong sign that ABM (and perhaps other non-traditional interventions) will likely have a role in future GAD research and treatment.

Repetitive transcranial magnetic stimulation. rTMS is a noninvasive procedure that involves the delivery of repetitive magnetic stimulation to the frontal or temporal lobes. A pilot trial of fMRI guided rTMS showed significant decreases of anxiety symptoms occurring in GAD in every enrolled participant, with some patients also reporting a reduction in treatment resistant depression and insomnia after just one session (Bystritsky et al., 2008). Despite these exciting preliminary findings, more testing is needed to determine how rTMS may be used in GAD treatment.

FUTURE DIRECTIONS IN THE UNDERSTANDING AND TREATMENT OF GENERALIZED ANXIETY DISORDER

Despite significant advances in research and practice, GAD is the *most treatment refractory anxiety disorder* (Newman et al., 2013). With this in mind, we recommend three specific ways the field can advance in better understanding and treating GAD.

Adopt Common Change Principles

For decades researchers and clinicians have called for rapprochement and a shift to "shared goals, change principles, and therapeutic processes" (Mennin et al., 2013, p. 234) as a major way to advance clinical research and practice. Goldfried (1980) argues that a meaningful consensus can be found by jointly developing empirically grounded *clinical strategies* or *principles of change* as heuristics to guide our practice. Contemporary treatments for GAD share theoretical origins (e.g. Barlow, 2000; Borkovec et al., 2004), but diverge on the conceptualization of targets and packaging of treatment components. However, these distinctions may reflect "faux-uniqueness" (Mennin et al., 2013) as the approaches commonly place a core emphasis on avoidance of overwhelming threatening and aversive internal experiences and target excessive worry as a maladaptive emotion regulation strategy (Borkovec et al., 2004). Adopting this common viewpoint allows for a principle of change that translates into therapeutic practice, in this case encouraging individuals with GAD to engage in what they previously avoided (e.g. to sit with uncomfortable emotions, to cope with uncertainty, to tolerate emotional/motivational contrasts) and providing therapeutic support and training that allows these individuals to eventually master this change.

Use and Extend the Research Domain Criteria

The research domain criteria (RDoC) framework is a promising way for the field to have greater focus on mechanisms underlying the etiology and maintenance of GAD that cut across diagnostic categories and that have durable, testable biobehavioral substrates (e.g., behavioral tasks, functional magnetic resonance imaging, psychophysiology; Insel et al., 2010). Combined with insights gained from categorical frameworks (e.g. the DSM and ICD), the RDoC framework may lead to better understanding and treating psychopathology. For example, Brown and Barlow (2009) discuss an intriguing "diagnostic profile" that combines categorical (e.g. DSM-V) with dimensional (e.g. RDoC) data as a way to merge insights gained from these two frameworks and better capture important phenomena related to GAD. Mennin and Fresco (2013) encourage an extension of both categorical and dimensional frameworks to better understand and treat mechanisms central to GAD etiology and maintenance (e.g. negative self-referential processing; NSRP). The testing of these ideas will undoubtedly lead to important advances in the understanding and treatment of GAD and may be an important way to establish common change principles.

Listen to Patients

Clients with GAD often are reliant upon therapists' interventions and insight in hopes of ameliorating psychological symptoms. Historically, however, some of our most important advances in psychotherapy research and practice have occurred by carefully listening to clients' experiences and insights (Bohart, 2007). Cougle (2012) suggests that one important way we may listen to our clients is by adopting a "quality-oriented" approach to clinical research and practice. This includes requesting and assessing feedback from clients on the parsimony, ease, and efficiency of interventions when evaluating their effectiveness. For example, people with GAD have responded positively to computer and/or app-based interventions (e.g. Amir and Taylor, 2012; Dennis and O'Toole, 2014). However, while these approaches, in addition to technology-delivered interventions are likely to be popular or preferable for those who lack time and access for more extensive, in-person interventions, further data is needed to ensure that they produce strong and lasting effects for refractory patients such as those with GAD. In an effort to establish balance between best practice and client preferences, we as mental health professionals must figure out how to best listen to individuals with GAD so that we are able to help achieve the greatest treatment gains possible.

CONCLUSION

The past thirty years have seen a surge in the understanding of GAD. The field has produced a reliable knowledge and skill base of which advances in understanding and treatment of GAD have grown, thus elucidating the core features of one of the most prevalent, costly, and treatment resistant anxiety disorder. The current chapter has highlighted these advances and suggested how these advances can potentially be integrated in conceptualization and intervention in order to help further propel research on GAD forward. It is our hope that the information highlighted in this chapter will foster improvements in research, treatment, communication, and collaboration—towards the common value of helping those who are suffering from the debilitating symptoms associated with GAD.

DISCLOSURE STATEMENTS

Emmanuel Garcia is funded by NIH MBRS-RISE Program at Hunter College Grant# GM060665. Megan E. Renna and Douglas S. Mennin have no conflicts to disclose.

NOTES

1. http://www.nimh.nih.gov/research-priorities/rdoc/nimh-research-domain-criteria-rdoc. shtml#toc_matrix
2. http://www.psychologicaltreatments.org/
3. National Institute for Clinical Excellence in the United Kingdom; The Substance Abuse and Mental Health Services Administration (SAMHSA) also maintains a National Registry of Evidence-Based Programs and Practices that includes treatments for GAD; http://www.nrepp.samhsa.gov/

REFERENCES

American Psychiatric Association (2013). *Diagnostic and statistical manual of mental disorders* (5th ed.). Arlington, VA: American Psychiatric Publishing.

Amir, N., and Taylor, C. T. (2012). Combining computerized home-based treatments for generalized anxiety disorder: An attention modification program and cognitive behavioral therapy. *Behav Therapy*, 43 (3), 546–559.

Anderson, I. M., and Palm, M. E. (2006). Pharmacological treatments for worry: Focus on generalised anxiety disorder. In G. C. Davey, A. Wells (Eds.), *Worry and its psychological disorders: Theory, assessment and treatment* (305–334). Chichester, UK: John Wiley & Sons, Ltd.

Baldwin, D. S., and Polkinghorn, C. (2005). Evidence-based pharmacotherapy of generalized anxiety disorder. *Int J Neuropsychopharmacol*, 8 (02), 293–302.

Bar-Haim, Y. (2010). Attention bias modification (ABM): A novel treatment for anxiety disorders. *J Child Psychol Psychiatry*, 51 (8), 859–870.

Barlow, D. H. (2000). Unraveling the mysteries of anxiety and its disorders from the perspective of emotion theory. *Am Psychol*, 55 (11), 1247.

Barrett, J. E., Barrett, J. A., Oxman, T. E., and Gerber, P. D. (1988). The prevalence of psychiatric disorders in a primary care practice. *Arch Gen Psychiatry*, 45 (12), 1100–1106.

Beekman, A. T., Bremmer, M. A., Deeg, D. J., Van Balkom, A. J., Smit, J. H., De Beurs, E., . . . Van Tilburg, W. (1998). Anxiety disorders in later life: A report from the Longitudinal Aging Study Amsterdam. *Int J Geriatr Psychiatry*, 13 (10), 717–726.

Behar, E., DiMarco, I. D., Hekler, E. B., Mohlman, J., Staples, A. M. (2009). Current theoretical models of generalized anxiety disorder (GAD): Conceptual review and treatment implications. *J Anxiety Disord*, 23 (8), 1011–1023.

Bohart, A. C. (2007). An alternative view of concrete operating procedures from the perspective of the client as active self-healer. *J Psychother Integration*, 17 (1), 125.

Borkovec, T. D., Alcaine, O., and Behar, E. (2004). Avoidance theory of worry and generalized anxiety disorder. In R. G. Heimberg, C. L. Turk, and D. S. Mennin (Eds.), *Generalized anxiety disorder: Advances in research and practice* (pp. 77–108). New York: Guilford Press.

Borkovec, T. D., Newman, M. G., Pincus, A. L., and Lytle, R. (2002). A component analysis of cognitive-behavioral therapy for generalized anxiety disorder and the role of interpersonal problems. *J Consult Clin Psychol*, 70(2), 288.

Brown, T. A., and Barlow, D. H. (2009). A proposal for a dimensional classification system based on the shared features of the DSM-IV anxiety and mood disorders: Implications for assessment and treatment. *Psycholl Assess*, 21 (3), 256.

Bruce, S. E., Machan, J. T., Dyck, I., and Keller, M. B. (2001). Infrequency of "pure" GAD: Impact of psychiatric comorbidity on clinical course. *Depress Anxiety*, 14 (4), 219–225.

Bystritsky, A., Kaplan, J. T., Feusner, J. D., Kerwin, L. E., Wadekar, M., Burock, M., . . . and Iacoboni, M. (2008). A preliminary study of fMRI-guided rTMS in the treatment of generalized anxiety disorder. *J Clin Psychiatry*, 69 (7), 1092–1098.

Cougle, J. R. (2012). What makes a quality therapy? A consideration of parsimony, ease, and efficiency. *Behav Therapy*, 43 (3), 468–481.

Covin, R., Ouimet, A. J., Seeds, P. M., and Dozois, D. J. (2008). A meta-analysis of CBT for pathological worry among clients with GAD. *J Anxiety Disorders*, 22 (1), 108–116.

Crits-Christoph, P., Newman, M. G., Rickels, K., Gallop, R., Gibbons, M. B. C., Hamilton, J. L., . . . and Pastva, A. M. (2011). Combined medication and cognitive therapy for generalized anxiety disorder. *J Anxiety Disorders*, 25 (8), 1087–1094.

Cuijpers, P., Sijbrandij, M., Koole, S., Huibers, M., Berking, M., and Andersson, G. (2014). Psychological treatment of generalized anxiety disorder: A meta-analysis. *Clin Psychol Rev, 34* (2), 130–140.

Dennis, T. A., and O'Toole, L. J. (2014). Mental health on the go: Effects of a gamified attention-bias modification mobile application in trait-anxious adults. *Clin Psychol Sci*, 2, 576–590. doi: 10.1177/2167702614522228

Durham, R. C. (2007). Treatment of generalized anxiety disorder. *Psychiatry*, 6 (5), 183–187.

Fisher, P. L. (2007). Psychopathology of generalized anxiety disorder. *Psychiatry*, 6 (5), 171–175.

Goldfried, M. R. (1980). Toward the delineation of therapeutic change principles. *Am Psychol*, 35 (11), 991–999.

Greenberg, P. E., Sisitsky, T., Kessler, R. C., Finkelstein, S. N., Berndt, E. R., Davidson, J. R., . . . Fyer, A. J. (1999). The economic burden of anxiety disorders in the 1990s. *J Clin Psychiatry*, 60 (7), 427–435.

Hakamata, Y., Lissek, S., Bar-Haim, Y., Britton, J. C., Fox, N. A., Leibenluft, E., . . . Pine, D. S. (2010). Attention bias modification treatment: A meta-analysis toward the establishment of novel treatment for anxiety. *Biol Psychiatry*, 68 (11), 982–990.

Hayes-Skelton, S. A., Orsillo, S. M., & Roemer, L. (2013). An acceptance-based behavioral therapy for individuals with generalized anxiety disorder. *Cog Behav Pract*, 20 (3), 264–281.

Hunt, C. (2000). The treatment of generalised anxiety disorder. *Clin Psychol*, 5 (2), 41–48.

Hunt, C., Slade, T., and Andrews, G. (2004). Generalized anxiety disorder and major depressive disorder comorbidity in the National Survey of Mental Health and Well-Being. *Depress Anxiety, 20* (1), 23–31.

Huppert, J. D., and Sanderson, W. C. (2002). Psychotherapy for generalized anxiety disorder. In D. J. Stein, and E. Hollander (Eds.), *Textbook of anxiety disorders* (pp. 219–238). Washington: American Psychiatric Publishing, Inc.

Hyman, S. E. (2007). Can neuroscience be integrated into the DSM-V? *Nature Rev Neurosci, 8*(9), 725–732.

Insel, T., Cuthbert, B., Garvey, M., Heinssen, R., Pine, D. S., Quinn, K., . . . Wang, P. (2010). Research domain criteria (RDoC): Toward a new classification framework for research on mental disorders. *Am J Psychiatry, 167* (7), 748–751.

Judd, L. L., Kessler, R. C., Paulus, M. P., Zeller, P. V., Wittchen, H. U., and Kunovac, J. L. (1998). Comorbidity as a fundamental feature of generalized anxiety disorders: Results from the National Comorbidity Study (NCS). *Acta Psychiatrica Scandinavica, 98* (s393), 6–11.

Kazdin, A. E., and Blase, S. L. (2011). Rebooting psychotherapy research and practice to reduce the burden of mental illness. *Perspect Psychol Sci, 6* (1), 21–37.

Kessler, R. C., and Wittchen, H. U. (1999). Anxiety, mood, and substance abuse disorders: Patterns and correlates of comorbidity. *Eur Neuropsychopharmacol, 9*, 142–144.

Kessler, R. C., Berglund, P., Demler, O., Jin, R., Merikangas, K. R., and Walters, E. E. (2005a). Lifetime prevalence and age-of-onset distributions of DSM-IV disorders in the National Comorbidity Survey Replication. *Arch Gen Psychiatry, 62* (6), 593–602.

Kessler, R. C., Brandenburg, N., Lane, M., Roy-Byrne, P., Stang, P. D., Stein, D. J., and Wittchen, H. U. (2005b). Rethinking the duration requirement for generalized anxiety disorder: Evidence from the National Comorbidity Survey Replication. *Psychol Med, 35* (07), 1073–1082.

Kessler, R. C., Walters, E. E., and Wittchen, H. U. (2004). Epidemiology. In R. G. Heimberg, C. L. Turk, and D. S. Mennin (Eds.), *Generalized anxiety disorder: Advances in research and practice* (pp. 29–50). New York: Guilford Press.

Llera, S. J., and Newman, M. G. (2014). Rethinking the role of worry in generalized anxiety disorder: Evidence supporting a model of emotional contrast avoidance. *Behav Ther, 45* (3), 283–299.

Mennin, D. S., Ellard, K. K., Fresco, D. M., and Gross, J. J. (2013). United we stand: Emphasizing commonalities across cognitive-behavioral therapies. *Behav Ther, 44* (2), 234–248.

Mennin, D. S., and Fresco, D. M. (2013). What, me worry and ruminate about DSM-5 and RDoC? The importance of targeting negative self-referential processing. *Clin Psychol Sci Pract, 20* (3), 258–267.

Mennin, D. S. and Fresco, D. M. (2014). Emotion regulation therapy. In J. J. Gross (Ed.) *Handbook of emotion regulation* (pp. 469–490), 2nd ed. New York, NY: Guilford Press.

Mennin, D. S., and Heimberg, R. G. (2004). Clinical presentation and diagnostic features. In R. G. Heimberg, C. L. Turk, & D. S. Mennin (Eds.), *Generalized anxiety disorder: Advances in research and practice* (pp. 3–28). New York: Guilford Press.

Moffitt, T. E., Caspi, A., Taylor, A., Kokaua, J., Milne, B. J., Polanczyk, G., and Poulton, R. (2010). How common are common mental disorders? Evidence that lifetime prevalence rates are doubled by prospective versus retrospective ascertainment. *Psychol Med, 40* (06), 899–909.

Newman, M. G., and Erickson, T. M. (2010). Generalized anxiety disorder. In J. G. Beck (Ed.), *Interpersonal processes in the anxiety disorders: Implications for understanding psychopathology and treatment* (pp. 235–259). Washington, DC: American Psychological Association.

Newman, M. G., Jacobson, N. C., and Castonguay, L. G. (2014). Interpersonal and emotion-focused processing psychotherapy. In P. Emmelkamp, T. Ehring (Eds.), *The Wiley handbook of anxiety disorders* (840–851). Chichester, UK: John Wiley & Sons, Ltd.

Newman, M. G., Llera, S. J., Erickson, T. M., Przeworski, A., and Castonguay, L. G. (2013). Worry and generalized anxiety disorder: A review and theoretical synthesis of evidence on nature, etiology, mechanisms, and treatment. *Annu Rev Clin Psychol, 9*, 275–297.

Robichaud, M., and Dugas, M. J. (2006). A cognitive-behavioral treatment targeting intolerance of uncertainty. In G. C. Davey, A. Wells (Eds.), *Worry and its psychological disorders: Theory, assessment and treatment* (289–304). Chichester, UK: John Wiley & Sons, Ltd.

Roemer, L., Orsillo, S. M., and Salters-Pedneault, K. (2008). Efficacy of an acceptance-based behavior therapy for generalized anxiety disorder: Evaluation in a randomized controlled trial. *J Consult Clin Psychol, 76* (6), 1083.

Tyrer, P., and Baldwin, D. (2006). Generalised anxiety disorder. *Lancet, 368*(9553), 2156–2166.

Wells, A., and King, P. (2006). Metacognitive therapy for generalized anxiety disorder: An open trial. *J Behav Ther Exp Psychiatry, 37* (3), 206–212.

Whisman, M. A., Sheldon, C., and Goering, P. (2000). Psychiatric disorders and dissatisfaction with social relationships: Does type of relationship matter? *J Abnorm Psychol, 109* (4), 803.

Wittchen, H.-U., Krause, P., Hoyer, J., Beesdo, K., Jacobi, F., Hofler, M., and Winter, S. (2001). Prävalenz und Korrelate Generalisierter Angststo rungen in der Allgemeinarztpraxis [Prevalence and correlates of generalized anxiety disorder in primary care]. *Fortschritte der Medizin,* 119 (Suppl. 1), 17–25.

World Health Organization. (1992). *International Statistical Classification of Diseases and Related Health Problems, 10th Revision (ICD-10).* Geneva: WHO.

Yonkers, K. A., Dyck, I. R., Warshaw, M., and Keller, M. B. (2000). Factors predicting the clinical course of generalised anxiety disorder. *Br J Psychiatry, 176* (6), 544–549.

/// 23 /// ANXIETY AND SUICIDE

JESSICA D. RIBEIRO AND MATTHEW K. NOCK

INTRODUCTION

As one of the leading causes of injury and death worldwide, suicidal behavior is a tremendous public health problem. The scope and urgency of the problem is clearly reflected in the high rates of morbidity and mortality associated with suicidal behavior. Each year, suicide contributes substantially to the global burden of disease, accounting nearly one million deaths worldwide (World Health Organization [WHO], 2012)—a figure that is outnumbered by nonfatal attempts, which independently confer risk of significant injury and associated distress (Centers for Disease Control and Prevention [CDC], 2012).

Mental disorders have been identified as significant risk factors for suicide (Harris and Barraclough, 1997). More than 90% of suicide decedents are estimated to have been suffering from a mental disorder at the time of their death (Henriksson et al., 1993; Arsenaul-Lapierre, Kim, and Turecki, 2004). This chapter focuses exclusively on the nature of the association between anxiety disorders and suicidal behavior. To this end, the chapter first presents a brief overview of the nature and epidemiology of suicidal behavior. Following this, the chapter reviews evidence documenting the association between anxiety and suicidal behavior, proposed mechanisms for these associations, and empirically informed interventions. The chapter closes with an overview of several gaps in the literature and recommendations for future research.

SUICIDE AND SUICIDAL BEHAVIOR

Despite several efforts to establish a common nomenclature for describing suicidal behaviors (e.g., Silverman, Berman, Sanddal, O'Carroll, and Joiner, 2007), a standard classification system has yet to be widely adopted. Generally, however, *suicide* refers to death caused by self-inflicted injury enacted with any intent to die as a result of the injury. *Suicide attempt* refers to a non-fatal, self-directed, potentially injurious behavior enacted with any intent to die as a result of the behavior. *Suicidal behavior* is an inclusive term that describes suicide death, suicide attempts, and any preparatory behaviors; *suicide ideation* is a term that describes thoughts of suicidal behaviors. Nonsuicidal self-injury (NSSI) refers to the deliberate, self-inflicted destruction of body tissue without suicidal intent and for non-socially sanctioned purposes (Nock, 2010). Of note, although a comprehensive discussion of NSSI is beyond the scope of this chapter, emerging evidence indicates there is a link between NSSI and anxiety (Chartrand, Sareen, Toews, and Bolton, 2012). The body of literature is small, however; as such, more research is needed to refine our understanding of the association.

The prevalence of suicidal thoughts and behaviors varies by gender, race/ethnicity, and age. With respect to gender, men are approximately four times more likely than women to die by suicide in virtually every country around the world (Nock et al., 2008). By contrast, women have significantly higher rates of suicidal thoughts and nonfatal attempts (Nock et al., 2008). In terms of race/ethnicity in the United States, American Indian/Alaskan Native as well as non-Hispanic Whites have the highest rates of death by suicide (CDC, 2012). With respect to age-of-onset and course, the risk of initial onset of suicidal ideation increases dramatically during early adolescence and young adulthood (Nock et al., 2008; Nock et al., 2013). Moreover, about one-third of those who report suicidal ideation later transition to making a suicide plan, and about the same percentage go on to make a suicide attempt (Kessler, Borges, and Walters, 1999). These transitions appear occur most frequently within the first year after the initial onset of suicidal ideation among adults (Kessler et al., 1999) and adolescents (Nock et al., 2013). Persistent suicidal ideation in the absence of a suicide plan or attempt has also been reported to be associated with decreasing risk of later plans or attempts (Borges, Angst, Nock, Ruscio, and Kessler, 2008).

ASSOCIATIONS BETWEEN ANXIETY AND SUICIDAL THOUGHTS AND BEHAVIORS

Although it has been widely shown that mental disorders confer significant risk of suicidal thoughts and behavior, anxiety disorders have received less empirical attention than other disorders (e.g., mood disorders, alcohol/substance use disorders). Early efforts examining the role of anxiety disorders in suicide resulted in inconsistent findings (Sareen et al., 2011). However, converging evidence resulting from continued research appears to largely support the role of anxiety disorders as risk factors for suicidal thoughts and behaviors.

Cross-sectional community and clinical studies have repeatedly documented associations between anxiety disorders and suicidal ideation, attempts, and death (Kanwar et al., 2013). Though fewer studies have employed longitudinal designs, several prospective studies have indicated that anxiety disorders confer risk for later suicidal thoughts and behaviors, even after accounting for the co-occurrence of other mental disorders (Boden, Fergusson, and Horwood, 2007; Bolton, Pagura, Enns, Grant, and Sareen, 2007; Borges et al., 2008; Nepon, Belik, Bolton, and Sareen, 2010; Sareen et al., 2005a; Sareen, Houlahan, Cox, and Asmundson, 2005b). Further substantiating the link, a recent meta-analysis reported a greater likelihood of suicidal ideation, attempts, and death associated with anxiety disorders (Kanwar et al., 2013). Research also suggests that the effects of anxiety disorders may be particularly strong among those with comorbid mood disorders, as the co-occurrence of anxiety and mood disorders appear to confer higher risk of serious suicidal behavior, as compared to either anxiety or mood disorders alone (Sareen et al., 2005a).

Although the presence of any anxiety disorder appears to be associated with increased risk of suicide attempts (Sareen et al., 2005a; Nepon et al., 2010), this does not necessarily imply that every anxiety disorder independently confers risk. Several large epidemiological studies support the independent associations with several conditions (Cougle et al., 2009; Nepon et al., 2010; Thibodeau et al., 2010). Associations with post-traumatic stress disorder appear to be most consistent (Cougle et al., 2009; Nepon et al., 2010; Sareen et al., 2005a; Thibodeau et al., 2010). Other conditions, including generalized anxiety disorder, obsessive-compulsive disorder, panic disorder, specific phobia, and social anxiety disorder have also demonstrated associations with suicidal thoughts and behaviors; however, when considered in the context of sociodemographic variables and other Axis I and II conditions, the effects appear to be less stable (Cougle et al., 2009; Nepon et al., 2010; Sareen et al., 2005a; et al., 2005b).

Among anxiety disorders, the association between panic disorder and suicidal behavior has garnered the greatest research attention. This is likely due to frequent discrepant results across large-scale studies (Sareen, 2011). Findings from an initial study conducted by Weissman and colleagues (1989) reported that those diagnosed with panic disorder have significantly elevated risk of suicidal thoughts and attempts, even after accounting for the effects of mood and substance and alcohol use disorders. However, several subsequent studies reported that the association between panic disorder and suicidal behavior are fully accounted for by the presence of co-morbid conditions, such as depression, alcohol use disorders, and borderline personality disorder (Hornig and McNally, 1995; Vickers and McNally, 2004). More recent studies have indicated that co-morbidity only partially accounts for the effects. For instance, data from the National Comorbidity Survey Replication suggest that although comorbid conditions accounted for a substantial proportion of the variance in suicide outcomes, effects of panic remained significant (though attenuated), when predicting later suicide attempts (Nock et al., 2009).

In sum, converging evidence drawn from large, representative samples indicate anxiety disorders are associated with increased risk of suicidal thoughts and behavior. Inconsistencies in the literature have raised questions about the validity of anxiety disorders as independent risk factors, however. Methodological differences across studies, including heterogeneity in predictors, outcomes, study timelines, and nature of the populations studied, are likely resulting in the discrepant findings (Thibodeau et al., 2013; Kanwar et al., 2013). Continued research focused on definitively characterizing the independent effects of specific anxiety disorders would be fruitful. To this end, studies involving large, representative samples and prospective designs would likely prove most informative.

ANXIETY AS AN INDICATOR OF IMMINENT SUICIDAL BEHAVIOR

Beyond the risk anxiety may confer for eventual death by suicide, anxiety may also be an important indicator of imminent or short-term suicidal behavior. In particular, severe anxiety, agitation, and panic attacks have been identified as key "warning signs" for imminent suicidal behavior by expert clinical consensus (Rudd et al., 2006).

Consistent with expert clinical consensus, a small but growing literature provides further support for the importance of these states during times of imminent risk. Retrospective studies of inpatient (Busch, Fawcett and Jacobs, 2003) and inmate (Way, Miraglia, Sawyer, Beer, and Eddy, 2005) suicide deaths report rates of agitation and severe anxiety close to 80% in the weeks before death. Similarly, a psychological autopsy study of suicide decedents found that "tension" and "nervousness" emerged as two of the most frequently reported symptoms observed in decedents in the days before their deaths, across individuals suffering from a range of mental disorders (Robins, 1981).[1] Pronounced rates of agitation have also been associated with near-lethal attempts. A study of emergency room patients admitted following a suicide attempt revealed that close to 90% of patient reported experiencing "severe psychic anxiety" during the month preceding the attempt, and nearly 80% endorsed panic attacks during that same time period (Hall, Platt, and Hall, 1999). Agitation has been found to discriminate between suicidal patients determined to be at acute risk versus those more chronic, with agitation being more pronounced among individuals who were acutely suicidal (Conrad et al., 2009; Jobes, Jacoby, Cimbolic, and Hustead, 1997).

Though empirical evidence in this area has drawn largely from retrospective and cross-sectional studies, there is emerging evidence supporting the longitudinal effects of these states. Among a large sample a mood disorder patients, panic attacks and agitation (i.e., "severe psychic anxiety") emerged as a significant predictor of short-term (i.e., within 1-year follow-up) but not long-term (i.e., more than 1-year follow-up) suicide (Fawcett et al., 1990). Britton and colleagues (2012) examined predictors of suicide death present one month before death in a group of military veterans. Consistent with previous evidence, anxiety was found to be a significant predictor of suicide within a month.

MECHANISMS UNDERLYING THE ASSOCIATION BETWEEN ANXIETY AND SUICIDE

Although a number of etiological mechanisms have been proposed to explain the nature of the relationship between anxiety and suicide, research systematically evaluating mechanisms underlying the nature of the associations has been scant. Anxiety may have a direct effect on the occurrence of suicidal behavior via several potential mechanisms. In line with escape based models of suicide (e.g., Psycheache Theory; Shneidman, 1993), high anxiety may result in increased motivation to escape distress, and, suicide may be considered as one means of doing so. Consistent with this perspective, Nock and colleagues (2008) have reported findings suggesting that anxiety disorders may facilitate suicidal behavior whereas affective disorders may confer risk to developing suicidal ideation. Considering the additional evidence suggesting that the presence of anxiety disorder may potentiate suicide risk among individuals suffering from mood disorders (Sareen et al., 2005a), it is possible that anxiety symptoms may function to facilitate the transition from suicidal thoughts to engaging in suicidal behavior.

With respect to imminent risk, it has been proposed that acute and heightened states of arousal, like severe agitation, may emerge as a result of planning for lethal suicidal behavior in the near future, given the daunting prospect of the behavior (Ribeiro et al., 2012). It has also been suggested that these states may have differential effects on suicidal risk depending on an individual's capability for suicide, which is characterized in part by a sense of fearlessness about pain, injury and death. Among suicidal individuals low on capability for suicide, who remain averse or fearful of pain, injury, and death, increased arousal may serve to facilitate further avoidance of potentially lethal means and behaviors. However, among suicidal individuals high on suicidal capability, increased states of arousal may promote further approach to the means necessary to engage in potentially lethal suicidal behavior. To date, two studies have supported this proposition (Ribeiro et al., 2014; Ribeiro, Silva, and Joiner, 2014), though neither study provided prospective evidence.

It also is possible that anxiety indirectly contributes to suicide risk. For instance, anxiety disorders may increase the likelihood of later development of a mood or substance use disorder, which in turn may contribute additional risk of suicidal ideation and behaviors. This possibility is consistent with evidence suggesting that accounting for comorbidity attenuates effects of anxiety disorder of suicidal thoughts and behaviors. However, given that many studies have indicated that independent associations

A. ESCAPE-BASED PERSPECTIVE

Anxiety Symptoms → Desire to Escape Distress → Suicidal Behavior

B. CAPABILITY-BASED PERSPECTIVE

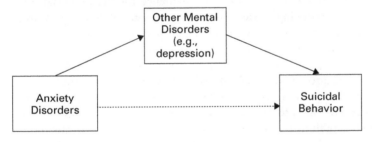

Capability for Suicide

Planning/ Preparing for suicide → ↑Anxiety/ Arousal Symptoms

High Capability → Approach toward Suicidal Stimuli

Low Capability → Avoidance of Suicidal Stimuli

C. INDIRECT EFFECTS OF ANXIETY

Other Mental Disorders (e.g., depression)

Anxiety Disorders → Suicidal Behavior

D. SHARED ETIOLOGY

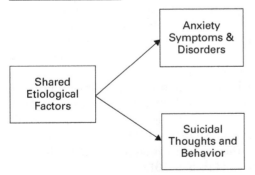

Anxiety Symptoms & Disorders

Shared Etiological Factors

Suicidal Thoughts and Behavior

FIGURE 23.1 Potential mechanisms through which anxiety may affect suicidal behavior.

remain even after accounting for comorbidity, the explanation may not fully account for the relationship. Others have suggested that factors shared by both anxiety disorders and suicidal behavior may account for the relationship (Hawton and van Heeringen, 2009). For instance, anxiety disorders and suicidal behavior have both demonstrated associations between certain common biological factors (e.g., low levels of serotonin metabolites in the cerebrospinal fluid; Fawcett, Busch, Jacobs, Kravitz, and Fogg, 1997), personality features (e.g., self-criticism; Cox, Enns, and Clara, 2004), and environmental factors (e.g., childhood maltreatment; Molnar, Berkman, and Buka, 2001; Molnar, Buka, and Kessler, 2001, trauma; Bruce et al., 2001). These shared factors may independently predispose individuals to develop both anxiety disorders and suicidal behavior (Hawton and van Heeringen, 2009). See Figure 23.1 for a graphical depiction of the possible mechanisms through which anxiety may effect suicidal behavior discussed here.

TREATMENT

Anxiety has been proposed as a potentially modifiable risk factor for suicide (Fawcett et al., 1990). Despite this, no anxiety-focused treatments have been identified as empirically-established interventions for the treatment of suicidal thoughts or behaviors. Given the established links between anxiety and suicidal thoughts and behaviors and the availability of effective anxiety disorder treatments, this area may represent an extremely viable domain for continued research. Systematic efforts to evaluate the effectiveness of anxiety-focused interventions on suicidal thoughts and behaviors have been rare, however.

Recent research has provided some preliminary evidence for the potential utility of interventions focused on reducing anxiety sensitivity symptoms (Schmidt, Capron, Raines, and Allan, 2014). Anxiety sensitivity has been proposed as one viable target for reducing risk of suicidal ideation, given recent evidence supporting the link between domains of anxiety sensitivity and suicide-relevant outcomes (Capron, Cougle, Ribeiro, Joiner, & Schmidt, 2012; Capron et al., 2012). Based on findings from Schmidt and colleagues (2014), a novel intervention, which is referred to cognitive anxiety sensitivity treatment (CAST), was developed to reduce the cognitive concerns domain of anxiety sensitivity. According to a preliminary study examining the efficacy of the intervention, CAST was found to be associated with reductions in anxiety sensitivity cognitive concerns symptoms, which in turn were found to mediate reductions in suicidal ideation at one-month follow-up (Schmidt et al., 2014). Although encouraging, a significant limitation of the study was that the range of suicidality in the sample was fairly circumscribed with mean levels of self-report suicidal ideation measures falling close to 0, indicating very minimal risk. As such, questions remain about the utility of the treatment among individuals evidencing clinically significant suicide risk.

Some existing treatments for suicidal behaviors also incorporate the treatment and management of anxiety symptoms. For instance, in dialectical behavior therapy (DBT; Linehan, 1993a) learning to manage, cope with, and change distressing emotions, like anxiety, is a fundamental aspect of the intervention. Further, DBT has also recently been adapted to incorporate Prolonged Exposure therapy for treating suicidal individuals suffering from PTSD (Harned, Korslund, Foa, and Linehan, 2012).

With respect to individuals at imminent suicide risk, acute management of agitation and severe anxiety is often recommended. Recommendations typically involve the time-limited use of pharmacological agents like benzodiazepines, antipsychotics or their combination (Kleespies and Dettmer, 2000). Importantly, however, despite being common practice, there is no clear empirical evidence that reducing acute agitation prevents serious suicidal behavior (Youssef and Rich, 2008).

FUTURE DIRECTIONS

Anxiety has emerged as an important risk factor for suicidal thoughts and behaviors. Despite growing research interest, our understanding of the nature of the relationship between anxiety and suicide remains underdeveloped. Several gaps in the literature remain that warrant additional research attention and point toward directions for future research.

Given repeated inconsistencies in the literature regarding the nature of the association between anxiety and suicidal behavior, future research efforts should aim to clarifying which anxiety disorders increase the risk of subsequent suicidal behavior, and which part of the pathway to suicide they may be affecting. To this end, large meta-analytic efforts examining the overall and unique effects of anxiety disorders and anxiety features would be informative. It would be particularly useful to further refine our understanding of the effects of anxiety on suicide, especially as anxiety relates to imminent versus lifetime risk of suicidal thoughts, nonfatal attempts and death. In pursuing such efforts, care should be taken to account for methodological differences across studies, which likely contribute to the existing inconsistencies in the literature.

Another major point in need of clarification is whether it is individual anxiety disorders that are predictive of suicidal behavior per se, or whether there are specific features of anxiety disorders that are associated with elevated risk. Studying features of anxiety may allow for a finer-grained analysis that may prove more informative than examining discrete diagnoses. With respect to anxiety, first considering which disorders independently confer risk and then identifying which features are common across these conditions would provide some direction of what features to home in on. Also, given that post-traumatic stress disorder has been most consistently linked to suicide, prominent features of that condition may be particularly salient.

With respect to the role of anxiety in imminent suicide risk, existing research and a growing clinical consensus makes clear that acute anxiety-like states (e.g., agitation, panic attacks) may represent extremely informative indicators of imminent and serious suicidal behavior. Despite its importance, this domain of research has remained woefully understudied. Advances can be made in a number of domains. First, this area of research is significantly limited by the lack of prospective research—our understanding largely draws from a relatively small pool of retrospective and cross-sectional studies. As such, pursuing prospective studies that provide insight into the narrow window of time (i.e., days, hours) immediately preceding serious suicidal behavior would be one means of substantially improving our understanding in this area. Secondly, should evidence continue to accrue supporting the role of these states as indicators of imminent suicidal behavior, it would also be informative to determine what interventions may be most useful to implement when these states are observed among high risk individuals.

A final recommendation for future research involves work focused on evaluating the utility of anxiety-focused interventions for reducing suicidal thoughts and behaviors. Anxiety may be a malleable treatment target; however, questions remain about whether reducing anxiety will result in corresponding reductions in suicide-relevant outcomes. Although a promising avenue of future research, some concerns remain, especially when considering that some suicide experts have argued that treating suicidal behavior may not be effectively addressed by treating the disorders associated with suicide (Miller et al., 2007). Even so, further research is necessary to conclusively address whether anxiety-focused interventions may be useful in reducing suicide risk, either directly or indirectly. As such, studies focused on the utility and feasibility of anxiety-focused suicide interventions would be fruitful.

SUMMARY

Converging evidence supports a link between anxiety disorders and suicidal behavior; however, many questions remain about the specific nature of this association. Cross-sectional as well as prospective studies drawing from community and clinical populations suggest that the presence of any anxiety disorder confers increased risk of suicidal thoughts and behaviors. Although findings have been mixed, several studies have indicated that these effects, though attenuated, persist beyond the effects of co-morbidity and sociodemographic variables (Kanwar et al., 2013; Thibodeau et al., 2013). This is especially true in the case of post-traumatic stress disorder, which shown the most robust association with suicidal behavior of all anxiety disorders. Acute states of heightened arousal (e.g., agitation, panic) have also been identified by expert clinical consensus and a small but growing empirical literature as important "warning signs" for imminent and serious suicidal behavior (Rudd et al., 2006). Unfortunately, systematic empirical research examining *why* anxiety is associated with this increase risk has been scant, though a few etiological mechanisms have been proposed.

Treatment approaches were also discussed. Anxiety has been identified as a potentially modifiable target for suicide intervention (Fawcett et al., 1990); however, to date, there have been no empirically-established treatments of anxiety that have demonstrated significant effects on suicidal thoughts and behaviors.

Taken together, the role of anxiety in suicidal behavior appears to be a viable area for continued research. Many questions remain about the nature of the relationship, the mechanisms that account for the associations, and the utility and feasibility of anxiety-focused suicide interventions as a means of reducing suicidal thoughts and behaviors. Continued research will likely prove useful in making meaningful inroads on our understanding of the nature and prevention of suicidal behaviors.

DISCLOSURE STATEMENT

The authors report no competing interests.

NOTE

1. Of note, psychological autopsy is a method used to determine the antecedents of a suicide death. This is done by collecting information about a decedent from a range of sources, including health care and psychiatric records, personal documents, forensic examinations, and structured interviews of surviving friends and relatives. A notable advantage of this method is its focus on suicide death as opposed to nonfatal attempts and other suicidal-relevant outcomes, as there may be meaningful differences between fatal and nonfatal suicidal behaviors.

REFERENCES

Arsenault-Lapierre, G., Kim, C., and Turecki, G. (2004). Psychiatric diagnoses in 3275 suicides: a meta-analysis. *BMC Psychiatry*, 4(1), 37.

Boden, J. M., Fergusson, D. M., and John Horwood, L. (2007). Anxiety disorders and suicidal behaviours in adolescence and young adulthood: findings from a longitudinal study. *Psychological Medicine*, 37(03), 431–440.

Borges, G., Angst, J., Nock, M. K., Ruscio, A. M., and Kessler, R. C. (2008). Risk factors for the incidence and persistence of suicide-related outcomes: a 10-year follow-up study using the National Comorbidity Surveys. *Journal of Affective Disorders*, 105(1), 25–33.

Britton, P. C., Ilgen, M. A., Rudd, M. D., & Conner, K. R. (2012). Warning signs for suicide within a week of healthcare contact in Veteran decedents. *Psychiatry Research*, 200(2), 395–399.

Bruce, S. E., Weisberg, R. B., Dolan, R. T., Machan, J. T., Kessler, R. C., Manchester, G., . . . Keller, M. B. (2001). Trauma and posttraumatic stress disorder in primary care patients. *Primary care companion to the Journal of clinical psychiatry*, 3(5), 211.

Busch, K. A., Fawcett, J., and Jacobs, D. G. (2003). Clinical correlates of inpatient suicide. *Journal of Clinical Psychiatry*, 64(1), 13–19.

Capron, D. W., Cougle, J. R., Ribeiro, J. D., Joiner, T. E., and Schmidt, N. B. (2012). An interactive model of anxiety sensitivity relevant to suicide attempt history and future suicidal ideation. *Journal of Psychiatric Research*, 46(2), 174–180.

Capron, D. W., Fitch, K., Medley, A., Blagg, C., Mallott, M., and Joiner, T. (2012). Role of anxiety sensitivity subfactors in suicidal ideation and suicide attempt history. *Depression and Anxiety*, 29(3), 195–201.

Centers for Disease Control and Prevention. (2012). *Web-based injury statistics query and reporting system (WISQARS). Fatal injury reports and nonfatal injury reports*. Atlanta, GA: National Center for Injury Prevention and Control. Available at: http://www.cdc.gov/injury/wisqars/index.html.

Chartrand, H., Sareen, J., Toews, M., and Bolton, J. M. (2012). Suicide attempts versus nonsuicidal self-injury among individuals with anxiety disorders in a nationally representative sample. *Depression and anxiety*, 29(3), 172–179.

Conrad, A. K., Jacoby, A. M., Jobes, D. A., Lineberry, T. W., Shea, C. E., Arnold Ewing, T. D., . . . Kung, S. (2009). A psychometric investigation of the Suicide Status Form II with a psychiatric inpatient sample. *Suicide and Life-Threatening Behavior*, 39(3), 307–320.

Cougle, J. R., Keough, M. E., Riccardi, C. J., and Sachs-Ericsson, N. (2009). Anxiety disorders and suicidality in the National Comorbidity Survey-Replication. *Journal of Psychiatric Research*, 43(9), 825–829.

Cox, B. J., McWilliams, L. A., Enns, M. W., and Clara, I. P. (2004). Broad and specific personality dimensions associated with major depression in a nationally representative sample. *Comprehensive psychiatry*, 45(4), 246–253.

Fawcett, J., Busch, K. A., Jacobs, D., Kravitz, H. M., and Fogg, L. (1997). Suicide: A four-pathway clinical-biochemical model. *Annals of the New York Academy of Sciences*, 836(1), 288–301.

Fawcett, J., Scheftner, W. A., Fogg, L., Clark, D. C., Young, M. A., Hedeker, D., and Gibbons, R. (1990). Time-related predictors of suicide in major affective disorder. *The American Journal of Psychiatry*, 147, 1189–1194.

Hall, R. C., Platt, D. E., and Hall, R. C. (1999). Suicide risk assessment: a review of risk factors for suicide in 100 patients who made severe suicide attempts: evaluation of suicide risk in a time of managed care. *Psychosomatics*, 40(1), 18–27.

Harned, M. S., Korslund, K. E., Foa, E. B., and Linehan, M. M. (2012). Treating PTSD in suicidal and self-injuring women with borderline personality disorder: Development and preliminary evaluation of a dialectical behavior therapy prolonged exposure protocol. *Behaviour Research and Therapy*, 50(6), 381–386.

Harris, E. C., and Barraclough, B. (1997). Suicide as an outcome for mental disorders. A meta-analysis. *The British Journal of Psychiatry*, 170(3), 205–228.

Hawton, K., and van Heeringen, K. (2009). Suicide. *Lancet*, 9672, 1372–1381.

Henriksson, M. M., Aro, H. M., Marttunen, M. J., Heikkinen, M. E., Isometsa, E. T., Kuoppasalmi, K. I., and Lonnqvist, J. K. (1993). Mental disorders and comorbidity in suicide. *American journal of Psychiatry*, 150, 935–935.

Hornig, C. D., and McNally, R. J. (1995). Panic disorder and suicide attempt. A reanalysis of data from the epidemiologic catchment area study. *The British Journal of Psychiatry, 167*(1), 76–79.

Jobes, D. A., Jacoby, A. M., Cimbolic, P., and Hustead, L. A. T. (1997). Assessment and treatment of suicidal clients in a university counseling center. *Journal of counseling psychology, 44*(4), 368.

Kanwar, A., Malik, S., Prokop, L. J., Sim, L. A., Feldstein, D., Wang, Z., and Murad, M. H. (2013). The association between anxiety disorders and suicidal behaviors: a systematic review and meta-analysis. *Depression and Anxiety, 30*(10), 917–929.

Kessler, R. C., Borges, G., and Walters, E. E. (1999). Prevalence of and risk factors for lifetime suicide attempts in the National Comorbidity Survey. *Archives of General Psychiatry, 56*(7), 617–626.

Kleespies, P. M., and Dettmer, E. L. (2000). An evidence-based approach to evaluating and managing suicidal emergencies. *Journal of Clinical Psychology, 56*(9), 1109–1130.

Linehan, M. (1993a). *Cognitive-behavioral treatment of borderline personality disorder.* New York, NY: Guilford Press.

Miller, A., Rathus, J., and Linehan, M. (2007). *Dialectical behavior therapy with adolescents.* New York: Guilford Press.

Molnar, B. E., Berkman, L. F., and Buka, S. L. (2001). Psychopathology, childhood sexual abuse and other childhood adversities: relative links to subsequent suicidal behaviour in the US. *Psychological medicine, 31*(06), 965–977.

Molnar, B. E., Buka, S. L., and Kessler, R. C. (2001). Child sexual abuse and subsequent psychopathology: results from the national comorbidity survey. *American Journal of Public Health, 91*(5), 753.

Nepon, J., Belik, S. L., Bolton, J., and Sareen, J. (2010). The relationship between anxiety disorders and suicide attempts: findings from the national epidemiologic survey on alcohol and related conditions. *Depression and Anxiety, 27*(9), 791–798.

Nock, M. K. (2010). Self-injury. *Annual Review of Clinical Psychology, 6*, 339–363.

Nock, M. K., Borges, G., Bromet, E. J., Cha, C. B., Kessler, R. C., and Lee, S. (2008). Suicide and suicidal behavior. *Epidemiologic reviews, 30*(1), 133–154.

Nock, M. K., Green, J. G., Hwang, I., McLaughlin, K. A., Sampson, N. A., Zaslavsky, A. M., and Kessler, R. C. (2013). Prevalence, correlates, and treatment of lifetime suicidal behavior among adolescents: results from the National Comorbidity Survey Replication Adolescent Supplement. *JAMA Psychiatry, 70*(3), 300–310.

Nock, M. K., Hwang, I., Sampson, N. A., and Kessler, R. C. (2009). Mental disorders, comorbidity and suicidal behavior: results from the National Comorbidity Survey Replication. *Molecular Psychiatry, 15*(8), 868–876.

Ribeiro, J. D., Bender, T. W., Buchman, J. M., Nock, M. K., Rudd, M. D., Bryan, C. J., . . . Joiner, T. E. (2014). An investigation of the interactive effects of the capability for suicide and acute agitation on suicidality in a military sample. *Depression and Anxiety, 32*(1), 25–31.

Ribeiro, J. D., Silva, C., and Joiner, T. E. (2014). Overarousal interacts with a sense of fearlessness about death to predict suicide risk in a sample of clinical outpatients. *Psychiatry Research, 218*(1–2), 106–112.

Robins, E. (1981). *The final months: A study of the lives of 134 persons who committed suicide.* New York: Oxford University Press.

Rudd, M. D., Berman, A. L., Joiner, T. E., Nock, M. K., Silverman, M. M., Mandrusiak, M., . . . Witte, T. (2006). Warning signs for suicide: Theory, research, and clinical applications. *Suicide and Life-Threatening Behavior, 36*(3), 255–262.

Sareen, J., Cox, B. J., Afifi, T. O., de Graaf, R., Asmundson, G. J., ten Have, M., and Stein, M. B. (2005a). Anxiety disorders and risk for suicidal ideation and suicide attempts: A population-based longitudinal study of adults. *Archives of General Psychiatry, 62*(11), 1249–1257.

Sareen, J., Houlahan, T., Cox, B. J., and Asmundson, G. J. (2005b). Anxiety disorders associated with suicidal ideation and suicide attempts in the National Comorbidity Survey. *The Journal of Nervous and Mental Disease, 193*(7), 450–454.

Sareen, J. (2011). Anxiety disorders and risk for suicide: Why such controversy? *Depression and Anxiety,* *28*(11), 941–945.

Schmidt, N. B., Capron, D. W., Raines, A. M., and Allan, N. P. (2014). Randomized clinical trial evaluating the efficacy of a brief intervention targeting anxiety sensitivity cognitive concerns. *Journal of Consulting and Clinical Psychology, 82*(6), 1023–1033.

Shneidman, E. S. (1993). *Suicide as psychache: A clinical approach to self-destructive behavior.* Northvale, NJ: Jason Aronson.

Silverman, M. M., Berman, A. L., Sanddal, N. D., O'Carroll, P. W., and Joiner, T. E. (2007). Rebuilding the tower of babel: A revised nomenclature for the study of suicide and suicidal behaviors part 2: Suicide-related ideations, communications, and behaviors. *Suicide and Life-Threatening Behavior, 37*(3), 264–277.

Thibodeau, M. A., Welch, P. G., Sareen, J., and Asmundson, G. J. (2013). Anxiety disorders are independently associated with suicide ideation and attempts: Propensity score matching in two epidemiological samples. *Depression and Anxiety, 30*(10), 94–954.

Vickers, K., and McNally, R. J. (2004). Panic disorder and suicide attempt in the national comorbidity survey. *Journal of Abnormal Psychology, 113*(4), 582.

Way, B. B., Miraglia, R., Sawyer, D. A., Beer, R., and Eddy, J. (2005). Factors related to suicide in New York state prisons. *International Journal of Law and Psychiatry, 28*(3), 207–221.

World Health Organization. (2012). Mental health: Suicide prevention (SUPRE). Retrieved from http://www.who.int/mental_health/prevention/suicide/suicideprevent/en/index.html. Accessed August 1, 2014.

Weissman, M. M., Klerman, G. L., Markowitz, J. S., and Ouellette, R. (1989). Suicidal ideation and suicide attempts in panic disorder and attacks. *New England Journal of Medicine, 321*(18), 1209–1214.

Youssef, N. A., and Rich, C. L. (2008). Does acute treatment with sedatives/hypnotics for anxiety in depressed patients affect suicide risk? A literature review. *Annals of Clinical Psychiatry, 20*(3), 157–169.

COGNITIVE AND EXPOSURE-BASED TREATMENTS OF ANXIETY DISORDERS

24

NEURAL CIRCUIT MECHANISMS OF FEAR EXTINCTION

BLAKE L. ROSENBAUM, KARA K. COVER, HUIJIN SONG, AND MOHAMMED R. MILAD

INTRODUCTION

Pavlovian fear conditioning is commonly used to study emotional learning and memory (Pavlov 1927, Bouton and King 1983, Quirk 2002). In this paradigm, a neutral conditioned stimulus (CS; e.g., a light or a tone) is paired with an aversive unconditioned stimulus (US; e.g., a mild electrical shock). After several pairings, the participant exhibits conditioned fear responses (CRs) when the now-conditioned cue is presented. This type of fear conditioning is known as "cued conditioning." A second type of conditioning, known as contextual conditioning, occurs when multimodal cues (i.e., visual, auditory, olfactory) are present within an environment (i.e., a cage of animal or a room) and are collectively paired with the US (Figure 24.1).

In humans, fear conditioning can be achieved using ecologically relevant stimuli (such as images of negative or fearful faces, or innately fear-provoking animals) or neutral stimuli (e.g., shapes, neutral images). Fear learning in rodents may be quantified with several measures. *Freezing*, a hallmark fear response, is the absence of all movement except respiration and is measured during the CS presentation (Fanselow 1980, Davis 1986). *Fear potentiated startle* describes the increase in the reflexive startle response with a loud unexpected noise that occurs in the presence of the CS versus a neutral stimulus (Davis 1986). Lastly, *conditioned suppression* of feeding behaviors is defined by a reduction of food intake, or the behaviors leading to obtaining food, when the CS is present (Cryan and Holmes 2005), typically measured through bar presses inside the rodent cage. In human fear conditioning studies, skin-conductance responses (SCRs) on the fingers or wrist, and fear-potentiated startle responses of the orbicularis eye blink response, are the most commonly used psychophysiological measures of fear (Milad, Rauch et al. 2006).

Conditioned fear responses diminish through extinction training (See Figure 24.2). During fear extinction, the animal is repeatedly presented with the CS without the US,

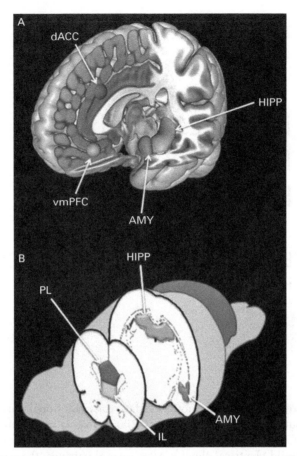

FIGURE 24.1 Highlighting the core brain regions in the fear network, homologous across rodent, and human brains. (A) Human brain: dACC, dorsal anterior cingulate cortex; vmPFC, ventromedial prefrontal cortex; AMY, amygdala; HIPP, hippocampus. (B) Rodent brain: PL, prelimbic; IL, infralimbic; AMY, amygdala; HIPP, hippocampus.

that is, in the absence of any negative reinforcement. After several presentations, conditioned fear responses gradually decline as the subject learns that the stimulus no longer predicts the aversive outcome. This reduction in conditioned fear responses during extinction training is known as "within-session extinction training," or "extinction learning" (Garcia 2002, Myers and Davis 2007). The memory of this extinction learning is tested after a time delay, typically 24 hours. During this *extinction retention* or *recall* test, the previously extinguished CS is presented again without any negative reinforcement. Good extinction recall is indexed by low levels of conditioned responding, consistent with ongoing suppression of the prior fear response. In contrast, poor extinction recall is indexed by recovered conditioned fear responses.

Extinction was initially defined by Pavlov as diminished response to nonreinforced cues over time. However, it was debated whether this behavioral process represented a forgetting or erasure of the initial fear memory, or whether in contrast, it represented a learning of a new inhibitory memory trace that competed with the original fear memory, thereby suppressing expression of that prior fear behavior. Several behavioral observations

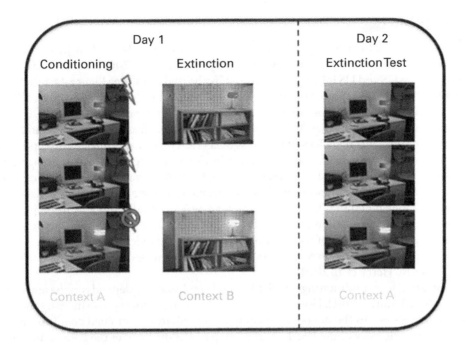

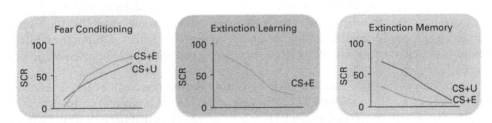

FIGURE 24.2 A schematic breakdown of a fear conditioning paradigm and standardized responding as measure by skin conductance. *Conditioning*: The CS– and two CS+ are presented within a conditioning context, the CS+ are paired with a US, in this case an electric shock. *Extinction*: In a novel extinction context, the CS– and one CS+ (CS+E) are presented with no US reinforcement. The remaining CS+ (CS+U) is not presented and remains unextinguished. *Extinction Test*: On the next day, all three CS are presented once again in the initial conditioning context without a US to test the extinction memory from the previous day.

suggested that the latter was the case (Bouton, Westbrook et al. 2006), which have since been further verified with modern molecular behavioral neuroscience approaches. First it was shown that extinguished cued fear response would return upon restressing the animal with an unconditioned footshock, known as *reinstatement*. Second, the process of *spontaneous recovery*, was observed when animals would over time, with no interceding intervention, gradually recover some of the initially extinguished cued fear responding. Third, *renewal* of the cued fear response is seen when the animal is tested in a context different from that in which it was originally extinguished. These findings suggest that the original cued fear memory trace persists after the learning of a new extinction memory, which suppresses the prior fear response.

RODENT STUDIES

Mechanisms by which fear is acquired have been extensively studied in the rodent (Charney and Redmond 1983, Garcia 2002, Myers and Davis 2007). Sensory information about the CS and US is initially processed by the thalamus (See Figure 24.1 for brain regions involved in fear and extinction). The basolateral nucleus of the amygdala (BLA) receives and directs this information to produce a specific representation of the CS-US association (LeDoux 2007). Any expression of conditioned fear requires a BLA induced activation of the central nucleus of the amygdala (CeA). The experimental disruption of BLA function either through lesions, inactivation, or administration of drug antagonists impairs fear conditioning (Maren and Quirk 2004). BLA activation of the CeA activates downstream structures involved in species-specific defensive responses (e.g., freezing via the periaqueductal gray). Although the CeA was originally thought to be primarily involved in the expression of fear, more recent evidence has suggested that it is also involved in the acquisition of fear memories, as functional inactivation of the CeA prior to fear conditioning disrupts the formation of such memories (Wilensky, Schafe et al. 2006, Ciocchi, Herry et al. 2010).

Contextual fear conditioning, much like cued conditioning, depends on the amygdala (Goosens and Maren 2001). However, contextual fear conditioning also involves the hippocampus. Lesions to the dorsal hippocampus immediately after cued conditioning do not affect the memory of the cue, but rather impair the memory of the context in which the cued conditioning occurred (Anagnostaras, Maren et al. 1999). This suggests that the hippocampus is necessary for conditioning to diffuse, multimodal and contextual cues, but not to discrete stimuli. Based on these findings, it has been suggested that the hippocampus is responsible for integrating the various sensory information about the context into one unified representation, which is then converged with the US representation in the BLA.

There is also evidence that amygdala activation during the recall of fear conditioning is regulated by the prelimbic (PL) division of the medial prefrontal cortex (mPFC). Expression of both contextual and cued fear conditioning is disrupted following PL inactivation, and conversely, microstimulation of PL increases conditioned fear responses and hinders extinction (Vidal-Gonzalez, Vidal-Gonzalez et al. 2006, Corcoran and Quirk 2007).

Rodent studies have also established that, similar to fear conditioning, fear extinction also involves interactions between the mPFC and limbic structures. Specifically, it has been suggested that during extinction consolidation and recall, the infralimbic (IL) region of the mPFC inhibits conditioned responding by activating the inhibitory interneurons of the BLA, as well as potentially activating the inhibitory intercalated cell masses between the BLA and CeA. Both populations of inhibitory interneurons then prevent activation of the output neurons of the CEA, further preventing downstream activation of specific fear responses (Quirk and Mueller 2008). Again, the hippocampus is thought to be involved in the contextual regulation of extinction memories by activating the IL only when the extinguished CS is presented within the extinction context (Corcoran and Maren 2001).

MOLECULAR MECHANISMS OF FEAR EXTINCTION

Investigation of the molecular mechanisms underlying fear extinction learning and memory retrieval implicate the mitogen-activated protein kinase/extracellular signal-regulated kinase (MAPK/ERK) signaling pathway (See Figure 24.3). Inhibiting this pathway in the BLA with MAPK inhibitors prior to extinction training blocks fear extinction learning (Lu, Walker et al. 2001, Herry, Trifilieff et al. 2006), while post-training inhibitor infusions to the vmPFC impair extinction retrieval (Hugues, Deschaux, and Garcia, 2004). Conversely, extinction training and reconsolidation alter MAPK/ERK signaling activity in the amygdala, PFC, and hippocampus (Hugues, Chessel et al. 2006). Increased phosphorylated ERK immunoreactivity has been detected in the IL(Kim, Li et al. 2011), BLA (Herry, Trifilieff et al. 2006), and hippocampus (Fischer, Radulovic et al. 2007) following extinction learning. Additionally, consolidation of fear extinction depends on MAPK/ERK signaling and protein synthesis in the medial PFC (Santini, Ge et al. 2004, Hugues, Chessel et al. 2006). Enhancing extinction learning with pretraining administration of D-serine, an NMDA receptor agonist, correlates with ERK phosphorylation in the hippocampus during extinction training and in the BLA during recall (Matsuda, Matsuzawa et al. 2010). Taken together, these data highlight the critical role of the MAPK/ERK signaling pathway in fear learning, as reviewed in detail elsewhere (Cestari, Rossi-Arnaud et al. 2014).

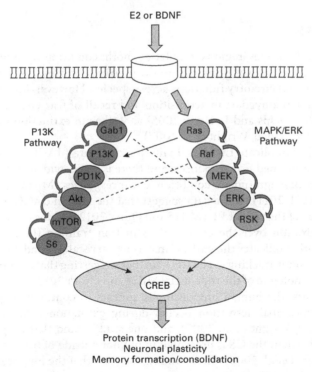

FIGURE 24.3 An illustration of two molecular pathways that are implicated in fear extinction. PI3K (*left*) and MAPK/ERK (*right*) protein cascades may be activated by E2 or BDNF-bound membrane receptors. Both pathways phosphorylate CREB, resulting in protein transcription, neuronal plasticity, and memory formation and consolidation. Some examples of intrapathway crosstalk are also illustrated, with facilitative actions represented by *solid arrows* and inhibitory actions by *dashed lines*. Republished with permission from *Translation Psychiatry* (Aug 2014). 4(8): e422 doi: 10.1038/tp.2014.67.

One downstream outcome of MAPK/ERK signaling is activation of CREB, a cellular transcription factor, which increases the transcription of the brain-derived neurotrophic factor (BDNF) gene. BDNF is a neurotrophin that critically supports long-term potentiation, spine genesis, and dendritic plasticity, mechanisms that underlie learning and memory. Binding of BDNF to the TrkB receptor activates MAPK/ERK and PI3K pathways (Carbone and Handa 2013). BDNF and TrkB are expressed abundantly in the PFC, hippocampus, and amygdala, consistent with a role in modulation of fear extinction (Peters, Dieppa-Perea et al. 2010, Do-Monte, Rodriguez-Romaguera et al. 2013). BDNF facilitates extinction consolidation in the amygdala, and supports cue-dependent extinction in the hippocampus (Andero and Ressler 2012, Inslicht, Metzler et al. 2013). Rosas-Vidal and colleagues (Rosas-Vidal, Do-Monte et al. 2014) recently demonstrated that IL-localized BDNF was "sufficient and necessary" for fear extinction and that extinction training increased BDNF levels in the ventral hippocampus. Moreover, infusing BDNF in the ventral hippocampus results in enhanced neuronal excitability in the IL and induces extinction. This provides support for BDNF's role in hippocampal-IL connectivity, which mediates fear extinction. Given the extensive role of BDNF in synaptic plasticity, learning, and memory, this pathway has proved to be an attractive target for potential therapies aimed at improving extinction. (Andero and Ressler 2012, Andero, Choi et al. 2014).

HUMAN STUDIES

Imaging studies highlight regions regulating both conditioning and extinction in humans. This chapter focuses primarily on the prefrontal cortex, reflecting remarkable preservation of neural circuitry functions across species. However, imaging studies also implicate the human amygdala in acquisition and recall of fear conditioning (Knight, Smith et al. 2004, Phelps and LeDoux 2005) as well as in extinction learning (LaBar, Gatenby et al. 1998, Milad, Wright et al. 2007).

Imaging studies implicate the dorsal anterior cingulate (dACC) in acquisition and expression of conditioned fear responses, and there is some evidence that dACC thickness correlates with magnitude of conditioned fear responses (Milad, Quirk et al. 2007, Hartley, Fischl et al. 2011). These data suggest that the human dACC may be the functional homologue of the rodent PL (Milad and Quirk 2012), as does evidence of increasing vmPFC activation over the course of extinction training (Gottfried and Dolan 2004). Other work implicates the vmPFC in extinction recall (Milad, Quinn et al. 2005, Linnman, Rougemont-Bucking et al. 2011), further suggesting that the human vmPFC is the functional homologue of the rodent IL (Milad and Quirk 2012).

As with rodents, the human hippocampus appears to contextually gate extinction memories. Hippocampal activation occurs during extinction recall (Knight, Smith et al. 2004, Milad, Wright et al. 2007), and one study found that hippocampal activity increases only when the CS is presented in but not outside of the extinction context (Kalisch, Korenfeld et al. 2006). These findings suggest that the hippocampus gates the "when and where" of extinction memory expression.

THE PATHOPHYSIOLOGY OF ANXIETY DISORDERS

Fear conditioning and extinction are relevant to anxiety disorder pathophysiology, because they mimic clinical features of anxiety, such as heightened arousal and physiological responses. In fact, fear conditioning and extinction models form the basis of many exposure-based therapies (Graham and Milad 2011, Milad, Rosenbaum et al. 2014, Morrison and Ressler 2014). The use of this model also enables the development of novel therapeutic approaches, such as prolonged exposure (Shin and Liberzon 2009, Rabinak, Holman et al. 2013, Marin, Camprodon et al. 2014). Additionally, the primary measures for conditioning and extinction in humans, e.g fear potentiated startle and SCRs (Jovanovic and Ressler 2010), reduce concerns about bias in subjective reports. Moreover, the reliability of psychophysiological measures, specifically SCR, as an index of fear has been shown consistently across fear conditioning, extinction and extinction recall, at least in healthy adults (Zeidan, Lebron-Milad et al. 2012). This has led fear-based physiological to represent important intermediate phenotypes highlighted in the NIMH RDoC initiative (see chapter 2).

In addition, fear conditioning and extinction behaviors appear to be heritable phenotypes, based on data from animal studies (Hefner, Whittle et al. 2008), and the few available studies in humans; Hettema and colleagues (Hettema, Annas et al. 2003) show that genetics accounts for 35-45% of this variance. Similarly in rodents, Shumake and colleagues tested the offspring of good and poor extinguishers, and found that heritability explained 36% of the variance in extinction recall, consistent with human studies (Shumake, Furgeson-Moreira et al. 2014). Given that most phobias are usually triggered by ecologically relevant stimuli (Ohman and Mineka 2001), the use of such stimuli in laboratory tasks may be optimally suited to detect genetic substrates of the conditioning/ extinction processes that are relevant to the etiology of anxiety. Together, these studies support the notion that associative learning, the theorized cognitive mechanism underlying conditioning and extinction, is at least somewhat heritable.

The etiology of some anxiety and fear-based disorders may be linked to processes related to associative learning and memory, highlighting another reason why conditioning paradigms serve as a useful experimental model for studying these disorders. There are data to suggest that fear and anxiety are associated with heightened conditionability and/or impaired extinction. A meta-analysis that reviewed 20 studies of laboratory conditioning and extinction tasks in a range of anxiety disorders demonstrated enhanced conditioned responding during fear acquisition and extinction in people with anxiety disorders relative to healthy controls (Lissek, Baas et al. 2005). Other studies comparing responses to a conditioned cue versus a "safety" cue (i.e., a cue that was never reinforced) have revealed that participants with posttraumatic stress disorder (PTSD) show higher levels of conditioned responding to both the conditioned cue as well as a non-US-reinforced cue, suggesting a diminished ability amongst people with PTSD to discriminate between aversive and safe cues (Orr, Metzger et al. 2000, Peri, Ben Shakhar et al. 2000, Blechert, Michael et al. 2007, Norrholm, Jovanovic et al. 2011). These studies also reported delays in subsequent extinction, although that may reflect the heightened acquisition during conditioning, rather than an additional impairment in fear extinction.

There are also reports indicating that patients with anxiety disorders exhibit deficient fear extinction. Recent studies have reported specific failures in extinction learning or extinction recall in patients with anxiety disorders, despite there being no differences in fear conditioning when compared to healthy controls. This has been demonstrated in people with panic disorder using both SCRs and self-report valence ratings as indices of conditioned fear (Michael, Blechert et al. 2007). Similarly, participants with PTSD exhibit impairments in extinction recall, despite there being no differences in conditioning or extinction learning compared to trauma-exposed controls (Milad, Orr et al. 2008, Milad, Pitman et al. 2009). Compared to healthy controls, participants with PTSD exhibited reduced suppression of potentiated startle in trials that included the conditioned inhibitor (Jovanovic, Norrholm et al. 2009). Furthermore, patients with PTSD show impaired fear inhibition, a model of fear that examines the ability to suppress fear responses when a CS is presented in the presence of a conditioned inhibitor (i.e., a safety signal) (Jovanovic and Ressler 2010).

The degree of impairment in conditioning and extinction appears to be related to symptom severity, with greater severity correlating with more heightened fear conditioning, and/or greater impairment of extinction ability (Milad, Pitman et al. 2009, Norrholm, Jovanovic et al. 2011). In addition, these deficits are associated with differences in the underlying neural circuitry. For example, using PET, Bremner and colleagues (Bremner, Vermetten et al. 2005) demonstrated that people with PTSD exhibited heightened behavioral responses that were associated with increased resting metabolic activity in the left amygdala during fear acquisition, and decreased resting metabolic activity in the ventromedial prefrontal cortex during extinction, when compared to healthy controls. Impaired extinction recall observed in PTSD populations is associated with reduced activity in the vmPFC and hippocampus, but heightened dACC activity (Milad, Pitman et al. 2009). These data suggest that behavioral and psychophysiological measures of conditioning and extinction ability in anxious populations may tap into underlying dysfunctions in cortical and limbic regions that mediate emotion regulation.

DEFICIENT FEAR EXTINCTION: CAUSE OR CONSEQUENCE?

The data reviewed provide evidence indicating that dysfunctions in acquisition and extinction of fear are associated with anxiety disorders across a number of experimental tasks. However, it remains unclear if these dysfunctions represent genetic vulnerabilities or represent a consequence of developing a pathological emotional response. Such questions can be answered with data on the degree to which fear conditioning/extinction phenotypes and anxiety disorders "co-segregate" in family members (Gottesman and Gould 2003).

One study examined genetic covariation between psychophysiological measures of conditioning/extinction profiles and self-reported phobic fears in monozygotic and dizygotic twins (Hettema, Annas et al. 2003). A negative correlation was reported between psychophysiological fear responses and self-reported phobic fears. However, the genetic factors underlying fear conditioning/extinction accounted for only 9% of individual differences in self-reported phobic fears. The authors suggested that their data should caution against the use of fear conditioning as a behavioral phenotype for specific phobia. In a study of monozygotic twins discordant for trauma exposure and PTSD, extinction recall was impaired in PTSD participants but not in their nontrauma exposed co-twin, relative to non-PTSD twins discordant for trauma exposure (Milad, Orr et al. 2008). These data suggest that impaired extinction may not be a preexisting genetic factor, and further, that it is not a consequence of trauma exposure per se. Rather, impaired extinction may be a specific consequence of the development of a fear or anxiety based psychopathology.

SUMMARY AND CONCLUSIONS

As the domain of fear extinction research continues to grow, further basic and translation efforts will contribute to understanding of fear-based and anxiety disorders. Nevertheless, there remains doubt about broad clinical applicability. Perhaps fear conditioning and extinction represent intermediate phenotypes reflecting only one component of anxiety disorders, which are complex phenotypes spanning other negative valence domains as well. That said, they remain some of the best understood behavioral processes spanning rodents to humans, and thus provide a great deal of promise with regards to translational research.

Furthermore, while this chapter focuses primarily on the amygdala, vmPFC, hippocampus, and dACC, there is a burgeoning field of research implicating other brain regions such as the thalamus, striatum, and cerebellum. Complimentary research should help address these concerns, especially through the use of additional approaches in reconsolidation and avoidance paradigms. With recent developments in neurogenesis and genetics, the molecular underpinnings of fear extinction are attractive targets for potential therapies. Ultimately, researchers and clinicians alike will be best served by a confluence of these approaches, and a greater emphasis on collaborative research. While early skepticism about the validity of the model may have delayed clinical applications, it has become increasingly clear that the neural circuitry underlying the etiology of anxiety disorders can be assessed through fear extinction paradigms.

DISCLOSURE STATEMENT

M. R. Milad received funding from the NIMH R01 MH097964-01 and R01 MH097880-01.

ACKNOWLEDGMENTS

The authors would like to acknowledge the members of the Behavioral Neuroscience Program for their assistance in the production of this chapter.

REFERENCES

Anagnostaras, S. G., S. Maren, J. R. Sage, S. Goodrich and M. S. Fanselow (1999). "Scopolamine and Pavlovian fear conditioning in rats: dose-effect analysis." *Neuropsychopharmacology* 21(6): 731–744.

Andero, R., D. C. Choi and K. J. Ressler (2014). "BDNF-TrkB receptor regulation of distributed adult neural plasticity, memory formation, and psychiatric disorders." *Prog Mol Biol Transl Sci* 122: 169–192.

Andero, R. and K. J. Ressler (2012). "Fear extinction and BDNF: translating animal models of PTSD to the clinic." *Genes Brain Behav* 11(5): 503–512.

Blechert, J., T. Michael, N. Vriends, J. Margraf and F. H. Wilhelm (2007). "Fear conditioning in posttraumatic stress disorder: Evidence for delayed extinction of autonomic, experiential, and behavioural responses." *Behav Res Ther, 45*(9): 2019–2033.

Bouton, M. E. and D. A. King (1983). "Contextual control of the extinction of conditioned fear: tests for the associative value of the context." *J Exp Psychol Anim Behav Process* 9(3): 248–265.

Bouton, M. E., R. F. Westbrook, K. A. Corcoran and S. Maren (2006). "Contextual and temporal modulation of extinction: behavioral and biological mechanisms." *Biol Psychiatry* 60(4): 352–360.

Bremner, J. D., E. Vermetten, C. Schmahl, V. Vaccarino, M. Vythilingam, N. Afzal, C. Grillon and D. S. Charney (2005). "Positron emission tomographic imaging of neural correlates of a fear acquisition and extinction paradigm in women with childhood sexual-abuse-related post-traumatic stress disorder." *Psychol Med* 35(6): 791–806.

Carbone, D. L. and R. J. Handa (2013). "Sex and stress hormone influences on the expression and activity of brain-derived neurotrophic factor." *Neuroscience* 239: 295–303.

Cestari, V., C. Rossi-Arnaud, D. Saraulli and M. Costanzi (2014). "The MAP(K) of fear: from memory consolidation to memory extinction." *Brain Res Bull* 105: 8–16.

Charney, D. S. and D. E. Redmond, Jr. (1983). "Neurobiological mechanisms in human anxiety. Evidence supporting central noradrenergic hyperactivity." *Neuropharmacology* 22(12B): 1531–1536.

Ciocchi, S., C. Herry, F. Grenier, S. B. Wolff, J. J. Letzkus, I. Vlachos, I. . . . A. Luthi (2010). "Encoding of conditioned fear in central amygdala inhibitory circuits." *Nature* 468(7321): 277–282.

Corcoran, K. A. and S. Maren (2001). "Hippocampal inactivation disrupts contextual retrieval of fear memory after extinction." *J Neurosci* 21(5): 1720–1726.

Corcoran, K. A. and G. J. Quirk (2007). "Recalling safety: cooperative functions of the ventromedial prefrontal cortex and the hippocampus in extinction." *CNS Spectr* 12(3): 200–206.

Cryan, J. F. and A. Holmes (2005). "The ascent of mouse: advances in modeling human depression and anxiety." *Nat Rev Drug Discov* 4(9): 775–790.

Davis, M. (1986). "Pharmacological and anatomical analysis of fear conditioning using the fear-potentiated startle paradigm." *Behav Neurosci* 100(6): 814–824.

Do-Monte, F. H., J. Rodriguez-Romaguera, L. E. Rosas-Vidal and G. J. Quirk (2013). "Deep brain stimulation of the ventral striatum increases BDNF in the fear extinction circuit." *Front Behav Neurosci* 7: 102.

Fanselow, M. S. (1980). "Conditioned and unconditional components of post-shock freezing." *Pavlov J Biol Sci* 15(4): 177–182.

Fischer, A., M. Radulovic, C. Schrick, F. Sananbenesi, J. Godovac-Zimmermann and J. Radulovic (2007). "Hippocampal Mek/Erk signaling mediates extinction of contextual freezing behavior." *Neurobiol Learn Mem* 87(1): 149–158.

Garcia, R. (2002). "Stress, synaptic plasticity, and psychopathology." *Rev Neurosci* 13(3): 195–208.

Goosens, K. A. and S. Maren (2001). "Contextual and auditory fear conditioning are mediated by the lateral, basal, and central amygdaloid nuclei in rats." *Learn Mem* 8(3): 148–155.

Gottesman, II and T. D. Gould (2003). "The endophenotype concept in psychiatry: etymology and strategic intentions." *Am J Psychiatry* 160(4): 636–645.

Gottfried, J. A. and R. J. Dolan (2004). "Human orbitofrontal cortex mediates extinction learning while accessing conditioned representations of value." *Nat Neurosci* 7(10): 1144–1152.

Graham, B. M. and M. R. Milad (2011). "The study of fear extinction: Implications for anxiety disorders." *Am J Psychiatry* 168(12): 1255–1265.

Hartley, C. A., B. Fischl and E. A. Phelps (2011). "Brain structure correlates of individual differences in the acquisition and inhibition of conditioned fear." *Cereb Cortex* 21(9): 1954–1962.

Hefner, K., N. Whittle, J. Juhasz, M. Norcross, R. M. Karlsson, L. M. Saksida, T. J. Bussey, N. Singewald and A. Holmes (2008). "Impaired fear extinction learning and cortico-amygdala circuit abnormalities in a common genetic mouse strain." *J Neurosci* 28(32): 8074–8085.

Herry, C., P. Trifilieff, J. Micheau, A. Luthi and N. Mons (2006). "Extinction of auditory fear conditioning requires MAPK/ERK activation in the basolateral amygdala." *Eur J Neurosci* 24(1): 261–269.

Hettema, J. M., P. Annas, M. C. Neale, K. S. Kendler and M. Fredrikson (2003). "A twin study of the genetics of fear conditioning." *Arch Gen Psychiatry* 60(7): 702–708.

Hugues, S., A. Chessel, I. Lena, R. Marsault and R. Garcia (2006). "Prefrontal infusion of PD098059 immediately after fear extinction training blocks extinction-associated prefrontal synaptic plasticity and decreases prefrontal ERK2 phosphorylation." *Synapse* 60(4): 280–287.

Hugues, S., Deschaux, O. and Garcia, R. (2004). Postextinction infusion of a mitogen-activated protein kinase inhibitor into the medial prefrontal cortex impairs memory of the extinction of conditioned fear. *Learn Mem*, 11: 540–543. doi:10.1101/lm.77704

Inslicht, S. S., T. J. Metzler, N. M. Garcia, S. L. Pineles, M. R. Milad, S. P. Orr, C. R. Marmar and T. C. Neylan (2013). "Sex differences in fear conditioning in posttraumatic stress disorder." *J Psychiatr Res* 47(1): 64–71.

Jovanovic, T., S. D. Norrholm, J. E. Fennell, M. Keyes, A. M. Fiallos, K. M. Myers, M. Davis and E. J. Duncan (2009). "Posttraumatic stress disorder may be associated with impaired fear inhibition: relation to symptom severity." *Psychiatry Res.* 167(1–2): 151–160.

Jovanovic, T. and K. J. Ressler (2010). "How the neurocircuitry and genetics of fear inhibition may inform our understanding of PTSD." *Am J Psychiatry* 167(6): 648–662.

Kalisch, R., E. Korenfeld, K. E. Stephan, N. Weiskopf, B. Seymour and R. J. Dolan (2006). "Context-dependent human extinction memory is mediated by a ventromedial prefrontal and hippocampal network." *J Neurosci* 26(37): 9503–9511.

Kim, J. H., S. Li and R. Richardson (2011). "Immunohistochemical analyses of long-term extinction of conditioned fear in adolescent rats." *Cereb Cortex* 21(3): 530–538.

Knight, D. C., C. N. Smith, D. T. Cheng, E. A. Stein and F. J. Helmstetter (2004). "Amygdala and hippocampal activity during acquisition and extinction of human fear conditioning." *Cogn Affect Behav Neurosci* 4(3): 317–325.

LaBar, K. S., J. C. Gatenby, J. C. Gore, J. E. Ledoux and E. A. Phelps (1998). "Human amygdala activation during conditioned fear acquisition and extinction: a mixed-trial fMRI study." *Neuron* 20(5): 937–945.

LeDoux, J. (2007). "The amygdala." *Curr Biol* 17(20): R868–R874.

Linnman, C., A. Rougemont-Bucking, J. C. Beucke, T. A. Zeffiro and M. R. Milad (2011). "Unconditioned responses and functional fear networks in human classical conditioning." *Behav Brain Res* 221(1): 237–245.

Lissek, S., J. M. Baas, D. S. Pine, K. Orme, S. Dvir, M. Nugent, E. Rosenberger, E. Rawson and C. Grillon (2005). "Airpuff startle probes: an efficacious and less aversive alternative to white-noise." *Biol Psychol* 68(3): 283–297.

Lu, K. T., D. L. Walker and M. Davis (2001). "Mitogen-activated protein kinase cascade in the basolateral nucleus of amygdala is involved in extinction of fear-potentiated startle." *J Neurosci* 21(16): RC162.

Maren, S. and G. J. Quirk (2004). "Neuronal signalling of fear memory." *Nat Rev Neurosci* 5(11): 844–852.

Marin, M. F., J. A. Camprodon, D. D. Dougherty and M. R. Milad (2014). "Device-based brain stimulation to augment fear extinction: implications for PTSD treatment and beyond." *Depress Anxiety* 31(4): 269–278.

Matsuda, S., D. Matsuzawa, K. Nakazawa, C. Sutoh, H. Ohtsuka, D. Ishii, H. Tomizawa, M. Iyo and E. Shimizu (2010). "d-serine enhances extinction of auditory cued fear conditioning via ERK1/2 phosphorylation in mice." *Prog Neuropsychopharmacol Biol Psychiatry* 34(6): 895–902.

Michael, T., J. Blechert, N. Vriends, J. Margraf and F. H. Wilhelm (2007). "Fear conditioning in panic disorder: Enhanced resistance to extinction." *J Abnorm Psychol* 116(3): 612–617.

Milad, M. R., S. P. Orr, N. B. Lasko, Y. Chang, S. L. Rauch and R. K. Pitman (2008). "Presence and acquired origin of reduced recall for fear extinction in PTSD: results of a twin study." *J Psychiatr Res* 42(7): 515–520.

Milad, M. R., R. K. Pitman, C. B. Ellis, A. B. Gold, L. M. Shin, N. B. Lasko, K. Handwerger, S. P. Orr and S. L. Rauch (2009). "Neurobiological basis for failure to recall extinction memory in posttraumatic stress disorder." *Biol Psychiatry* 66(12): 1075–1082.

Milad, M. R., B. T. Quinn, R. K. Pitman, S. P. Orr, B. Fischl and S. L. Rauch (2005). "Thickness of ventromedial prefrontal cortex in humans is correlated with extinction memory." *Proc Natl Acad Sci USA* 102(30): 10706–10711.

Milad, M. R. and G. J. Quirk (2012). "Fear extinction as a model for translational neuroscience: ten years of progress." *Annu Rev Psychol* 63: 129–151.

Milad, M. R., G. J. Quirk, R. K. Pitman, S. P. Orr, B. Fischl and S. L. Rauch (2007). "A role for the human dorsal anterior cingulate cortex in fear expression." *Biol Psychiatry* 62(10): 1191–1194.

Milad, M. R., S. L. Rauch, R. K. Pitman and G. J. Quirk (2006). "Fear extinction in rats: Implications for human brain imaging and anxiety disorders." *Biol Psychol*

Milad, M. R., B. L. Rosenbaum and N. M. Simon (2014). "Neuroscience of fear extinction: Implications for assessment and treatment of fear-based and anxiety related disorders." *Behav Res Ther* 62: 17–23.

Milad, M. R., C. I. Wright, S. P. Orr, R. K. Pitman, G. J. Quirk and S. L. Rauch (2007). "Recall of fear extinction in humans activates the ventromedial prefrontal cortex and hippocampus in concert." *Biol Psychiatry* 62(5): 446–454.

Morrison, F. G. and K. J. Ressler (2014). "From the neurobiology of extinction to improved clinical treatments." *Depress Anxiety* 31(4): 279–290.

Myers, K. M. and M. Davis (2007). "Mechanisms of fear extinction." *Mol Psychiatry* 12(2): 120–150.

Norrholm, S. D., T. Jovanovic, I. W. Olin, L. A. Sands, I. Karapanou, B. Bradley and K. J. Ressler (2011). "Fear extinction in traumatized civilians with posttraumatic stress disorder: relation to symptom severity." *Biol Psychiatry* 69(6): 556–563.

Ohman, A. and S. Mineka (2001). "Fears, phobias, and preparedness: toward an evolved module of fear and fear learning." *Psychol Rev* 108(3): 483–522.

Orr, S. P., L. J. Metzger, N. B. Lasko, M. L. Macklin, T. Peri and R. K. Pitman (2000). "De novo conditioning in trauma-exposed individuals with and without posttraumatic stress disorder." *J Abnorm Psychol* 109(2): 290–298.

Pavlov, I. (1927). *Conditioned Reflexes*. London, Oxford University Press.

Peri, T., G. Ben Shakhar, S. P. Orr and A. Y. Shalev (2000). "Psychophysiologic assessment of aversive conditioning in posttraumatic stress disorder." *Biol Psychiatry* 47(6): 512–519.

Peters, J., L. M. Dieppa-Perea, L. M. Melendez and G. J. Quirk (2010). "Induction of fear extinction with hippocampal-infralimbic BDNF." *Science* 328(5983): 1288–1290.

Phelps, E. A. and J. E. LeDoux (2005). "Contributions of the amygdala to emotion processing: from animal models to human behavior." *Neuron* 48(2): 175–187.

Quirk, G. J. (2002). "Memory for extinction of conditioned fear is long-lasting and persists following spontaneous recovery." *Learn Mem* 9(6): 402–407.

Quirk, G. J. and D. Mueller (2008). "Neural mechanisms of extinction learning and retrieval." *Neuropsychopharmacology* 33(1): 56–72.

Rabinak, C. A., A. Holman, M. Angstadt, A. E. Kennedy, G. Hajcak and K. L. Phan (2013). "Neural response to errors in combat-exposed returning veterans with and without post-traumatic stress disorder: a preliminary event-related potential study." *Psychiatry Res* 213(1): 71–78.

Rosas-Vidal, L. E., F. H. Do-Monte, F. Sotres-Bayon and G. J. Quirk (2014). "Hippocampal—prefrontal BDNF and memory for fear extinction." *Neuropsychopharmacology* 39(9): 2161–2169.

Santini, E., H. Ge, K. Ren, S. Pena de Ortiz and G. J. Quirk (2004). "Consolidation of fear extinction requires protein synthesis in the medial prefrontal cortex." *J Neurosci* 24(25): 5704–5710.

Shin, L. M. and I. Liberzon (2009). "The Neurocircuitry of Fear, Stress, and Anxiety Disorders." *Neuropsychopharmacology* 35: 165–191.

Shumake, J., S. Furgeson-Moreira and M. H. Monfils (2014). "Predictability and heritability of individual differences in fear learning." *Anim Cogn* 17(5): 1207–1221.

Vidal-Gonzalez, I., B. Vidal-Gonzalez, S. L. Rauch and G. J. Quirk (2006). "Microstimulation reveals opposing influences of prelimbic and infralimbic cortex on the expression of conditioned fear." *Learn Mem* 13(6): 728–733.

Wilensky, A. E., G. E. Schafe, M. P. Kristensen and J. E. LeDoux (2006). "Rethinking the fear circuit: the central nucleus of the amygdala is required for the acquisition, consolidation, and expression of Pavlovian fear conditioning." *J Neurosci* 26(48): 12387–12396.

Zeidan, M. A., K. Lebron-Milad, J. Thompson-Hollands, J. J. Im, D. D. Dougherty, D. J. Holt, S. P. Orr and M. R. Milad (2012). "Test-retest reliability during fear acquisition and fear extinction in humans." *CNS Neurosci Ther* 18(4): 313–317.

25

LEARNING THEORY AND COGNITIVE BEHAVIORAL THERAPY

MICHAEL TREANOR,
LINDSAY K. STAPLES-BRADLEY, AND
MICHELLE G. CRASKE

INTRODUCTION

Behavioral and cognitive behavioral therapies (CBT) for anxiety disorders represent one of the successes of modern clinical psychology. However, despite the efficacy of these interventions, a substantial number of individuals either fail to respond to treatment or demonstrate a return of symptoms (Arch & Craske, 2009). Elucidating and targeting the mechanisms that underlie treatment may increase the efficacy of CBT and mitigate relapse as well as increase our understanding of these disorders.

Associative learning and memory processes were once at the core of conceptualizations of anxiety disorders. Recently, there has been renewed interest in a modern learning theory account of pathological anxiety and CBT (see Craske, Kircanski, Zelikowsky, Mystkowski, Chowdhury, & Baker 2008; Craske, Liao, Brown, & Vervliet, 2012; Craske, Treanor, Conway, Zbozinek, & Vervliet, 2014). This approach has numerous advantages, including providing a more parsimonious account of clinical interventions based in animal, human, and neurobiological research.

A modern learning theory conceptualization of pathological anxiety is based on the notion that a previously neutral cue (conditioned stimulus or CS) elicits a conditioned response (e.g., fear or anxiety) after being paired with an aversive stimulus (unconditioned stimulus or US). Modern learning theory emphasizes the predictive nature of CS-US relations, such that conditioned responding occurs as a result of the CS being predictive of the US. For example, in the case of social anxiety disorder an individual may display anxiety when confronted with social interactions (CS) after instances of social rejection or exclusion (US). Initial criticisms of associative learning as an account of clinical anxiety were often based on a misunderstanding of the CS-US relationship, including the assumption that the primary association was a stimulus-response (social interaction is associated with anxiety) rather than a stimulus-stimulus relationship (social interaction predicts rejection). However, a wealth of experimental evidence suggests that the primary association that is formed during conditioning relates to the CS and US (Rescorla & Wagner, 1972). Thus, the core of an associative account of clinical anxiety is based on the formation of a predictive association between a CS and US.

In addition, it was assumed that learning theory could not account for anxiety disorders that did not seem to involve a direct conditioning experience. However, research has demonstrated that these associations can be formed via modeling and even verbal transmission of information (Olsson & Phelps, 2007). Once a CS-US association has been established, it can generalize to other stimuli that share perceptual or conceptual features with the original CS through a process known as stimulus generalization (Lissek et al., 2010).

Repeatedly presenting the CS in the absence of the US leads to a reduction in conditioned responding through a process known as extinction learning. For example, by repeatedly engaging in social interactions in the absence of rejection or humiliation, an individual who previously feared social situations will report decreased anxiety. This is because the individual learns that the CS (social interaction) is no longer a good predictor of the US (rejection).

Conceptualizing CBT from a learning theory perspective allows the integration of psychological and neurobiological research aimed at facilitating learning processes that target the CS-US relationship. This may be particularly important for individuals with anxiety disorders, as the extant literature suggests that they demonstrate deficits in associative learning processes (Craske et al., 2012). The present chapter will outline a conceptualization of CBT that is based in modern learning theory with attention to the wealth of animal and human research that supports associative learning processes.

EXPOSURE-BASED PROCEDURES

Exposure therapy, or repeated and systematic confrontation with a CS, is at the core of most efficacious treatments for anxiety disorders. Although current conceptualizations of exposure therapy based in modern learning theory share some similarities with information processing models (Foa & Kozak, 1986) and behavioral experiments (Clark & Beck, 2010), there are several important differences between these approaches and an associative learning account of exposure. First and foremost is that exposure from a learning theory perspective mirrors the components of extinction including the initial acquisition, consolidation, and later retrieval and generalization of new learning. Various procedures are designed to target these processes and optimize new inhibitory learning. Second, although information processing models propose that either within, or between, session decreases in fear are necessary for successful treatment, a wealth of research suggests that these are neither necessary nor sufficient (see Craske et al., 2008 for a review). This is consistent with the broader literature on learning, which states that performance during training (e.g., within session decreases in anxiety) is not commensurate with actual learning when tested at a later point in time. Rather, performance at test (e.g., confronting a feared stimulus following treatment) is influenced by factors such context, time, and generalization of learning (Craske et al., 2008). In fact, there is some evidence that maintaining arousal throughout exposure (versus habituation of arousal) may be beneficial, as glucocorticoids enhance extinction consolidation (Quirk & Mueller, 2008).

Acquisition of Extinction

Inasmuch as extinction is thought to operate via an error correction mechanism, exposure from a learning theory perspective is designed to violate expectancies regarding the frequency or intensity of aversive outcomes. Indeed, research suggests that learning, or in this case extinction learning, is enhanced when there is a greater discrepancy between what is predicted and what actually occurs (Rescorla & Wagner, 1972). Thus, for a client with panic disorder who predicts that elevated heart rate is likely to lead to a heart attack, exposures are designed to repeatedly violate this expectancy through inducing increased heart rate, reducing any safety behaviors or avoidance, and including contexts or occasion setters that moderate the likelihood that the US will occur. Research in humans has found that this approach yielded as much long-term benefit at follow-up with just one trial of exposure per day (for two days) compared to repeated trials of exposure each day for acrophobia (Baker et al., 2010) while Deacon et al. (2013) found that interoceptive exposure that continued until the patient's expectancy of an aversive outcome reached less than 5% was superior to standard interoceptive exposure. Using this approach of expectancy violation, the end of a given exposure trial is determined by the violation in expectancy or the stated behavioral goal, rather than fear reduction.

Prediction can be enhanced by combining two conditioned stimuli simultaneously during extinction. The associative strength of the CSs summate or combine to "overpredict" the occurrence of the US. When the US does not occur, there is a greater discrepancy between what was predicted and what actually occurred and extinction learning is enhanced. For example, for a client with panic disorder, combining hyperventilation and spinning may increase the expectation that a given physical catastrophe, such as passing out, is likely to happen. Several studies in animals and humans have found that this "deepened extinction" enhances learning (Culver, Vervliet, and Craske, 2014; Rescorla, 2006), while others have failed to replicate these effects (Vervliet, Vansteenwegen, Hermans, & Eelen, 2007). The failure to replicate these effects may be due to the nature of extinction learning and the need to balance the attentional salience of the target CS with other stimuli during exposure. During a learning trial all stimuli that are present affect the degree of associative change that occurs, and stimuli essentially "compete" to acquire this change (Rescorla & Wagner, 1972). Changes in associative strength are directed toward stimuli with the greatest attentional salience. Thus, when two or more stimuli are equally salient, any net change in associative strength is divided equally between them thereby negating any potential benefit in combined extinction (Rescorla 2006). This can be overcome by either conducting extinction to both stimuli separately prior to combining them, or by conducting extinction to one stimulus prior to combining it with the target CS (Rescorla, 2000; 2006).

Inasmuch as extinction is affected by all stimuli present during a given trial, the presence of inhibitory stimuli can negatively impact extinction. Conditioned inhibitors, or "safety signals," are stimuli that predict the nonoccurrence of the US and therefore reduce the expectation that a US will occur. Numerous studies in both animal and human samples have demonstrated the deleterious effects of safety signals on extinction learning (Lovibond, 2004). Examples of safety signals include anxiolytic medication in panic disorder or hygienic wipes in obsessive-compulsive disorder. However, recent evidence suggests that safety signals may not always negatively impact exposure. For example, Deacon and colleagues have failed to replicate the deleterious effect of engaging in safety behaviors during exposure in claustrophobic fear (Deacon et al., 2010). The ability of safety signals to mitigate extinction learning likely varies depending on the ratio of inhibition and excitation in a given trial. The impact of inhibitory stimuli on extinction learning will therefore depend on the number and strength of inhibitory stimuli versus the number and strength of excitatory stimuli (i.e., stimuli that predict the US; Rescorla & Wagner, 1972). For example, in the Deacon et al. (2010) study, safety signals were only present during some exposures, ensuring the ratio of excitation to inhibition was greater throughout treatment.

An important component of extinction learning is maintaining the salience of the target CS. As mentioned previously, error-correction models posit an important role for the salience of the CS such that any change in associative strength (e.g., extinction learning) will be directed to the cue that is most salient (Mackintosh, 1975; Pearce & Hall, 1980). In addition, inasmuch as extinction represents learning that a CS no longer is the best predictor of the US, awareness of both the CS and the nonoccurrence of the US is essential. Thus, during an exposure trial it is important that the client fully attend to the target CS. For a client with social anxiety, this may entail directing eye contact toward the individual she is speaking with and not rehearsing perceived negative aspects of the situation (e.g., "postevent processing") following the exposure. The former strategy reduces CS salience while the later mitigates awareness of the nonoccurrence of the US. The clinical application of attentional manipulation requires a thorough understanding of learning theory and a functional analysis of a given exposure trial. For example, while the client may be maintaining eye contact with the individual (CS), it is important that she not use this focus as a means of distracting from other possible conditioned stimuli, such as physiological signs of anxiety, that may increase her expectation of negative evaluation. The decision as to which CS to "focus on" will likely vary from client to client, and exposure to exposure, depending upon which target CS elicits the greatest amount of expectancy.

Consolidation of Extinction

Learning, once acquired, is then consolidated into long-term memory. Although this involves neurobiological processes including protein synthesis and system level reorganization (Wang & Morris, 2010) it can potentially be enhanced through behavioral and pharmacological manipulations. For example, the extant literature on memory suggests that mental rehearsal is an important component of memory consolidation (Joos, 2011; Meeter & Murre, 2004). Consistent with this notion, following a given exposure trial, the client and therapist should engage in an interactive discussion designed to repeatedly rehearse the noncontingent relationship between the CS and US. This is accomplished by detailed discussion and asking participants to judge what they learned regarding the nonoccurrence of the feared event, discrepancies between what was predicted and what occurred, and the degree of "surprise" from the exposure practice (e.g., Rescorla & Wagner, 1972).

Consolidation of extinction learning relies in part on N-methyl-D-aspartate (NMDA) receptors within the basolateral nucleus of the amygdala (Royer & Pare, 2002). The antibiotic D-cycloserine (DCS), a partial NMDA receptor agonist, may therefore offer an advantage in strengthening consolidation of the inhibitory memories developed during exposure (Walker, Rattiner, & Davis, 2002). Indeed, a recent body of literature suggests that DCS may bolster the effects of exposure therapy for anxiety disorders when taken before or up to four hours after treatment sessions (e.g., Ressler et al., 2004). A recent meta analysis (Rodrigues et al., 2014) has confirmed that d-cycloserine stands to improve current exposure therapy when administered at low doses and close in time to exposures.

Some evidence suggests that, while DCS administration may increase the pace at which treatment gains are achieved, it is not associated with overall improved outcomes compared to placebo controls. This has been demonstrated in snake phobia, obsessive compulsive disorder, and social anxiety (Nave, Tolin, & Stevens, 2012; Kushner et al., 2007, Hofmann et al., 2013, respectively). Other studies have failed to find any effect of DCS on treatment outcomes, both when administered prior to (Tart et al., 2013) and following exposures (Mataix-Cols et al., 2014). Ceiling effects due to favorable response to CBT in placebo groups may account for these results. Similarly, in one study of DCS enhancement of exposure for posttraumatic stress disorder, no effects were observed for the overall sample; however, a subsample of patients who showed a delayed response to CBT showed greater improvement than placebo (de Kleine et al., 2012). Augmentation of exposure therapy using DCS may therefore be a viable option for severe or treatment-resistant populations.

Notably, certain events during exposure with DCS may be associated with less favorable outcomes than CBT alone (Vervliet, 2008). Aversive experiences such as exposure to a US or unsuccessful exposure sessions may limit or reverse the effects of DCS on extinction memories (Langton and Richardson, 2010; Smits et al., 2013). This is in keeping with our understanding of the mechanism behind DCS: that it enhances memory consolidation, such that when a successful exposure occurs the extinction memory is enhanced; however, when exposure to an unsuccessful exposure occurs, DCS may also enhance consolidation of the aversive memory instead of the targeted extinction memory. However, there is less data on the latter, and in animal studies DCS appears to enhance extinction memories more strongly than aversive memories (Bolkan & Lattal, 2014). Therefore, future research is needed in order to identify specific populations for whom DCS augmentation of exposure therapy may be indicated.

Generalization and Retrieval of Extinction Learning

If extinction learning is the primary mechanism behind exposure therapy, then success can be measured by the extent to which this learning prevails over time and across contexts. Gains achieved in therapy are only as successful as they are generalizable to environments outside of therapy. Unfortunately some patients experience a return of fear following exposure (Craske and Mystkowski, 2006). This may be due to the nature of extinction learning, as research suggests that extinction is highly context dependent. Despite the use of the term "extinction," decades of research has demonstrated that following extinction the original excitatory association is neither lost nor erased. New learning occurs. The CS takes on a new, inhibitory meaning in addition to the original excitatory fear meaning. The organism relies on the context to disambiguate the situation; the context (e.g., the therapist's office vs. a feared social situation) determines which of these two memories is activated (Bouton, 1993). Strategies including occasional reinforced trials during extinction, stimulus variability, multiple contexts, and retrieval cues may be viable methods for bolstering the effects of exposure therapy against the passage of time and novel situations.

Recent studies have explored occasional reinforced trials during extinction as a strategy for limiting return of fear. This counterintuitive strategy involves pairing the US with the CS on a small proportion (2:8) of extinction trials and has been effective in limiting spontaneous recovery in rats (Bouton, Woods, & Pineno, 2004). The Rescorla-Wagner model offers an explanation for this phenomenon. During extinction, the more the organism expects the US during any given CS presentation, the more learning takes place on trials where the US is absent (Rescorla & Wagner, 1972). Occasionally pairing the US with the CS keeps the expectancy of the US elevated during trials in which the CS is presented alone, thus allowing more extinction learning to take place. Alternatively, the procedure of occasional reinforcement during extinction may enhance salience of the CS which in turn contributes to new learning about the CS (Pearce & Hall, 1980). For example, in a single exposure session for social phobia, a client may be asked to start conversations with five different individuals. During some of the conversations, she may engage in strategies that elicit a high likelihood of negative evaluation (such as asking strange questions), while during others she would engage in typical behavior. This strategy may be associated with increased fear at the end of the exposure session but less return of fear at follow-up. Some limitations to this procedure include ethical issues inherent in exposing certain anxious populations to their unconditioned stimulus (e.g., exposing snake-phobic clients to snake bites), and may be better suited to other anxiety disorders such as social phobia.

Anxiety develops in part due to overgeneralization of fear memories to situations and stimuli in which the fear response is inappropriate or disproportional (e.g., Lissek et al., 2014). In turn, introducing variation into exposure sessions may help individuals with anxiety disorders to generalize their extinction memories to novel stimuli and situations. Strategies for introducing this variation include: varying the feared stimuli used in exposures, conducting exposures from different places on the fear hierarchy, ensuring the patient experiences a variety of fear levels throughout exposure, and conducting exposure in multiple contexts (Craske et al., 2012). It is possible that this variation in exposure allows patients to identify a rule that will translate to similar stimuli to be encountered in the future or may serve as a retrieval cue for the extinction memory (Schmidt and Bjork, 1992, Vervliet, Baker & Craske, 2012). Research on the use of multiple contexts has presented mixed findings; however, studies that produced null results may have used contexts that were too similar to one another or used contexts that served as discrete stimuli and not "environments" per se. Issues of feasibility may limit use of multiple contexts in session, however research on their effect on extinction retention should inform therapists developing homework assignments over the course of exposure therapy.

The therapeutic strategy of mental reinstatement may help to prevent recurrence of symptoms in novel contexts without the feasibility concerns of conducting exposures in several different environments. In this strategy, patients are instructed to recall what they learned during exposures *and* the environment in which therapy took place upon encountering their feared stimulus outside of the treatment setting. For example, a spider-phobic individual may experience a return of fear encountering a spider outdoors if exposure sessions were conducted in a therapist's office. Equipping the patient with instructions to think about not only what they learned during exposure but also the setting of the therapist's office may serve to attenuate this context renewal effect. Indeed, use of this approach has been supported by research on phobic populations (Mystkowski et al., 2006).

In addition, one can use a "retrieval cue," or a cue that was present during extinction and is used once extinction is over. Usually a small object such as a wrist band, retrieval cues serve to remind patients of what they learned in exposure and increase the likelihood that inhibitory extinction memories will prevail over fear memories (Brooks & Bouton, 1994; Vansteenwegen et al., 2006). While this may prove a useful strategy in relapse prevention, it is important that the retrieval cue not develop inhibitory properties and function as a safety signal. In order to decrease the likelihood that a retrieval cue functions as a safety signal, one can present the cue prior to the target CS, include the cue on only a small percentage of trials, or ensure that the cue is less salient than the target CS (Brooks & Bouton, 1994). Inasmuch as retrieval cues reduce the expectation of the US, this strategy may not be indicated early in treatment when the focus is on acquiring extinction learning, but rather as a strategy to maintain treatment gains after therapy.

COGNITIVE STRATEGIES

Although cognitive interventions are traditionally conceptualized from within a Beckian framework, they too can be conceptualized from within a learning theory perspective offering a parsimonious and unifying framework from which to situate CBT. For example, the extant literature suggests that conditioned responding can be altered following acquisition as a result of behavioral experiences or knowledge regarding the US through a process known as US-revaluation. In a typical US-revaluation procedure presenting a less intense US, or modifying the valence of the US, reduces conditioned responding to the original CS (Davey, 1989). Conversely, reinterpreting the US as more aversive than originally experienced can increase responding due to US-inflation (Davey, De Jong, & Tallis, 1993). Cognitive strategies, such as "decatastrophizing" may help to mitigate conditioned responding, such as fear and anxiety, through reinterpretation of the intensity or valence of the US (Lovibond, 2004). For example, in social phobia the experience of rejection can be reinterpreted as less aversive ("It wasn't that bad") or less indicative of additional rejection by others ("Just because it didn't work out with one person, doesn't mean I can't make other friends").

Cognitive strategies may also be helpful in generalizing extinction learning to additional stimuli. Individuals with anxiety disorders demonstrate heighted stimulus generalization, or generalization of fear to stimuli that resemble the CS (Lissek et al., 2010). Extinction is much more stimulus specific and does not generalize as readily to related stimuli (Vervliet, Vansteenwegen, & Eelen, 2006). However, extinction can generalize to perceptually and categorically related stimuli under specific conditions (Vervoort, Vervliet, Bennett, & Baeyens, 2014). Cognitive interventions may help to facilitate this process, by generating rules that link stimuli, or directing attentional resources to shared perceptual or categorical features (and making explicit what was learned during exposure). For example, following exposure to a "contaminated" toilet in obsessive-compulsive disorder, Socratic questioning may assist the individual in noticing the similarities between the target stimulus (e.g., toilet) and other feared items (door handle, bathroom sink, etc.).

Although cognitive interventions may be helpful in reducing fear, they may also have deleterious consequences if used in conjunction with some extinction strategies. Inasmuch as extinction relies on a violation of expectancy, using traditional cognitive restructuring of threat overestimation prior to exposure may reduce US-expectancy and mitigate extinction learning. Similarly, reducing the aversiveness of the US through decatastrophizing may also reduce any net change in associative strength thereby mitigating extinction. Thus, while cognitive interventions are important treatment strategies, care must be used when combining them with exposure procedures. Additional research is needed to determine the effect of combining cognitive strategies with exposure procedures on extinction learning.

CASE STUDY

Maria is a 43-year-old, Mexican-American, mother of two who sought treatment due to frequent panic attacks. She reported fear that her rapid heart rate, dizziness, and shortness of breath were predictive of a heart attack and had begun to avoid numerous activities as a result of her anxiety, including exercise, playing with her children, and drinking caffeine. She reported numerous safety behaviors, including carrying her cell phone with her at all times and not exerting herself when her husband was not present.

Therapy began with a discussion regarding the nature of associative learning and how avoidance and safety behaviors can interfere with exposure by preventing violation in expectancy. In addition, Maria and her therapist developed a list of avoided situations along with the feared outcome associated with these situations. Although the hierarchy contained distress and expectancy ratings, exposures did not proceed in a linear fashion consistent with the concept of variability discussed previously.

Exposures began shortly thereafter without training in cognitive restructuring. Initial exposures focused on interoceptive sensations, including inducing increased heart rate through vigorous exercise, shortness of breath through "straw breathing," and dizziness by spinning rapidly in a circle. Prior to each exposure, Maria learned to describe her feared outcome in order to facilitate expectancy violation. Following each in-session exposure exercise, Maria and her therapist engaged in lengthy discussion regarding the nonoccurrence of her feared event. This represented an attempt to consolidate extinction learning. Open-ended questions such as "What did you fear would happen as a result of the exposure?" "What happened?" "How was that surprising?" and "What did you learn?" were used as part of an interactive discussion. Maria was given monitoring sheets for between-session practices where she could list the anticipated negative outcome prior to exposure (e.g., having a heart attack) and engage in postexposure consolidation. Exposures continued until Maria's expectancy had been violated or until the agreed-upon behavioral goal was reached, regardless of fear level.

Treatment included various extinction enhancement strategies such as deepened extinction (e.g., combining vigorous exercise and spinning after conducting extinction to both in isolation), maintaining attentional salience of the target CS, reducing safety behaviors, and varying the contexts in which exposures were conducted.

Following several weeks of exposure sessions, Maria and her therapist discussed the similarities between many of the exposures, in an attempt to generalize the extinction learning among perceptually and categorically related stimuli. For example, her recognition that increased heart rate did not lead to a heart attack was discussed in relation to how other physical symptoms, such as pressure in her chest, might be benign.

Prior to termination, Maria's therapist discussed the context dependent nature of extinction learning, and suggested several relapse prevention strategies. Specifically, Maria practiced "mentally reinstating" previous extinction contexts by imagining, in detail, an exposure session that went well (i.e., her expectation was violated). She practiced this during several exposure trials during her last week of therapy, but was cautioned not to do this too often, nor to rely on it as a safety signal.

SUMMARY AND FUTURE DIRECTIONS

Modern learning theory provides a parsimonious and unifying framework from which to situate both behavioral and cognitive treatments for anxiety disorders (Table 25.1 provides an overview of these strategies). Research in both animal and human populations

TABLE 25.1 Behavioral and Cognitive Strategies for Targeting Associative Learning

ASSOCIATIVE LEARNING PROCESS	STRATEGY	DESCRIPTION
Acquisition of Extinction	Expectancy violation	*Design exposures to violate specific expectations*
	Deepened extinction	*Present two cues during the same exposure after conducting initial extinction with at least one of them*
	Remove safety behaviors	*Decrease the use of safety signals and behaviors*
	Attentional focus	*Maintain attention on the target CS during exposure*
Consolidation of Extinction	Postexposure discussion	*Discuss, in detail the nonoccurrence of the US*
	Pharmacological agents	*D-cycloserine may aid in the consolidation of learning*
Generalization/Retrieval of Extinction	Reinforced extinction	*Occasionally present the US during exposures*
	Variability	*Vary stimuli and contexts*
	Mental reinstatement/ retrieval cues	*Use a cue present during extinction or imaginally reinstate previous successful exposures*
	Cognitive generalization	*Generate rules that link stimuli, or direct attentional resources to shared perceptual or categorical features of stimuli*
US-Revaluation	Decatastrophizing	*Reinterpret the intensity or valence of the US*

has provided support for the processes of extinction learning and suggests behavioral and pharmacological avenues for enhancing treatment. However, additional research is needed to determine the best methods for employing these procedures in clinical settings as well as further elucidating methods for generalizing inhibitory learning across contexts and stimuli.

REFERENCES

Arch, J. J., & Craske, M. G. (2009). First-line treatment: a critical appraisal of cognitive behavioral therapy developments and alternatives. *Psychiatric Clinics of North America, 32*(3), 525–547. doi: 10.1016/j.psc.2009.05.001

Baker, A., Mystkowski, J., Culver, N., Yi, R., Mortazavi, A., Craske, M.G. (2010). Does habituation matter? Emotional processing theory and exposure therapy for acrophobia. *Behaviour Research and Therapy, 48*, 1139–1143. doi: 10.1016/j.brat.2010.07.009

Bolkan, S. S., & Lattal, K. M. (2014). Opposing effects of D-cycloserine on fear despite a common extinction duration: Interactions between brain regions and behavior. *Neurobiology of Learning and Memory, 113*, 25–34. doi: 10.1016/j.nlm.2013.12.009

Bouton, M. E. (1993). Context, time, and memory retrieval in the interference paradigms of Pavlovian learning. *Psychological Bulletin, 114*, 80–99. doi: 10.1037/0033-2909.114.1.80

Bouton, M. E., Woods, A. M., & Pineño, O. (2004). Occasional reinforced trials during extinction can slow the rate of rapid reacquisition. *Learning and Motivation, 35*(4), 371–390. doi: 10.1016/j.lmot.2004.05.001

Brooks, D. C., & Bouton, M. E. (1994). A retrieval cue for extinction attenuates response recovery (renewal) caused by a return to the conditioning context, *Journal of Experimental Psychology: Animal Behavior Processes, 20*, 366–379. doi: 10.1037/0097-7403.20.4.366

Clark, D. A., & Beck, A. T. (2010). *Cognitive Therapy of Anxiety Disorders: Science and Practice*. New York, NY: Guilford Press.

Craske, M. G., Kircanski, K., Zelikowsky, M., Mystkowski, J., Chowdhury, N., & Baker, A. (2008). Optimizing inhibitory learning during exposure therapy. *Behaviour Research and Therapy, 46*, 5–27. doi: 10.1016/j.brat.2007.10.003

Craske, M. G., Liao, B., Brown, L., & Verliet, B. (2012). Role of inhibition in exposure therapy. *Journal of Experimental Psychopathology, 3*, 322–345. doi:10.5127/jep.026511

Craske, M. G., & Mystkowski, J. (2006). Exposure therapy and extinction: clinical studies. In M. G. Craske, D. Hermans, & D. Vansteenwegen (Eds.), *Fear and Learning: Basic Science to Clinical Application*. Washington, DC: APA Books.

Craske, M. G., Treanor, M., Conway, C. Zbozinek, T., & Vervliet, B. (2014). Maximizing exposure therapy: An inhibitory learning approach. *Behaviour Research and Therapy, 58*, 10–23. doi: 10.1016/j.brat.2014.04.006

Culver, N. C., Vervliet, B., & Craske, M. G. (2014). Compound extinction: Using the Rescorla-Wagner model to maximize exposure therapy for anxiety disorders. *Clinical Psychological Science, 18*, 1–14. doi: 10.1177/2167702614542103.

Davey, G. C. L. (1989). UCS revaluation and conditioning models of acquired fears. *Behaviour Research and Therapy, 27*, 521–528. doi:10.1016/0005-7967(89)90086-7.

Davey, G. C. L., De Jong, P. J., & Tallis, F. (1993). UCS inflation in the aetiology of anxiety disorders: Some case histories. *Behaviour Resarch and Therapy, 5*, 495–498. doi:10.1016/0005-7967(93)90130-M.

Deacon, B., Kemp, J. J., Dixon, L. J., Sy, J. T., Farrell, N. R., & Zhang, A. R. (2013). Maximizing the efficacy of interoceptive exposure by optimizing inhibitory learning: A randomized controlled trial. *Behaviour Research and Therapy, 51*, 588–596. doi: 10.1016/j.brat.2013.06.006

Deacon, B. J., Sy, J., Lickel, J. J., & Nelson, E. O. (2010). Does the judicious use of safety behaviors improve the efficacy and acceptability of exposure therapy for claustrophobic fear? *Journal of Behavior Therapy and Experimental Psychiatry, 41*, 71–80. doi: 10.1016/j.jbtep.2009.10.004

De Kleine, R.A., Hendriks, G., Kusters, W.J.C., Broekman, T.G., van Minnen, A. (2012) A randomized placebo-controlled trial of d-cycloserine to enhance exposure therapy for posttraumatic stress disorder. *Biological Psychiatry, 71*:962–968. doi: 10.1016/j.biopsych.2012.02.033

Foa, E. B., & Kozak, M. J. (1986). Emotional processing of fear: exposure to corrective information. *Psychological Bulletin, 99*, 2–35. doi: 10.1037/0033-2909.99.1.20

Hofmann, S.G., Smits, J.A.J., Rosenfield, D., Simon, N., Otto, M.W., Meuret, A.E., Marques, L., Fang, A., Tart, C., Pollack, M.H. (2013). D-cycloserine as an augmentation strategy with cognitive-behavioral therapy for social anxiety disorder. *American Journal of Psychiatry, 170*, 751–758. doi:10.1176/appi.ajp.2013.12070974

Joos, E. (2011). *Repetitive thought in human (fear) conditioning: Strengthening the acquisition and extinction memory*. Unpublished doctoral dissertation, KU Leuven.

Kushner, M.G., Kim, S.W., Donahue, C., Thuras, P., Adson, D., Kotlyar, M., McCabe, J., Peterson, J., Foa, E.B. (2007). D-cycloserine augmented exposure therapy for obsessive-compulsive disorder. *Biological Psychiatry, 62*, 835–838. doi: 10.1016/j.biopsych.2006.12.020

Langton, J.M., Richardson, R. (2010). The effect of D-cycloserine on immediate vs. delayed extinction of learned fear. *Learning and Memory*, 17:547–551. doi:10.1101/lm.1927310

Lissek, S., Kaczkurkin, A.N., Rabin, S., Geraci, M., Pine, D.S., Grillon, C. (2014). Generalized anxiety disorder is associated with overgeneralization of classically conditioned fear. *Biological Psychiatry*, 75, 909–915. doi: 10.1016/j.biopsych.2013.07.025

Lissek, S., Rabin, S., Heller, R. E., Lukenbaugh, D., Geraci, M., Pine, D. S., & Grillon, C. (2010). Overgeneralization of conditioned fear as a pathogenic marker of panic disorder. *The American Journal of Psychiatry*, 167, 47–55. doi:10.1176/appi.ajp.2009.09030410

Lovibond, P. F. (2004). Cognitive processes in extinction. *Learning & Memory*, 11, 495–500. doi: 10.1101/lm.79604

Mackintosh, N. J. (1975). A theory of attention: Variations in the associability of stimuli with reinforcement. *Psychological Review*, 82(4), 276. doi: 10.1037/h0076778

Mataix-Cols, D., Turner, C., Monzani, B., Isomura, K., Murphy, C., Krebs, G., & Heyman, I. (2014). Cognitive-behavioural therapy with post-session d-cycloserine augmentation for paediatric obsessive-compulsive disorder: Pilot randomized controlled trial. *The British Journal of Psychiatry*, 204, 77–78. doi: 10.1192/bjp.bp.113.126284

Meeter, M., & Murre, J. M. J. (2004). Consolidation of long-term memory: Evidence and alternatives. *Psychological Bulletin*, 130, 843–857. doi: 10.1037/0033-2909/130.6.843

Mystkowski, J. L., Craske, M. G., Echiverri, A. M., & Labus, J. S. (2006). Mental reinstatement of context and return of fear in spider-fearful participants. *Behavior Therapy*, 37, 49–60. doi: 10.1016/j.beth.2005.04.001

Nave, A.M., Tolin, D.F., Stevens, M.C. (2012). Exposure therapy, d-cycloserine, and functional magnetic resonance imaging in patients with snake phobia: A randomized pilot study. *Journal of Clinical Psychiatry*, 73(9)1179–1186.

Olsson A., & Phelps, E. A. (2007). Social learning of fear. *Nature Neuroscience*, 10, 1095–1102. doi:10.1038/nn1968

Pearce, J. M., & Hall, G. (1980). A model for Pavlovian learning: variations in the effectiveness of conditioned but not of unconditioned stimuli. *Psychological review*, 87(6), 532.doi:10.1037/0033-295X.87.6.532

Quirk, G. J., & Mueller, D. (2008). Neural mechanisms of extinction learning and retrieval. *Neuropsychopharmacology*, 33, 56–72. doi:10.1038/sj.npp.1301555

Rescorla, R.A. (2000). Extinction can be enhanced by a concurrent excitor. *Journal of Experimental Psychology*, 26, 251–260.

Rescorla, R. A. (2006). Deepened extinction from compound stimulus presentation. *Journal of Experimental Psychology: Animal Behavior Processes*, 32, 135–144. doi: 10.1037/0097-7403.32.2.135. 135

Rescorla R. A. & Wagner A. R. (1972). A theory of Pavlovian conditioning: Variations in the effectiveness of reinforcement and non-reinforcement. In A. H. Prokasy (Ed.), *Classical Conditioning II: Current Research and Theory* (64–99). New York, NY: Appleton-Century-Croft.

Ressler, K. J., Rothbaum, B. O., Tannenbaum, L., Anderson, P., Graap, K., Zimand, E., . . . Davis, M. (2004). Cognitive enhancers as adjuncts to psychotherapy: Use of D-cycloserine in phobic individuals to facilitate extinction of fear. *Archives of General Psychiatry*, 61, 1136–1144. doi:10.1001/archpsyc.61.11.1136

Rodrigues, H., Figueira, I., Lopes, A., Goncalves, R., Mendlowicz, M.V., Coutinho, E. S., Ventura, P. (2014). Does d-cycloserine enhance exposure therapy for anxiety disorders in humans? A meta-analysis. *PLoS One*, 9(7): e93519. doi: 10.1371/journal.pone.0093519

Royer, S., and Pare, D. (2002). Bidirectional synaptic plasticity in intercalated amygdala neurons and the extinction of conditioned fear responses. *Neuroscience*, 115(2) 455–462. doi: 10.1016/S0306-4522(02)00455-4

Schmidt, R. A., & Bjork, R. A. (1992). New conceptualization of practice: Common principles in three paradigms suggest new concepts for training. *Psychological Science*, 3, 207–217.

Smits, J. A. J., Rosenfield, D., Otto, M. W., Powers, M. B., Hofmann, S. G., Telch, M. J., Pollack, M. H., Tart, C. D. (2013). D-cycloserine enhancement of fear extinction is specific to successful exposure sessions: Evidence from the treatment of height phobia. *Biological Psychiatry*, 73, 1054–1058. doi: 10.1016/j.biopsych.2012.12.009

Tart, C. D., Handelsman, P. R., DeBoer, L. B., Rosenfield, D., Pollack, M., Hofmann, S. G., Powers, M. B., Otto, M. W., Smits, J. A. J. (2013). Augmentation of exposure therapy with post-session administration of d-cycloserine. *Journal of Psychiatric Research*, 47, 168–174.

Vansteenwegen, D., Vervliet, B., Hermans, D., Beckers, T., Baeyens, F., & Eelen, P. (2006). Stronger renewal in human fear conditioning when tested with an acquisition retrieval cue than with an extinction retrieval cue. *Behaviour Research and Therapy*, 44(12), 1717–1725. doi: 10.1016/j.brat.2005.10.014

Vervliet, B. (2008). Learning and memory in conditioned fear extinction: effects of D-cycloserine. *Acta Psychologica*, 127, 601–613. doi: 10.1016/j.actpsy.2007.07.001

Vervliet, B., Baker, A., & Craske, M. G. (2012). Fear conditioning in animals and humans. In N. M. Seel & D. Quinones (Eds.), *Encyclopedia of the sciences of learning*. New York: Springer Science + Business Media.

Vervliet, B., Vansteenwegen, D., & Eelen, P. (2006). Generalization gradients for acquisition and extinction in human contingency learning. *Experimental Psychology*, 53, 132–142. doi:10.1027/1618-3169.53.2.132

Vervliet, B., Vansteenwegen, D., Hermans, D., & Eelen, P. (2007). Concurrent excitors limit the extinction of conditioned fear in humans. *Behaviour Research and Therapy*, 45, 375–383. doi: 10.1016/j.brat.2006.01.009

Vervoort, E., Vervliet, B., Bennett, M., & Baeyens, F. (2014). Generalization of human fear acquisition and extinction within a novel arbitrary stimulus category. *PLoS One*, 9, e9656. doi: 10.1371/journal.pone.0096569

Walker, D. L., Rattiner, L. M., & Davis, M. (2002). Group II metabotropic glutamate receptors within the amygdala regulate fear as assessed with potentiated startle in rats. *Behavioral Neuroscience*, 116, 1075–1083.

Wang, S. H., & Morris, R. G. M. (2010). Hippocampal-neocortical interactions in memory formation, consolidation and reconsolidation. *Annual Review of Psychology*, 61, 49–79. doi: 10.1146/annurev.psych.093008.100523

/// 26 /// PHARMACOLOGICAL MECHANISMS OF MODULATING FEAR AND EXTINCTION

BOADIE W. DUNLOP, KERRY J. RESSLER, AND BARBARA O. ROTHBAUM

INTRODUCTION

Fear is an emotional experience shared across humans and other mammals. Fear reactions are valuable for life; without fear, individuals would not avoid dangerous objects and situations, thereby exposing themselves to potential injury or death. Fears can be innate (e.g., acrophobia, the fear of heights) or learned (e.g., electrophobia, fear of electricity). Because fear facilitates survival, the neurobiology of fear processing has been evolutionarily conserved among mammals and can reliably be identified in both wild and laboratory animals. This shared biology allows researchers to study how fears are formed and modified, thereby providing potential means to intervene when fear experiences become pathologically excessive.

People experience fear when they sense that a significant danger is imminent. Fear is distinguished from anxiety in that it arises in response to a *specific* threat that is *immediately present*. Fear manifests rapidly and involves sympathetic activation (e.g., increases in heart rate, blood pressure, sweating), heightened processing of threats, and a desire to flee. Because survival in dangerous situations requires a rapid reaction, fear-related behaviors typically manifest automatically with minimal deliberation of options. In settings of true threat, such as encountering a venomous snake along a trail, such reactions are appropriate. However, people with fear disorders experience excessive fear in settings that are safe or at least manageable. Such conditions involve perturbed fear learning or expression.

Research over the last two decades defines the neurobiology of fear learning in ways that inform therapeutics. Research is particularly notable on mechanisms involved in overcoming fear, referred to as fear extinction. This chapter first summarizes knowledge in these areas and then describes how this knowledge is being used to evaluate pharmacological methods to enhance extinction.

The Fear-Related Disorders

Pathological fear causes extreme distress or avoidance, as reflected in the psychiatric nosology (see Table 26.1). Specific phobias and social anxiety disorder are considered fear disorders since they involve excessive fear of particular objects or situations. People suffering from these conditions typically avoid the focus of their fear. For some specific phobias, such as snake phobia, the avoidance may minimally impact a person's daily life, but the disorder can still be considered pathological because the excessive fear reactivity indicates a deficit in emotion regulatory systems. Indeed, specific phobia may represent a risk factor for later development of major depressive disorder (Pine et al., 2001). Additionally, pervasive conditions, such as social anxiety disorder, more significantly impact functioning through avoidance, which can limit career choices and social relationships.

Panic disorder is unique in that fear appears to manifest spontaneously. However, through associative learning, fear-triggering cues becoming generalized to contexts and internal physical stimuli (e.g., sweating, heart racing), such that the patient becomes very afraid of future attacks, often known as "the fear of fear." The settings in which the attacks occurred become feared themselves, resulting in avoidance of those situations, known as agoraphobia. Panic attacks are strictly defined fear episodes of high intensity and rapid onset. The intensity of the physical symptoms and apparent inexplicability of panic attacks often lead their sufferers to feel as if they are "going crazy" or having a medical emergency and thus to proceed to an emergency room for a medical evaluation. Panic attacks represent an excessive somatic expression of fear.

Posttraumatic stress disorder (PTSD) is a fear disorder with features that complicate treatment. At its core, PTSD emerges due to excessively powerful learning of the dangers associated with traumatic events or by failure to recover after the initial traumatic episode, which can occur through lack of extinction learning. In addition to excessive fear and avoidance of the objects and settings associated with the trauma, PTSD involves re-experiencing symptoms, persistent hyperarousal, and prominent negative thoughts about one's self, others, or one's future.

TABLE 26.1 Fear-Related Disorders

DSM-5 DISORDER	NATURE OF FEAR	12-MONTH PREVALENCE*
Specific phobia	Circumscribed fear of a specific object or situation	9.1%
Social anxiety disorder	Fear of negative evaluation while being observed by others	7.1%
Panic disorder	Fear of attacks of sudden intense fear characterized by multiple physical and mental symptoms	2.7%
Posttraumatic stress disorder	Fear of harm or death associated with the people, objects, or situations that remind the individual of a previously experienced traumatic event	3.6%

*National Comorbidity Survey Replication, 2005.

The fear-related disorders are of significant public health concern, affecting approximately 19% of Americans (National Comorbidity Survey Replication, 2005) and costing society in excess of $40 billion annually (Kessler and Greenberg, 2002). Without treatment, fear disorders can persist, particularly when avoidance precludes extinction learning. In fact, avoidance can even act as a rewarding cue in further convincing the patient that by avoiding the situation, the feared bad outcome did not occur. Thus, successful treatment of fear disorders must focus on confronting avoidance behaviors.

TREATMENT OF FEAR DISORDERS VIA EXPOSURE

Within the emotional processing theory proposed by Foa and Kozak (1986), fear becomes pathologic when associations among stimuli, responses, and meaning are not accurate, i.e., harmless stimuli or responses assume threat meaning. Cognitive behavior therapy (CBT), which is highly effective, represents a first line treatment. Most CBT approaches for anxiety and fear disorders involve (1) exposure and (2) anxiety management.

Exposure therapy has its basis in the animal literature examining the process of fear extinction, which began with Pavlov over a century ago. Extinction learning refers to the reduction of fear to a cue previously paired with an aversive event when that cue is presented repeatedly in the absence of the aversive event. By presenting the feared stimuli repeatedly with no aversive consequences, the fear decreases over time, until ideally, the stimuli no longer engender fear. In general, exposure therapy involves confrontation with feared stimuli in a therapeutic manner. For the exposure to be therapeutic, the anxiety must be activated and changed. In exposure therapy, presumably patients learn (1) what they fear will not occur, and (2) the fear will decrease even while they are exposed to their feared stimuli. Desired changes include decreased symptoms of anxiety and arousal (i.e., responses), and decreased estimates of danger (i.e., meaning). Stimuli can be presented in imagination, in vivo (in real life), or in virtual reality, among others. Elsewhere in this volume, chapters discuss what is learned in exposure therapy, especially via inhibitory learning (*see chapter 25*) and in PTSD (*see chapter 10*), which may be the epitome of a learned fear disorder.

Another major CBT approach includes anxiety management training (AMT). Exposure addresses avoidance, while AMT addresses excessive arousal. The two most popular components of AMT include cognitive restructuring and relaxation. In cognitive restructuring, the patient's cognitive errors are made explicit and means to correct these errors are taught. Relaxation often includes breathing retraining and/or deep muscle relaxation.

Subtle variations in applications of CBT occur for specific fear disorders. Specific phobias are most efficiently treated with exposure therapy targeting the feared object, usually delivered in vivo, in imagination, or in virtual reality. CBT treatment of social anxiety disorder (see *chapter 14*) relates closely to a cognitive model (Rapee and Heimberg, 1997; Clark and Wells, 1995) and typically includes exposure to social situations in vivo or in virtual reality. CBT treatment of panic disorder (see *chapter 15)* targets erroneous interpretations of physiological responses associated with panic and associated avoidance behavior, often including cognitive restructuring to correct misinterpretations and exposure to interoceptive cues as well as external situations if agoraphobia is present. CBT for obsessive-compulsive disorder (OCD) (*see chapter 12*) involves exposure and response prevention, whereby patients are exposed to feared situations, thoughts, or images without being allowed to engage in rituals or avoidance. PTSD responds well to CBT (*see chapter 10*). Prolonged exposure (PE) is the form of CBT with the strongest empirical support. Other related, effective psychological interventions include eye movement desensitization and reprocessing (EMDR) and cognitive processing therapy (CPT), both of which involve exposure to traumatic memories, although to a much lesser extent in CPT. Treatment of PTSD with PE involves (1) exposure to the memory of the trauma in imagination, (2) in vivo exposure to situations that act as triggers of the traumatic memory or that are avoided, (3) breathing retraining, and (4) processing of the traumatic material to make the new learning explicit.

NEUROBIOLOGY OF FEAR LEARNING AND EXTINCTION

Successful exposure therapy involves extinction learning. Indeed, the fear disorders may offer the best example of translational methods in psychiatry, in that animal models directly inform treatment. Although neural circuitry is more fully examined in *chapter 24*, we briefly outline relevant translational neuroscience in this chapter.

Decades of work has demonstrated that the amygdala is the hub of the fear "reflex" across mammals. Neural inputs representing the sensory conditioned stimuli (CS, the previously neutral cues and contexts) and unconditioned stimuli (US, the aversive cues) are combined within the lateral and basolateral nuclei of the amygdala (Figure 26.1A). Processed information from these regions is sent to the central nucleus and then to multiple subcortical areas that mediate the fear reflex reaction. In addition to receiving inputs from sensory areas, amygdala processing of fear is modulated by contextual information

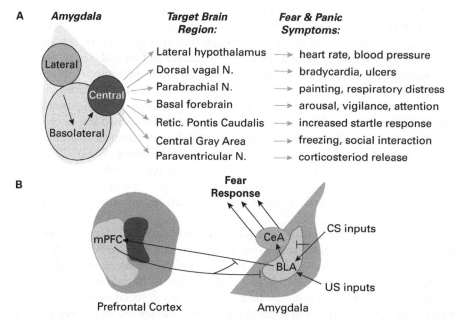

FIGURE 26.1 Amygdala Mediated Expression of Fear and Circuit Modulation of Amygdala Function. (A) This schematic demonstrates subregions of the amygdala (lateral and basolateral) which receive CS and US sensory information, and which activate the central nucleus of the amygdala (CeA). CeA activation leads to neural circuit activation of a broad range of fear symptoms (which overlay onto the symptoms of Panic Attacks), via specific subcortical target brain regions. (B) More broadly, the basolateral nucleus of the amygdala (BLA) receives CS and US inputs and is modulated by hippocampal and medial prefrontal cortex (mPFC) projections which are involved in the learning to inhibit previously acquired fear memories.

from the hippocampus and regulated by medial prefrontal cortex (mPFC) projections (Figure 26.1B) (Herry et al., 2010; Jovanovic and Ressler, 2010).

The acquisition of fear involves the co-occurrence of neutral CS with aversive US, leading to increased conditioned fear responses, such as freezing, with repetitive pairings (Figure 26.2A, left). Extinction then involves exposure to the CS in the absence of the US (Figure 26.2A, middle). Drugs that enhance the extinction process or the consolidation of extinction lead to decreased memory when the CS is presented again at later times (Figure 26.2A, right).

In contrast, reconsolidation allows prior memories to be changed when reactivated in a transient, labile state. Thus, the primary difference between extinguishing a prior aversive memory and reconsolidating that memory is whether the reminder is short (reconsolidation prevails) or repetitive/long (extinction prevails) when no US is present (Figure 26.2B and Table 26.2). The extra- and intracellular circuitry involved in reconsolidation provide several potential targets for pharmacological manipulation. Therefore, the nascent neurobiological understanding of fear inhibition/extinction and fear enhancement/reconsolidation are leading to new approaches to targeted modulation of fear memory manipulation.

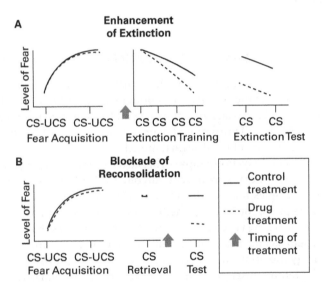

FIGURE 26.2 Schematic of Behavioral Expression of Extinction Enhancement and Reconsolidation Blockade. This schematic demonstrates the process by which memories are altered when extinction of fear is enhanced or reconsolidation of fear memories are blocked with drug treatment. (A) The left panel demonstrates how conditioned stimulus (CS)—unconditioned stimulus (UCS) pairing leads to increased level of fear expression. Upon extinction training, wherein the CS is presented repeatedly in the absence of an UCS, the fear to the CS gradually diminishes. When retested at a later date, animals that have had extinction learning enhanced with drug treatment show lower levels of fear, also known as retention of the extinction memory. (B) With Blockade of Reconsolidation designs, the fear acquisition is similar, but upon re-exposure to the CS, only a single, or very brief, exposure is performed, as opposed to the prolonged and repeated CS reexposure that occurs with extinction. The now vulnerable memory reconsolidation process is now interfered with by memory disruptor drug treatment, leading to decreased memory of the original fear when retested at a later date. For further information, see Parsons and Ressler (2013).

TABLE 26.2 Enhancing Extinction versus Disrupting Memory

	ENHANCE EXTINCTION	MEMORY DISRUPTION
Goal	Form new fear-inhibiting memories	Weaken original fear memory
Effect on reconsolidation	Increase synaptic strength of newly formed memories of fear extinction	Weaken synaptic strength of activated fear memories
Duration of fear memory retrieval	Long: Sufficient duration to obtain reduction in experienced fear	Short: Sufficient to activate fear experience, without developing habituation to fear.
Clinical effect of extinction augmentation (e.g., DCS)	Positive: Reduced fear by strengthening extinction learning	Negative: Enhanced fear due to strengthened reconsolidation of original fear memory
Effect of reconsolidation blockade (e.g., propranolol)	Negative: No reduction in fear due to disrupting extinction learning	Positive: Reduced fear due to disruption of reconsolidation of original fear memory

PHARMACOLOGICAL APPROACHES TO ENHANCING EXPOSURE THERAPY

Currently, the primary FDA approved first-line treatments for fear-related anxiety disorders are antidepressants of the selective serotonin reuptake inhibitor (SSRI) class. These and other currently used medications dampen symptoms, but do not target the underlying causes of the disorders. Translational neuroscience generates treatments that target such causes, identified in preclinical animal models.

Medication-enhanced psychotherapy is a broad term, encompassing the use of medications to improve psychotherapy treatment outcomes (Dunlop et al., 2012). Medications used to enhance therapies for fear disorders can be categorized as "cognitive enhancers," "memory disrupters," or "therapy facilitators." Cognitive enhancers are thought to improve extinction learning via effects on the cellular machinery that determine synaptic strength, and include agents modulating glutamate, norepinephrine, and glucocorticoid signaling, or energy metabolism, genetic expression, or post-transcriptional processing (See Table 26.3). Memory disrupters aim to weaken the reconsolidation process. Some of the same biological targets of cognitive enhancers are also targets of memory disrupters, but in the direction of blockade rather than enhancement of signaling. Therapy facilitators act to increase the patient's engagement with the feared memories, thereby increasing their accessibility for modification through therapy.

Cognitive Enhancement of Extinction

Enhancement of fear extinction requires increasing the synaptic strength of inhibitory inputs to the amygdala and other fear circuit pathways that process the specific feared object or situation. This remodeling of synaptic structure requires the formation of new proteins. Thus, pharmacologic interventions to enhance extinction must ultimately act to increase the expression of synaptic proteins. These interventions may also act well upstream of protein expression via activating specific signal transduction cascades and

TABLE 26.3 Mechanisms of Action of Pharmacological Agents Combined with Psychotherapy

MEDICATION	PRIMARY MECHANISM	EFFECT
COGNITIVE ENHANCERS		
D-cycloserine	Partial agonist at glycine site of NMDA receptor	Increases glutamatergic signaling of NMDA receptor in presence of glutamate release
Yohimbine	Antagonist at adrenergic α2 receptor	Enhances noradrenergic signaling via inhibiting negative feedback or norepinephrine
Methylene Blue	Mitochondrial respiration	Enhances metabolic capacity of mitochondria in activated neurons
Dronabinol	Cannabinoid type 1 receptor	Gating BLA activity via presynaptic inhibition
Hydrocortisone	Glucocorticoid receptor	Enhances gene transcription; increases endocannabinoid synthesis in cell membrane; increase trafficking of AMPA and NMDA receptors to cell membrane
MEMORY DISRUPTERS		
Propranolol	Adrenergic β receptors	Antagonize noradrenergic signaling, thereby reducing cAMP formation
Mifepristone	Glucocorticoid receptor	Antagonize glucocorticoid receptor, reducing gene transcription
Rapamycin (Sirolimus)	mTOR	Antagonize mTOR, thereby reducing post-transcriptional protein synthesis
THERAPY FACILITATORS		
MDMA	Serotonin and Norepinephrine transporters; Oxytocin release	Diminished fear and increased openness to memory engagement

gene expression, as reviewed elsewhere (Herry et al., 2010; Jovanovic and Ressler, 2010; Holmes and Singewald, 2013).

Pharmacologic enhancement of extinction learning has been demonstrated in clinical trials in which all participants receive exposure-based CBT and are randomized to receive pre-session doses of the active drug or a placebo. Several outcomes have been examined, including: (1) subjective fear when exposed to the feared object or situation; (2) physiologic reactivity upon exposure; and (3) self-reported real-world engagement with feared objects or situations.

Glutamate

The glutamate system by far has received the most intensive focus in human trials of cognitive enhancers. D-cycloserine (DCS) was the first agent shown to enhance extinction learning for a fear disorder based on animal models of glutamate's critical role in extinction memory formation (Falls et al., 1992; Walker et al., 2002). In the first clinical trial, it was found to improve outcomes more than placebo when given prior to exposure therapy sessions for acrophobia (Ressler et al., 2004). DCS acts as a partial agonist at the glycine binding site on NMDA receptors, thereby enhancing the NMDA receptor response upon binding glutamate. Thus the active learning process initiated by exposure therapy is enhanced via this increase in NMDA receptor signaling. Since the original study was published, more than 20 additional trials have been conducted. The studies have not consistently demonstrated enhanced outcomes with DCS versus placebo, but meta-analyses across disorders have quantified a small, non-heterogeneous effect indicating benefit with DCS augmentation (Rodrigues et al., 2014; Norberg et al., 2008). A small trial in panic disorder patients of a glycine transporter 1 inhibitor (which raises synaptic glycine levels) did not improve exposure therapy treatment outcomes over placebo augmentation (Nations, et al., 2012). As additional work has examined these processes, a more nuanced view of important considerations in the pharmacological enhancement of emotional learning has begun to develop.

DCS has been used successfully in research on specific phobia (5 trials), social anxiety disorder (4 trials), and panic disorder (2 trials). For PTSD (6 trials), results are inconsistent, with two positive studies, other studies finding greater benefit with placebo treatment, and still others finding positive effects only on secondary outcomes (e.g., Rothbaum et al., 2014). Similarly, despite two initial positive trials, most efficacy studies of DCS in OCD find no enhancement, although improvements at mid-treatment have been seen (McGuire et al., 2014); and an ongoing large pediatric trial should be informative (McGuire et al., 2012). DCS demonstrates excellent tolerability, with no consistent side effects that could diminish blinding of patients or investigators.

Further investigation of these studies suggests that DCS enhances emotional learning regardless of the emotional valence. Thus, in sessions in which the fear exposure does not result in substantial fear reduction, DCS (and other cognitive enhancers) may create the potential risk of enhancing the strength of the reconsolidated fear memory. Indeed, in one trial of PTSD, outcomes with DCS were worse than with placebo augmentation (Litz et al., 2012). Review of data from this and other PTSD trials indicate the importance of within-session habituation to fear and between-session fear learning (Rothbaum et al., 2014). Nearly all studies using DCS have dosed the medication 30 minutes or one hour prior to the exposure session, with the aim of having peak blood levels at the time of exposure; two studies which dosed patients following exposure were negative (Tart et al., 2013; Mataix-Cols et al., 2014). Dosing prior to exposure precludes the ability to dose the patient only after successful exposure sessions, which would eliminate the potential for enhancing fear learning if the session is unsuccessful.

Norepinephrine

The norepinephrine and glutamate systems are the key processes activated in states of new learning. In rodent models, successful extinction of conditioned fears is associated with increased concentrations of norepinephrine in the mPFC (Hugues et al., 2007), and interventions that diminish norepinephrine concentrations reduce fear extinction (Mueller and Cahill, 2010). The most extensively studied agent to boost norepinephrine concentrations in humans is yohimbine, which acts as an antagonist at α2 autoreceptors in the locus coeruleus. By blocking these inhibitory autoreceptors, yohimbine produces an increase in locus coeruleus firing and norepinephrine synaptic release. Although yohimbine may have important effects beyond the norepinephrine system (Holmes and Quirk, 2010), the increased activation of β1 receptors resulting from increased synaptic norepinephrine is believed to be the most relevant action of yohimbine's ability to enhance extinction.

To date, yohimbine-enhanced exposure therapy has only been studied in three small trials (social anxiety, claustrophobia, fear of flying). Two trials indicated reductions in fear during the short (1–3 week) follow-up periods used. Methylphenidate is another catecholamine-enhancing agent being investigated for possible extinction enhancement effects. Although activation of β receptors enhances long term potentiation, use of the non-selective β-agonist isoproterenol has not been shown to alter extinction learning in preclinical models. The failure of direct β-agonists and of more selective α2-antagonists to enhance extinction suggest that yohimbine's extinction-enhancing effects are achieved, at least in part, by non-noradrenergic mechanisms. Another caveat to yohimbine's use is that some pre-clinical data suggest that the fear-reducing effects of yohimbine are context-dependent (Morris and Bouton, 2007), which would limit the generalizability of benefit beyond the treatment setting.

Glucocorticoids

Fear experiences trigger the release of glucocorticoids (GCs) that activate glucocorticoid receptors (GRs), which are widely distributed in the brain. The best established effect of GCs is their effect on gene expression. GRs, once bound with GC, translocate to the nucleus and bind to glucocorticoid responsive elements, acting as transcription factors in the promoter regions of GC-responsive genes. GCs also have non-genomic effects that are relevant to memory formation by (1) inducing the synthesis of endocannabinoids from membrane phospholipids after GR binding; (2) presynaptically increasing the number of glutamate vesicles available for rapid release; (3) post-synaptically increasing the trafficking of N-methyl D-aspartate receptors (NMDAR) and α-amino-3 -hydroxy-5-methyl-4-isoxazolepropionic acid receptors (AMPAR) from intracellular pools to the cell membrane surface; (4) activating intracellular signaling cascades via the ERK/MAPK pathways (de Kloet, 2013). In contrast to these acute effects of GCs, chronic exposure to GCs in rodent models reduces the surface expression of NMDAR and AMPAR (Gourley et al., 2009).

Emerging evidence suggests that co-activation of both GC and NMDA receptors facilitates new learning, perhaps by inducing histone-level epigenetic modifications that permits transcription of the genes necessary for new memory consolidation (Reul, 2014). Disrupting GC production impairs the consolidation of extinction learning (de Kloet, 2013). Reducing emotional arousal (and presumably GC release) inhibits these epigenetic histone modifications (Singewald, et al., 2003). Conversely, administering dexamethasone, a synthetic glucocorticoid, before exposure facilitates consolidation of extinction memories (Yang et al., 2006).

A strong preclinical evidence base generates interest in manipulating cortisol to enhance extinction. Small studies suggest that GC-augmented exposure-based CBT improves fear extinction in specific (acrophobia, arachnophobia) and social phobias. In the arachnophobia study, 20 mg of hydrocortisone or matching placebo was given by mouth 1 hour before two group exposure sessions to spider stimuli. Reduction of fear versus placebo was not evident immediately after the second exposure session, but was detected at the follow-up one month later, suggesting an effect of activating the GR system on enhancing long-term extinction retention (Soravia, et al., 2014).

Endocannabinoids

The endogenous ligands for cannabinoid receptors (endocannabinoids) include anandamide and 2-arachidonoylglycerol. In preclinical studies, activation of the CB-1 receptor by endocannabinoids contributes to both the formation and expression of extinction memories, probably by gating BLA excitability through induction of synaptic plasticity and inhibition of glutamate release. Although no studies in fear disorder patients exist, healthy volunteers undergoing fear conditioning who received exogenous cannabinoid agonists demonstrated increases in both fear extinction and resistance to reinstatement (Das et al., 2013; Rabinak et al., 2013). An alternative approach to giving agonists at CB receptors is to enhance endogenous endocannabinoid concentrations via administration of a fatty acid amide hydroxylase (FAAH) inhibitor. FAAH degrades endogenous cannabinoids, and inhibition of FAAH enhances retention of fear extinction in animal models (Gunduz-Cinar, et al., 2013).

Methylene Blue

Methylene blue (MB) is best known in medicine for its value in treating methemoglobinemia, a state of high levels of methemoglobin. In the CNS, metabolically active neurons preferentially accumulate MB, with resultant increases in neuronal metabolism due to MB's role in mitochondrial energy production. For extinction learning, this effect is relevant because activated mitochondria increase transcription of nuclear- and mitochondria-genes that contribute to synaptic strengthening. In rats, administration of MB facilitates memory consolidation of both fear learning and extinction. In the only human trial conducted to date, patients with claustrophobia who received MB improved extinction learning over placebo after 5 sessions of prolonged exposure therapy, an effect maintained at one-month follow-up (Telch et al., 2014). If these studies hold-up, a possible advantage of using MB as opposed to previously discussed extinction enhancing medications is that it can be administered *after* an exposure therapy session. After-the-session dosing permits the therapist to judge whether adequate extinction to the fear occurred during the session. If the session was unsuccessful in reducing fear, MB administration could be withheld, thus avoiding the risk of enhanced reconsolidation of an inadequately extinguished memory. There are, however, unique concerns that affect MB's clinical and research use. First, conducting placebo-controlled studies is challenging because MB changes urine color, leading to a loss of blinding of participants. Secondly, methylene blue can induce hemolysis in individuals with certain types of glucose-6-phosphate dehydrogenase deficiency, and it can inhibit monoamine oxidase, with cases of serotonin syndrome documented when MB was combined with an SSRI.

Epigenetic Modification

The methods for enhancing extinction learning all involve altering signal transduction cascades that impact gene expression. In contrast, epigenetics refers to changes in aspects of gene transcription that occur through DNA modification, but are not related to the regulation of specific encoded DNA sequence via the signaling cascades we have discussed. Epigenetic mechanisms control the accessibility of DNA to the to the proteins involved in transcription, thereby regulating which genes are available or unavailable for transcription, and the length of time transcription occurs. For genes to be available for transcription, the dense structure of chromatin must be relaxed to allow the transcriptional machinery access to the DNA. Chromatin can be relaxed by diminishing the electrostatic bonding of positively charged histone proteins, around which DNA is tightly wrapped, with negatively charged DNA. This effect is achieved by acetylation of histone lysine residues by histone acetyltransferases (HATs). Opposing HATs are histone deacetylases (HDACs), which act as repressors to inhibit gene transcription (Monti, 2013).

Preclinical research suggests that acetylation of a histone in the promoter region of the brain derived neurotrophic factor (*bdnf*) gene can enhance fear extinction, and agents that enhance fear extinction may act by enhancing histone acetylation. Similarly inhibitors of HDAC, such as valproic acid (which has very broad effects including HDAC inhibition) increase histone acetylation in promoter regions of genes associated with fear extinction (Whittle and Singewald, 2014). Histone acetylation modifying agents have not yet been tested as augmenting agents for exposure therapy, in part because there are many HATs of potential importance. Further preclinical work is necessary before human studies can commence.

Two additional epigenetic regulatory mechanisms are likely to become increasingly relevant to extinction learning studies. DNA methylation involves the covalent bonding of a methyl ($-CH_3$) group to a cytosine side-chain. DNA methylation of the *bdnf* gene in mice has been found in extinction-resistant female mice (Baker-Andresen et al., 2013). Because DNA methylation is reversible, targeting this epigenetic mechanism may also emerge in the future as a means of enhancing extinction learning with exposure therapy. Finally non-coding RNAs, including micro-RNAs (miRNAs), are involved in post-transcriptional regulation of genes associated with synaptic plasticity. Although miRNAs typically act to suppress mRNA translation (and thus new protein synthesis), the brain-specific miRNA, miR-128b, may act to facilitate the formation of fear-extinction memories (Lin et al., 2011).

MEMORY DISRUPTORS

As opposed to strengthening extinction learning after exposure treatment, an alternative approach to weakening fear memories is to disrupt the reconsolidation of the fear memory after it is activated. Essentially, this process targets the same systems as those involved in extinction learning. However, instead of enhancing synaptic strength of fear-inhibition circuits through generation of synaptic proteins, memory disruption aims to weaken the synaptic strength of fear expression memories. The same systems that are involved in extinction learning are also targeted in memory disruption; the difference is the emotional state of the person at the time the medications are designed to work. In contrast to extinction learning, when the emotional state at the time of drug activity should be one of low fear, in memory disruption the emotional state should be high fear, thus weakening the fear memory representation.

To date, memory disruption approaches have only been studied in patients with PTSD, targeting the recurrent intrusive memories of the original trauma. Three systems have been identified as potential targets in humans: β-adrenergic receptors, glucocorticoid receptors, and RNA translation. The β-blocker propranolol given to rats prior to brief reactivation of a fear memory inhibits expression of fear behavior (Debiec and Ledoux, 2004), and propranolol reduces physiologic reactivity compared to placebo among chronic PTSD patients who listen to a recorded script of their traumatic event (Brunet et al., 2008; Brunet et al., 2014). However, β-blocker administration in the aftermath of a traumatic event does not reduce likelihood of developing PTSD in subsequent months, suggesting this approach does not prevent the consolidation of a fearful memory (Hoge et al., 2012). Ongoing studies are evaluating whether propranolol when given prior to exposure therapy can serve as a memory disrupter. Propranolol is also being studied in PTSD patients as an as-needed treatment to be taken whenever hyperarousal in response to a traumatic memory occurs.

The GR antagonist mifepristone may have potential as a blocker of reconsolidation; this drug is currently being studied as a monotherapy, not in conjunction with exposure therapy. Finally, rapamycin (sirolimus) is an agent that inhibits the mammalian target of rapamycin (mTOR) protein. mTOR is a serine/threonine kinase that is required for synaptic remodeling. By inhibiting mTOR, rapamycin can disrupt both consolidation and reconsolidation of fear memories (Blundell, et al., 2008), and is currently under study for patients with PTSD. In the realm of epigenetic regulation, using p300 inhibitors to block the pro-transcription effects of genes important for reconsolidation by the histone acetyltransferase p300 may also emerge as future memory disruption approach (Marek et al., 2011).

THERAPY FACILITATORS

A unique agent in the area of pharmacologically enhanced extinction research is methylenedioxymethamphetamine (MDMA), better known as "Ecstasy." MDMA induces feelings of euphoria, relaxation, empathy, emotional openness, and reduced inhibition, but the cellular mechanisms are less clear at this point. By inducing a calmer state, MDMA is thought to reduce patient's fear of engaging with fearful memories, thus allowing them to be fully activated with less avoidance in a therapeutic setting, although the drug may also act to enhance extinction learning. A key component of use of MDMA in this way is the appropriate setting: the situation needs to be one of peace and acceptance. In the studies to date, this has involved long (>8 hour sessions) of psychotherapy on the days MDMA is administered. Also unique to this approach is that the therapy administered is not standard exposure-based psychotherapy. Rather, it is a non-directive approach of empathic listening, inquiry, and relaxation, aimed at overcoming avoidance and engaging the patient in processing the trauma.

MDMA peak effects are achieved approximately 1–1.5 hours after ingestion. The drug likely reverses the direction of transport of the monoamines serotonin, norepinephrine, and dopamine, consistent with the action of amphetamines generally (Liechti and Vollenweider, 2000). MDMA also increases circulating levels of glucocorticoids and induces release of oxytocin (Johansen and Krebs, 2009). It is possible that by increasing norepinephrine and glucocorticoid signaling, the previously discussed mechanisms of synaptic remodeling during extinction learning may also be produced by MDMA.

An initial proof-of-principle study in 20 patients with PTSD demonstrated dramatic benefits of two sessions of MDMA-augmented psychotherapy versus placebo-augmented therapy (these experimental sessions were followed by several integration sessions without medication augmentation; Mithoefer et al., 2011). Three-year follow-up showed continued benefit in the majority of patients, with none developing drug abuse (Mithoefer et al., 2013). A similarly designed study also found substantial benefit of MDMA versus placebo augmentation of psychotherapy for PTSD (Oehen, et al., 2013).

Challenges to the use of MDMA include that it is classed as a Schedule 1 drug by the US Drug Enforcement Agency due to its abuse potential. Like methylene blue, MDMA is also an inhibitor of MAO-A. A long-standing concern about MDMA is that its primary metabolite, 3,4-methylenedioxyamphetamine (MDA), can induce degeneration of serotonergic nerve terminals, presumably through the generation of free radicals (Sprague and Nichols, 1995). Some data suggest this neurotoxicity is associated with dosing frequency and quantity and is most significant in settings of hyperthermia. Thus, limited dosing in controlled therapeutic situations may mitigate this risk. Still to be determined is the optimal number of sessions and minimum necessary dose required to achieve the enhanced outcomes.

FUTURE

The future of medication-enhanced treatment of prolonged exposure therapy is bright. We have outlined a number of different approaches using either enhancers of extinction memory formation or blockade of fear reconsolidation to illustrate how an understanding of the neuroscience of fear modulation can lead to rationally designed translationally informed treatments (Figure 26.3). It is exciting to anticipate the direct translation of highly applicable animal models of extinction learning to the clinical care of patients. However, before medications become routinely used to enhance exposure therapy treatments, several outstanding questions remain to be addressed. By clarifying issues around treatment effectiveness, patient selection, and safety, the probability of successful application of pharmacologically enhanced psychotherapy will be increased.

The first question to address is whether cognitive enhancers improve only the speed of extinction learning rather than overall outcomes of patients. Because exposure therapy is highly effective for fear disorders, trials examining the efficacy of extinction enhancing agents have often used an abbreviated number of treatment sessions, shorter than the usual course of 9–12 sessions, in order to demonstrate that extinction learning is being enhanced. Nearly all the trials that demonstrated improvements with DCS and yohimbine employed abbreviated courses of exposure therapy (1–5 sessions), and several of the negative trials revealed early time-point benefits of DCS that were not evident at the end of a full course of exposure. Although shorter treatment trials are an efficient way to test a drug's efficacy, it is not necessarily the best test of the overall effectiveness of the intervention. For example, if patients receiving active drug demonstrate greater extinction of fear after four sessions than placebo-treated patients, the ability of the drug to enhance the speed of extinction learning has been demonstrated, but it does not necessarily follow that fear extinction would have been greater among drug-treated patients if all patients had received the full 12 sessions of exposure. Thus, it is possible that extinction-enhancing drugs may only enhance extinction among individuals capable of benefitting from exposure-based CBT.

While shortening time in treatment may provide savings and reduce patient drop-out (Chasson et al., 2010), the more important questions are (1) whether cognitive enhancers can convert patients who would be non-responders to standard exposure therapy into responders; and (2) is the extinction learning achieved while taking a cognitive enhancer more durable (less liable to reinstatement and recovery) than non-enhanced extinction learning. Answering these questions will require new study designs and longer periods of follow-up with more frequent assessments than have been conducted to date.

Another key question regards the appropriate patients for this intervention. Some individuals benefit fully from exposure therapy without pharmacological enhancement;

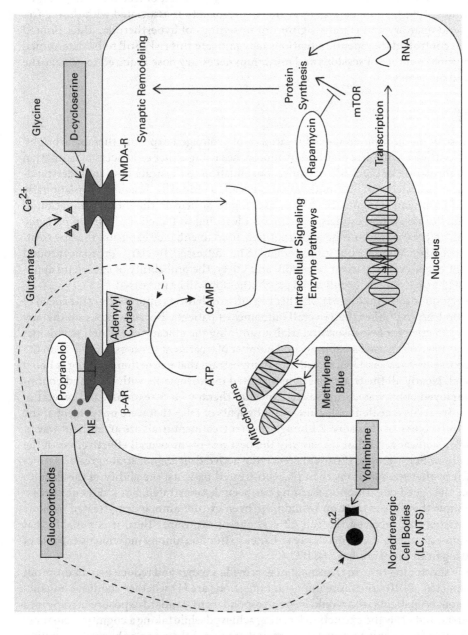

FIGURE 26.3 Schematic of Cellular Mechanisms of Pharmacological Translational Approaches to Fear-Related Disorders. The figure shows sites of action of medications being evaluated to enhance psychotherapy for fear disorders. Medications in rectangles act to enhance extinction learning; medications in ovals disrupt reconsolidation. Reprinted with permission from Dunlop et al. (2012).

conversely, there are individuals who cannot benefit from exposure therapy even with drug-enhancement. In one of the few attempts to identify predictors of outcome, a study of 67 patients with PTSD who received DCS or placebo enhancement found that the personality variables of high conscientiousness and low extraversion emerged as specific characteristics that predicted better outcomes with DCS than placebo (de Kleine et al., 2014). Previous work has suggested that healthy individuals higher in extraversion retain extinction learning better than individuals low in extraversion (Rauch et al., 2005). It is possible that low extraversion is a psychological marker for deficits in extinction learning, which may be overcome by DCS. Biomarkers may also have value in selecting patients and identifying need for additional treatment. Startle response, neuroendocrine, and psychophysiological measures may all be informative to these questions and should be measured in future studies.

An important safety issue yet to be resolved is the risk for increased fear learning. All cognitive enhancers have the potential for increasing the intensity of the fear memory if reconsolidation of an activated memory occurs without the patient achieving an improved level of fear habituation by the end of the treatment session. Determining whether cognitive enhancers can improve extinction learning when dosed after the exposure session (as has been done with methylene blue) would enable the therapist to determine whether the patient has shown sufficient improvement in the session to be safely dosed. It is possible that as extinction learning processes are fully mapped, we will be able to combine two or more pharmacologic mechanisms that act at different stages of signal transduction and gene expression to maximize extinction.

A major challenge to be overcome is the reluctance of patients to engage in exposure therapy due to the aversive experience of confronting the fears. To maximize the number of patients who could benefit from exposure therapy, it may be necessary to find agents that reduce the intensity of fear experience without interfering with new synapse formation associated with extinction. Benzodiazepines are not recommended and in some studies have been associated with worse response when combined with virtual reality exposure therapy for PTSD (Rothbaum et al., 2014).

SUMMARY

Medication-enhancement of extinction learning to treat fear disorders has been demonstrated for several drugs that modulate aspects of extinction learning. There is evidence supporting the use of the cognitive enhancers DCS, yohimbine, and glucocorticoids, and some data indicate the therapy facilitator MDMA may also be beneficial for PTSD. Although these initial findings are highly encouraging and represent a potential breakthrough for clinical care, more work needs to be done before these approaches are used in general practice. Specifically, clarification is needed to determine optimal dosing regimens, risk of adverse outcomes, durability of benefits, optimal patient selection, as well as determining whether medication-induced enhancement of extinction learning represents merely a shortening of time to benefit or an improvement in overall response rates. These issues will need to be addressed in larger trials using longer periods of exposure therapy to resolve.

DISCLOSURE STATEMENTS

Dr. Dunlop has receives research support from Assurex, Forest, GlaxoSmithKline, NIMH, Otsuka, Pfizer, Takeda. Dr. Ressler is a founding member of Extinction

Pharmaceuticals/Therapade Technologies, which exist to develop d-Cycloserine for use to augment the effectiveness of psychotherapy. He has received no equity or income from this relationship within the last 3 years. Dr. Rothbaum and Emory University own equity in *Virtually Better, Inc.*, which is developing products related to virtual reality research, and Dr. Rothbaum is a consultant for *Virtually Better, Inc.* The terms of this arrangement have been reviewed and approved by Emory University in accordance with its conflict of interest policies.

ACKNOWLEDGMENTS

Support was provided by NIH (R01MH071537; R01MH096764; 1R01MH094757-01; U19 MH069056), the Burroughs Wellcome Fund, NIH/NCRR base grant (P51RR000165) to Yerkes National Primate Research Center, the Department of Defense (Clinical Trial Grant No.W81XWH-10-1-1045), the Brain and Behavior Research Foundation (NARSAD) Distinguished Investigator Grant, "Optimal Dose of early intervention to prevent PTSD," and the McCormick Foundation "Brave Heart: MLB's Welcome Back Veterans South East Initiative."

REFERENCES

Baker-Andresen D., Flavell, C. R., Li, X., and Bredy, T. W. (2013) Activation of BDNF signaling prevents the return of fear in female mice. *Learning and Memory 20* (5), 237–240.

Blundell, J., Kouser, M., and Powell, C. M. (2008). Systemic inhibition of mammalian target of rapamycin inhibits fear memory reconsolidation. *Neurobiology of Learning and Memory, 90*, 28–35.

Brunet, A., Orr, S. P., Tremblay, J., Robertson, K., Nader, K., and Pitman, R. K. (2008). Effect of post-retrieval propranolol on psychophysiological responding during subsequent script-driven traumatic imagery in post-traumatic stress disorder. *Journal of Psychiatric Research, 42*, 503–506.

Brunet, A., Thomas, É., Saumier, D., Ashbaugh, A. R., Azzoug, A., Pitman, R. K., Orr, S. P., and Tremblay, J. (2014). Trauma reactivation plus propranolol is associated with durably low physiological responding during subsequent script-driven traumatic imagery. *Canadian Journal of Psychiatry, 59*, 228–232.

Chasson, G. S., Buhlmann, U., Tolin, D. F., Rao, S. R., Reese, H. E., Rowley, T., Welsh, K. S., and Wilhelm, S. (2010). Need for speed: evaluating slopes of OCD recovery in behavior therapy enhanced with d-cycloserine. *Behaviour Research and Therapy, 48*, 675–679.

Clark, D. M., and Wells, A. (1995). A cognitive model of social phobia. In Heimberg, R.G., Liebowitz, M.R., Hope, D.A., Schneier, F.R. (Eds.), *Social Phobia: Diagnosis, assessment and treatment* (pp. 69–93). New York, NY: Guilford Press.

Das, R. K., Kamboj, S. K., Ramadas, M., Yogan, K., Gupta, V., Redman, E., Curran, H. V., and Morgan, C. J. (2013). Cannabidiol enhances consolidation of explicit fear extinction in humans. *Psychopharmacology, 226*, 781–792.

Debiec, J., and Ledoux, J. E. (2004). Disruption of reconsolidation but not consolidation of auditory fear conditioning by noradrenergic blockade in the amygdala. *Neuroscience, 129*, 267–272.

de Kleine, R. A., Hendriks, G. J., Smits, J. A., Broekman, T. G., and van Minnen, A. (2014). Prescriptive variables for d-cycloserine augmentation of exposure therapy for posttraumatic stress disorder. *Journal of Psychiatric Research, 48*, 40–46.

de Kloet, E. R. (2013) Functional profile of the binary brain corticosteroid receptor system: mediating, multitasking, coordinating, integrating. *European Journal of Pharmacology, 719*(1–3):53–62.

Dunlop, B. W., Mansson, E., and Gerardi, M. (2012). Pharmacological innovations for posttraumatic stress disorder and medication-enhanced psychotherapy. *Current Pharmaceutical Design, 18*, 5645–5658.

Falls, W. A., Miserendino, M. J., and Davis, M. (1992). Extinction of fear-potentiated startle: blockade by infusion of an NMDA antagonist into the amygdala. *Journal of Neuroscience, 12,* 854–863.

Foa, E. B., and Kozak, M. J. (1986). Emotional processing of fear: exposure to corrective information. *Psychological Bulletin, 99,* 20–35.

Gourley, S. L., Kedves, A. T., Olausson, P., and Taylor, J. R. (2009). A history of corticosterone exposure regulates fear extinction and cortical NR2B, GluR2/3, and BDNF. *Neuropsychopharmacology, 34,* 707–716.

Gunduz-Cinar, O., MacPherson, K.P., Cinar, R., Gamble-George, J., Sugden, K., Williams, B., ... Holmes, A. (2013). Convergent translational evidence of a role for anandamide in amygdala-mediated fear extinction, threat processing and stress-reactivity. *Molecular Psychiatry, 18,* 813–823.

Herry C., Ferraguti F., Singewald N., Letzkus J. J., Ehrlich I., and Lüthi A. (2010). Neuronal circuits of fear extinction. *European Journal of Neuroscience, 31*(4), 599–612.

Hoge, E.A., Worthington, J. J., Nagurney, J. T., Chang, Y., Kay, E. B., Feterowski, C. M., ... Pitman, R.K. (2012). Effect of acute posttrauma propranolol on PTSD outcome and physiological responses during script-driven imagery. *CNS Neuroscience and Therapeutics, 18,* 21–27.

Holmes, A., and Quirk, G. J. (2010). Pharmacological facilitation of fear extinction and the search for adjunct treatments for anxiety disorders—the case of yohimbine. *Trends in Pharmacological Sciences, 31,* 2–7.

Holmes, A., and Singewald, N. (2013). Individual differences in recovery from traumatic fear. *Trends in Neuroscience36*(1):23–31.

Hugues, S., Garcia, R., and Léna, I. (2007). Time course of extracellular catecholamine and glutamate levels in the rat medial prefrontal cortex during and after extinction of conditioned fear. *Synapse, 61,* 933–937.

Johansen, P. O., and Krebs, T. S. (2009). How could MDMA (ecstasy) help anxiety disorders? A neurobiological rationale. *Journal of Psychopharmacology, 23,* 389–391.

Jovanovic T., and Ressler K. J. (2010) How the neurocircuitry and genetics of fear inhibition may inform our understanding of PTSD. *American Journal of Psychiatry, 167*(6):648–62.

Kessler, R. C., and Greenberg, P. E. (2002). The economic burden of anxiety and stress disorders. In In K. L. Davis, D. Charney, J. T. Coyle, and C. Nemeroff (Eds.), *Neuropsychopharmacology: The fifth generation of progress* (pp. 981–992). Philadelphia, PA: Lippincott, Williams and Wilkins.

Liechti, M. E., and Vollenweider, F. X. (2000). The serotonin uptake inhibitor citalopram reduces acute cardiovascular and vegetative effects of 3,4-methylenedioxymethamphetamine ("Ecstasy") in healthy volunteers. *Journal of Psychopharmacology, 14,* 269–274.

Lin, Q., Wei, W., Coelho, C.M., Li, X., Baker-Andresen, D., Dudley, K., ... Bredy, T. W. (2011). The brain-specific microRNA miR-128b regulates the formation of fear-extinction memory. *Nature Neuroscience, 14,* 1115–1117.

Litz, B. T., Salters-Pedneault, K., Steenkamp, M. M., Hermos, J. A., Bryant, R. A., Otto, M. W., and Hofmann, S. G. (2012). A randomized placebo-controlled trial of D-cycloserine and exposure therapy for posttraumatic stress disorder. *Journal of Psychiatric Research, 46,* 1184–1190.

Marek, R., Coelho, C. M., Sullivan, R. K., Baker-Andresen, D., Li, X., Ratnu, V., ... Bredy, T. W. (2011). Paradoxical enhancement of fear extinction memory and synaptic plasticity by inhibition of the histone acetyltransferase p300. *Journal of Neuroscience, 31,* 7486–7491.

Mataix-Cols, D., Turner, C., Monzani, B., Isomura, K., Murphy, C., Krebs, G., and Heyman, I. (2014). Cognitive-behavioural therapy with post-session D-cycloserine augmentation for paediatric obsessive-compulsive disorder: pilot randomised controlled trial. *British Journal of Psychiatry, 204,* 77–78.

McGuire, J. F., Lewin, A. B., Geller, D. A., Brown, A., Ramsey, K., Mutch, J., ... Storch, E. A. (2012). Advances in the treatment of pediatric obsessive–compulsive disorder: rationale and design for the evaluation of D-cycloserine with exposure and response prevention. *Neuropsychiatry 2,* 4.

McGuire, J. F., Lewin, A. B., and Storch, E. A. (2014). Enhancing exposure therapy for anxiety disorders, obsessive-compulsive disorder and post-traumatic stress disorder. *Expert Reviews Neurotherapeutics, 14,* 893–910.

Mithoefer, M. C., Wagner, M. T., Mithoefer, A. T., Jerome, L., and Doblin, R. (2011). The safety and efficacy of {+/-}3,4-methylenedioxymethamphetamine-assisted psychotherapy in subjects with chronic, treatment-resistant posttraumatic stress disorder: the first randomized controlled pilot study. *Journal of Psychopharmacology, 25*, 439–452.

Mithoefer, M. C., Wagner, M. T., Mithoefer, A. T., Jerome, L., Martin, S. F., Yazar-Klosinski, B., ... Doblin, R. (2013). Durability of improvement in post-traumatic stress disorder symptoms and absence of harmful effects or drug dependency after 3,4-methylenedioxymethamphetamine-assisted psychotherapy: a prospective longterm follow-up study. *Journal of Psychopharmacology, 27*, 28–39.

Monti, B. (2013). Histone post-translational modifications to target memory-related diseases. *Current Pharmaceutical Design, 19*, 5065–5075.

Morris, R. W., and Bouton, M. E. (2007). The effect of yohimbine on the extinction of conditioned fear: a role for context. *Behavioral Neuroscience, 121*, 501–514.

Mueller, D., and Cahill, S. P. (2010). Noradrenergic modulation of extinction learning and exposure therapy. *Behavioural Brain Research, 208*, 1–11.

National Comorbidity Survey Replication. (2005). 12-month prevalence of DSM-IV/WMH-CIDI disorders by sex and cohort. Retrieved from http://www.hcp.med.harvard.edu/ncs/ftpdir/table_ncsr_12monthprevgenderxage.pdf.

Nations, K. R., Smits, J. A., Tolin, D. F., Rothbaum, B. O., Hofmann, S. G., Tart, C. D., ... Otto, M. W. (2012). Evaluation of the glycine transporter inhibitor Org 25935 as augmentation to cognitive-behavioral therapy for panic disorder: a multicenter, randomized, double-blind, placebo-controlled trial. *Journal of Clinical Psychiatry, 73*, 647–653.

Norberg, M. M., Krystal, J. H., and Tolin, D. F. (2008). A meta-analysis of D-cycloserine and the facilitation of fear extinction and exposure therapy. *Biological Psychiatry, 63*, 118–1126.

Oehen, P., Traber, R., Widmer, V., and Schnyder, U. (2013). A randomized, controlled pilot study of MDMA (± 3,4-Methylenedioxymethamphetamine)-assisted psychotherapy for treatment of resistant, chronic post-traumatic stress disorder (PTSD). *Journal of Psychopharmacology, 27*, 40–52.

Parsons R. G., and Ressler K. J. (2013) Implications of memory modulation for post-traumatic stress and fear disorders. *Nature Neuroscience, 16*(2):146–153.

Pine, D. S., Cohen, P., and Brook, J. (2001). Adolescent fears as predictors of depression. *Biological Psychiatry, 50*, 721–724.

Rabinak, C. A., Angstadt, M., Sripada, C. S., Abelson, J. L., Liberzon, I., Milad, M. R., & Phan, K. L. (2013). Cannabinoid facilitation of fear extinction memory recall in humans. *Neuropharmacology, 64*, 396–402.

Rapee, R. M., and Heimberg, R. G. (1997). A cognitive-behavioral model of anxiety in social phobia. *Behaviour Research and Therapy, 35*, 741–756.

Rauch, S. L., Milad, M. R., Orr, S. P., Quinn, B. T., Fischl, B., and Pitman, R. K. (2005) Orbitofrontal thickness, retention of fear extinction, and extraversion. *Neuroreport, 16*, 1909–1912.

Ressler, K. J., Rothbaum, B. O., Tannenbaum, L., Anderson, P., Grapp, K., Zimand, E., Hodges, L., and Davis, M. (2004). Cognitive enhancers as adjuncts to psychotherapy: use of D-cycloserine in phobic individuals to facilitate extinction of fear. *Archives of General Psychiatry, 61*, 1136–1144.

Reul, J. M. (2014). Making memories of stressful events: a journey along epigenetic, gene transcription, and signaling pathways. *Frontiers in Psychiatry, 5*, 5.

Rodrigues, H., Figueira, I., Lopes, A., Gonçalves, R., Mendlowicz, M. V., Coutinho, E. S., and Ventura, P. (2014). Does D-cycloserine enhance exposure therapy for anxiety disorders in humans? A meta-analysis. *PLoS One, 9*, e93519.

Rothbaum, B. O., Price, M., Jovanovic, T., Norrholm, S. D., Gerardi, M., Dunlop, B. W., ... Ressler, K. J. (2014). Randomized, double-blind evaluation of D-cycloserine or alprazolam combined with virtual reality exposure therapy for posttraumatic stress disorder (PTSD) in OEF/OIF war veterans. *American Journal of Psychiatry, 171*, 640–648.

Singewald, N., Salchner, P., and Sharp, T. (2003). Induction of c-Fos expression in specific areas of the fear circuitry in rat forebrain by anxiogenic drugs. *Biological Psychiatry, 53*, 275–283.

Soravia, L. M., Heinrichs, M., Winzeler, L., Fisler, M., Schmitt, W., Horn, H., Dierks, T., Strik, W., Hofmann, S.G., and de Quervain, D. J. (2014). Glucocorticoids enhance in vivo exposure-based therapy of spider phobia. *Depression and Anxiety, 31*, 429–435.

Sprague, T. D., and Nichols, D. E. (1995). The monoamine oxidase-B inhibitor L-deprenyl protects against 3,4-methylenedioxymethamphetamineinduced lipid peroxidation and long-term serotonergic deficits. *Journal of Pharmacology and Experimental Therapeutics, 273*, 667–673.

Tart, C. D., Handelsman, P. R., DeBoer, L. B., Rosenfield, D., Pollack, M. H., Hofmann, S. G., . . . Smits, J. A. (2013). Augmentation of exposure therapy with post-session administration of D-cycloserine. *Journal of Psychiatric Research, 47*, 168–174.

Telch, M. J., Bruchey, A. K., Rosenfield, D., Cobb, A. R., Smits, J., Pahl, S., and Gonzalez-Lima, F. (2014). Effects of post-session administration of methylene blue on fear extinction and contextual memory in adults with claustrophobia. *American Journal of Psychiatry, 171*, 1091–1098.

Walker, D. L., Ressler, K. J., Lu, K. T., and Davis, M. (2002). Facilitation of conditioned fear extinction by systemic administration or intra-amygdala infusions of D-cycloserine as assessed with fear-potentiated startle in rats. *Journal of Neuroscience, 22*, 2343–2351.

Whittel, N., and Singewald, N. (2014). HDAC inhibitors as cognitive enhancers in fear, anxiety and trauma therapy: where do we stand? *Biochemical Society Transactions, 42*, 569–581.

Yang, Y. L. Chao, P. K., and Lu, K. T. (2006). Systemic and intra-amygdala administration of glucocorticoid agonist and antagonist modulate extinction of conditioned fear. *Neuropsychopharmacology, 31*, 912–924.

NEUROTRANSMITTER PATHWAYS AND PHARMACOLOGICAL TREATMENTS OF ANXIETY DISORDERS

27

STRESS, ANXIETY, AND DEPRESSION AND THE ROLE OF GLUTAMATE NEUROTRANSMISSION

WENDOL WILLIAMS AND GERARD SANACORA

INTRODUCTION

The mechanisms underlying neurotransmitter dysfunction in mental illness are shaped by environmental and genetic factors. The former, serving as a potential accelerant or unmasking influence, and the latter, serving as a vulnerability factor in the evolution of neuropsychiatric disease. Significant advances have been made in our understanding of the functional neuroanatomy and physiology of neuronal pathways as related to reward, fear, arousal, and cognition. Yet there still remains much to be learned about the molecular mechanisms and the intricate interdependent network of neuronal signaling processes that govern these circuits, and how these systems contribute to the pathogenesis and pathophysiology of mood and anxiety.

Currently, neuropsychiatric research is undergoing a paradigm shift from a simplified neurochemical framework of mood and anxiety psychopathology (the monoamine hypothesis) to a more highly integrated neuroplasticity model. With this neuroplasticity model in mind, it's difficult to think of any one neurotransmitter system in isolation as being the primary pathogenic factor in the development of mood and anxiety disorders. However, glutamate, as a principal neurotransmitter system involved in the regulation of neuroplastic change in the brain, has gained significant interest in the last few decades. The interest in glutamate as a target for study in relation to mood and anxiety disorders has recently been fueled by the exciting new evidence showing that glutamate function modulating drugs can produce rapid and robust antidepressant and anxiolytic effects. This chapter will present a brief overview of glutamate's potential contributions to the pathogenesis, pathophysiology and treatment of mood and anxiety disorders.

THE BRAIN: A GLUTAMATE MACHINE

When considering central nervous system physiology as a whole, it would be difficult to imagine any complex neuropathological process that does not involve the glutamatergic system at some level. Glutamate mediates the vast majority of fast excitatory transmission in the brain, while γ-aminobutyric acid (GABA), another amino acid neurotransmitter synthesized from a glutamate molecule, mediates the vast majority of fast inhibitory transmission. Glutamate neurons and synapses by far outnumber all other neurotransmitter systems in the brain, and the metabolic processes related to maintaining homeostatic levels of glutamate neurotransmission in the brain are estimated to consume up to 80% of the cortex's energy consumption (Hyder, Rothman, and Bennett, 2013). Thus, the brain is largely a glutamatergic machine, regulated by a relatively smaller GABAergic inhibitory component and modulated by a much smaller number of neurons releasing a variety of other neurotransmitters, including monoamines. With those facts in mind, it follows that glutamate likely plays a critical role in the regulation of most aspects of brain function.

EVIDENCE FOR GLUTAMATERGIC CONTRIBUTIONS TO THE PATHOGENESIS AND PATHOPHYSIOLOGY OF MOOD AND ANXIETY-RELATED PHENOTYPES IN NONHUMAN MODELS

Compared to medical disorders such as ischemic cardiac disease, we know very little of the pathogenic factors contributing to the development of mood and anxiety disorders. This places us at a tremendous disadvantage in prescribing preventative measures and in developing novel therapeutic strategies. However, there is general agreement within the field that varying intensities and durations of psychosocial stress exposure are associated with the onset and exacerbation of mood and anxiety disorders. Considering this, we review the relationship between stress, glutamatergic neurotransmission and the pathogenesis of these disorders.

EVIDENCE OF A STRESS, GLUTAMATE, AND PSYCHOPATHOLOGY INTERACTION FROM PRECLINICAL STRESS MODELS

Effects of stress on structural remodeling in the brain have been investigated in detail over the last several decades (McEwen, 2012; Pittenger and Duman, 2008). Different forms of stress can induce remodeling of dendrites and are associated with significant changes in dendritic spine density in hippocampal and mPFC regions (Radley et al., 2008). Chronic stress is associated with retraction and reduced spine density along with impairment of cognitive functions and reduced plasticity in hippocampal and mPFC synapses (Cerqueira, Mailliet, Almeida, Jay, and Sousa, 2007; Liston, McEwen, and Casey, 2009). These findings suggest a possible link to the brain volume abnormalities and functional changes commonly reported in association with mood and anxiety disorders (Koolschijn, van Haren, Lensvelt-Mulders, Hulshoff Pol, and Kahn, 2009).

Stress has been shown to have large effects on glutamatergic synapses in both hippocampal and prefrontal cortical regions. It has been hypothesized that changes in glutamatergic synaptic transmission are critical components responsible for dendritic remodeling and, in turn, tissue morphological changes seen in mood and anxiety disorders (Popoli, Yan, McEwen, and Sanacora, 2012). More specifically, glutamate synapses undergo structural and functional change in response to experience, learning and memory, and emotion processing (Sudhof and Malenka, 2008). These same changes in glutamate synaptic neurotransmission mediate further effects on synaptic terminals, spines and dendritic branches. Through these mechanisms, environmental stress is capable of influencing brain tissue morphology and likely serves as a risk factor for mood/anxiety disorders. However, stress responses are incompletely understood; a continuum is thought to exist between physiological mechanisms of plasticity ensuring survival and changes in structure and function that lead to pathological change.

Understanding glutamate's critical role in modulating the brain's response to environmental stimuli, and the relatively narrow window between glutamate's role in adaptive neuroplasticity vs. potentially neurotoxic effects, it is understandable that the system would be tightly regulated in the CNS for optimal brain function. If regulatory processes are encroached upon by stress or other factors, this may trigger alterations in synaptic connections and circuits that may play a decisive role in the development of mood or anxiety disorders.

Glutamate neurotransmission can be regulated at several points including presynaptic synthesis and release, postsynaptic activation and signaling, and through mechanisms of clearance to ensure optimal brain function and response to stimuli (see Figure 27.1). The following is a brief review of what is known about stress effects at these various control points.

At the **presynaptic level**, early *in vivo* microdialysis studies demonstrated that rats exposed to different stressors or administered corticosterone, rapidly show marked increases in the level of extracellular glutamate in different brain regions (Moghaddam, 2002). More recent studies further identified marked, rapid changes in the depolarization-evoked release of glutamate related to glucocorticoid effects on the regulation of vesicular membrane fusion. Interestingly, chronic administration of most classes of antidepressant agents have been found to dampen this effect in *in vitro* studies (Musazzi et al., 2010), suggesting that the control of stress-related glutamate release may provide a mechanism of antidepressant drug action.

As already mentioned, mechanisms of **postsynaptic plasticity** in hippocampus and frontal cortex are rapidly activated by stress. The postsynaptic changes are hypothesized to help ensure memory of the conditions related to stressful events (Joels and Baram, 2009). The major mechanism underlying postsynaptic plasticity involves an increase in the ionotropic α-amino-3-hydroxy-methyl-4-isoxazolepropionic acid receptors (AMPAR) within the postsynaptic density, driven by activity-dependent changes in AMPAR trafficking (Citri and Malenka, 2008). Electrophysiological recordings have shown that both N-methyl-D-aspartate receptor (NMDAR)- and AMPAR-mediated synaptic currents are markedly increased in PFC pyramidal neurons in various models of acute stress (Yuen et al., 2009). This effect can be sustained for 24 hours after the cessation of stress and can be mimicked by short-term corticosterone treatment in vitro, consistent with increased levels of AMPAR and NMDAR surface expression during this time. In contrast, chronic stress exposure had opposing effects, significantly reducing AMPAR- and NMDAR-mediated synaptic transmission and glutamate receptor expression in the PFC of animals (Yuen et al., 2012). Thus, these studies suggest that the effects of stress on glutamate mediated synaptic plasticity may vary based on the duration, and possibly the intensity of the stressor. Moreover, the studies also highlight the potentially divergent effects of stress on brain function, and how chronic stress could ultimately dampen glutamate transmission and inhibit glutamate mediated plasticity.

Stress has also been found to have effects on **glutamate clearance**. Glial cells play a critical role in modulating glutamatergic neurotransmission by rapidly clearing

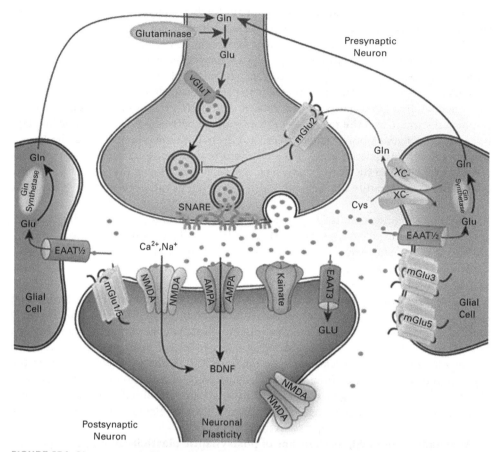

FIGURE 27.1 Glutamatergic Neurotransmission: Due to the delicate balance between optimal brain function and excito-toxicity, the glutamate synapse remains under precise physiological control with multiple levels of regulation. Glutamate (Glu) is synthesized within neurons when Glutamine (Gln) is converted to glutamate (Glu) by glutaminase [glutamate may also be derived from the TCA cycle (not shown)]. Cytosolic Glu is packaged into presynaptic vesicles for use as a neurotransmitter by vesicular Glu transporter (VGLUT) proteins. Glu is released synaptically in a voltage-dependent manner through vesicular interactions with SNARE proteins. Glu is recycled from the extracellular space by excitatory amino acid transporters (EAATs) expressed predominantly on astroglia and converted to Gln by Gln synthetase present in the glial cells. It is then exported through the extracellular space, to be taken up again by neurons. Additionally, system x-C is a cystine/glutamate antiporter also expressed on glia that also contributes to Glu recycling and serves as a target for N-acetylcysteine. Glu receptors are present on presynaptic and postsynaptic neurons as well as on glial cells. These include both ionotropic receptors (NMDA, AMPA/KA) and metabotropic receptors (mGluRs). The signal transduction effect of Glu is determined by the receptor subtype, localization (synaptic, peri-synaptic and extrasynaptic), and interactions with various scaffolding and signaling proteins (not shown) in the postsynaptic density. Glu receptor stimulation results not only in rapid ionotropic effects but also synaptic plasticity, e.g. long-term potentiation (LTP) and long-term depression (LTD), via cognate signal transduction cascades.

glutamate from the extracellular space through the two most abundant excitatory amino acid transporters (EAAT1 and EAAT2). The rapid clearance of glutamate into the glial cells limits the duration of synaptic transmission and prevents extrasynaptic spillover. Glia also serve a central role in amino acid neurotransmitter metabolism by converting glutamate to glutamine for the glutamate/glutamine cycle, and providing the majority of the glutamine precursor required for GABA synthesis.

Several recent studies have characterized the effects of stress on glial cell structure and function. Chronic stress results in a variety of effects on glial function that are likely tied to alterations in glutamate neurotransmission including: reduced proliferation of glial progenitor cells, reduced levels of excitatory amino acid transporters, and reduced rates of glutamate/glutamine cycling (G. Sanacora and Banasr, 2013). Interestingly, riluzole, a drug shown to modulate both glutamate release and uptake, was demonstrated to be effective in attenuating or reversing many of the behavioral, structural and metabolic changes seen with chronic stress (Banasr et al., 2010).

In sum, these studies suggest that stress can have marked effects on the glutamate synapse that appear to be critical in modulating and regulating neuroplasticity. Chronic stress appears to alter normal glutamatergic neurotransmission through effects on presynaptic release, postsynaptic receptor trafficking and glial mediated glutamate clearance. The results of these changes are hypothesized to lead to an enhanced ratio of extrasynaptic to synaptic glutamate receptor activation, an effect believed to be associated with impaired neuroplasticity and even in promoting neuronal toxicity in several degenerative neuropsychiatric disorders (Hardingham and Bading, 2010).

EVIDENCE FOR GLUTAMATERGIC CONTRIBUTIONS TO THE PATHOPHYSIOLOGY OF MOOD AND ANXIETY DISORDERS: CLINICAL EVIDENCE

Several pathophysiological findings have been described with regard to glutamatergic neurotransmission in individuals with mood disorders. Broadly scattered reports of altered glutamate levels have been observed in the plasma, serum, and cerebrospinal fluid (CSF) of individuals with mood disorders. Postmortem studies have reported increased glutamate levels in several brain regions in individuals with mood disorders (Hashimoto, Sawa, and Iyo, 2007). Several magnetic resonance spectroscopy studies have also identified regional- and state-related alterations of glutamate metabolites associated with mood disorders (Luykx et al., 2012); but before attempting to draw any pathophysiological meaning from the MRS and postmortem findings, it is important to clearly understand that these studies provide measures of total tissue metabolite content. The overwhelming majority of the metabolites being measured are intracellular, with an exceedingly small fraction reflecting synaptic glutamate. Thus, it is very difficult to draw any conclusions about glutamatergic neurotransmitter function directly from these findings. However, the fact that tissue glutamate, glutamine and even GABA content appear to be abnormal in several brain regions, and likely even in plasma of individuals afflicted with various forms of mood disorder, suggests that dysregulation of amino acid neurotransmitter system metabolism in some form is likely to be associated with the disorders. Consistent with this hypothesis, a recent ^{13}C-Magnetic resonance spectroscopy study of depressed subjects found evidence of reduced metabolism in glutamatergic neurons in the occipital cortex (Abdallah et al., 2014).

As noted previously, glial cells, especially astroglia, play a critical role in the regulation of glutamate and GABA metabolism. Consistent with the idea that changes in glial cell function may be related to the reports of abnormal glutamatergic function in patients with mood disorders, reduced numbers and density of glial cells have been reported in a number of postmortem studies examining individuals with mood disorders compared to non-mood disorder controls (Rajkowska and Stockmeier, 2013). Other studies have demonstrated reduced expression of EAAT1 and EAAT2, and glutamine synthetase, the enzyme responsible for the conversion of glutamate to glutamine within glia, in several brain regions from depressed individuals (G. Sanacora and Banasr, 2013). The reduced astrocytic function can result in impaired glutamate clearance from the extrasynaptic space and altered rates of glutamate/glutamine and GABA/glutamine cycling. Thus, many of the observed differences in amino acid neurotransmitter content between mood disorder and healthy comparison subjects could be related to glial pathology.

THE GLUTAMATERGIC SYSTEM IN THE TREATMENT OF MOOD AND ANXIETY DISORDERS

The roots of a "glutamate hypothesis of mood disorders" suggesting the system as a target for antidepressant drug development, can be traced back to the early 1990s when Trullas and Skolnick first reported that NMDAR antagonists possess antidepressant-like action in rodent models (Trullas and Skolnick, 1990). The hypothesis has broadened over the years, integrating research from many different fields, showing both that chronic administration of classical monoaminergic antidepressant medications modulate NMDAR function, and that a variety of drugs that directly target various parts of the glutamatergic system can produce antidepressant- and anxiolytic-like effects in both rodent models and in the clinical setting (G. Sanacora, Zarate, Krystal, and Manji, 2008). There is now a growing list of studies demonstrating antidepressant- and anxiolytic-like properties belonging to drugs that modulate glutamate release, uptake, and receptor transmission.

TREATMENTS TARGETING THE GLUTAMATERGIC SYSTEM

The complexity and the multiple levels of regulatory control maintained over glutamatergic neurotransmission renders the system rich with potential pharmacological targets. However, the critical need to maintain tight physiological control over the system creates a significant challenge when attempting to safely introduce these drugs into the clinic. Several sites within the glutamatergic system are actively being pursued as potential targets for antidepressant drug development.

MODULATORS OF GLUTAMATE RELEASE AND UPTAKE

Increasing evidence suggests several drug classes with antidepressant action have effects on the regulation of neuronal glutamate release, raising the possibility that this could be a shared mechanism of antidepressant action (Bonanno et al., 2005). There are also data suggesting drugs with known direct effects on glutamate release, such as lamotrigine, are effective in treating mood disorders (Bowden et al., 2003). Riluzole, a drug currently indicated for the treatment of amyotrophic lateral sclerosis, is known to modulate both glutamate release and uptake. In addition to its documented neuroprotective effects, riluzole has been shown to have antidepressant and anxiolytic effects in a variety of rodent models (Pittenger et al., 2008). Moreover, preliminary results from a number of small open-label clinical trials exploring riluzole's efficacy in the treatment of severe mood, anxiety, and impulsive disorders are encouraging (C. A. Zarate and Manji, 2008).

However, more recently published small pilot studies did not find riluzole to be effective in preventing the relapse of depressive symptoms following the use of another glutamatergic drug, ketamine (Mathew et al., 2009). Other, preclinical studies also suggest that ceftriaxone, a ß-lactam antibiotic known to increase glutamate clearance, has antidepressant and anxiolytic properties and may have use in preventing relapse in a variety of substance abuse disorders (G. Sanacora and Banasr, 2013).

MODULATORS OF GLUTAMATE SIGNAL TRANSDUCTION

Metabotropic Glutamate Receptors

G protein-coupled metabotropic glutamate receptors (mGluRs) are divided into three groups on the basis of structure and function (Figure 27.2). Group I (mGluR1 and mGluR5) are located primarily on postsynaptic neurons and glial cells where they are believed to play a major role in regulating postsynaptic excitability. Groups II (mGluR 2 and 3) and III (mGluR4, mGluR6-8) receptors are largely present on the presynaptic membrane where they act by regulating transmitter release. Group I modulating drugs, especially mGluR5 antagonists, have recently come under intense study owing to the receptors' role in modulating synaptic plasticity and the potential to modify developmental illnesses such as Fragile X syndrome. The drugs also have strong anxiolytic- and potential antidepressant-like activity in preclinical animal models (Palucha and Pilc, 2007; Witkin, Marek, Johnson, and Schoepp, 2007). Although early phase clinical trials are now in progress for a variety of disorders, no clinical studies demonstrating the effectiveness of this class of drug in mood or anxiety disorders have been reported to date.

Other evidence suggests the group II metabotropic receptors, especially mGluR2, also serve important roles in modulating glutamate neurotransmission and the mechanisms of neuroprotection and neurodegeneration, thus making them extremely interesting targets for antidepressant drug development. Preclinical studies show drugs targeting the

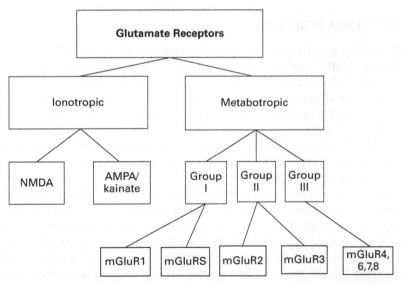

FIGURE 27.2 Outline of Glutamate Receptors: Shown in schematic form are the relative relationships between the functional and structural classes of different glutamate receptors.

group II metabotropic receptors possess both antidepressant and anxiolytic properties in preclinical models (see Palucha and Pilc, 2007; Witkin et al., 2007 for reviews). An early phase clinical trial supports the hypothesis that mGluR2/3 receptor agonists may be efficacious in the treatment of anxiety, but raises some concern over the safety of the specific agent tested due to findings of convulsions in preclinical studies (Dunayevich et al., 2008). No clinical studies have yet been reported exploring the antidepressant efficacy of mGluR2/3 receptor drugs.

IONOTROPIC AMPA AND KAINATE RECEPTORS

Adaptations in synaptic AMPAR signal transmission are recognized to be a critically important mechanism regulating various forms of synaptic plasticity. Studies showing that the receptors are altered in animal models of mood disorders and in some depressed individuals (Bleakman, Alt, and Witkin, 2007; Laje et al., 2007) suggest that the receptors may contribute to the underlying pathophysiology of the disorders. Additional studies showing that AMPA receptor function is modified by many classes of existing mood stabilizers and antidepressant agents suggest a potential common mechanism of action for the drugs (Du et al., 2007). This idea has been further supported by evidence showing AMPAR activation is a critical component of mechanism of antidepressant action associated with the NMDAR antagonist drugs (Duman and Aghajanian, 2012) (see next section).

There is a growing interest in targeting AMPA receptors, by employing a new class of compounds referred to as AMPA potentiators that indirectly modulate AMPA signaling through effects on receptor desensitization and deactivation, for a variety of indications ranging from impaired cognition to Parkinson's disease. Several preclinical studies suggest AMPA potentiators possess antidepressant properties (Bleakman et al., 2007). A single phase Ib clinical trial examining the safety of one of these drugs showed the drug to have good tolerability in depressed patients, but was inadequately powered to provide any meaningful test of efficacy (Nations et al., 2012).

IONOTROPIC NMDA RECEPTORS

NMDARs exist primarily as multi-subunit complexes composed of NR1, NR2, and NR3 subunits. Multiple splice variants of each of the subunits result in a variety of NMDARs with slightly varied properties. In addition to glutamate, the NMDARs have binding sites for other neuromodulators including glycine, which serves as an obligatory co-agonist. Magnesium and zinc concentrations also modulate NMDA receptor function, providing other potential means of modifying the receptors' signal transduction properties. As alluded to earlier, the NMDAR serves complex roles in the regulation of brain function, and NMDARs are known to both promote neuronal survival and cell death (Hardingham and Bading, 2010).

Case reports noting antidepressant-like effects associated with the NMDAR active drug cycloserine can be found dating back as early as the late 1950s (Crane, 1959) (long predating the knowledge that glutamate was even a neurotransmitter). However, the first widely recognized reports of NMDAR antagonists having antidepressant-like effects in rodent models date to the early 1990s (Trullas and Skolnick, 1990). The hypothesis that NMDARs could be targeted for the development of antidepressant medications experienced a surge in interest from academics and the pharmaceutical industry following a report by Berman et al. showing a single sub-anesthetic dose ketamine, a non-competitive NMDA antagonist, delivered intravenously over a period of 40 minutes, resulted in a dramatic improvement in depressive symptoms lasting for several days in a group of 7 depressed subjects (Berman et al., 2000). The finding of a rapid and sustained improvement in depressive symptoms following a single dose of ketamine was later replicated by Zarate et al. (C. A. Zarate, Jr., Singh, Carlson, et al., 2006). In that study, over 70% of the subjects showed at least a 50% reduction in depression severity, and 29% of the subjects met criteria for remission within 24 hours of dosing. This finding has now been replicated with a high level of consistency in multiple clinical trials and case reports (McGirr et al., 2014). Moreover, ketamine and other NMDAR antagonists have also been demonstrated to have antidepressant-like and anxiolytic effects in a variety of rodent models (Browne and Lucki, 2013). Rapidly accumulating evidence suggests the mechanism of ketamine's action involves changes in glutamatergic signaling through non-NMDA glutamate receptors (most notably AMPA), and down-stream effects on neuroplasticity involving brain derived neurotrophic factor (BDNF) activity (Duman and Aghajanian, 2012). However, other mechanisms have also been proposed (see G. Sanacora and Schatzberg, 2015 for review).

Despite the large effect-sizes associated with ketamine's efficacy in the treatment of mood disorders, the unwanted short-term physiological and psychological effects of ketamine limit its potential clinical utility at present. Considering those limitations, the potential ability to take advantage of the complex NMDAR pharmacology affords some promise that it may be possible to capture some of the antidepressant properties of ketamine while avoiding the major unwanted short-term physiological and psychological effects seen with ketamine. Using this approach, Preskorn et al. presented preliminary evidence that an NMDA NR2B selective drug (CP101,606) was effective in treating depressed patients who had failed to respond to an SSRI (Preskorn et al., 2008). Another recently published study of 151 depressed subjects found evidence that repeated intravenous administration of lanicemine, a low trapping non-selective NMDAR antagonist, produced sustained antidepressant effects (G. Sanacora et al., 2013). However, this finding was not replicated in a recent multi-national follow-up study (G Sanacora et al., 2014). Memantine, another low-to-moderate-affinity noncompetitive NMDAR antagonist failed to show any antidepressant advantage at doses of up to 20mg/day compared to placebo in a double blind randomized placebo controlled trial of 32 subjects over a period of 8 weeks (C. A. Zarate, Jr., Singh, Quiroz, et al., 2006).

There is also interest surrounding the potential of exploiting drugs that modulate glycine's effects on NMDA receptor activation for use in treating various mood and anxiety disorders. D-cycloserine (DCS), a glycine partial agonist, has been shown in several rodent studies and small clinical trials to facilitate fear extinction (Davis, Ressler, Rothbaum, and Richardson, 2006), offering the hope that it may be possible to use partial NMDA agonists to expedite and enhance the effectiveness of exposure/extinction therapies in treating anxiety disorders. Despite the early reports of cycloserine's antidepressant-like activities previously mentioned (Crane, 1959), recent studies examining the antidepressant effects of DCS in depressed subjects although somewhat encouraging, have been mixed (Heresco-Levy et al., 2013; Heresco-Levy et al., 2006).

In conclusion, there is a rapidly increasing interest in glutamate's potential contributions to the pathogenesis, pathophysiology and treatment of mood and anxiety disorders. The role of glutamate as a modulator of stress response in the CNS provides a strong mechanistic link to the long recognized association of stress and psychopathology. The emerging evidence suggesting ketamine and other glutamate targeting drugs have robust effects in the treatment of mood and anxiety disorders suggests that the system may indeed provide a fruitful target for future drug development. However, additional studies are required to determine the true clinical meaningfulness of this approach.

DISCLOSURE STATEMENT

Dr. Sanacora has received consulting fees from AstraZeneca, Avanier Pharmaceuticals, Bristol-Myers Squibb, Eli Lilly and Co., Hoffman La-Roche, Janssen Pharmaceuticals, Lundbeck, Merck & Co, Naurex, Noven Pharmaceuticals, and Takeda over the last 24 months. He has also received additional research contracts from AstraZeneca, Bristol-Myers Squibb, Eli Lilly & Co., Janssen Pharmaceuticals, Hoffman La-Roche, Merck & Co., Naurex and Servier over the last 24 months. Free medication was provided to Dr. Sanacora for an NIH sponsored study by Sanofi-Aventis. In addition Dr. Sanacora holds shares in BioHaven Pharmaceuticals Holding Company and is a co-inventor on a US patent (#8,778,979) held by Yale University.

Dr. Williams has no interests to disclose.

ACKNOWLEDGMENTS

We would like to thank Lisa Roach for her assistance with the preparation of this chapter and Dr. Benjamin Kelmendi for his assistance with the preparation of the figures.

REFERENCES

Abdallah, C. G., Niciu, M. J., Fenton, L. R., Fasula, M. K., Jiang, L., Black, A., . . . Sanacora, G. (2014). Decreased occipital cortical glutamate levels in response to successful cognitive-behavioral therapy and pharmacotherapy for major depressive disorder. *Psychother Psychosom*, 83(5), 298–307.

Banasr, M., Chowdhury, G. M., Terwilliger, R., Newton, S. S., Duman, R. S., Behar, K. L., and Sanacora, G. (2010). Glial pathology in an animal model of depression: reversal of stress-induced cellular, metabolic and behavioral deficits by the glutamate-modulating drug riluzole. *Mol Psychiatry*, 15(5), 501–511.

Berman, R. M., Cappiello, A., Anand, A., Oren, D. A., Heninger, G. R., Charney, D. S., and Krystal, J. H. (2000). Antidepressant effects of ketamine in depressed patients. *Biol Psychiatry*, 47(4), 351–354.

Bleakman, D., Alt, A., and Witkin, J. M. (2007). AMPA receptors in the therapeutic management of depression. *CNS Neurol Disord Drug Targets*, 6(2), 117–126.

Bonanno, G., Giambelli, R., Raiteri, L., Tiraboschi, E., Zappettini, S., Musazzi, L., . . . Popoli, M. (2005). Chronic antidepressants reduce depolarization-evoked glutamate release and protein interactions favoring formation of SNARE complex in hippocampus. *J Neurosci*, 25(13), 3270–3279.

Bowden, C. L., Calabrese, J. R., Sachs, G., Yatham, L. N., Asghar, S. A., Hompland, M., . . . DeVeaugh-Geiss, J. (2003). A placebo-controlled 18-month trial of lamotrigine and lithium maintenance treatment in recently manic or hypomanic patients with bipolar I disorder. *Arch Gen Psychiatry*, 60(4), 392–400.

Browne, C. A., and Lucki, I. (2013). Antidepressant effects of ketamine: mechanisms underlying fast-acting novel antidepressants. *Front Pharmacol*, 4, 161.

Cerqueira, J. J., Mailliet, F., Almeida, O. F., Jay, T. M., and Sousa, N. (2007). The prefrontal cortex as a key target of the maladaptive response to stress. *J Neurosci*, 27(11), 2781–2787.

Citri, A., and Malenka, R. C. (2008). Synaptic plasticity: multiple forms, functions, and mechanisms. *Neuropsychopharmacology*, 33(1), 18–41.

Crane, GE. (1959). Cycloserine as an antidepressant agent. *American Journal of Psychiatry*, 115, 1025–1026.

Davis, M., Ressler, K., Rothbaum, B. O., and Richardson, R. (2006). Effects of D-cycloserine on extinction: translation from preclinical to clinical work. *Biol Psychiatry*, 60(4), 369–375.

Du, J., Suzuki, K., Wei, Y., Wang, Y., Blumenthal, R., Chen, Z., . . . Manji, H. K. (2007). The anticonvulsants lamotrigine, riluzole, and valproate differentially regulate AMPA receptor membrane localization: relationship to clinical effects in mood disorders. *Neuropsychopharmacology, 32*(4), 793–802.

Duman, R. S., and Aghajanian, G. K. (2012). Synaptic dysfunction in depression: potential therapeutic targets. *Science, 338*(6103), 68–72.

Dunayevich, E., Erickson, J., Levine, L., Landbloom, R., Schoepp, D. D., and Tollefson, G. D. (2008). Efficacy and tolerability of an mglu2/3 agonist in the treatment of generalized anxiety disorder. *Neuropsychopharmacology,* Jun;33(7):1603–1610

Hardingham, G. E., and Bading, H. (2010). Synaptic versus extrasynaptic NMDA receptor signalling: implications for neurodegenerative disorders. *Nat Rev Neurosci, 11*(10), 682–696.

Hashimoto, K., Sawa, A., and Iyo, M. (2007). Increased levels of glutamate in brains from patients with mood disorders. *Biol Psychiatry, 62*(11), 1310–1316.

Heresco-Levy, U., Gelfin, G., Bloch, B., Levin, R., Edelman, S., Javitt, D. C., and Kremer, I. (2013). A randomized add-on trial of high-dose D-cycloserine for treatment-resistant depression. *Int J Neuropsychopharmacol, 16*(3), 501–506.

Heresco-Levy, U., Javitt, D. C., Gelfin, Y., Gorelik, E., Bar, M., Blanaru, M., and Kremer, I. (2006). Controlled trial of D-cycloserine adjuvant therapy for treatment-resistant major depressive disorder. *J Affect Disord, 93*(1–3), 239–243.

Hyder, F., Rothman, D. L., and Bennett, M. R. (2013). Cortical energy demands of signaling and nonsignaling components in brain are conserved across mammalian species and activity levels. *Proc Natl Acad Sci USA, 110*(9), 3549–3554. doi: 10.1073/pnas.1214912110

Joels, M., and Baram, T. Z. (2009). The neuro-symphony of stress. *Nat Rev Neurosci, 10*(6), 459–466.

Koolschijn, P. C., van Haren, N. E., Lensvelt-Mulders, G. J., Hulshoff Pol, H. E., and Kahn, R. S. (2009). Brain volume abnormalities in major depressive disorder: a meta-analysis of magnetic resonance imaging studies. *Hum Brain Mapp, 30*(11), 3719–3735.

Laje, G., Paddock, S., Manji, H., Rush, A. J., Wilson, A. F., Charney, D., and McMahon, F. J. (2007). Genetic markers of suicidal ideation emerging during citalopram treatment of major depression. *Am J Psychiatry, 164*(10), 1530–1538.

Liston, C., McEwen, B. S., and Casey, B. J. (2009). Psychosocial stress reversibly disrupts prefrontal processing and attentional control. *Proc Natl Acad Sci USA, 106*(3), 912–917.

Luykx, J. J., Laban, K. G., van den Heuvel, M. P., Boks, M. P., Mandl, R. C., Kahn, R. S., and Bakker, S. C. (2012). Region and state specific glutamate downregulation in major depressive disorder: a meta-analysis of (1)H-MRS findings. *Neurosci Biobehav Rev, 36*(1), 198–205.

Mathew, S. J., Murrough, J. W., Aan Het Rot, M., Collins, K. A., Reich, D. L., and Charney, D. S. (2009). Riluzole for relapse prevention following intravenous ketamine in treatment-resistant depression: a pilot randomized, placebo-controlled continuation trial. *Int J Neuropsychopharmacol, 13*(1), 71–82.

McEwen, B. S. (2012). Brain on stress: how the social environment gets under the skin. *Proc Natl Acad Sci USA, 109 Suppl 2*, 17180–17185.

McGirr, A., Berlim, M. T., Bond, D. J., Fleck, M. P., Yatham, L. N., and Lam, R. W. (2014). A systematic review and meta-analysis of randomized, double-blind, placebo-controlled trials of ketamine in the rapid treatment of major depressive episodes. *Psychol Med, 10*, 1–12.

Moghaddam, B. (2002). Stress activation of glutamate neurotransmission in the prefrontal cortex: implications for dopamine-associated psychiatric disorders. *Biol Psychiatry, 51*(10), 775–787.

Musazzi, L., Milanese, M., Farisello, P., Zappettini, S., Tardito, D., Barbiero, V. S., . . . Popoli, M. (2010). Acute stress increases depolarization-evoked glutamate release in the rat prefrontal/frontal cortex: the dampening action of antidepressants. *PLoS One, 5*(1), e8566.

Nations, K. R., Dogterom, P., Bursi, R., Schipper, J., Greenwald, S., Zraket, D., . . . Ereshefsky, L. (2012). Examination of Org 26576, an AMPA receptor positive allosteric modulator, in patients diagnosed with major depressive disorder: an exploratory, randomized, double-blind, placebo-controlled trial. *J Psychopharmacol, 26*(12), 1525–1539.

Palucha, A., and Pilc, A. (2007). Metabotropic glutamate receptor ligands as possible anxiolytic and antidepressant drugs. *Pharmacol Ther, 115*(1), 116–147.

Pittenger, C., Coric, V., Banasr, M., Bloch, M., Krystal, J. H., and Sanacora, G. (2008). Riluzole in the treatment of mood and anxiety disorders. *CNS Drugs, 22*(9), 761–786.

Pittenger, C., and Duman, R. S. (2008). Stress, depression, and neuroplasticity: a convergence of mechanisms. *Neuropsychopharmacology, 33*(1), 88–109.

Popoli, M., Yan, Z., McEwen, B. S., and Sanacora, G. (2012). The stressed synapse: the impact of stress and glucocorticoids on glutamate transmission. *Nat Rev Neurosci, 13*(1), 22–37.

Preskorn, S. H., Baker, B., Kolluri, S., Menniti, F. S., Krams, M., and Landen, J. W. (2008). An innovative design to establish proof of concept of the antidepressant effects of the NR2B subunit selective N-methyl-D-aspartate antagonist, CP-101,606, in patients with treatment-refractory major depressive disorder. *J Clin Psychopharmacol, 28*(6), 631–637.

Radley, J. J., Rocher, A. B., Rodriguez, A., Ehlenberger, D. B., Dammann, M., McEwen, B. S., . . . Hof, P. R. (2008). Repeated stress alters dendritic spine morphology in the rat medial prefrontal cortex. *J Comp Neurol, 507*(1), 1141–1150.

Rajkowska, G., and Stockmeier, C. A. (2013). Astrocyte pathology in major depressive disorder: insights from human postmortem brain tissue. *Curr Drug Targets, 14*(11), 1225–1236.

Sanacora, G, Johnson, M, Khan, A, Atkinson, SD, Riesenberg, R, Schronen, J, . . . Pathak, S. (2014). *Adjunctive lanicemine (AZD6765) in patients with major depressive disorder and a history of inadequate response to antidepressants: primary results from a randomized, placebo controlled study (PURSUIT).* Paper presented at the American Society of Clinical Psychiatry, Hollywood FL.

Sanacora, G., and Banasr, M. (2013). From pathophysiology to novel antidepressant drugs: glial contributions to the pathology and treatment of mood disorders. *Biol Psychiatry, 73*(12), 1172–1179.

Sanacora, G., and Schatzberg, A. F. (2015). Ketamine: Promising Path or False Prophecy in the Development of Novel Therapeutics for Mood Disorders? *Neuropsychopharmacology, 40*(2), 259–267.

Sanacora, G., Smith, M. A., Pathak, S., Su, H. L., Boeijinga, P. H., McCarthy, D. J., and Quirk, M. C. (2013). Lanicemine: a low-trapping NMDA channel blocker produces sustained antidepressant efficacy with minimal psychotomimetic adverse effects. *Mol Psychiatry, 19*(9), 978–985.

Sanacora, G., Zarate, C. A., Krystal, J. H., and Manji, H. K. (2008). Targeting the glutamatergic system to develop novel, improved therapeutics for mood disorders. *Nat Rev Drug Discov, 7*(5), 426–437.

Sudhof, T. C., and Malenka, R. C. (2008). Understanding synapses: past, present, and future. *Neuron, 60*(3), 469–476.

Trullas, R., and Skolnick, P. (1990). Functional antagonists at the NMDA receptor complex exhibit antidepressant actions. *Eur J Pharmacol, 185*(1), 1–10.

Witkin, J. M., Marek, G. J., Johnson, B. G., and Schoepp, D. D. (2007). Metabotropic glutamate receptors in the control of mood disorders. *CNS Neurol Disord Drug Targets, 6*(2), 87–100.

Yuen, E. Y., Liu, W., Karatsoreos, I. N., Feng, J., McEwen, B. S., and Yan, Z. (2009). Acute stress enhances glutamatergic transmission in prefrontal cortex and facilitates working memory. *Proc Natl Acad Sci U S A, 106*(33), 14075–14079.

Yuen, E. Y., Wei, J., Liu, W., Zhong, P., Li, X., and Yan, Z. (2012). Repeated stress causes cognitive impairment by suppressing glutamate receptor expression and function in prefrontal cortex. *Neuron, 73*(5), 962–977.

Zarate, C. A., Jr., Singh, J. B., Carlson, P. J., Brutsche, N. E., Ameli, R., Luckenbaugh, D. A., . . . Manji, H. K. (2006). A randomized trial of an N-methyl-D-aspartate antagonist in treatment-resistant major depression. *Arch Gen Psychiatry, 63*(8), 856–864.

Zarate, C. A., Jr., Singh, J. B., Quiroz, J. A., De Jesus, G., Denicoff, K. K., Luckenbaugh, D. A., . . . Charney, D. S. (2006). A double-blind, placebo-controlled study of memantine in the treatment of major depression. *Am J Psychiatry, 163*(1), 153–155.

Zarate, C. A., and Manji, H. K. (2008). Riluzole in psychiatry: a systematic review of the literature. *Expert Opin Drug Metab Toxicol, 4*(9), 1223–1234.

28

THE ROLE OF THE HYPOTHALAMIC–PITUITARY–ADRENAL AXIS IN ANXIETY DISORDERS

LUMINITA LUCA AND CHARLES B. NEMEROFF

INTRODUCTION

The current understanding of the neurobiological underpinnings of all severe psychiatric disorders, including anxiety disorders, is evolving as advances in neuroscience are realized. Of particular importance is a growing body of evidence suggesting that early life trauma induces vulnerability to stress later in life, manifested by increased risk for mood and anxiety disorders (Heim and Nemeroff, 2001; Nemeroff and Valle, 2005). More recent stress in adulthood is also known to precipitate anxiety symptoms in genetically vulnerable individuals. The substrate of such vulnerability is, at least in part, persistent sensitization of stress-responsive neural circuits. This review explores the role of the hypothalamic–pituitary–adrenal (HPA) axis in stress regulation and in the pathogenesis of anxiety disorders, by conceptualizing the combination of genetic factors, early life stressors, and ongoing trauma that regulate an individual's vulnerability to syndromal anxiety disorders. Posttraumatic stress disorder (PTSD) has been the most intensively studied, and the cardinal symptoms likely reflect, in part, changes in the activity of the HPA axis and other systems that regulate the response to stress.

Fear-evoking stimuli are processed in the thalamus, amygdala, and other limbic and cortical circuits inducing the classic "fight or flight response." The thalamus sends efferents to the brain stem for automatic reflexes, to basolateral amygdala, via a "short loop," and to associative cortex, insula, prefrontal cortex, and back to amygdala via a "long loop" (Amiel et al., 2009). The sympathetic nervous system is activated via the lateral hypothalamus, whereas the parasympathetic nervous system receives excitatory input via the dorsal motor nucleus of the vagus nerve; the endogenous opioid system, as well as circuits mediated by norepinephrine and dopamine are activated, as well. These circuits offer protection from threat, yet, when dysregulated, they may play a role in the pathophysiology of anxiety disorders.

The HPA axis is the major neuroendocrine mediator of the response to stress and, with the sympathetic nervous system, comprises the sympathoadrenal system, the major peripheral regulators of the stress response. The HPA axis is represented by neurons in the paraventricular nucleus (PVN) of the hypothalamus which contain corticotropin-releasing factor (CRF) a so-called hypothalamic releasing factor that is secreted from nerve endings in the median eminence into hypothalamo-hypophyseal portal system and then humorally transported to the anterior pituitary gland. CRF, in turn, stimulates the secretion of adrenocorticotrophic hormone (ACTH), from adenohypophyseal corticotrophs. Upon release into the systemic circulation, ACTH stimulates the synthesis and release of cortisol from the adrenal cortex.

The activity of the HPA axis is influenced by other limbic structures: the amygdala input enhances the activity of HPA axis, whereas the hippocampus, which is rich in mineralocorticoid receptors, suppresses HPA axis activity (see Figure 28.1).

The activity of the HPA axis can be assessed clinically in humans with a variety of methods including the dexamethasone (DEX) suppression test (DST), the CRF stimulation test, and the combined DEX/CRF test. DEX, a synthetic glucocorticoid administered systemically, decreases plasma ACTH and cortisol concentration via negative feedback at the level of the anterior pituitary. In the CRF stimulation test, CRF is administered intravenously stimulating CRF1 receptors in the anterior pituitary, inducing elevations in ACTH, ß-endorphin and cortisol concentrations. The combined DEX/CRF test (Heuser et al., 1994) is arguably the most sensitive measure of HPA axis activity: CRF is administered after pretreatment with DEX. In normal healthy volunteers CRF does not induce cortisol secretion in DEX-pretreated subjects; "escape" from suppression in patients with hyperactivity of the HPA axis is observed as for example in depressive disorders.

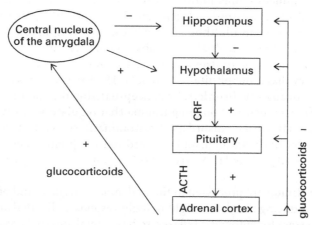

FIGURE 28.1 The extended HPA axis. HPA axis activity is stimulated by the central nucleus of amygdala and inhibited by the hippocampus. CRF is synthesized in the hypothalamus and, upon release, induces secretion of ACTH from the anterior pituitary gland. ACTH stimulates the production of glucocorticoids, which, in turn, exert inhibitory feedback on the pituitary, hypothalamus, and hippocampus and facilitate the activity of the amygdala. Adapted, with permission, from Martin et al., 2010.

CRF AND CRF RECEPTORS

The CRF system comprises four endogenous ligands (CRF, urocortin 1, urocortin 2, and urocortin 3) and two receptors (Binder and Nemeroff, 2010). CRF is a 41-amino acid neuropeptide expressed mostly in the CNS—hypothalamus, amygdala, cerebrocortical areas, hippocampus, and septum—and in certain peripheral organs, as well. Urocortins are structurally similar to CRF; urocortin 1 is expressed mostly in the periphery, while urocortin 2 is found in hypothalamus, locus coeruleus and brain stem, with an expression pattern similar to that of CRF. Urocortin 3 is localized in the median preoptic area, and the medial nucleus of the amygdala. Outside the CNS, the urocortins are found in cardiovascular structures (urocortin 2), the gastrointesinal tract and adrenal gland (urocortin 3). The availability of CRF in blood and brain is regulated by a CRF-binding protein (CRFBP), which reduces the free fraction of CRF and urocortins.

The CRF family of peptides binds to two identified receptors—CRF_1 and CRF_2. CRF and urocortin 1 preferentially bind to $CRFR_1$, while urocortins 1, 2 and 3 preferentially bind to $CRFR_2$. Both receptors are G-protein coupled receptors, distributed largely in cortical and subcortical areas: the cerebral cortex, cerebellum, hippocampus, amygdala and pituitary (CRF_1), and in subcortical areas (CRF_2). In the *rhesus* monkey, CRF_2 receptors, but not CRF_1 receptors, are found in certain hypothalamic nuclei and the bed nucleus of the stria terminalis (Sanchez et al., 1999). The CRF_1 receptor is widely distributed in cortical regions, and its expression appears to predominate over CRF_2 receptors. High CRF_1 receptor expression was observed in pituitary and cerebellum, but CRF receptor immunoreactivity was also described in cerebral cortex, forebrain, limbic regions, basal ganglia and thalamus (Kostick et al., 2004). This suggests that the CRF1 receptor may play roles in attention processing, processing of sensory and motor information (via modulation of thalamus) and in defensive or anxious responses (by modulation of activity of the amygdala, hippocampus, hypothalamus; Risbrough and Stein, 2006). The role of CRF_1 and CRF_2 receptors was inferred initially from laboratory animal studies, which showed that pharmacological blockade of CRF_1 receptors or deletion of the $CRFR_1$ gene resulted in attenuation of the neuroendocrine response to stress (Reul and Hoelsboer, 2002).

THE ROLE OF CRF IN STRESS RESPONSIVITY

It is well-established that CRF is the primary regulator of ACTH release and synthesis, therefore controlling the activity of the HPA axis. ACTH stimulates the synthesis and release of adrenal glucocorticoids from the adrenal cortex (Tsatanis et al., 2007). The CRF system modulates the activity of CNS noradrenergic and sympathetic nervous system activity by CRF projections to the locus coeruleus (Valentino et al., 1983). The many effects of CRF are summarized in Figure 28.2.

CRF has been hypothesized to play a seminal role in the pathogenesis of anxiety-related behaviors as it has been reported to induce fear, alertness, and anxiety in laboratory animals (Reul and Holsboer, 2002) and activation of the "fight or flight response." These functions appear to be dysregulated in anxiety and depressive disorders (Binder and Nemeroff, 2010). CRF activates CRF_1 receptors to produce depressive-like and anxiogenic behaviors, which are blocked by CRF_1 receptor antagonists in animal studies and in a clinical trial (Holsboer and Ising, 2008). In fact, various antagonists of the CRF_1 receptor have been found to exert anxiolytic effects in rodent studies (Lelas et al., 2004, Dzierba et al., 2004). In a clinical trial, pretreatment with the CRF_1 receptor antagonist NBI-34041 attenuated stress-induced plasma ACTH and cortisol elevations (Hoelsboer

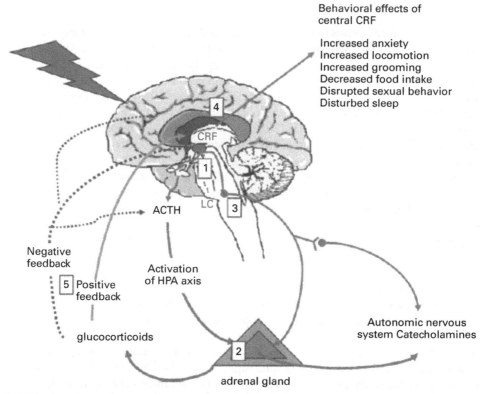

FIGURE 28.2 The actions of CRF at different levels of stress response. (1) Hypothalamic para-ventricular CRF-containing neurons release CRF into the hypothalamo-hypophyseal portal system, stimulating ACTH release from the anterior pituitary. (2) CRF directly stimulates corti-sol and cathecholamine synthesis from the adrenal cortex and medulla, respectively. (3) CRF stimulates noradrenergic neurons in the locus coeruleus. (4) CRF mediates behaviors through actions on cortical and limbic brain regions. (5) CRF transcription is negatively regulated by glucocorticoids in the hypothalamus and positively regulated in limbic brain regions (adapted with permission from Binder and Nemeroff, 2010).

and Issing, 2008). However, this compound did not diminish the CRF-induced secre-tion of ACTH, suggesting that chronic CRF_1 receptor antagonist treatment did not com-pletely suppress HPA axis responsiveness.

THE HPA AXIS IN ANXIETY DISORDERS

Panic Disorder

There is evidence suggesting alterations in the HPA axis in panic disorder (PD) (Kent et al., 2002). Plasma cortisol levels were found to be elevated in patients with PD at base-line (Roy-Byrne et al., 1986; Abelson et al., 2007) and prior to infusion of an anxiogenic compound, lactate (Coplan et al., 1998). Other studies reported normal diurnal levels of cortisol, but increased levels overnight (Abelson and Curtis, 2006). Elevated cortisol levels were reported to correlate with baseline indices of fear, suggesting that this may represent a marker for anticipatory anxiety (Coplan et al., 1998).

Studies measuring CSF CRF concentrations (Risbrough and Stein, 2006) found no differences in CRF levels in CSF of patients with panic disorder versus no disorder (Fossey et al., 1996). However, the stressful lumbar puncture procedure may mask PD-associated elevations (Risbrough and Stein 2006).

Salivary cortisol levels were recently found to be lower upon awakening in a large sample of patients with anxiety disorders than in healthy comparisons, suggesting a blunting of the HPA response (Hek et al., 2013). This effect was most prominent in patients with a diagnosis of GAD. However, salivary cortisol levels upon awakening were found to be elevated in patients with acute anxiety disorders, an effect driven largely by patients with PD; no changes in salivary cortisol, evening cortisol or on cortisol suppression after DEX were noted (Vreeburg et al., 2010). In contrast, abnormalities in HPA axis activity and ACTH response have been described, e.g. blunted ACTH response in a CRF stimulation test (Roy-Byrne et al., 1986).

Panic can be provoked by various agents (caffeine, lactate, CO_2) without apparent HPA axis activation, raising questions on the degree to which HPA activity relates specifically to anticipatory anxiety as opposed to the acute panic attack. In an experimental design aimed to describe the HPA axis response in panic disorder, several paradigms have been used: doxapram (panic inducer known not to stimulate the HPA axis); pentagastrin, a cholecystokinin agonist well known to stimulate HPA axis activity; and cognitive interventions to reduce the novelty factor were administered to a subgroup of PD patients. Patients with PD had elevated baseline cortisol and ACTH levels, consistent with anticipatory anxiety, and exhibited an exaggerated ACTH response. Patients exposed to pentagastrin also showed an elevated HPA axis response; however, the patients who received the cognitive intervention prior to pentagastrin infusion demonstrated a normalized ACTH response. These findings suggest that novelty and threat contribute to HPA axis hyperactivation and that HPA axis hypersensitivity may represent a trait exhibited by patients with PD (Abelson et al., 2007).

Generalized Anxiety Disorder

Few studies have examined HPA axis reactivity in patients with GAD; among those, the results are mostly negative. Fossey et al. (1996) found no changes in CSF concentrations of CRF in patients with GAD, or in other anxiety disorders, compared to controls. Review of the existent data failed to show either basal hypercortisolism or abnormalities in the DEX suppression test (Martin and Nemeroff, 2010). In contrast, as noted above, a recent study (Hek et al., 2013) describes a blunting of the stress-related HPA axis response in patients with GAD, as reflected in salivary cortisol concentrations. A randomized controlled trial of a CRF R_1 antagonist (pexacerfont) in GAD failed to demonstrate efficacy (Coric et al., 2010). Whether this result and the negative trial results in major depression are due to inadequate CRF R_1 receptor occupancy, poor brain penetrability, or inherent lack of efficacy is unclear. The HPA axis does not appear to play an important role in the pathophysiology of GAD, despite evidence of its involvement in other anxiety disorders. The small number of studies does not rule out a role for HPA axis disruption in GAD.

Posttraumatic Stress Disorder

Considerable evidence reveals HPA axis alterations in patients with PTSD. CSF concentrations of CRF were found to be elevated in PTSD in two studies (Bremner et al., 1997 and Baker et al., 1999), and the ACTH response to CRF is blunted (Smith et al.,

1989). Another study found police officers with PTSD symptoms to exhibit lower levels of salivary cortisol upon awakening compared to their colleagues without PTSD (Neylan et al., 2005); low 24 hour urinary cortisol was also found in a study of military veterans with PTSD (Yehuda et al., 1990). It was suggested that subjects with PTSD show inhibition of HPA axis activity through exaggerated negative feedback (Yehuda et al., 2004) as demonstrated by the super-suppression observed with low doses of DEX; however, HPA axis deregulation in PTSD might also be due to hyporeactivity of the adrenal cortex or "low adrenal output"(Yehuda et al., 2004). In a seminal study in which the ACTH and cortisol response to DEX were measured in medically healthy veterans, patients with PTSD showed greater ACTH and cortisol suppression (Yehuda et al., 2004), although the ratio of ACTH to cortisol did not differ between groups. These findings further suggest that a possible mechanism for dysregulation in HPA axis in PTSD is enhanced negative feedback inhibition—DEX inhibition of ACTH release at the pituitary rather than low cortisol output; DEX hypersupprésion may result from central glucocorticoid receptors being sensitized under the influence of chronically hypersecreted CRF (Martin et al., 2010). In a recent study, Pacella et al. (2014) measured the salivary cortisol awakening response in PTSD patients at baseline and after treatment with prolonged exposure therapy or sertraline. Female but not male treatment non-responders displayed higher cortisol reactivity than female responders.

Social Anxiety Disorder

Data on HPA axis regulation in patients with social phobia, also known as social anxiety disorder (SAD), were initially negative. In an early study of girls with social phobia exposed to a social stress test, pretest elevations of salivary cortisol were found in both patients with SAD and healthy comparisons, with no differences among groups at post-test (Martel et al., 1999). Another study found patients with SAD to exhibit elevated plasma cortisol after a psychological stress, while pretask levels of cortisol and ACTH were no different from controls (Condren et al., 2002). A trend toward increased ACTH levels was noted in patients with SAD, but the difference did not attain statistical significance. The authors posited that elevations of serum cortisol seen after a stressor suggest a hyperactive HPA axis in SAD, in line with previously described elevations in cortisol levels in patients with phobic anxiety (Nesse et al., 1985). Elevated cortisol levels in healthy subjects exposed to public speaking correlated with temperamental traits of low self-esteem and negative mood (Kirksbaum et al., 1995)

NEUROBIOLOGY OF CHILD ABUSE AND NEGLECT

Childhood trauma has been repeatedly shown to increase the risk for adulthood mood and anxiety disorders—major depression, bipolar disorder, GAD, PD, and PTSD (Heim and Nemeroff, 2001; Nemeroff and Vale, 2005); one pioneering study suggested that traumatic events during childhood increase risk for suicide later in life (Dube et al., 2001). Adverse childhood experiences increased the risk of attempted suicide two- to five-fold, and there was a graded relationship between the number of early adverse life events and the risk of attempted suicide; the risk was, in part, mediated by substance abuse and depressed mood. Another study suggested that childhood trauma influences outcome in depression, bipolar disorder, and anxiety, with childhood abuse predicting longer, protracted episodes of depression (Zlotnick et al., 2001).

CHANGES IN THE HPA AXIS AFTER EARLY LIFE TRAUMA

Traumatic events early in life have been unequivocally demonstrated to produce a myriad of long-term neurobiological alterations including persistent alterations of stress-responsive neural circuits. Current evidence suggests that early life stressors are associated with multiple HPA axis disturbances in depressed patients (Heim et al., 2002). A blunted cortisol response in the ACTH stimulation test was found in depressed women and in women with childhood trauma (Heim et al., 2001); this blunted cortisol response is possibly mediated by hypersecretion of CRF, further resulting in downregulation of CRF receptors. This blunted cortisol secretion may also be due to glucocorticoid receptor resistance. The hypothesis of glucocorticoid resistance may, in part, be tested by the combined DEX-CRH test (Heim et al., 2008). As noted earlier, DEX, a synthetic glucocorticoid, suppresses endogenous cortisol by inhibiting ACTH secretion from the anterior pituitary. When CRF is administered in DEX-treated subjects, the next day little or no cortisol secretion is observed in normal subjects; in contrast, an "escape" of cortisol secretion is often seen in depressed patients and patients with childhood trauma. This suggests a relative glucocorticoid receptor resistance after early life trauma. Other studies have consequently shown that early adverse life events are associated with elevations of CSF CRF concentrations (Carpenter et al., 2004; Heim et al., 2008), as well as decreased CSF levels of oxytocin (Heim et al., 2009). These changes suggest increased activity of CRF-containing neural circuits in patients with early life trauma. Due to these and other neurobiological alterations, Heim et al. (2008) and Saveanu and Nemeroff (2012) proposed that depression and anxiety with early life trauma may represent distinct endophenotypes.

GENETIC AND EPIGENETIC FACTORS REGULATING THE ACTIVITY OF THE HPA AXIS

Keck et al. (2008) reported an association of CRHR1 polymorphisms with panic disorder. These authors described variants at the CRHR1 locus and variants at the AVPR1b (encoding the vasopressin 1B receptor), associated with panic disorder. Thus, polymorphisms at the CRHR1 and AVPR1B genes appear to render vulnerability to panic disorder. The CRH1R polymorphism was studied in relation to response to antidepressant treatment by Licinio et al. (2004), who identified $CRHR_1$ alleles associated with better response to antidepressants (fluoxetine or desipramine) in patients with depression and anxious traits. There is also evidence supporting an interaction of these and related genes with stressful life events, and susceptibility to develop psychiatric disorders. A strong association was found between a SNP of CRFR1 and suicide attempts in a sample of depressed adults exposed to low levels of stress (Wasserman et al., 2008). Moreover, in a sample of inner city African American individuals, polymorphisms at $CRHR_1$ gene interacted strongly with child abuse, as certain haplotypes rendered susceptibility to depression after exposure to childhood abuse, while other haplotypes were described as protective (Bradley et al., 2008). Ressler et al. (2010) reported a complex gene x gene x environment interaction in the same population: CRHR1 polymorphism interacted with the serotonin transporter-linked polymorphic region (5-HTTLPR) and with childhood trauma, to predict development of depression in adults.

A large body of work has been conducted with FKBP5, a co-chaperone protein that regulates the activity of the glucocorticoid receptor, by modulating its translocation to the nucleus. Binder et al. (2008) reported that polymorphisms of the *FKBP5* gene interacted with the severity of child abuse and neglect to predict the diathesis for PTSD in adults. Adult trauma, coupled with child abuse and neglect, further increases risk for PTSD and predicts disease severity. The PTSD patients with the FKBP5 risk alleles demonstrated enhanced cortisol suppression to DEX. Recently, the molecular mechanism of the *FKBP5* gene polymorphism has been elucidated, and it involves epigenetic processes (Klengel et al., 2013). In contrast to the recent success of genome-wide association studies (GWAS) in bipolar disorder and schizophrenia, the studies thus far have not been informative in anxiety or depressive disorders.

EPIGENETIC FACTORS IN EARLY LIFE TRAUMA

Recent evidence from postmortem and preclinical studies supports the idea that childhood trauma induces epigenetic changes in hippocampus. McGowan et al. (2009) identified differences in the methylation pattern of the promoter region (NR3C1) of the glucocorticoid receptor gene in the hippocampus of suicide victims: altered cytosine methylation was seen in samples of former victims of childhood trauma but not in samples of those without childhood abuse. The methylation of the promoter induces silencing of the glucocorticoid receptor gene and consequently decreases expression of the glucocorticoid receptor protein, changes that may reflect an increase in the stress response. Moreover, early trauma has been found to decrease DNA methylation at a regulatory element of the *FKBP5* gene, resulting in increased expression of the FKBP5 protein and attenuated HPA axis negative feedback (Klengel et al., 2013).

CONCLUSION

Compared to the vast literature in mood disorders, there are fewer studies on the neurobiology of and, more specifically, the role of neuroendocrine function in the various anxiety disorders. Indeed, rigorous and well-powered studies of GAD, SAD, or panic disorder are urgently needed. There is considerably more information available on PTSD. The lack of a CRFR1 PET ligand has hampered efforts to assess alterations in extra-hypothalamic CRF-containing circuits in anxiety disorders. This obstacle has also precluded assessment of the receptor occupancy of CRFR1 receptor antagonists in clinical trials of mood and anxiety disorders. Finally, as noted previously, few well-powered GWAS studies of syndromal anxiety disorders, as compared to bipolar disorder or schizophrenia, have been conducted.

DISCLOSURE STATEMENT

To my knowledge, all of my possible conflicts of interest and those of my coauthors, financial or otherwise, including direct or indirect financial or personal relationships, interests, and affiliations, whether or not directly related to the subject of the chapter, are listed below:

Research/Grants: National Institutes of Health (NIH)

Consulting (last three years): Xhale, Takeda, SK Pharma, Shire, Roche, Lilly, Allergan, Mitsubishi Tanabe Pharma Development America, Taisho Pharmaceutical Inc., Lundbeck, Prismic Pharmaceuticals, Clintara LLC, Total Pain Solutions (TPS)

Stockholder: Xhale, Celgene, Seattle Genetics, Abbvie, Titan Pharmaceuticals

Scientific Advisory Boards: American Foundation for Suicide Prevention (AFSP), Brain and Behavior Research Foundation (BBRF; formerly named National Alliance for Research on Schizophrenia and Depression, NARSAD), Xhale, Anxiety Disorders Association of America (ADAA), Skyland Trail, Clintara LLC, RiverMend Health LLC.

REFERENCES

Abelson JL, Curtis GC. Hypothalamic-pituitary-adrenal axis activity in panic disorder. 24-hour secretion of corticotropin and cortisol. Arch Gen Psychiatry. 1996. 4:323–331.

Abelson JL, Khan S, Liberzon I, Young EA. HPA axis activity in patients with panic disorder: review and synthesis of four studies. Depress Anxiety. 2007. 24(1):66–76.

Amiel et al. "Neurobiology of Anxiety Disorders" in Textbook of Psychopharmacology, ed. Alan Schatzberg and Charles B. Nemeroff, vol. 4, Arlington, VA: American Psychiatric Association Press, 2009, p. 965.

Baker DG, West SA, Nicholson WE, Ekhator NN, Kasckow JW, Hill KK, Bruce AB, Orth DN, Geracioti TD Jr. Serial CSF corticotropin-releasing hormone levels and adrenocortical activity in combat veterans with posttraumatic stress disorder. Am J Psychiatry. 1999. 156(4):585–588. Erratum in: Am J Psychiatry 1999.156(6):986.

Binder EB, Bradley RG, Liu W, Epstein MP, Deveau TC, Mercer KB, Tang Y, Gillespie CF, Heim CM, Nemeroff CB, Schwartz AC, Cubells JF, Ressler KJ. Association of FKBP5 polymorphisms and childhood abuse with risk of posttraumatic stress disorder symptoms in adults. JAMA. 2008. 299(11):1291–1305.

Binder EB, Nemeroff CB. The CRF system, stress, depression and anxiety-insights from human genetic studies. Mol Psychiatry. 2010. 15(6):574–588.

Bradley RG, Binder EB, Epstein MP, Tang Y, Nair HP, Liu W, . . . Ressler KJ. Influence of child abuse on adult depression: moderation by the corticotropin-releasing hormone receptor gene. Arch Gen Psychiatry. 2008. 65(2):190–200.

Bremner JD, Licinio J, Darnell A, Krystal JH, Owens MJ, Southwick SM, Nemeroff CB, Charney DS. Elevated CSF corticotropin-releasing factor concentrations in posttraumatic stress disorder. Am J Psychiatry. 1997. 154(5):624–629.

Carpenter LL, Tyrka AR, McDougle CJ, Malison RT, Owens MJ, Nemeroff CB, Price LH. Cerebrospinal fluid corticotropin-releasing factor and perceived early-life stress in depressed patients and healthy control subjects.,Neuropsychopharmacology. 2004. 29(4):777–784.

Condren RM, O'Neill A, Ryan MC, Barrett P, Thakore JH. HPA axis response to a psychological stressor in generalised social phobia. Psychoneuroendocrinology. 2002. 27(6):693–703.

Coplan JD, Goetz R, Klein DF, Papp LA, Fyer AJ, Liebowitz MR, Davies SO, Gorman JM. Plasma cortisol concentrations preceding lactate-induced panic. Psychological, biochemical, and physiological correlates. Arch Gen Psychiatry. 1998. 55(2):130–136.

Coric V, Feldman HH, Oren DA, Shekhar A, Pultz J, Dockens RC, Wu X, Gentile KA, Huang SP, Emison E, Delmonte T, D'Souza BB, Zimbroff DL, Grebb JA, Goddard AW, Stock EG. Multicenter, randomized, double-blind, active comparator and placebo-controlled trial of a corticotropin-releasing factor receptor-1 antagonist in generalized anxiety disorder. Depress Anxiety. 2010. 27(5):417–425.

Dube SR, Anda RF, Felitti VJ, Chapman DP, Williamson DF, Giles WH. Childhood abuse, household dysfunction, and the risk of attempted suicide throughout the life span: findings from the Adverse Childhood Experiences Study. JAMA. 2001. 286(24):3089–3096.

Dzierba CD, Takvorian AG, Rafalski M, Kasireddy-Polam P, Wong H, Molski TF, Zhang G, Li YW, Lelas S, Peng Y, McElroy JF, Zaczek RC, Taub RA, Combs AP, Gilligan PJ, Trainor GL. Synthesis, structure-activity relationships, and in vivo properties of 3,4-dihydro-1H-pyrido[2,3-b] pyrazin-2-ones as corticotropin-releasing factor-1 receptor antagonists. J Med Chem. 2004. 47(23):5783–5790.

Fossey MD, Lydiard RB, Ballenger JC, Laraia MT, Bissette G, Nemeroff CB. Cerebrospinal fluid corticotropin-releasing factor concentrations in patients with anxiety disorders and normal comparison subjects. Biol Psychiatry. 1996. 39(8):703–707.

Heim C, Nemeroff CB. The role of childhood trauma in the neurobiology of mood and anxiety disorders: preclinical and clinical studies. Biol Psychiatry. 2001.49(12):1023–1039.

Heim C, Newport DJ, Bonsall R, Miller AH, Nemeroff CB. Altered pituitary-adrenal axis responses to provocative challenge tests in adult survivors of childhood abuse. Am J Psychiatry. 2001. 158(4):575–581.

Heim C, Newport DJ, Mletzko T, Miller AH, Nemeroff CB. The link between childhood trauma and depression: insights from HPA axis studies in humans. Psychoneuroendocrinology. 2008. 33(6):693–710.

Heim C, Newport DJ, Wagner D, Wilcox MM, Miller AH, Nemeroff CB. The role of early adverse experience and adulthood stress in the prediction of neuroendocrine stress reactivity in women: a multiple regression analysis. Depress Anxiety. 2002. 15(3):117–125.

Heim C, Young LJ, Newport DJ, Mletzko T, Miller AH, Nemeroff CB. Lower CSF oxytocin concentrations in women with a history of childhood abuse. Mol Psychiatry. 2009. 14(10):954–958.

Hek K, Direk N, Newson RS, Hofman A, Hoogendijk WJ, Mulder CL, Tiemeier H. Anxiety disorders and salivary cortisol levels in older adults: a population-based study. Psychoneuroendocrinology. 2013. 38(2):300–305.

Heuser I, Yassouridis A, Holsboer F. The combined dexamethasone/CRH test: A refined laboratory test for psychiatric disorders. J Psychiatr Res. 1994. 28:341–356.

Holsboer F, Ising M. Central CRH system in depression and anxiety—evidence from clinical studies with CRH1 receptor antagonists. Eur J Pharmacol. 2008. 583(2–3):350–357.

Keck ME, Kern N, Erhardt A, Unschuld PG, Ising M, Salyakina D, . . . Binder EB. Combined effects of exonic polymorphisms in CRHR1 and AVPR1B genes in a case/control study for panic disorder. Am J Med Genet B Neuropsychiatr Genet. 2008. 147B(7):1196–1204.

Kent JM, Mathew SJ, Gorman JM. Molecular targets in the treatment of anxiety. Biol Psychiatry. 2002. 52(10):1008–1030.

Kirschbaum C, Prüssner JC, Stone AA, Federenko I, Gaab J, Lintz D, Schommer N, Hellhammer DH. Persistent high cortisol responses to repeated psychological stress in a subpopulation of healthy men. Psychosom Med. 1995. 57(5):468–474.

Klengel T, Mehta D, Anacker C, Rex-Haffner M, Pruessner JC, Pariante CM, Pace TW, Mercer KB, Mayberg HS, Bradley B, Nemeroff CB, Holsboer F, Heim CM, Ressler KJ, Rein T, Binder EB. Allele-specific FKBP5 DNA demethylation mediates gene-childhood trauma interactions. Nat Neurosci. 2013. 16(1):33–41.

Kostich WA, Grzanna R, Lu NZ, Largent BL. Immunohistochemical visualization of corticotropin-releasing factor type 1 (CRF1) receptors in monkey brain. J Comp Neurol. 2004. 478(2):111–125.

Lelas S, Wong H, Li YW, Heman KL, Ward KA, Zeller KL, Sieracki KK, Polino JL, Godonis HE, Ren SX, Yan XX, Arneric SP, Robertson DW, Hartig PR, Grossman S, Trainor GL, Taub RA, Zaczek R, Gilligan PJ, McElroy JF. Anxiolytic-like effects of the corticotropin-releasing factor1 (CRF1) antagonist DMP904 [4-(3-pentylamino)-2,7-dimethyl-8-(2-methyl-4-methoxyphenyl)-pyrazolo-[1,5-a]-pyrimidine] administered acutely or chronically at doses occupying central CRF1 receptors in rats. J Pharmacol Exp Ther. 2004. 309(1):293–302.

Licinio J, O'Kirwan F, Irizarry K, Merriman B, Thakur S, Jepson R, Lake S, Tantisira KG, Weiss ST, Wong ML. Association of a corticotropin-releasing hormone receptor 1 haplotype and antidepressant treatment response in Mexican-Americans. Mol Psychiatry. 2004. 9(12):1075–1082.

Martel FL, Hayward C, Lyons DM, Sanborn K, Varady S, Schatzberg AF. Salivary cortisol levels in socially phobic adolescent girls. Depress Anxiety. 1999. 10(1):25–27.

Martin E and Nemeroff CB, The biology of generalized anxiety disorder and major depressive disorder, commonalities and distinguishing features, in "Diagnostic Issues in Depression and Generalized Anxiety Disorder." Eds. Goldberg, Kendler, Sirovatka and Regier (American Psychiatric Association Press), 2010.

Martin EI, Ressler KJ, Binder E, Nemeroff CB. The neurobiology of anxiety disorders: brain imaging, genetics, and psychoneuroendocrinology. Clin Lab Med. 2010. 30(4):865–891.

McGowan PO, Sasaki A, D'Alessio AC, Dymov S, Labonté B, Szyf M, Turecki G, Meaney MJ Epigenetic regulation of the glucocorticoid receptor in human brain associates with childhood abuse. Nat Neurosci. 2009.12(3):342–348.

Nemeroff CB and Vale WW. The neurobiology of depression: inroads to treatment and new drug discovery. J Clin Psychiatry. 2005. 66 Suppl. 7:5–13.

Nesse RM, Curtis GC, Thyer BA, McCann DS, Huber-Smith MJ, Knopf RF. Endocrine and cardiovascular responses during phobic anxiety. Psychosom Med. 1985. 47(4):320–332.

Neylan TC, Brunet A, Pole N, Best SR, Metzler TJ, Yehuda R, Marmar CR. PTSD symptoms predict waking salivary cortisol levels in police officers. Psychoneuroendocrinology. 2005. 30(4):373–381.

Pacella ML, Feeny N, Zoellner L, and Delahanty D. The impact of PTSD treatment on the cortisol awakening response. Depression and Anxiety. 2014. 31: 862–869.

Ressler KJ, Bradley B, Mercer KB, Deveau TC, Smith AK, Gillespie CF, Nemeroff CB, Cubells JF, Binder EB. Polymorphisms in CRHR1 and the serotonin transporter loci: gene x gene x environment interactions on depressive symptoms. Am J Med Genet B Neuropsychiatr Genet. 2010. 153B(3):812–824.

Reul JM, Holsboer F. On the role of corticotropin-releasing hormone receptors in anxiety and depression. Dialogues Clin Neurosci. 2002. 4(1):31–46.

Risbrough VB, Stein MB. Role of corticotropin releasing factor in anxiety disorders: a translational research perspective. Horm Behav. 2006. 50(4):550–561.

Roy-Byrne PP, Uhde TW, Post RM, Gallucci W, Chrousos GP, Gold PW. The corticotropin-releasing hormone stimulation test in patients with panic disorder. Am J Psychiatry. 1986. 143(7):896–899.

Sánchez MM, Young LJ, Plotsky PM, Insel TR. Autoradiographic and in situ hybridization localization of corticotropin-releasing factor 1 and 2 receptors in nonhuman primate brain. J Comp Neurol. 1999. 408(3):365–377.

Saveanu RV, Nemeroff CB. Etiology of depression: genetic and environmental factors. Psychiatr Clin North Am. 2012. 35(1):51–71.

Smith MA, Davidson J, Ritchie JC, Kudler H, Lipper S, Chappell P, Nemeroff CB. The corticotropin-releasing hormone test in patients with posttraumatic stress disorder. Biol Psychiatry. 1989.26(4):349–355.

Tsatsanis C, Dermitzaki E, Venihaki M, Chatzaki E, Minas V, Gravanis A, Margioris AN. The corticotropin-releasing factor (CRF) family of peptides as local modulators of adrenal function. Cell Mol Life Sci. 2007. 64(13):1638–1655.

Valentino RJ, Aston-Jones G. Activation of locus coeruleus neurons in the rat by a benzazocine derivative (UM 1046) that mimics opiate withdrawal. Neuropharmacology. 1983. 22(12A):1363–1368.

Vreeburg SA, Zitman FG, van Pelt J, Derijk RH, Verhagen JC, van Dyck R, Hoogendijk WJ, Smit JH, Penninx BW. Salivary cortisol levels in persons with and without different anxiety disorders. Psychosom Med. 2010. 72(4):340–347.

Wasserman D, Sokolowski M, Rozanov V, Wasserman J. The CRHR1 gene: a marker for suicidality in depressed males exposed to low stress. Genes Brain Behav. 2008. 7(1):14–19.

Yehuda R, Southwick SM, Nussbaum G, Wahby V, Giller EL Jr, Mason JW. Low urinary cortisol excretion in patients with posttraumatic stress disorder. J Nerv Ment Dis. 1990. 178(6):366–369.

Yehuda R, Golier JA, Halligan SL, Meaney M, Bierer LM. The ACTH response to dexamethasone in PTSD. Am J Psychiatry. 2004. 161(8):1397–1403.

Zlotnick C, Mattia J, Zimmerman M. Clinical features of survivors of sexual abuse with major depression. Child Abuse Negl. 2001. 25(3):357–367.

/// 29 /// PHARMACOLOGICAL INTERVENTIONS FOR ADULT ANXIETY DISORDERS

RYAN J. KIMMEL AND PETER P. ROY-BYRNE

INTRODUCTION

Use of benzodiazepines for the treatment of anxiety dates back almost 60 years, and the efficacy of monoamine-reuptake inhibition-based interventions in anxiety disorders has been established for over 50 years. Currently, a more specific type of monoamine reuptake inhibitor, the SSRI, is now well accepted as a first line treatment. Though the DSM-5 divides anxiety disorders, obsessive compulsive disorders, and trauma-related disorders into separate chapters (American Psychiatric Association, 2013), serotonergic compounds still demonstrate efficacy across this spectrum of anxiety, in contrast to the more limited efficacy of benzodiazepines. The value of medications that target other receptor systems varies by diagnosis, as do pharmacologic augmentation strategies and overall rates of response to the SSRIs. Given the breadth of published data now available, only randomized, controlled trials are discussed in this chapter. Any medication failing to separate from placebo in a randomized controlled trial is unlikely to be effective for more than a minority of patients, if it is effective at all.

PANIC DISORDER AND AGORAPHOBIA

Unlike the fourth edition, wherein panic disorder was specified by the presence or absence of agoraphobia, the fifth edition of the *Diagnostic and Statistical Manual of Mental Disorders* (American Psychiatric Association, 2013) gives agoraphobia its own diagnosis. However, most medication trials for panic included patients with agoraphobia, and most trials included phobic avoidance as an outcome measure; moreover, very few studies examined patients with agoraphobia without panic attacks. Thus, prior studies of antipanic agents are likely applicable to patients with panic disorder and agoraphobia or panic disorder alone.

SSRIs

Fluoxetine, paroxetine, and sertraline are FDA approved for panic and there are numerous trials to support their use. In addition, there are abundant, placebo-controlled trials of fluvoxamine, citalopram, and escitalopram. The Number Needed to Treat (NNT) for SSRIs during the acute phase of treatment in panic disorder is 5–8 (Kumar and Malone, 2008).

Early data suggested that one may need to employ higher SSRI doses, relative to those employed for major depressive disorder, when treating panic (Michelson et al., 2001). However, in a more recent trial, patients with continued panic symptoms after 6 weeks of sertraline at max dose 100 mg or escitalopram at max dose 15 mg were randomized to either continue or double these doses for another 6 weeks (Simon et al., 2009). With greater duration of treatment, increased dose did not increase efficacy. This is an especially important finding for citalopram, given the preference to use low doses in light of the Black Box Warning regarding dose-dependent QTc prolongation.

It is possible that, relative to major depressive disorder, panic disorder requires longer trials before patients reach maximal benefit. For example, in naturalistic studies, some patients have their SSRI dose increased after six weeks (mirroring the standard, major depressive disorder algorithms), with improved efficacy eventually noted. However, the same efficacy might have been seen with more patience, rather than more milligrams, as clinical trials show a subset of patients who respond at 9 and 12 weeks (Michelson et al., 2001; Oehrberg et al., 1995). In fact, patients who respond continue to improve and demonstrate benefit in trials lasting 29–52 weeks (especially for anticipatory anxiety and phobic avoidance).

Not every analysis has shown separation among SRIs, tricyclics, and benzodiazepines (Bakker, van Balkom, and Spinhoven, 2002), and drug-related differences in efficacy may be small. However, SSRIs are better tolerated than tricyclics, as evidenced by a much higher completer percentage (82% vs. 69%) (Bakker et al., 2002). SSRI withdrawal, with symptoms that can include headache, nausea, dizziness, and irritability, can be seen in cases of rapid dose reduction. Stimulation of anxiety symptoms with initiation of SSRIs is rare, and is seen in only 2.5% of patients on sertraline, for example (Pohl, Wolkow, and Clary, 1998). When clinically observed, marked overstimulation should also prompt consideration of an atypical bipolar disorder, especially since panic attacks are commonly comorbid in bipolar illness.

When SSRI efficacy is seen, current recommendations are to continue treatment for 1–2 years based on follow-up studies, lasting 8–52 weeks, documenting an odds ratio of 0.35 for recurrence when remaining on antidepressants compared to randomized switch to placebo (Donovan, Glue, Kolluri, and Emir, 2010).

SNRIs

The SNRI, venlafaxine, is also approved by the FDA for panic, based on several, placebo-controlled trials. In the principal, flexible-dose, placebo-controlled trial of extended-release venlafaxine, a mean daily dose of 163 mg/day yielded a significant reduction in panic frequency (Bradweijn, Stein, Salinas, G.Emlien, and T.Whitaker, 2005). This again argues that, for panic disorder, dosing well within the FDA recommended range is appropriate.

Benzodiazepines

Two benzodiazepines, alprazolam and clonazepam, carry FDA indications for panic. Sedation and memory impairment can be significant issues, but are more common in older individuals, as well as younger patients taking more than 1 mg of clonazepam or 2 mg of alprazolam. Panic patients on long-term treatment do not develop tolerance to the anxiolytic effects of benzodiazepines, do not escalate their doses over time, and abuse is rare in the absence of comorbid substance use disorders (Garvey and Tollefson, 1986). Risk of physiologic dependence and withdrawal symptoms on discontinuation are the greatest clinical concern. This risk, along with the risk of breakthrough anxiety between doses, is greater with short half-life benzodiazepines such as alprazolam, making clinicians usually prefer clonazepam over alprazolam (Roy-Byrne, Dager, Cowley, Vitaliano, and Dunner, 1989). While patients discontinuing clonazepam often experience a re-emergence of their symptoms (Moroz and Rosenbaum, 1999), it is unclear if this is any different from the reemergence of panic symptoms that one sees after SSRI taper.

Other Medications

Numerous trials support the antipanic efficacy of tricyclic antidepressants, especially the more serotinergic agents in this spectrum. The effect size of TCAs and SSRIs is equal (Mitte, 2005). Overstimulation and weight gain are common reasons for discontinuation of tricyclics in panic patients (Noyes, Garvey, Cook, and Samuelson, 1989). However, sedation, orthostatic hypotension, and anticholinergic effects are also seen, varying by tricyclic.

A recent, randomized, blinded study of tranycylpromine showed efficacy for co-morbid panic and social anxiety disorder at a 60 mg daily dose (Nardi et al., 2010). There is extensive, though somewhat dated, evidence for efficacy using the MAOI, phenelzine (Mountjoy, Roth, Garside, and Leitch, 1977). Though overstimulation is seldom reported, the need for a low-monoamine diet, as well as notable rates of insomnia, sexual dysfunction, and weight gain, often limit the use of MAO inhibitors.

The anti-panic efficacy of nefazodone is supported by one controlled trial in patients selected for comorbid depression (Zajecka, 1996). Buspirone (Sheehan, Raj, Sheehan, and Soto, 1990), bupropion (Sheehan, Davidson, Manschreck, and Van Wyck Fleet, 1983), propranolol (Munjack et al., 1989), and clonidine (Uhde et al., 1989) are no more efficacious than placebo, nor are anaticonvulsants, though gabapentin showed efficacy in a secondary analysis confined to high-frequency panic subjects (Pande et al., 2000). There are no placebo-controlled trials of pregabalin or atypical antipsychotics. One very small trial suggested efficacy for verapamil (Klein and Uhde, 1988), but this has never been replicated and may constitute type-1 statistical error due to small sample size. D-cycloserine has been used to augment cognitive behavioral therapy trials, though the outcomes have been mixed (Siegmund et al., 2011).

GENERALIZED ANXIETY DISORDER

The DSM-5 did not make significant changes to the diagnostic criteria for generalized anxiety disorder. However, the defining symptoms of this disorder have been much more fluid in prior DSM iterations. Generalized anxiety disorder also has an extremely high rate of mood and anxiety disorder co-morbidities. Relative to other anxiety disorders, a broader range of pharmacologic mechanisms of action have demonstrated efficacy.

SSRIs

Paroxetine and escitalopram are FDA-approved for generalized anxiety disorder, with paroxetine's NNT at 10 (average doses 24 mg/day) (K. Rickels, Rynn, Iyengar, and Duff,

2006). Escitalopram at 10 mg/day (Goodman, Bose, and Wang, 2005) and sertraline at 50–150 mg/day are efficacious (Allgulander et al., 2004). As with panic disorder, SSRI dosing for GAD often need not approach the FDA maximum. The first head-to-head trial of paroxetine vs. sertraline found no difference in tolerability or efficacy (Ball, Kuhn, Wall, Shekhar, and Goddard, 2005). A subsequent study of escitalopram vs. paroxetine also showed no separation in efficacy, but did suggest that paroxetine's side effect burden was greater (Bielski, Bose, and Chang, 2005), consistent with speculation that escitalopram may, for some patients, be more tolerable than other SSRIs.

SNRIs

Venlafaxine and duloxetine are FDA-approved for generalized anxiety disorder, and do not differ in terms of efficacy or tolerability (Allgulander et al., 2008). Similarly, in meta-analysis, there appears to be no difference in efficacy between venlafaxine extended-release and SSRIs (Mitte, 2005). Though the data are not as extensive, duloxetine and venlafaxine are generally considered first-line agents, alongside the SSRIs. Venlafaxine extended-release shows efficacy in the 75 mg/day to 225 mg/day range (see Figure 29.1), while duloxetine is used at 60 mg/day to 120 mg/day. Owing to a relapse rate of 60% when SSRIs or SNRIs are discontinued after the acute phase of treatment, longer-term antidepressant treatment has been recommended by meta-analysis (Donovan et al., 2010). Though antidepressants appear to continue to work over the first 6 months of treatment, little is known about the period beyond this.

Buspirone

Buspirone, a 5HT-1A receptor partial agonist, was FDA-approved for DSM-III's iteration of GAD. Given its age, most of the head-to-head buspirone trials are against benzodiazepines, where buspirone shows a slower response, but similar end-point efficacy. The azopirones' NNT has been calculated at 4.4 (Chessick et al., 2006). Meta-analyses have not demonstrated a significant difference in effect size between buspirone and venlafaxine (Mitte,

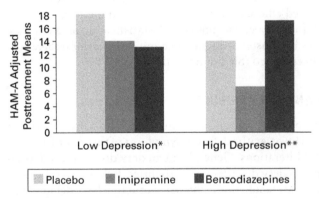

FIGURE 29.1 Generalized Anxiety Disorder with Depressive Symptoms: Understanding Adverse Effects of Benzodiazepine Monotherapy. The histograms show the difference in anxiety symptoms (Hamilton Anxiety Index) in groups treated with Imipramine, Benzodiazepines, and Placebo. *Imipramine/diazepam > placebo, $p < 0.05$; **Imipramine > diazepam, $p < 0.05$; BZD = benzodiazepine; Rickels K, Downing R, Schweizer E, Hassman H. *Arch Gen Psychiatry.* 1993(Nov);50(11):884–895.

2005). Common side effects of buspirone include headaches, nausea, and dizziness, but not usually sedation. Doses from 20–60 mg/day, divided BID or TID, have shown efficacy.

Other Agents

Pregabalin, with an effect that reaches its peak at 300 mg/day, demonstrates efficacy in GAD (Lydiard, Rickels, Herman, and Feltner, 2010). The discontinuation rate with pregabalin is low, with dizziness, dry mouth, and somnolence as the most common side effects. Head to head trials between pregabalin and benzodiazepines have not yielded a clear difference (Feltner et al., 2003; K. Rickels et al., 2005). Pregabalin, however, has been superior to venlafaxine in some measures in head-to-head trials (Kasper et al., 2009).

Several meta-analyses of quetiapine monotherapy trials show efficacy over placebo (Depping, Komossa, Kissling, and Leucht, 2010). The most common side effects of quetiapine are dry mouth, somnolence, dizziness, and nausea. Concerns about neurological and metabolic side effects with long-term use lead many clinicians to consider quetiapine to be a second-line treatment. A head-to-head trial of quetiapine vs. escitalopram demonstrated similar efficacy, though the antipsychotic-associated metabolic syndrome was evident with quetiapine use (Merideth, Cutler, She, and Eriksson, 2012). The metabolic side effects, in the absence of a clear difference in efficacy compared to SSRIs, keeps quetiapine from garnering FDA approval. Ziprasidone, an atypical antipsychotic with a lower metabolic burden, is not effective for GAD (Lohoff, Etemad, Mandos, Gallop, and Rickels, 2010).

Benzodiazepines are clearly efficacious for GAD (Shader and Greenblatt, 1993), but are less so in individuals with comorbid depressive symptoms, even if the symptoms are not sufficient to meet criteria for major depression (see Figure 29.2) (K. Rickels, Downing, Schweizer, and Hassman, 1993). The doses required for GAD are less than those required for panic disorder, though the side effects are similar. In the absence of co-morbid substance use, dose escalation is not a frequent occurrence (Karl Rickels, Case, Schweizer, Swenson, and Fridman, 1986).

There are no placebo-controlled trials of mirtazapine or bupropion. There are several studies that support the use of propranolol, including a large trial that showed propranolol's efficacy to be similar, but with less prominent side effects, to

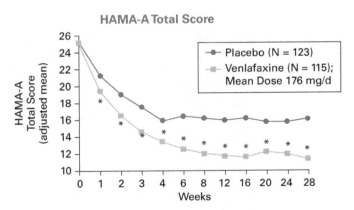

FIGURE 29.2 Anxiety response to Venlafaxine. The difference in anxiety symptoms (Hamilton Anxiety Total Score) across 28 weeks of treatment with flexible dose venlafaxine vs. placebo in Generalized Anxiety Disorder. *P < 0.5 vs. PBO. Observed-case analysis. Gelenberg et al. JAMA. 2000:283:3082.

chlordiazepoxide (Meibach, Mullane, and Binstok, 1987). A meta-analysis of five trials showed that hydroxyzine (several studies with doses of 25–50 mg/day and several with doses ≥100 mg/day) is efficacious (Guaiana, Barbui, and Cipriani, 2010), though its anticholinergic and antihistaminic side effects have limited its widespread use.

SPECIFIC PHOBIA

Compared to psychotherapy, there is a paucity of controlled data on pharmacologic interventions for specific phobia. Behavioral treatments continue to be the first line approach with meta-analyses demonstrating a moderate to large effect size (Wolitzky-Taylor, Horowitz, Powers, and Telch, 2008). A placebo-controlled trial of paroxetine showed some benefit over 4 weeks (Benjamin, Ben-Zion, Karbofsky, and Dannon, 2000).

Much of the current psychopharmacology research in specific phobia focuses on using d-cycloserine to augment desensitization therapy sessions. For example, d-cycloserine, given to acrophobic participants whose fear was low at the end of an exposure session, seemed to positively reinforce the psychotherapy benefit. Conversely, when given to acrophobic patients whose fear was high at the end of an exposure session, d-cycloserine might be detrimental (Smits, Rosenfield, Otto, Powers, et al., 2013). This is a promising approach that suggests tailoring administration according to the result of the session, that is, administering only if anxiety was reduced after the session.

A placebo-controlled study of quetiapine, delivered during an exposure session, showed only limited benefit. There is some older data suggesting that benzodiazepines may be counterproductive for exposure sessions (Wilhelm and Roth, 1997), though this remains controversial and has not been systematically investigated.

SOCIAL ANXIETY DISORDER

Though the DSM-5 has done away with the "generalized" specifier for this disorder, most of the medication trials in the DSM-IV era did not separate the sample by social anxiety disorder subtypes. Thus, the DSM-IV era pharmacologic recommendations ought to apply seamlessly to those patients meeting DSM-5 criteria.

SSRIs

Paroxetine and sertraline are approved for social anxiety disorder by the FDA. There are more than two-dozen placebo-controlled trials of SSRIs for this disorder, and multiple meta-analyses document the extent of their benefit (Hansen et al., 2008). As was suggested for panic disorder, SSRI nonresponders or partial-responders at 8 weeks may see additional benefit at 12 (see Figure 29.3) or 24 weeks (Pollack et al., 2014; D. J. Stein, Versiani, Hair, and Kumar, 2002). As in panic disorder, this suggests patience, rather than dosing above FDA maximum, may be an effective strategy. Usual dosing for paroxetine is 20–50 mg/day, with sertraline at 50–200 mg/day. Once effective and well-tolerated, the SSRIs appear to be indicated for at least 6 months, with studies suggesting over a third of patients demonstrate symptom relapse when their less-than-six-month SSRI trials are switched to placebo (D. J. Stein et al., 2002), and current guidelines suggest that effective antidepressants be continued for at least a year.

Though not formally FDA-approved, fluvoxamine (100–300 mg/day) and escitalopram (5–20 mg/day) have also demonstrated efficacy over placebo in multiple trials, with similar rates of efficacy as seen with paroxetine (J. Davidson et al., 2004; Lader, Stender,

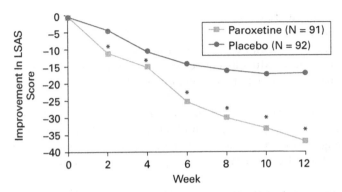

FIGURE 29.3 Anxiety response to Paroxetine. The difference in social anxiety symptoms (Liebowitz Social Anxiety Scale) across 12 weeks of treatment with paroxetine vs. placebo in Social Anxiety Disorder. *P< 0.5 vs. PBO. Mean dose = 36.6 mg/d at end point. Stein et al. *JAMA*. 1998:280:708.

Burger, and Nil, 2004). The data on fluoxetine's efficacy is less consistent, with a high placebo-response rate and complicated, psychotherapy-augmentation study designs, disrupting our ability to make definitive conclusions (Clark et al., 2003; Kobak, Greist, Jefferson, and Katzelnick, 2002).

SNRIs

Venlafaxine is FDA-approved for social anxiety disorder. Head-to-head trials versus paroxetine showed no difference in efficacy and no difference in side effect rates (Allgulander et al., 2004). Neither desvenlafaxine, nor duloxetine, have been the subject of placebo-controlled trials. Reflecting a theme in the anxiety disorders covered so far, comparisons of a range of venlafaxine doses (75 mg/day vs. 150–225 mg/day) yielded no difference in outcome, though both were effective, in a 28-week trial (M. B. Stein, Pollack, Bystritsky, Kelsey, and Mangano, 2005). This stands in contrast to some studies of venlafaxine in major depression, where there appears to be a greater effect with higher doses.

Other Agents

Among the irreversible MAO inhibitors, phenelzine has demonstrated efficacy for social anxiety disorder in multiple, placebo-controlled trials (Blanco et al., 2010). Phenelzine is often dosed in the range of 75 mg/day in social anxiety trials (Liebowitz et al., 1992). Unfortunately, phenelzine carries significant risks of hypertensive crisis, weight gain, and sexual dysfunction. Reversible MAO inhibitors, which have lower risk of hypertensive crisis, also have significant placebo-controlled evidence for efficacy in social anxiety disorder, but are not available in the United States.

Clonazepam is efficacious for social anxiety disorder, but the risk of abuse may be greater given the high rate of alcohol use disorders in patients with social anxiety disorder (Schneier, Johnson, Hornig, Liebowitz, and Weissman, 1992). When used as augmentation for patients with an insufficient response to sertraline, clonazepam was superior to continued sertraline monotherapy, and a switch to venlafaxine, as well (Pollack et al., 2014). However, the response rate to clonazepam monotherapy is no higher than that of cognitive behavioral therapy (Otto et al., 2000), which of course, has fewer risks.

Placebo-controlled trials of nefazodone (Van Ameringen et al., 2007), buspirone (van Vliet, den Boer, Westenberg, and Pian, 1997), and atomoxetine (Ravindran, Kim, Letamendi, and Stein, 2009) showed no benefit. Mirtazapine has one, positive, placebo-controlled trial (Muehlbacher et al., 2005). Tricyclics have not been the subject of a placebo-controlled trial, but an earlier open trial failed to find any benefit (Simpson et al., 1998).

Pregabalin demonstrates efficacy, but only at 600 mg/day, in placebo-controlled trials (Feltner, Liu-Dumaw, Schweizer, and Bielski, 2011). Gabapentin beat placebo in its lone trial, though with a response rate much lower than is typically seen in SSRI trials (Pande et al., 1999). Both pregabalin and gabapentin are associated with somnolence and dizziness.

Though olanzapine was superior to placebo in its one, small, placebo-controlled trial (Barnett, Kramer, Casat, Connor, and Davidson, 2002), the metabolic side effects of this medication may be prohibitive, especially when there are so many other effective, more metabolically neutral, options for treating social anxiety disorder. Quetiapine was ineffective in the only trial conducted (Donahue et al., 2009).

As with panic disorder, d-cycloserine is the subject of ongoing augmentation studies for exposure therapy in social anxiety disorder. Though the overall data has been mixed, the impact of targeting those who have had a more successful (i.e., low fear at the end) session may merit further study (Smits, Rosenfield, Otto, Marques, et al., 2013).

POSTTRAUMATIC STRESS DISORDER

Initial PTSD trials focused on male combat veterans. More recent studies have tried to define other cohorts, including one-time trauma exposures, sexual trauma, women, and minority ethnicities. The DSM-5 has also expanded the diagnosis to allow for symptoms arising from exposure that was not first-hand. It is not yet clear what can be generalized from population to population and from exposure to exposure(s). Moreover, not every medication appears to impact all three PTSD symptom clusters as defined in the DSM-IV. The cluster of negative cognitions and mood, added in the DSM-5, is poorly tracked in the current body of psychopharmacology literature. However, there is a high rate of comorbid depression in PTSD and many studies have demonstrated improvement in depressive symptoms with pharmacologic treatment, though other negative symptoms (e.g., anger) have not been assessed.

SSRIs

Paroxetine is FDA-approved for PTSD and, when used at 20–40 mg/day, shows a robust treatment response across all three of DSM-IV's symptom clusters (D. J. Stein, Davidson, Seedat, and Beebe, 2003). There has been at least one, positive, paroxetine, PTSD study that included a primarily minority population (Marshall et al., 2007), but there has not been a paroxetine trial that focused on women. This lack of gender-specific data may be an important distinction in PTSD. For example, the same author conducted two placebo-controlled trials with fluoxetine in PTSD, one demonstrating efficacy for fluoxetine in a cohort of male combat veterans (Martenyi, Brown, Zhang, Prakash, and Koke, 2002), and one showing no fluoxetine separation from placebo in a primarily female, noncombat cohort (Martenyi, Brown, and Caldwell, 2007). To be fair, not every fluoxetine study in PTSD has separated from placebo and it is not fully known what combinations of factors predict benefit.

Sertraline is FDA approved for PTSD. In a study focusing on childhood abuse and interpersonal trauma, with a mostly female cohort, sertraline demonstrated efficacy (J. R. Davidson, Rothbaum, van der Kolk, Sikes, and Farfel, 2001). However, the same author, with a mostly noncombat trauma cohort, did not find significant efficacy for sertraline (J. Davidson et al., 2006). Positive sertraline trials have employed doses of 50–200 mg/day, and there are significant gains at 6 months that are not evident at 2 months (Londborg et al., 2001).

Citalopram has been the subject of only one, placebo-controlled trial in PTSD, and the results were equivocal (Tucker et al., 2003). Escitalopram has not been the subject of a placebo-controlled trial for PTSD.

SNRIs

Venlafaxine ER shows benefit in PTSD, but perhaps not in every symptom cluster, nor every symptom within the same cluster. For example, avoidance, sleep disturbance, and nightmares did not respond as well, or as early, as did symptoms of irritability and intrusive memories (D. J. Stein et al., 2009). Duloxetine and desvenlafaxine have not yet been employed in a double-blind trial.

Other Agents

Though seldom used due to a higher side-effect rate without an apparently higher efficacy rate, tricyclics, such as imipramine, and MOA inhibitors, such as phenelzine, have separated from placebo in multiple trials (Frank, Kosten, Giller, and Dan, 1988). While limited in size (29 patients), there is one placebo-controlled trial that showed benefit for mirtazapine (J. R. Davidson et al., 2003). Like mirtazapine, nefazodone's benefits for sleep make it an attractive candidate for PTSD, and there is one, small (41 patients), placebo-controlled trial that notes benefit (Davis et al., 2004). Nefazodone's black-box warning for hepatotoxicity may preclude future studies.

Like several of the other anxiety disorders, d-cycloserine, a partial NMDA receptor agonist, has been evaluated as an augmentation strategy for exposure psychotherapy sessions. As with the other anxiety disorders, the overall results have been mixed, ranging from beneficial, to equivocal, to detrimental (de Kleine, Hendriks, Smits, Broekman, and van Minnen, 2014; Difede et al., 2014; Litz et al., 2012; Rothbaum et al., 2014). There are efforts to quantify predictive factors that would prospectively identify the patients who seem to benefit.

Prazosin, an alpha-1 adrenergic antagonist, was developed decades ago to treat hypertension. At a maximum dose of 5 mg mid-morning and 20 mg at bedtime for men, or 2 mg midmorning and 10 mg at bedtime for women, prazosin was evaluated over 15 weeks in active-duty soldiers returning from combat duty. Trauma nightmares and sleep quality were significantly improved. While hyperarousal cluster symptoms also showed significant improvement, improvements in reexperiencing and avoidance cluster symptoms did not reach significance (Raskind et al., 2013). In another small study, prazosin also demonstrated benefit for sleep and trauma nightmares in a civilian population (Taylor et al., 2008).

Risperidone and olanzapine, but not quetiapine, have been studied in numerous, placebo-controlled trials, both as monotherapy and augmentation for antidepressants, and in both military and civilian populations. A meta-analysis of these studies does demonstrate some overall benefit, albeit with a small effect size, for PTSD (Ahearn, Juergens,

Cordes, Becker, and Krahn, 2011). The effect may be especially pronounced in "intrusion" symptoms when these medications are used as augmentation. Monotherapy studies have been inconsistent (Pae et al., 2008). Not every placebo-controlled trial of antipsychotics has tracked weight gain, much less the full, atypical antipsychotic-associated, metabolic syndrome. Olanzapine trials, as expected, have noted weight gain. As noted earlier, the clinician should attend to the risks associated with long-term use of these medications.

Topiramate has shown benefit, especially in the reexperiencing and avoidance clusters, in a placebo-controlled trial among a civilian population (Yeh et al., 2011). A trial of topiramate amongst the veteran population found no benefit, but the high drop-out rate due to CNS symptoms in this study highlights the difficulties of employing topiramate (Lindley, Carlson, and Hill, 2007). Divalproex did not demonstrate efficacy in its lone, placebo-controlled trial (Davis, Davidson, et al., 2008). Tiagabine, similarly, showed no benefit (J. R. Davidson, Brady, Mellman, Stein, and Pollack, 2007).

A recently-published, randomized trial of citalopram augmentation with baclofen, a GABA-ergic medication, demonstrated some efficacy over citalopram plus placebo and may warrant future study (Manteghi, Hebrani, Mortezania, Haghighi, and Javanbakht, 2014). Another GABA-ergic agent, eszopiclone, also demonstrated some benefit for sleep and PTSD symptoms in a short, small, placebo-controlled trial (Pollack et al., 2011).

A one-time dose of intravenous ketamine, a NMDA receptor antagonist, was recently the subject of a small, double-blind, crossover trial that employed IV midazolam as a control (Feder et al., 2014). Ketamine yielded a significant reduction in PTSD symptoms that was durable over the first 24 hours. The benefit slowly wore off over the following days, though there were some patients who were still deriving benefit at two weeks postinfusion. As one might expect, transient, dissociative symptoms were seen in the first few hours after the infusion, but these side effects were not durable.

Benzodiazepines do not yield efficacy in PTSD (Braun, Greenberg, Dasberg, and Lerer, 1990). Moreover, there is some evidence that they can negatively impact the efficacy of psychotherapy for PTSD (Rothbaum et al., 2014).

Guanfacine did not show benefit in its placebo-controlled trial (Davis, Ward, et al., 2008). Buspirone has not been the subject of a placebo-controlled trial. Bupropion's only placebo-controlled trial was equivocal (Becker et al., 2007).

OBSESSIVE-COMPULSIVE DISORDER

The DSM-5 carved "obsessive-compulsive and related disorders" out from the "anxiety disorders" section, and then further carved an independent, hoarding diagnosis out of OCD. These moves reflect an OCD spectrum that is still in flux, both in definition and evidence-based treatment. There is wide diversity in the range of symptoms, stability of symptom presentation over time, and anxiety co-morbidities. Moreover, the remission rate seen with pharmacotherapy is lower in OCD compared to the other disorders described in this chapter. Cognitive behavioral therapy, with exposure and response prevention, is a first-line treatment for OCD and is slightly more effective than medication. Even more importantly, CBT appears to be superior to augmentation with atypical neuroleptics in SSRI nonresponders (Simpson et al., 2013).

SSRIs

Fluoxetine, fluvoxamine, and sertraline have FDA approval for OCD. The NNT for SSRIs for OCD is 6–12 (Soomro, Altman, Rajagopal, and Oakley-Browne, 2008), though the "treatment effect" is smaller than for other anxiety disorders. Even more so than for other anxiety disorders, a longer trial of medication (16 vs. 8–12 weeks) may be necessary before efficacy is seen. Unlike the other anxiety disorders, dosing of the SSRIs for OCD often needs to be at the top-end of FDA-maximum recommendations and there is a clear dose-response relationship (Bloch, McGuire, Landeros-Weisenberger, Leckman, and Pittenger, 2010). This impacts citalopram, where extra vigilance for QTc effects might be required when attempting to employ the 60 mg/day dosing schedule used by some of the studies.

Long-term trials of antidepressant treatment in OCD, including blinded discontinuation trials, show results that are more varied compared to the other anxiety disorders. Opinions on the duration of treatment after initial response, in the absence of multiple prior relapses coincident with medication cessation, vary from 3 months to 2 years (Fineberg and Gale, 2005). Some experts believe that persistent treatment may be required and that relapse in the absence of medication is higher for OCD than the other anxiety disorders.

SNRIs

The trials of venlafaxine for OCD have employed active controls (SSRIs and tricyclics), rather than placebo controls. Venlafaxine's efficacy, when used at doses as high as 300 mg/day, appears to be equal to that of paroxetine and clomipramine (Albert, Aguglia, Maina, and Bogetto, 2002; Denys, van Megen, van der Wee, and Westenberg, 2004). Nonetheless, the evidence for venlafaxine is not as extensive as that of the FDA-approved SSRIs. Duloxetine and desvenlafaxine have not been the subject of placebo-controlled trials.

Clomipramine

This agent merits its own OCD section, given the extent of evidence in favor of clomipramine that has accumulated over the nearly 40 years since Fernandez-Cordoba and Lopez-Ibor first systematically documented its efficacy. In a placebo-controlled trial of 520 patients whose symptoms had been evident for >1 year, the NNT for clomipramine was calculated at 2.5 ("Clomipramine in the treatment of patients with obsessive-compulsive disorder. The Clomipramine Collaborative Study Group," 1991). Though this NNT would suggest efficacy far exceeding that of SSRIs, clomipramine's superiority to SSRIs, while still evident, is actually much more modest when evaluated via meta-analysis of head-to-head trials (Greist, Jefferson, Kobak, Katzelnick, and Serlin, 1995). Nonetheless, it does seem to have a definitive edge in terms of efficacy. Unfortunately, when compared to SSRIs, clomipramine exhibits more side effects, especially anticholinergic effects.

Other Agents

Patient's with OCD that do not respond to an initial, 12-week, SSRI trial are often first switched to another agent (SSRI or clomipramine) if an ongoing pharmacologic strategy is pursued. However, augmentation strategies may ultimately be considered. A meta-analysis of twelve antipsychotic augmentation trials for treatment-resistant OCD, including studies employing aripiprazole, haloperidol, olanzapine, quetiapine, or risperidone, demonstrated a medium effect size, as a class, for this strategy (Dold,

Aigner, Lanzenberger, and Kasper, 2013), though antipsychotics appear most effective in the subgroup of patients with a history of a tic disorder (see Bloch et al. meta-analysis). Subgroup analysis in this review demonstrated that medium-dosed antipsychotics separated from placebo, whereas low-dose augmentation did not. The adverse event profiles in these studies reflect, in general, the usual adverse event profiles seen when antipsychotics are used for other diagnoses. Variable study design issues make it difficult to compare different antipsychotics head-to-head in a meta-analysis, but the risperidone data, at the moment, might be considered the most robust (Dold et al., 2013), consistent with most experts who prefer this agent as the initial augmenting medication of choice. In contrast, a recent augmentation trial with paliperidone, an active metabolite of risperidone, was ineffective (Storch et al., 2013).

Among the antiepileptics, lamotrigine augmentation of SSRIs (Bruno et al., 2012), as well as topiramate augmentation of SSRIs (Berlin et al., 2011), have separated from placebo. Among medications that modulate the NMDA system, ketamine (Rodriguez et al., 2013) and memantine augmentation (Ghaleiha et al., 2013) have some placebo-controlled evidence. Two serotonin 5-HT(3) receptor antagonists, granisetron and ondansetron, have shown benefit versus placebo, as well (Askari et al., 2012; Soltani et al., 2010). Though the mechanism of benefit is not understood, once-weekly morphine separated from placebo in a very small trial (Koran et al., 2005).

In placebo-controlled trials, clonazepam did not boost sertraline response (Crockett, Churchill, and Davidson, 2004), clonazepam was not effective as monotherapy (Hollander, Kaplan, and Stahl, 2003), and lorazepam was not effective as augmentation (Koran et al., 2005). Desipramine shows less efficacy and more side effects than sertraline (Hoehn-Saric et al., 2000). MAO inhibitors, bupropion, mirtazapine, and nefazodone have not been the subject of placebo-controlled trials. Buspirone's trials, both as monotherapy and as augmentation to an SSRI, failed to separate from placebo (McDougle et al., 1993; Pigott et al., 1992).

SUMMARY

Though the diagnostic criteria for the disorders in this chapter have evolved over successive iterations of the DSM, experts are still comfortable designating certain pharmacologic interventions as "first-line" within the DSM-5's nosology. However, the anxiety disorders cannot be lumped together and presumed to have an equal response, even to "first line" medications. For example, while one could consider SSRIs to be first-line agents for Panic Disorder, GAD, Social Anxiety Disorder, PTSD, and OCD, the data for SSRIs in PTSD and OCD is more variable and there may be a higher NNT for SSRIs in these disorders. Similarly, SNRIs have similar data for GAD, Social Anxiety Disorder, and Panic Disorder, but the results in PTSD have been more uneven, perhaps due to a heterogeneity in this disorder that requires further study. Buspirone might be considered a first-line option in GAD, but there is little data for the other disorders. Clomipramine has uniquely strong data for OCD.

For all of these disorders, with the exception of OCD, antidepressant dosing often need not approach the FDA maximum, though time to maximal effect lags behind what is often seen when treating major depressive disorder with antidepressants. OCD often requires high-end antidepressant dosing, as well as longer medication trials.

Similar to the variability seen in first-line medications, second-line and augmentation data varies by diagnosis. For example, TCAs lack data for Social Anxiety Disorder. Prazosin shows more and more promise as an augmentation strategy targeting trauma-related nightmares. Benzodiazepine's risk physiologic dependence and their utility, either as monotherapy or augmentation, varies greatly by diagnosis, with no efficacy seen in PTSD and OCD. The efficacy of augmentation with antipsychotics also varies by diagnosis, and, even at lower doses, there are still metabolic and dopamine blockade side effects.

Cognitive Behavioral Therapy shows significant benefit in all of the anxiety disorders, and has fewer side effects than pharmacotherapy. Augmentation of CBT exposure sessions with D-cycloserine has had mixed results in panic disorder and PTSD, has not been studied in GAD or OCD, but may be beneficial when given after positive (low fear) exposure sessions for specific phobia and social anxiety disorder. Reinforcing less effective (high fear) exposure sessions may be ineffective or even detrimental. More research needs to be done in order to understand which patients, and which therapy sessions, might benefit from this pharmacologic reinforcement.

The variability of response to various interventions amongst the disorders in the anxiety spectrum suggests that it is imperative to make a clear diagnosis, identify specific symptomatology that might be amenable to a specific treatment, and then track treatment results closely.

REFERENCES

Ahearn, E. P., Juergens, T., Cordes, T., Becker, T., & Krahn, D. (2011). A review of atypical antipsychotic medications for posttraumatic stress disorder. *Int Clin Psychopharmacol, 26*(4), 193–200.

Albert, U., Aguglia, E., Maina, G., & Bogetto, F. (2002). Venlafaxine versus clomipramine in the treatment of obsessive-compulsive disorder: a preliminary single-blind, 12-week, controlled study. *J Clin Psychiatry, 63*(11), 1004–1009.

Allgulander, C., Dahl, A. A., Austin, C., Morris, P. L., Sogaard, J. A., Fayyad, R., et al. (2004). Efficacy of sertraline in a 12-week trial for generalized anxiety disorder. *Am J Psychiatry, 161*(9), 1642–1649.

Allgulander, C., Nutt, D., Detke, M., Erickson, J., Spann, M., Walker, D., et al. (2008). A non-inferiority comparison of duloxetine and venlafaxine in the treatment of adult patients with generalized anxiety disorder. *J Psychopharmacol, 22*(4), 417–425.

American Psychiatric Association. (2013). *Desk reference to the diagnostic criteria from DSM-5.* Washington, DC: American Psychiatric Publishing.

Askari, N., Moin, M., Sanati, M., Tajdini, M., Hosseini, S. M., Modabbernia, A., et al. (2012). Granisetron adjunct to fluvoxamine for moderate to severe obsessive-compulsive disorder: a randomized, double-blind, placebo-controlled trial. *CNS Drugs, 26*(10), 883–892.

Bakker, A., van Balkom, A. J., & Spinhoven, P. (2002). SSRIs vs. TCAs in the treatment of panic disorder: a meta-analysis. *Acta Psychiatr Scand, 106*(3), 163–167.

Ball, S. G., Kuhn, A., Wall, D., Shekhar, A., & Goddard, A. W. (2005). Selective serotonin reuptake inhibitor treatment for generalized anxiety disorder: a double-blind, prospective comparison between paroxetine and sertraline. *J Clin Psychiatry, 66*(1), 94–99.

Barnett, S. D., Kramer, M. L., Casat, C. D., Connor, K. M., & Davidson, J. R. (2002). Efficacy of olanzapine in social anxiety disorder: a pilot study. *J Psychopharmacol, 16*(4), 365–368.

Becker, M. E., Hertzberg, M. A., Moore, S. D., Dennis, M. F., Bukenya, D. S., & Beckham, J. C. (2007). A placebo-controlled trial of bupropion SR in the treatment of chronic posttraumatic stress disorder. *J Clin Psychopharmacol, 27*(2), 193–197.

Benjamin, J., Ben-Zion, I. Z., Karbofsky, E., & Dannon, P. (2000). Double-blind placebo-controlled pilot study of paroxetine for specific phobia. *Psychopharmacology (Berl), 149*(2), 194–196.

Berlin, H. A., Koran, L. M., Jenike, M. A., Shapira, N. A., Chaplin, W., Pallanti, S., et al. (2011). Double-blind, placebo-controlled trial of topiramate augmentation in treatment-resistant obsessive-compulsive disorder. *J Clin Psychiatry, 72*(5), 716–721.

Bielski, R. J., Bose, A., & Chang, C. C. (2005). A double-blind comparison of escitalopram and paroxetine in the long-term treatment of generalized anxiety disorder. *Ann Clin Psychiatry, 17*(2), 65–69.

Blanco, C., Heimberg, R. G., Schneier, F. R., Fresco, D. M., Chen, H., Turk, C. L., et al. (2010). A placebo-controlled trial of phenelzine, cognitive behavioral group therapy, and their combination for social anxiety disorder. *Arch Gen Psychiatry, 67*(3), 286–295.

Bloch, M. H., McGuire, J., Landeros-Weisenberger, A., Leckman, J. F., & Pittenger, C. (2010). Meta-analysis of the dose-response relationship of SSRI in obsessive-compulsive disorder. *Mol Psychiatry, 15*(8), 850–855.

Bradweijn, J., Stein, A. A., Salinas, E., Emlien, G. & Whitaker, T. (2005). Venlafaxine extended-release capsules in panic disorder. *Br J Psychiatry, 187*, 352–359.

Braun, P., Greenberg, D., Dasberg, H., & Lerer, B. (1990). Core symptoms of posttraumatic stress disorder unimproved by alprazolam treatment. *J Clin Psychiatry, 51*(6), 236–238.

Bruno, A., Mico, U., Pandolfo, G., Mallamace, D., Abenavoli, E., Di Nardo, F., et al. (2012). Lamotrigine augmentation of serotonin reuptake inhibitors in treatment-resistant obsessive-compulsive disorder: a double-blind, placebo-controlled study. *J Psychopharmacol, 26*(11), 1456–1462.

Chessick, C. A., Allen, M. H., Thase, M., Batista Miralha da Cunha, A. B., Kapczinski, F. F., de Lima, M. S., et al. (2006). Azapirones for generalized anxiety disorder. *Cochrane Database Syst Rev*(3), CD006115.

Clark, D. M., Ehlers, A., McManus, F., Hackmann, A., Fennell, M., Campbell, H., et al. (2003). Cognitive therapy versus fluoxetine in generalized social phobia: a randomized placebo-controlled trial. *J Consult Clin Psychol, 71*(6), 1058–1067.

Clomipramine in the treatment of patients with obsessive-compulsive disorder. The Clomipramine Collaborative Study Group. (1991). *Arch Gen Psychiatry, 48*(8), 730–738.

Crockett, B. A., Churchill, E., & Davidson, J. R. (2004). A double-blind combination study of clonazepam with sertraline in obsessive-compulsive disorder. *Ann Clin Psychiatry, 16*(3), 127–132.

Davidson, J., Rothbaum, B. O., Tucker, P., Asnis, G., Benattia, I., & Musgnung, J. J. (2006). Venlafaxine extended release in posttraumatic stress disorder: a sertraline- and placebo-controlled study. *J Clin Psychopharmacol, 26*(3), 259–267.

Davidson, J., Yaryura-Tobias, J., DuPont, R., Stallings, L., Barbato, L. M., van der Hoop, R. G., et al. (2004). Fluvoxamine-controlled release formulation for the treatment of generalized social anxiety disorder. *J Clin Psychopharmacol, 24*(2), 118–125.

Davidson, J. R., Brady, K., Mellman, T. A., Stein, M. B., & Pollack, M. H. (2007). The efficacy and tolerability of tiagabine in adult patients with post-traumatic stress disorder. *J Clin Psychopharmacol, 27*(1), 85–88.

Davidson, J. R., Rothbaum, B. O., van der Kolk, B. A., Sikes, C. R., & Farfel, G. M. (2001). Multicenter, double-blind comparison of sertraline and placebo in the treatment of posttraumatic stress disorder. *Arch Gen Psychiatry, 58*(5), 485–492.

Davidson, J. R., Weisler, R. H., Butterfield, M. I., Casat, C. D., Connor, K. M., Barnett, S., et al. (2003). Mirtazapine vs. placebo in posttraumatic stress disorder: a pilot trial. *Biol Psychiatry, 53*(2), 188–191.

Davis, L. L., Davidson, J. R., Ward, L. C., Bartolucci, A., Bowden, C. L., & Petty, F. (2008). Divalproex in the treatment of posttraumatic stress disorder: a randomized, double-blind, placebo-controlled trial in a veteran population. *J Clin Psychopharmacol, 28*(1), 84–88.

Davis, L. L., Jewell, M. E., Ambrose, S., Farley, J., English, B., Bartolucci, A., et al. (2004). A placebo-controlled study of nefazodone for the treatment of chronic posttraumatic stress disorder: a preliminary study. *J Clin Psychopharmacol, 24*(3), 291–297.

Davis, L. L., Ward, C., Rasmusson, A., Newell, J. M., Frazier, E., & Southwick, S. M. (2008). A placebo-controlled trial of guanfacine for the treatment of posttraumatic stress disorder in veterans. *Psychopharmacol Bull, 41*(1), 8–18.

de Kleine, R. A., Hendriks, G. J., Smits, J. A., Broekman, T. G., & van Minnen, A. (2014). Prescriptive variables for d-cycloserine augmentation of exposure therapy for posttraumatic stress disorder. *J Psychiatr Res, 48*(1), 40–46.

Denys, D., van Megen, H. J., van der Wee, N., & Westenberg, H. G. (2004). A double-blind switch study of paroxetine and venlafaxine in obsessive-compulsive disorder. *J Clin Psychiatry, 65*(1), 37–43.

Depping, A. M., Komossa, K., Kissling, W., & Leucht, S. (2010). Second-generation antipsychotics for anxiety disorders. *Cochrane Database Syst Rev*(12), CD008120.

Difede, J., Cukor, J., Wyka, K., Olden, M., Hoffman, H., Lee, F. S., et al. (2014). D-cycloserine augmentation of exposure therapy for post-traumatic stress disorder: a pilot randomized clinical trial. *Neuropsychopharmacology, 39*(5), 1052–1058.

Dold, M., Aigner, M., Lanzenberger, R., & Kasper, S. (2013). Antipsychotic augmentation of serotonin reuptake inhibitors in treatment-resistant obsessive-compulsive disorder: a meta-analysis of double-blind, randomized, placebo-controlled trials. *Int J Neuropsychopharmacol, 16*(3), 557–574.

Donahue, C. B., Kushner, M. G., Thuras, P. D., Murphy, T. G., Van Demark, J. B., & Adson, D. E. (2009). Effect of quetiapine vs. placebo on response to two virtual public speaking exposures in individuals with social phobia. *J Anxiety Disord, 23*(3), 362–368.

Donovan, M. R., Glue, P., Kolluri, S., & Emir, B. (2010). Comparative efficacy of antidepressants in preventing relapse in anxiety disorders—a meta-analysis. *J Affect Disord, 123*(1–3), 9–16.

Feder, A., Parides, M. K., Murrough, J. W., Perez, A. M., Morgan, J. E., Saxena, S., et al. (2014). Efficacy of Intravenous Ketamine for Treatment of Chronic Posttraumatic Stress Disorder: A Randomized Clinical Trial. *JAMA Psychiatry.*

Feltner, D. E., Crockatt, J. G., Dubovsky, S. J., Cohn, C. K., Shrivastava, R. K., Targum, S. D., et al. (2003). A randomized, double-blind, placebo-controlled, fixed-dose, multicenter study of pregabalin in patients with generalized anxiety disorder. *J Clin Psychopharmacol, 23*(3), 240–249.

Feltner, D. E., Liu-Dumaw, M., Schweizer, E., & Bielski, R. (2011). Efficacy of pregabalin in generalized social anxiety disorder: results of a double-blind, placebo-controlled, fixed-dose study. *Int Clin Psychopharmacol, 26*(4), 213–220.

Fineberg, N. A., & Gale, T. M. (2005). Evidence-based pharmacotherapy of obsessive-compulsive disorder. *Int J Neuropsychopharmacol, 8*(1), 107–129.

Frank, J. B., Kosten, T. R., Giller, E. L., Jr., & Dan, E. (1988). A randomized clinical trial of phenelzine and imipramine for posttraumatic stress disorder. *Am J Psychiatry, 145*(10), 1289–1291.

Garvey, M. J., & Tollefson, G. D. (1986). Prevalence of misuse of prescribed benzodiazepines in patients with primary anxiety disorder or major depression. *Am J Psychiatry, 143*(12), 1601–1603.

Ghaleiha, A., Entezari, N., Modabbernia, A., Najand, B., Askari, N., Tabrizi, M., et al. (2013). Memantine add-on in moderate to severe obsessive-compulsive disorder: randomized double-blind placebo-controlled study. *J Psychiatr Res, 47*(2), 175–180.

Goodman, W. K., Bose, A., & Wang, Q. (2005). Treatment of generalized anxiety disorder with escitalopram: pooled results from double-blind, placebo-controlled trials. *J Affect Disord, 87*(2–3), 161–167.

Greist, J. H., Jefferson, J. W., Kobak, K. A., Katzelnick, D. J., & Serlin, R. C. (1995). Efficacy and tolerability of serotonin transport inhibitors in obsessive-compulsive disorder. A meta-analysis. *Arch Gen Psychiatry, 52*(1), 53–60.

Guaiana, G., Barbui, C., & Cipriani, A. (2010). Hydroxyzine for generalised anxiety disorder. *Cochrane Database Syst Rev*(12), CD006815.

Hansen, R. A., Gaynes, B. N., Gartlehner, G., Moore, C. G., Tiwari, R., & Lohr, K. N. (2008). Efficacy and tolerability of second-generation antidepressants in social anxiety disorder. *Int Clin Psychopharmacol, 23*(3), 170–179.

Hoehn-Saric, R., Ninan, P., Black, D. W., Stahl, S., Greist, J. H., Lydiard, B., et al. (2000). Multicenter double-blind comparison of sertraline and desipramine for concurrent obsessive-compulsive and major depressive disorders. *Arch Gen Psychiatry, 57*(1), 76–82.

Hollander, E., Kaplan, A., & Stahl, S. M. (2003). A double-blind, placebo-controlled trial of clonazepam in obsessive-compulsive disorder. *World J Biol Psychiatry, 4*(1), 30–34.

Kasper, S., Herman, B., Nivoli, G., Van Ameringen, M., Petralia, A., Mandel, F. S., et al. (2009). Efficacy of pregabalin and venlafaxine-XR in generalized anxiety disorder: results of a double-blind, placebo-controlled 8-week trial. *Int Clin Psychopharmacol, 24*(2), 87–96.

Klein, E., & Uhde, T. W. (1988). Controlled study of verapamil for treatment of panic disorder. *Am J Psychiatry, 145*(4), 431–434.

Kobak, K. A., Greist, J. H., Jefferson, J. W., & Katzelnick, D. J. (2002). Fluoxetine in social phobia: a double-blind, placebo-controlled pilot study. *J Clin Psychopharmacol, 22*(3), 257–262.

Koran, L. M., Aboujaoude, E., Bullock, K. D., Franz, B., Gamel, N., & Elliott, M. (2005). Double-blind treatment with oral morphine in treatment-resistant obsessive-compulsive disorder. *J Clin Psychiatry, 66*(3), 353–359.

Kumar, S., & Malone, D. (2008). Panic disorder. *Clin Evid (Online)*, 2008.

Lader, M., Stender, K., Burger, V., & Nil, R. (2004). Efficacy and tolerability of escitalopram in 12- and 24-week treatment of social anxiety disorder: randomised, double-blind, placebo-controlled, fixed-dose study. *Depress Anxiety, 19*(4), 241–248.

Liebowitz, M. R., Schneier, F., Campeas, R., Hollander, E., Hatterer, J., Fyer, A., et al. (1992). Phenelzine vs atenolol in social phobia. A placebo-controlled comparison. *Arch Gen Psychiatry, 49*(4), 290–300.

Lindley, S. E., Carlson, E. B., & Hill, K. (2007). A randomized, double-blind, placebo-controlled trial of augmentation topiramate for chronic combat-related posttraumatic stress disorder. *J Clin Psychopharmacol, 27*(6), 677–681.

Litz, B. T., Salters-Pedneault, K., Steenkamp, M. M., Hermos, J. A., Bryant, R. A., Otto, M. W., et al. (2012). A randomized placebo-controlled trial of D-cycloserine and exposure therapy for posttraumatic stress disorder. *J Psychiatr Res, 46*(9), 1184–1190.

Lohoff, F. W., Etemad, B., Mandos, L. A., Gallop, R., & Rickels, K. (2010). Ziprasidone treatment of refractory generalized anxiety disorder: a placebo-controlled, double-blind study. *J Clin Psychopharmacol, 30*(2), 185–189.

Londborg, P. D., Hegel, M. T., Goldstein, S., Goldstein, D., Himmelhoch, J. M., Maddock, R., et al. (2001). Sertraline treatment of posttraumatic stress disorder: results of 24 weeks of open-label continuation treatment. *J Clin Psychiatry, 62*(5), 325–331.

Lydiard, R. B., Rickels, K., Herman, B., & Feltner, D. E. (2010). Comparative efficacy of pregabalin and benzodiazepines in treating the psychic and somatic symptoms of generalized anxiety disorder. *Int J Neuropsychopharmacol, 13*(2), 229–241.

Manteghi, A. A., Hebrani, P., Mortezania, M., Haghighi, M. B., & Javanbakht, A. (2014). Baclofen add-on to citalopram in treatment of posttraumatic stress disorder. *J Clin Psychopharmacol, 34*(2), 240–243.

Marshall, R. D., Lewis-Fernandez, R., Blanco, C., Simpson, H. B., Lin, S. H., Vermes, D., et al. (2007). A controlled trial of paroxetine for chronic PTSD, dissociation, and interpersonal problems in mostly minority adults. *Depress Anxiety, 24*(2), 77–84.

Martenyi, F., Brown, E. B., & Caldwell, C. D. (2007). Failed efficacy of fluoxetine in the treatment of posttraumatic stress disorder: results of a fixed-dose, placebo-controlled study. *J Clin Psychopharmacol, 27*(2), 166–170.

Martenyi, F., Brown, E. B., Zhang, H., Prakash, A., & Koke, S. C. (2002). Fluoxetine versus placebo in posttraumatic stress disorder. *J Clin Psychiatry, 63*(3), 199–206.

McDougle, C. J., Goodman, W. K., Leckman, J. F., Holzer, J. C., Barr, L. C., McCance-Katz, E., et al. (1993). Limited therapeutic effect of addition of buspirone in fluvoxamine-refractory obsessive-compulsive disorder. *Am J Psychiatry, 150*(4), 647–649.

Meibach, R. C., Mullane, J. F., & Binstok, C. (1987). A placebo-controlled multicenter trial of propranolol and chlordiazepoxide in the treatment of anxiety. *Current Therapeutic Research, 41*, 65–76.

Merideth, C., Cutler, A. J., She, F., & Eriksson, H. (2012). Efficacy and tolerability of extended release quetiapine fumarate monotherapy in the acute treatment of generalized anxiety disorder: a randomized, placebo controlled and active-controlled study. *Int Clin Psychopharmacol, 27*(1), 40–54.

Michelson, D., Allgulander, C., Dantendorfer, K., Knezevic, A., Maierhofer, D., Micev, V., et al. (2001). Efficacy of usual antidepressant dosing regimens of fluoxetine in panic disorder: randomised, placebo-controlled trial. *Br J Psychiatry, 179*, 514–518.

Mitte, K. (2005). A meta-analysis of the efficacy of psycho- and pharmacotherapy in panic disorder with and without agoraphobia. *J Affect Disord, 88*(1), 27–45.

Moroz, G., & Rosenbaum, J. F. (1999). Efficacy, safety, and gradual discontinuation of clonazepam in panic disorder: a placebo-controlled, multicenter study using optimized dosages. *J Clin Psychiatry, 60*(9), 604–612.

Mountjoy, C. Q., Roth, M., Garside, R. F., & Leitch, I. M. (1977). A clinical trial of phenelzine in anxiety depressive and phobic neuroses. *Br J Psychiatry, 131*, 486–492.

Muehlbacher, M., Nickel, M. K., Nickel, C., Kettler, C., Lahmann, C., Pedrosa Gil, F., et al. (2005). Mirtazapine treatment of social phobia in women: a randomized, double-blind, placebo-controlled study. *J Clin Psychopharmacol, 25*(6), 580–583.

Munjack, D. J., Crocker, B., Cabe, D., Brown, R., Usigli, R., Zulueta, A., et al. (1989). Alprazolam, propranolol, and placebo in the treatment of panic disorder and agoraphobia with panic attacks. *J Clin Psychopharmacol, 9*(1), 22–27.

Nardi, A. E., Lopes, F. L., Valenca, A. M., Freire, R. C., Nascimento, I., Veras, A. B., et al. (2010). Double-blind comparison of 30 and 60 mg tranylcypromine daily in patients with panic disorder comorbid with social anxiety disorder. *Psychiatry Res, 175*(3), 260–265.

Noyes, R., Jr., Garvey, M. J., Cook, B. L., & Samuelson, L. (1989). Problems with tricyclic antidepressant use in patients with panic disorder or agoraphobia: results of a naturalistic follow-up study. *J Clin Psychiatry, 50*(5), 163–169.

Oehrberg, S., Christiansen, P. E., Behnke, K., Borup, A. L., Severin, B., Soegaard, J., et al. (1995). Paroxetine in the treatment of panic disorder. A randomised, double-blind, placebo-controlled study. *Br J Psychiatry, 167*(3), 374–379.

Otto, M. W., Pollack, M. H., Gould, R. A., Worthington, J. J., 3rd, McArdle, E. T., & Rosenbaum, J. F. (2000). A comparison of the efficacy of clonazepam and cognitive-behavioral group therapy for the treatment of social phobia. *J Anxiety Disord, 14*(4), 345–358.

Pae, C. U., Lim, H. K., Peindl, K., Ajwani, N., Serretti, A., Patkar, A. A., et al. (2008). The atypical antipsychotics olanzapine and risperidone in the treatment of posttraumatic stress disorder: a meta-analysis of randomized, double-blind, placebo-controlled clinical trials. *Int Clin Psychopharmacol, 23*(1), 1–8.

Pande, A. C., Davidson, J. R., Jefferson, J. W., Janney, C. A., Katzelnick, D. J., Weisler, R. H., et al. (1999). Treatment of social phobia with gabapentin: a placebo-controlled study. *J Clin Psychopharmacol, 19*(4), 341–348.

Pande, A. C., Pollack, M. H., Crockatt, J., Greiner, M., Chouinard, G., Lydiard, R. B., et al. (2000). Placebo-controlled study of gabapentin treatment of panic disorder. *J Clin Psychopharmacol, 20*(4), 467–471.

Pigott, T. A., L'Heureux, F., Hill, J. L., Bihari, K., Bernstein, S. E., & Murphy, D. L. (1992). A double-blind study of adjuvant buspirone hydrochloride in clomipramine-treated patients with obsessive-compulsive disorder. *J Clin Psychopharmacol, 12*(1), 11–18.

Pohl, R. B., Wolkow, R. M., & Clary, C. M. (1998). Sertraline in the treatment of panic disorder: a double-blind multicenter trial. *Am J Psychiatry, 155*(9), 1189–1195.

Pollack, M. H., Hoge, E. A., Worthington, J. J., Moshier, S. J., Wechsler, R. S., Brandes, M., et al. (2011). Eszopiclone for the treatment of posttraumatic stress disorder and associated insomnia: a randomized, double-blind, placebo-controlled trial. *J Clin Psychiatry, 72*(7), 892–897.

Pollack, M. H., Van Ameringen, M., Simon, N. M., Worthington, J. W., Hoge, E. A., Keshaviah, A., et al. (2014). A double-blind randomized controlled trial of augmentation and switch strategies for refractory social anxiety disorder. *Am J Psychiatry, 171*(1), 44–53.

Raskind, M. A., Peterson, K., Williams, T., Hoff, D. J., Hart, K., Holmes, H., et al. (2013). A trial of prazosin for combat trauma PTSD with nightmares in active-duty soldiers returned from Iraq and Afghanistan. *Am J Psychiatry, 170*(9), 1003–1010.

Ravindran, L. N., Kim, D. S., Letamendi, A. M., & Stein, M. B. (2009). A randomized controlled trial of atomoxetine in generalized social anxiety disorder. *J Clin Psychopharmacol, 29*(6), 561–564.

Rickels, K., Case, W. G., Schweizer, E., Swenson, C., & Fridman, R. B. (1986). Low-dose dependence in chronic benzodiazepine users: a preliminary report on 119 patients. *Psychopharmacology Bulletin, 22*(2), 407–415.

Rickels, K., Downing, R., Schweizer, E., & Hassman, H. (1993). Antidepressants for the treatment of generalized anxiety disorder. A placebo-controlled comparison of imipramine, trazodone, and diazepam. *Arch Gen Psychiatry, 50*(11), 884–895.

Rickels, K., Pollack, M. H., Feltner, D. E., Lydiard, R. B., Zimbroff, D. L., Bielski, R. J., et al. (2005). Pregabalin for treatment of generalized anxiety disorder: a 4–week, multicenter, double-blind, placebo-controlled trial of pregabalin and alprazolam. *Arch Gen Psychiatry, 62*(9), 1022–1030.

Rickels, K., Rynn, M., Iyengar, M., & Duff, D. (2006). Remission of generalized anxiety disorder: a review of the paroxetine clinical trials database. *J Clin Psychiatry, 67*(1), 41–47.

Rodriguez, C. I., Kegeles, L. S., Levinson, A., Feng, T., Marcus, S. M., Vermes, D., et al. (2013). Randomized controlled crossover trial of ketamine in obsessive-compulsive disorder: proof-of-concept. *Neuropsychopharmacology, 38*(12), 2475–2483.

Rothbaum, B. O., Price, M., Jovanovic, T., Norrholm, S. D., Gerardi, M., Dunlop, B., et al. (2014). A Randomized, Double-Blind Evaluation of d-Cycloserine or Alprazolam Combined With Virtual Reality Exposure Therapy for Posttraumatic Stress Disorder in Iraq and Afghanistan War Veterans. *Am J Psychiatry.*

Roy-Byrne, P. P., Dager, S. R., Cowley, D. S., Vitaliano, P., & Dunner, D. L. (1989). Relapse and rebound following discontinuation of benzodiazepine treatment of panic attacks: alprazolam versus diazepam. *American Journal of Psychiatry, 146*(7), 860–865.

Schneier, F. R., Johnson, J., Hornig, C. D., Liebowitz, M. R., & Weissman, M. M. (1992). Social phobia. Comorbidity and morbidity in an epidemiologic sample. *Arch Gen Psychiatry, 49*(4), 282–288.

Shader, R. I., & Greenblatt, D. J. (1993). Use of benzodiazepines in anxiety disorders. *N Engl J Med, 328*(19), 1398–1405.

Sheehan, D. V., Davidson, J., Manschreck, T., & Van Wyck Fleet, J. (1983). Lack of efficacy of a new antidepressant (bupropion) in the treatment of panic disorder with phobias. *J Clin Psychopharmacol, 3*(1), 28–31.

Sheehan, D. V., Raj, A. B., Sheehan, K. H., & Soto, S. (1990). Is buspirone effective for panic disorder? *J Clin Psychopharmacol, 10*(1), 3–11.

Siegmund, A., Golfels, F., Finck, C., Halisch, A., Rath, D., Plag, J., et al. (2011). D-cycloserine does not improve but might slightly speed up the outcome of in-vivo exposure therapy in patients with severe agoraphobia and panic disorder in a randomized double blind clinical trial. *J Psychiatr Res, 45*(8), 1042–1047.

Simon, N. M., Otto, M. W., Worthington, J. J., Hoge, E. A., Thompson, E. H., Lebeau, R. T., et al. (2009). Next-step strategies for panic disorder refractory to initial pharmacotherapy: a 3-phase randomized clinical trial. *J Clin Psychiatry, 70*(11), 1563–1570.

Simpson, H. B., Foa, E. B., Liebowitz, M. R., Huppert, J. D., Cahill, S., Maher, M. J., et al. (2013). Cognitive-behavioral therapy vs risperidone for augmenting serotonin reuptake inhibitors in obsessive-compulsive disorder: a randomized clinical trial. *JAMA Psychiatry, 70*(11), 1190–1199.

Simpson, H. B., Schneier, F. R., Campeas, R. B., Marshall, R. D., Fallon, B. A., Davies, S., et al. (1998). Imipramine in the treatment of social phobia. *J Clin Psychopharmacol, 18*(2), 132–135.

Smits, J. A., Rosenfield, D., Otto, M. W., Marques, L., Davis, M. L., Meuret, A. E., et al. (2013). D-cycloserine enhancement of exposure therapy for social anxiety disorder depends on the success of exposure sessions. *J Psychiatr Res, 47*(10), 1455–1461.

Smits, J. A., Rosenfield, D., Otto, M. W., Powers, M. B., Hofmann, S. G., Telch, M. J., et al. (2013). D-cycloserine enhancement of fear extinction is specific to successful exposure sessions: evidence from the treatment of height phobia. *Biol Psychiatry, 73*(11), 1054–1058.

Soltani, F., Sayyah, M., Feizy, F., Malayeri, A., Siahpoosh, A., & Motlagh, I. (2010). A double-blind, placebo-controlled pilot study of ondansetron for patients with obsessive-compulsive disorder. *Hum Psychopharmacol, 25*(6), 509–513.

Soomro, G. M., Altman, D., Rajagopal, S., & Oakley-Browne, M. (2008). Selective serotonin re-uptake inhibitors (SSRIs) versus placebo for obsessive compulsive disorder (OCD). *Cochrane Database Syst Rev*(1), CD001765.

Stein, D. J., Davidson, J., Seedat, S., & Beebe, K. (2003). Paroxetine in the treatment of post-traumatic stress disorder: pooled analysis of placebo-controlled studies. *Expert Opin Pharmacother*, *4*(10), 1829–1838.

Stein, D. J., Pedersen, R., Rothbaum, B. O., Baldwin, D. S., Ahmed, S., Musgnung, J., et al. (2009). Onset of activity and time to response on individual CAPS-SX17 items in patients treated for post-traumatic stress disorder with venlafaxine ER: a pooled analysis. *Int J Neuropsychopharmacol*, *12*(1), 23–31.

Stein, D. J., Versiani, M., Hair, T., & Kumar, R. (2002). Efficacy of paroxetine for relapse prevention in social anxiety disorder: a 24-week study. *Arch Gen Psychiatry*, *59*(12), 1111–1118.

Stein, M. B., Pollack, M. H., Bystritsky, A., Kelsey, J. E., & Mangano, R. M. (2005). Efficacy of low and higher dose extended-release venlafaxine in generalized social anxiety disorder: a 6-month randomized controlled trial. *Psychopharmacology (Berl)*, *177*(3), 280–288.

Storch, E. A., Goddard, A. W., Grant, J. E., De Nadai, A. S., Goodman, W. K., Mutch, P. J., et al. (2013). Double-blind, placebo-controlled, pilot trial of paliperidone augmentation in serotonin reuptake inhibitor-resistant obsessive-compulsive disorder. *J Clin Psychiatry*, *74*(6), e527–e532.

Taylor, F. B., Martin, P., Thompson, C., Williams, J., Mellman, T. A., Gross, C., et al. (2008). Prazosin effects on objective sleep measures and clinical symptoms in civilian trauma posttraumatic stress disorder: a placebo-controlled study. *Biol Psychiatry*, *63*(6), 629–632.

Tucker, P., Potter-Kimball, R., Wyatt, D. B., Parker, D. E., Burgin, C., Jones, D. E., et al. (2003). Can physiologic assessment and side effects tease out differences in PTSD trials? A double-blind comparison of citalopram, sertraline, and placebo. *Psychopharmacol Bull*, *37*(3), 135–149.

Uhde, T. W., Stein, M. B., Vittone, B. J., Siever, L. J., Boulenger, J. P., Klein, E., et al. (1989). Behavioral and physiologic effects of short-term and long-term administration of clonidine in panic disorder. *Arch Gen Psychiatry*, *46*(2), 170–177.

Van Ameringen, M., Mancini, C., Oakman, J., Walker, J., Kjernisted, K., Chokka, P., et al. (2007). Nefazodone in the treatment of generalized social phobia: a randomized, placebo-controlled trial. *J Clin Psychiatry*, *68*(2), 288–295.

van Vliet, I. M., den Boer, J. A., Westenberg, H. G., & Pian, K. L. (1997). Clinical effects of buspirone in social phobia: a double-blind placebo-controlled study. *J Clin Psychiatry*, *58*(4), 164–168.

Wilhelm, F. H., & Roth, W. T. (1997). Acute and delayed effects of alprazolam on flight phobics during exposure. *Behav Res Ther*, *35*(9), 831–841.

Wolitzky-Taylor, K. B., Horowitz, J. D., Powers, M. B., & Telch, M. J. (2008). Psychological approaches in the treatment of specific phobias: a meta-analysis. *Clin Psychol Rev*, *28*(6), 1021–1037.

Yeh, M. S., Mari, J. J., Costa, M. C., Andreoli, S. B., Bressan, R. A., & Mello, M. F. (2011). A double-blind randomized controlled trial to study the efficacy of topiramate in a civilian sample of PTSD. *CNS Neurosci Ther*, *17*(5), 305–310.

Zajecka, J. M. (1996). The effect of nefazodone on comorbid anxiety symptoms associated with depression: experience in family practice and psychiatric outpatient settings. *J Clin Psychiatry*, *57 Suppl 2*, 10–14.

NEW TECHNOLOGIES AND APPROACHES TO TREATMENT

/// 30 /// ADHERENCE TO PSYCHOTHERAPY AND PHARMACOTHERAPY FOR ANXIETY DISORDERS

ALYSON K. ZALTA, ELIZABETH C. KAISER, SHEILA M. DOWD, AND MARK H. POLLACK

INTRODUCTION

Psychotherapy and pharmacotherapy have been established as effective treatments for anxiety disorders; however, many patients fall short of attaining clinically significant improvements. Adherence is one important factor that affects whether patients benefit from anxiety treatment. The World Health Organization (2003) defines adherence as "the extent to which a person's behavior—taking medications, following a diet, and/or executing lifestyle changes—corresponds with agreed-upon recommendations from a health care provider" (p. 17). While terms such as concordance and compliance have been used to describe a similar concept, adherence is currently viewed as the preferred term because it implies a partnership between the patient and provider rather than viewing the patient as a passive follower of providers' recommendations. In this chapter, we discuss types of adherence problems that arise in the treatment of anxiety disorders, why these adherence issues occur, and potential solutions for improving adherence including innovative techniques using technology.

Anxiety disorders are the most common occurring class of mental disorders, and a major health burden on the population (Santana and Fontenelle, 2011). Cognitive behavioral therapy (CBT) and antidepressants including selective serotonin reuptake inhibitors (SSRIs) and serotonin norepinephrine reuptake inhibitors (SNRIs) are considered first-line treatments for anxiety disorders (Dowd and Janicak, 2009). Evidence suggests that approximately 50% of patients with anxiety disorders drop out of treatment prematurely (Santana and Fontenelle, 2011). Although dropout is obviously a critical barrier to treatment, adherence encompasses a wide range of behaviors that reflect whether patients follow treatment recommendations. In the context of CBT, nonadherence often involves failure to complete homework assignments. While there is no agreement on the extent to which patients are adherent to their homework assignments, some research places completion of homework at around 50% (Levensky, 2006). Medication nonadherence includes failing to fill the prescription right away or not at all, adjusting doses without physician consultation, taking the medication at the wrong times or not at all, not taking the medication consistently, or taking too much or too little at one time. Stein and colleagues (2006) report that only 57% patients with anxiety disorders adhere to SSRI or SNRI medication regimens at 6 months. These statistics suggest that nonadherence is a common issue in the treatment of anxiety disorders, which is likely to have a serious impact on clinical, functional, and economic outcomes (Santana and Fontenelle, 2011).

FACTORS ASSOCIATED WITH NONADHERENCE

Identifying key predictors of nonadherence is important to establish potential intervention strategies. Disappointingly, few studies are found in the treatment of anxiety disorders (Julius, Novitsky, and Dubin, 2009). Next we highlight the factors that have received the greatest empirical support across mental health disorders and, when available, describe the evidence as it relates to anxiety disorder treatment (see Table 30.1).

PATIENT FACTORS

Patient Beliefs

Patient beliefs are a central component of many theoretical models of health behavior prediction and a number of patient beliefs have been shown to influence adherence to anxiety treatment (Wagner et al., 2005). Those most frequently discussed and researched include patients' beliefs about whether they need to change, expect treatment will be beneficial, trust the provider will be helpful, and have confidence that they can carry out provider recommendations. Given the central role of fear and avoidance in maintaining anxiety pathology, fear-based beliefs related to the treatment and provider are also likely to impact treatment adherence.

Many patients who come to treatment express ambivalence about their desire to make changes in their life due to the perceived difficulty of making changes, the potential loss of current benefits that they receive from maladaptive behavior, and the fear of the unknown once change has been affected. Prochaska and DiClemente's (1992) transtheoretical model proposes five distinct steps that patients successively move through as they contemplate making a change in their behavior. The transtheoretical model posits that as patients move toward an acceptance of their need to change, treatment adherence will increase. Although the transtheoretical model was first applied in the context of alcohol abuse, its role in adherence in the treatment of anxiety disorders is thought to be just as pivotal. Several studies have shown that readiness to engage in treatment and level of motivation predict treatment adherence to CBT for anxiety disorders (e.g., Maher et al., 2012).

Patients also have a number of preexisting expectations concerning their treatment. Gunzburger and colleagues (1985) found that patients who terminated treatment early felt that their expectations were not met in the first session, demonstrating the importance of addressing these expectations at the beginning of treatment. One critical expectation is whether patients believe the treatment will be beneficial in reducing their anxiety. In a group of patients with obsessive-compulsive disorder (OCD), Mancebo et al (2008)

TABLE 30.1 Factors Influencing Adherence

Patient	• Low motivation or willingness to change
	• Poor expectations regarding treatment
	• Low self-efficacy regarding ability to comply with treatment
	• Fear of treatment approach
	• Other problematic health and treatment-related beliefs
	• Uncertainty about provider's ability to help
	• Lack of trust and/or comfort with provider
	• Nature of the illness: severity/comorbidity/insight
	• Difficulty discussing problems with treatment and/or adherence
	• Lack of self-management/coping skills (e.g., organizational ability, self-control, problem solving)
	• Low health literacy and language deficits
	• Cognitive deficits
Provider	• Poor therapeutic alliance
	• Poor communication between patient and provider
	• Inadequate assessment of problems with adherence
	• Provider and patient have differing conceptualization or expectations of problem and/or treatment
	• Limited clinician availability
Treatment	• Frequent and/or severe side effects
	• High complexity and demands of the treatment
	• Poor fit between treatment requirements and patient's lifestyle/daily activities
	• Long duration of the treatment
	• Treatment is unwelcome reminder of illness
Social/Environmental	• Stressful life events
	• Stigma of the disease
	• Inadequate social support
	• Family/caregiver factors
Resources	• Transportation
	• Trouble obtaining child care
	• Lack of time
	• Costs
	• Insurance
	• Drug availability
	• Stable housing

found that one of the top reasons for nonadherence was the belief that medication will not be helpful. Treatment expectations (e.g., that symptoms can change, that treatment will be helpful in reducing anxiety) have also been shown to predict homework compliance in CBT for patients with anxiety disorders (Westra and Dozois, 2006). Relatedly, patients who believe in the effectiveness of their provider (Barrett et al., 2008) are more likely to adhere to psychotherapy. Although low expectancy has received the most research attention, it is also possible that overly high patient expectancy may diminish adherence as patients may be disappointed that treatment benefits do not match their expectations.

In addition to having the motivation to change and a belief that the treatment will work, patients must also have confidence in their own ability engage in the recommended treatment (i.e., self-efficacy beliefs). In CBT for anxiety disorders, patients are expected to change their behavior and apply therapeutic skills outside of session. Patients who believe that they are incapable of using therapeutic strategies on their own are unlikely to adhere to homework assignments. Similarly, patients who don't believe they are capable of following physician instructions regarding medication regimens (e.g., dietary changes required with MAOI use) are less likely to adhere to treatment. Although there is research demonstrating the importance of self-efficacy beliefs in predicting adherence to medical regimens such as obesity treatment, there is no current evidence examining the effect of self-efficacy beliefs in adherence to anxiety treatment.

Given that fear and avoidance are core components of anxiety disorders, fear-related beliefs are also likely to have a significant impact on adherence to treatment. Patients may have fears related to becoming addicted to medication, adverse effects of the treatment (i.e., medication side effects), consequences of exposure, symptom exacerbation, experiencing negative emotions, or provider responses to nonadherence (e.g., anger, rejection). In a study of patients with OCD, 55% dropped out of CBT because they were fearful of the therapy and too anxious. One study reported that the three most frequent reasons expressed by participants for medication nonadherence were dislike of the side effects (78%), being too anxious or fearful of taking the medications (41%) and not believing in the utility of the medications (41%; Mancebo et al., 2008). Despite the apparent importance of these fear-related beliefs in determining adherence to anxiety treatment, few studies have examined this relationship, making this an important area for future research.

Patient Characteristics

Studies show that adherence is affected by a patient's ability to read and understand medical instructions. Health literacy reflects the ability to process and understand health information. In a study of 2500 English and Spanish speaking patients, 24–58% misunderstood directions to take medication on an empty stomach, 21–31% misunderstood when their next appointment was scheduled and 41–75% did not sufficiently understand a standardized informed consent (Williams et al., 1995). Studies show that many people forget medical instructions as soon as they leave the office (Martin, Williams, Haskard, and Dimatteo, 2005). Cognitive impairment such as poor working memory or inattention can also negatively affect adherence as it influences a patient's ability to follow complicated instructions, complete homework assignments and manage their appointments. These issues may be particularly relevant for patients with complicated medication regimens or homework assignments.

Illness severity and comorbidity have been proposed as predictors of treatment adherence; however the research literature on these factors is mixed (Issakidis and Andrews, 2004; Stein et al., 2006). Mitchell and Selmes (2007) propose a bimodal relationship with both the mildest and most severe disorders evidencing the highest rates of nonadherence. This would suggest that those who are not significantly impaired by their symptoms might not be invested in treatment and those with very severe symptoms might be suffering so greatly they are unable to organize themselves to adhere to a treatment plan.

Insight is the ability of a person to critically appraise one's own state of mind from the inside (Vigne, de Menezes, Harrison, and Fontenelle, 2014). Patients with lower levels of insight might not realize that their symptoms and impairments are as severe as they are and therefore have difficulties adhering to treatment recommendations (Vigne et al., 2014). Lower levels of insight have been shown to predict treatment drop out for patients with social anxiety disorder (Vigne et al., 2014) and OCD (Diniz et al., 2011).

PROVIDER FACTORS

Mental health treatment involves a patient-clinician partnership that relies on the therapeutic alliance between them. The therapeutic alliance incorporates two elements: (1) the patient feels an affective bond with the clinician and (2) the patient and provider agree on therapeutic goals and tasks (Bordin, 1979). Both aspects of the alliance are important predictors of adherence to treatment. By developing an emotional bond, patients are more likely to trust their provider and believe that the provider is capable of helping. Patent-provider agreement on the treatment approach is also important, given research showing that patients who receive their preferred treatment are less likely to drop out of treatment (Rokke, Tomhave, and Jocic, 1999) and are more likely to adhere to treatment recommendations (Hunot, Horne, Leese, and Churchill, 2007).

Psychotherapy research shows that having a strong therapeutic alliance is associated with patients' willingness to learn and willingness to practice new skills in and out of session (Chu et al., 2004). A study by Hayes and colleagues (2007) showed that having a strong therapeutic alliance not only increased patients' willingness to participate in anxiety-provoking exposures, but also increased their willingness to maintain the exposure over a longer period of time. Adherence to psychotropic medication has also been associated with the strength of the therapeutic alliance; however, this relationship has primarily been examined in the literature on pharmacotherapy for schizophrenia, bipolar, and depressive disorders. One study examining the effect of the therapeutic alliance in the treatment of PTSD showed that early therapeutic alliance more strongly predicted adherence to psychotherapy homework ($r = .32$) than medication adherence ($r = .23$), suggesting that the issue of therapeutic alliance may be more critical in psychotherapy than pharmacotherapy for anxiety disorders (Keller, Zoellner, and Feeny, 2010).

Although the therapeutic alliance has been shown to impact patient adherence, adherence is also likely to have an important impact on the therapeutic alliance as providers can become frustrated with patients who are nonadherent. In a primary care study, general practitioners formed negative opinions and sometimes "punished" patients after missing an appointment (Husain-Gambles, Neal, Dempsey, Lawlor, and Hodgson, 2004). This suggests that the relationship between treatment adherence and the therapeutic alliance is bidirectional.

TREATMENT FACTORS

There are multiple factors relating to the treatment itself that affect adherence. In pharmacotherapy, experience with side effects associated with taking SSRIs is a common reason for poor treatment adherence (Taylor, Abramowitz, and McKay, 2012). Other "unfriendly" aspects of medication treatments are also associated with nonadherence (Kardas, Lewek, and Matyjaszczyk, 2013), such as being unable to open the bottle, bad taste from the medication, large tablets that are difficult to swallow, and required dietary changes. Evidence indicates that less frequent dosing (e.g., daily or weekly), long acting formulations, and reduced frequency injectable medications are associated with a positive effect on adherence compared to more frequent dosing regiments.

Several aspects of psychotherapy interventions can impact patient adherence. In one study with anxiety disorder patients, those offered group therapy were more likely to decline or fail to start treatment than those offered individual therapy (Issakidis and Andrews, 2004). Reasons for nonadherence to homework include not understanding the homework, moving up the hierarchy too quickly, and fear of the consequences of conducting homework assignments (Huppert, Roth Ledley, and Foa, 2006). Evidence is mixed as to whether the concept of exposure itself may be a deterrent for patients; however, if the treatment is not properly tailored to the patient or exposures are occurring too early on, this may certainly affect adherence (White et al., 2010).

SOCIAL/ENVIRONMENTAL FACTORS

Family members and loved ones can serve both a supportive and a hindering role in patient adherence to treatment. Often, family members can help to motivate patients to engage in treatment. For example, a study of CBT for OCD reported that participants were more likely to drop out if they did not have someone close to them providing "pressure" to complete therapy (Hansen, Hoogduin, Schaap, and de Haan, 1992). However, it is also the case that family members can interfere with the therapeutic process by reinforcing maladaptive behaviors, being critical of the patient, expressing negative beliefs about mental illness and treatment, and undermining the patients' therapeutic gains because it disrupts the homeostasis of the family system. In anxiety disorder treatment, it is common for family members to unwittingly encourage avoidance because it decreases the patients' subjective distress in the short-term.

In addition to the impact of individuals in patients' immediate social network, broader community-based attitudes toward mental health treatment also impact treatment engagement and adherence. Stigma has been identified as an important environmental factor that affects adherence to treatment. Stigma discourages individuals from seeking and adhering to mental health treatments because of a potential loss of self-esteem or for fear of being publicly labeled as "mentally ill" (Corrigan, 2004). Specifically, patients may reject treatment because the act of receiving treatment reinforces the idea that they are weak, defective, or not well.

RESOURCES

Many perceived and actual barriers prevent individuals suffering from anxiety from receiving proper care. In a review of patients with depression and anxiety, Prins and colleagues (2008) concluded that the cost of treatment was one of the most important barriers to seeking professional treatment. Increasing copayments limit patients' ability to attend weekly therapy. Many insurance plans restrict the use of nongeneric medications, restrict the number of medications a patient can receive, and deny claims for prescriptions that exceed the dose approved by the Food Drug Administration. Notably, the literature on income and unemployment as predictors of adherence is inconsistent. One study of panic disorder found that patients with lower income were more likely to drop out, whereas, a study in OCD found that those who were unemployed remained in treatment longer (Grilo et al., 1998; Lívia Santana, Versiani, Mendlowicz, and Fontenelle, 2010). These disparate findings may in part be attributable to the relative impact of factors such as the ability of unemployed patients to be more available for treatment but also to face greater burden of attendance in terms of cost.

In addition to cost, other barriers that impact patients' ability to come for treatment sessions have been shown to impact adherence. For example, both patients' inability to obtain transportation and difficulty arranging childcare have been shown to predict drop out from treatment (Zayfert and Black, 2000). Santana and colleagues (2010) found that patients who reside in the same city as their treatment clinic stayed in treatment longer than those who did not. Homelessness and unstable housing have been identified as predictors of poorer medication adherence and attendance (e.g., Coe et al., 2012). Additionally, limited access to care such as inconvenient appointment times and/or long wait lists have a negative impact on treatment seeking and adherence (Kardas et al., 2013). Of note, not all resource barriers are likely to have an equal impact on adherence to psychotherapy and pharmacotherapy. One study examining adherence to treatment in economically disadvantaged patients with panic disorder reported that time and travel barriers were significantly related to adherence to psychotherapy, but not pharmacotherapy (Mukherjee et al., 2006).

CONCLUSIONS REGARDING FACTORS INFLUENCING ADHERENCE

The predictors described do not act independently to predict adherence; rather, it is a combination of patient, therapist, treatment, environmental, and resource factors that predict treatment adherence. For example, the health beliefs model (Becker and Maiman, 1975) specifies that patients need to be motivated to change, believe that treatment is likely to be beneficial, and that they are capable of completing treatment requirements in order to engage in the treatment. Further, these factors may interact synergistically. For example, a lack of resources may affect individual's beliefs that they are capable of complying with treatment demands. This suggests that providers must conduct a comprehensive examination of the factors that affect adherence in order to effectively intervene. In the following sections, we describe potential strategies for improving adherence with particular emphasis on the strategies that have been designed to target predictors adversely affecting adherence and that have the greatest research scrutiny.

STRATEGIES FOR IMPROVING ADHERENCE

A number of different strategies have been proposed to increase adherence to pharmacotherapy and psychotherapy; however the research literature on the advantage of these techniques in the treatment of anxiety disorders is sparse. In the following sections, we describe the general strategies that have been reported in the literature and their applications to the treatment of anxiety disorders. It is important to note that these strategies are not mutually exclusive and can be used concurrently. In fact, several of the adherence protocols shown to be effective combine multiple strategies (e.g., Sirey, Bruce, and Kales, 2010). Thus, the strategies described most likely represent elements that should be combined and tailored to the individual to achieve maximal benefit.

Addressing Practical Barriers to Care

As described, there are a number of practical reasons why patients have difficulty adhering to recommended psychotherapy and pharmacotherapy. Although practitioners may have limited ability to overcome some of these barriers, it is also the case that straightforward, practical interventions can help to improve treatment adherence. For example, letter and telephone prompts reminding patients of appointments have been shown to reduce dropout rates (Clough and Casey, 2011). Research shows that written homework assignments increase the extent to which patients recall and adhere to homework (Cox, Tisdelle, and Culbert, 1988). For patients who face barriers related to poverty, concurrent case management may be particularly effective in promoting treatment adherence. A randomized trial of CBT alone versus CBT plus case management for depressed low-income minority patients showed that patients who received case management were significantly less likely to terminate CBT early and significantly more likely to complete a therapeutic trial of CBT than those who did not receive case management (Miranda, Azocar, Organista, Dwyer, and Areane, 2003). Research also suggests that reducing the cost of medications via increased insurance coverage and refill assistance increases treatment adherence (Zullig, Peterson, and Bosworth, 2013).

Pretreatment Education

Another potential set of interventions to improve adherence provides patients with education to increase their knowledge, improve their expectations, and enhance patient-provider alignment. The early psychotherapy research literature dating back to the 1960's focused on pretreatment preparatory techniques that were designed to provide patients with a rationale for therapy, information regarding the therapy process, realistic expectations for change, prognosis, and examples of therapist behavior and "good" patient behaviors (e.g., self-disclosure, reflection, regular attendance; Walitzer, Dermen, and Connors, 1999). Evidence from this early literature suggests that these pretreatment interventions improve adherence to psychotherapy (Walitzer et al., 1999). However, most CBT interventions for anxiety disorders involve a description of the treatment rationale, the therapy process, and typical treatment barriers, such as avoidance. Thus, it is unclear whether educational interventions would add to existing CBT treatments.

In the context of pharmacotherapy, it is generally believed to be important for physicians to educate patients about how medications are expected to improve symptoms, common side effects, therapeutic dosage, proper administration, and required time on medications to establish therapeutic benefit. Several studies have attempted to increase adherence to medications by providing further education using a variety of strategies including informational leaflets, personalized mailings, pharmacy-based coaching, and educational group sessions. Two reviews of adherence enhancement programs for antidepressant medications conclude that providing patients with education materials alone rarely improves patient adherence to antidepressants (van Servellen, Heise, and Ellis, 2011; Vergouwen, Bakker, Katon, Verheij, and Koerselman, 2003).

Shared Decision Making

Involving patients in the treatment decision-making process is another potential strategy for promoting adherence. Patients can be involved in many aspects of decision making including selecting which treatment they will receive and defining their goals for treatment. By participating in the decision-making, patients may be more likely to express which treatments they believe will be helpful to them, work on mutually agreed upon goals, have positive beliefs about their provider, and take an active role in treatment. Shared decision-making (SDM) also gives providers an opportunity to address unrealistic expectations for treatment that may lead to patient disappointment and drop out.

A body of evidence indicates that SDM is beneficial in the treatment of depression and corresponds to patient receiving pharmacotherapy or psychotherapy that is consistent with treatment guidelines (Clever et al., 2006). Loh and colleagues (2007) developed and tested a shared decision-making (SDM) intervention among individuals newly diagnosed with depression; relative to usual care, the SDM intervention increased patient-rated involvement and patient satisfaction without increasing consultation time. To our knowledge, there is no current research examining whether SDM approaches improve adherence to CBT for anxiety disorders, perhaps because the concept of patient-provider collaboration is a hallmark feature of CBT for anxiety. In exposure treatments, SDM often involves collaboration between the patient and therapist to select exposures; therapists are more involved in this process early in treatment and decrease their role over the course of treatment to the point where patients ultimately select exposures on their own. Although anecdotal evidence suggests that patients will be more likely to complete collaboratively selected or self-selected exposures as opposed to therapist-selected exposures, to our knowledge, there is no empirical research on this topic.

Motivational Interviewing

Motivational interviewing (MI) has been applied to promote treatment adherence for a number of health and mental health problems. MI is designed to build patients' intrinsic motivation and strengthen their commitment to change by helping them to explore and resolve ambivalent feelings about treatment. The intervention follows four overarching principles: 1) expressing empathy via reflective listening and acceptance, 2) developing a perceived discrepancy between the patient's current state and ideal state, 3) rolling with resistance, and 4) building confidence in the patient's ability to create change. MI strategies may be particularly beneficial for promoting adherence to anxiety treatment given the way in which anxiety pathology can promote feelings of ambivalence and fear of change.

Of the various strategies designed to promote adherence to CBT for anxiety disorders, MI has the greatest research evidence in support of its efficacy. MI has now been tested as an adjunctive intervention for CBT for generalized anxiety disorder (GAD), obsessive-compulsive disorder (OCD), and mixed anxiety disorders (Slagle and Gray, 2007). Three randomized trials have examined the extent to which MI pretreatment improved adherence to CBT for GAD, panic disorder, and social phobia relative to no pretreatment (Slagle and Gray, 2007). Results from these trials suggest that MI can reduce early treatment resistance and increase homework compliance. By contrast, studies examining MI to support adherence to CBT for OCD have shown more mixed results (Maltby and Tolin, 2005; Simpson et al., 2011), suggesting that MI may not be as beneficial for this population. MI has also been identified as a potentially useful adjunctive treatment for improving adherence to antidepressant medications; however the research literature on this topic is sparse (e.g., Interian, Lewis-Fernández, Gara, and Escobar, 2013).

Cognitive-Behavioral Techniques

Cognitive behavioral techniques have the potential to address a number of factors that contribute to poor adherence including the use of problem solving to overcome practical barriers to treatment, skill building to improve organizational abilities, chain analysis to gain insight into habitual patterns that contribute to poor adherence, and cognitive restructuring to modify maladaptive patient beliefs that interfere with adherence. Given that these strategies are already an integral part of CBT treatment for anxiety, cognitive-behavioral techniques are most likely to be beneficial in facilitating additional adherence to pharmacotherapy.

Several studies have shown that CBT can be used to support medication adherence in patients with serious mental illness and physical disorders such as HIV (Soroudi et al., 2008) and diabetes. To our knowledge, no studies have examined CBT as a strategy for medication adherence for individuals with anxiety disorders. Studies on combined CBT and antidepressant treatment for depression have shown that individuals in the combined treatment are less likely to drop out than individuals receiving antidepressants alone (Hollon et al., 2014). However, it is unclear whether reduced dropout rates are specifically due to CBT techniques or whether patients are more likely to receive their treatment preference in the combined treatment.

Family and Social Interventions

Family and social interventions have the potential to improve adherence to anxiety disorder treatment in numerous ways. Educating family members about mental illness and its treatment can help to enhance empathy for the patients, decrease antagonism between family members that is provoked by patient symptoms, and reduce misconceptions and stigma regarding the disorder and treatment. By joining in the therapy process, family members can learn how to promote patients' use of therapeutic strategies and how to decrease behaviors that reinforce patients' avoidance. Working with family members can also help to problem solve practical barriers to treatment adherence including family roles and responsibilities that might impact the patient's ability to adhere to treatment recommendations. Further, helping families to learn effective communication strategies more generally can improve family functioning, which is known to have an impact on adherence. However, family/social interventions also have the potential to decrease adherence due to greater logistic difficulties in scheduling appointments that include all relevant family members, externalization of motivation for treatment, and decreased self-efficacy on the part of the patient.

Family interventions have been applied in the context of psychotherapy for agoraphobia, OCD, and PTSD (Carr, 2009; Sherman et al., 2009). These interventions include the involvement of family members as therapy-aids as well as couples-based interventions that are meant to simultaneously target the couple's functioning and the identified patient's mental illness. However, the primary aim of these interventions has been to improve treatment outcome rather than specifically enhance treatment adherence. To our knowledge, none of these studies have reported on the extent to which family involvement impacts attendance, homework compliance, or other factors that predict adherence. One family intervention specifically designed to promote engagement in PTSD treatment is the REACH intervention (Sherman et al., 2009) designed by investigators at the Veteran's Administration. One study examining patient interest and engagement with REACH showed that almost half of patients with PTSD were interested in learning about the family intervention but only a quarter of patients actually followed through with a family session (Sherman et al., 2009). This suggests that further work is needed to determine how to maximize these interventions and the extent to which they can improve treatment adherence. To our knowledge, no studies have explored the benefits of family interventions to support medication adherence in anxiety disorders.

CONCLUSIONS REGARDING STRATEGIES TO IMPROVE ADHERENCE

At present, there is little systematic research on interventions that aim to improve adherence to CBT and pharmacotherapy for anxiety disorders. Much of the support for the intervention strategies we describe draw from populations with other psychiatric disorders. Furthermore, much of the psychotherapy research has focused on group treatment and much of the pharmacotherapy literature has examined mental health treatment in primary care practices. We believe that addressing practical barriers to care, providing pre-treatment education, and promoting shared decision-making should be standard aspects of quality care. Motivational interviewing, cognitive behavioral, and family/social interventions appear to have potential for improving treatment adherence to anxiety disorder treatment, but more research is required. Figure 30.1 illustrates how providers should

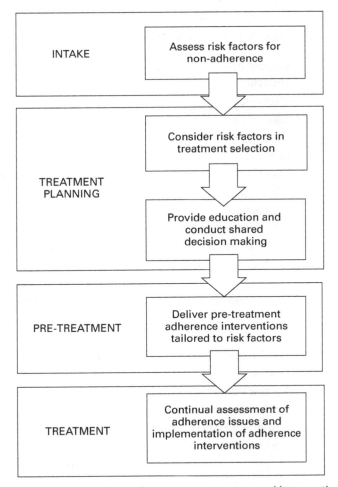

FIGURE 30.1 Strategies for integrating adherence assessments and interventions.

consider issues related to adherence at all phases of treatment and match adherence interventions to factors driving nonadherence.

USING TECHNOLOGY TO IMPROVE ADHERENCE

The use of technology to improve the delivery of mental health treatment is a burgeoning field. Tools such as Internet websites, phone or video conferencing, text messages, and mobile applications, have the potential to overcome a number of factors that impact adherence to treatment. There is nascent body of literature examining technological adjuncts for anxiety treatment to improve dissemination and outcome (Newman, Szkodny, Llera, and Przeworski, 2011); however, these studies have not yet explored technological adjuncts designed to improve adherence to anxiety treatment. We describe here the primary benefits of technology and how technological solutions can be used to improve adherence (see Table 30.2).

One important benefit of technology is its convenience. Research shows that 90% of adults in the United States have a cell phone and 58% have smartphones ("Mobile Technology Fact Sheet"). Additionally, 70% of all cell-phone users report that they have used their phone in the previous 30 days to receive "just-in-time information" such as

TABLE 30.2 Technology Solutions for Improving Treatment Adherence

ADHERENCE APPLICATION	TECHNOLOGY SOLUTION	BENEFITS
Practical Barriers	Text messages, alarms	Provides convenient reminders
	Telehealth, technology-delivered self-help	Allows for treatment without an office visit
Education	Video presentations, websites, mobile applications	Tailored content, allows for patients to easily reference materials
Communication	Telemonitoring system, mobile applications	Alerts clinicians of patient adherence
Family/Social Involvement	Self-help interventions for the family, involvement of social networks, online support groups	Involve family members who can't attend appointments, offers social support and accountability
Treatment Acceptability	Virtual reality exposures, homework assignments via mobile technology	Increases convenience of treatment procedures, decreases fear of procedures, increases information security
Perceived Stigma	Virtual therapist, technology-delivered self-help	Patient anonymity, help is received outside of the medical setting
Just-in-time Interventions	Real-time interventions delivered via mobile technology based on information that is acquired actively or passively	In the moment support when patients most need help, therapeutic information provided in context of patient's day-to-day life, intervention can be individualized based on adaptive algorithms

coordinating a meeting or looking up the score of a sporting event (Rainie and Fox, 2012). Investigators have attempted to take advantage of this convenience by sending intervention reminders and developing intervention tools that can be accessed via mobile technology. For example, text message reminders have been shown to increase medication adherence (Foreman et al., 2012) and can support adherence to therapy and therapeutic concepts (Aguilera and Muñoz, 2011).

Technology also has the potential to improve treatment adherence by offering a new medium for patient-provider communication. Tools can be developed that alerts clinicians when patients engage in (or fail to engage in) treatment behaviors. For example, Frangou and colleagues (2005) developed a telemonitoring system that alerts providers when their patients fail to take their medications based on an electronic dispenser. Investigators are also developing mobile applications that patients and providers are meant to use together in psychotherapy sessions to support treatment activities (e.g., Reger et al., 2013). These mobile applications can help providers to assess treatment adherence by logging when and for how long therapeutic tools were used.

In addition to improving patient-provider communication, technology can also help patients to connect with other individuals who can help to support treatment adherence. As described earlier, family and social interventions have the potential to increase adherence; however, it can be difficult to get families involved in treatment due to scheduling constraints. Technology can help to involve family members who cannot attend regular sessions. For example, Comer and colleagues (2014) developed an Internet-based family intervention for OCD. Perhaps an even more promising application of technology is to harness social networks to support treatment adherence. Research shows that 74% of Internet users access social networking sites and 28% of adults with cell phones access social network sites on their phone in a typical day ("Social Networking Fact Sheet," 2014). This suggests that social networks can serve as a powerful reinforcement for patient behaviors. The use of social networks to support treatment adherence has been applied to other health behaviors, such as online support groups for weight loss or communities of individuals using wearable devices to track steps, sleep, and nutrition. However, the use of social networks to support treatment adherence for mental health disorders is still in the early phases of development.

Given the potential impact of stigma on adherence, another critical advantage of technology is that it allows patients to engage in treatment anonymously. Technology-delivered self-help interventions enable patients to receive treatment without going to a medical setting (i.e., decreasing self-stigma of being "sick"). At the frontier of research in this area, investigators have developed a virtual therapist that can interact with patients without any human input. Lucas and colleagues (2014) showed that participants were more willing to disclose to a virtual therapist that they believed was operated by a computer than a virtual therapist that they believed was being operated by a human. Although this type of intervention is still in the early development stages, these findings suggest that technology-based interventions may be particularly useful in improving adherence for patients who experience stigma related to psychiatric care.

Finally, patients are more likely to adhere to treatment if they find it to be helpful when they need it most. Mobile technology offers the potential of giving patients individualized interventions in real-time. These "just-in-time" interventions are based on learning algorithms that use information provided by the patient (data collected actively) or information that is inferred from mobile technology without user entry (data collected passively). The ultimate goal of these algorithms is to identify when patients need an intervention and what type/dose of an intervention should be offered. Although these interventions are still under development, these real time interventions could have a significant impact on the extent to which patients use therapeutic tools outside of session.

SUMMARY

It is perhaps not surprising that adherence issues are extensive in the treatment of anxiety disorders given that fear and avoidance are core components of anxiety pathology. However, the research literature in this area is sparse, indicating that more work is needed to identify which strategies are likely to improve adherence for a given individual. At present, motivational interviewing, cognitive-behavioral, and family/social interventions appear to have the greatest potential to improve adherence to anxiety treatment. Research on the use of technology in mental health treatment may invigorate this field by offering a plethora of novel solutions to adherence issues. Some of most exciting work in this area focuses on ways to deliver interventions when patients need them the most in their daily lives. This type of personalized approach is likely to have the greatest impact on improving treatment adherence and ultimately decreasing the burden of mental illness.

DISCLOSURE STATEMENT

Alyson Zalta receives grant support from NIH. Elizabeth Kaiser receives grant support from NIH. Sheila Dowd receives grant support from NIMH, Neuronetics, Cervel Neurotech, Otsuka, and the Research Foundation for Mental Hygiene and is a consultant for the Women's Interagency HIV Study. Mark Pollack is on the advisory board and is a consultant for Concert Pharmaceuticals, Edgemont Pharmaceuticals, Ironwood Pharmaceuticals, Palo Alto Health Sciences, and Project Plus and receives grant support from NIH. He also has equity in Doyen Medical, Medavante, Mensante Corporation, Mindsite, Targia Pharmaceuticals, and receives royalty/patent from the SIGH-A, SAFER interviews.

REFERENCES

Aguilera, A., and Muñoz, R. F. (2011). Text messaging as an adjunct to CBT in low-income populations: A usability and feasibility pilot study. *Professional Psychology: Research and Practice, 42*(6), 472–478. doi: 10.1037/a0025499

Barrett, M. S., Chua, W., Crits-Christoph, P., Gibbons, M. B., Casiano, D., and Thompson, D. (2008). Early withdrawal from mental health treatment: Implications for psychotherapy practice. *Psychotherapy (Chic), 45*(2), 247–267.

Becker, M. H., and Maiman, L. A. (1975). Sociobehavioral determinants of compliance with health and medical care recommendations. *Medical Care, 13*(1), 10–24.

Bordin, E. S. (1979). The generalizability of the psychoanalytic concept of the working alliance. *Psychotherapy: Theory, Research & Practice, 16*(3), 252–260. doi: 10.1037/h0085885.

Carr, A. (2009). The effectiveness of family therapy and systemic interventions for adult-focused problems. *Journal of Family Therapy, 31*(1), 46–74. doi: 10.1111/j.1467-6427.2008.00452.x.

Chu, B. C., Choudhury, M. S., Shortt, A. L., Pincus, D. B., Creed, T. A., and Kendall, P. C. (2004). Alliance, technology, and outcome in the treatment of anxious youth. *Cognitive and Behavioral Practice, 11*(1), 44–55. doi: 10.1016/S1077-7229(04)80006-3.

Clever, S. L., Ford, D. E., Rubenstein, L. V., Rost, K. M., Meredith, L. S., Sherbourne, C. D., . . . Cooper, L. A. (2006). Primary care patients' involvement in decision-making is associated with improvement in depression. *Medical Care, 44*(5), 398–405. doi: 10.1097/01.mlr.0000208117.15531.da

Clough, B. A., and Casey, L. M. (2011). Technological adjuncts to increase adherence to therapy: a review. *Clinical Psychology Review*, *31*(5), 697–710. doi: 10.1016/j.cpr.2011.03.006

Coe, A. B., Moczygemba, L.R., Gatewood, S.B., Osborn, R.D., Matzke, G.R., and Goode, J.V. (2012). Medication adherence challenges among patients experiencing homelessness in a behavioral health clinic. *Research in Social and Administrative Pharmacy*. Advance online publication. Retrieved from http://www-ncbi-nlm-nih-gov.ezproxy.rush.edu/pmc/articles/PMC3733792/pdf/nihms427755.pdf.

Comer, J. S., Furr, J. M., Cooper-Vince, C. E., Kerns, C. E., Chan, P. T., Edson, A. L., . . . Freeman, J. B. (2014). Internet-delivered, family-based treatment for early-onset OCD: A preliminary case series. *Journal of Clinical Child and Adolescent Psychology*, *43*(1), 74–87. doi: 10.1080/15374416.2013.855127.

Corrigan, P. (2004). How stigma interferes with mental health care. *American Psychologist*, *59*(7), 614–625. doi: 10.1037/0003-066x.59.7.614

Cox, D. J., Tisdelle, D. A., and Culbert, J. P. (1988). Increasing adherence to behavioral homework assignments. *Journal of Behavioral Medicine*, *11*(5), 519–522.

Diniz, J. B., Malavazzi, D. M., Fossaluza, V., Belotto-Silva, C., Borcato, S., Pimentel, I., . . . Shavitt, R. G. (2011). Risk factors for early treatment discontinuation in patients with obsessive-compulsive disorder. *Clinics (Sao Paulo)*, *66*(3), 387–393.

Dowd, S. M., and Janicak, P. G. (2009). *Integrating Psychological and Biological Therapies*. Wolters Kluwer Health/Lippincott Williams & Wilkins.

Foreman, K. F., Stockl, K. M., Le, L. B., Fisk, E., Shah, S. M., Lew, H. C., . . . Curtis, B. S. (2012). Impact of a text messaging pilot program on patient medication adherence. *Clinical Therapeutics*, *34*(5), 1084–1091. doi: 10.1016/j.clinthera.2012.04.007

Frangou, S., Sachpazidis, I., Stassinakis, A., and Sakas, G. (2005). Telemonitoring of Medication Adherence in Patients with Schizophrenia. *Telemedicine and e-Health*, *11*(6), 675–683.

Grilo, C. M., Money, R., Barlow, D. H., Goddard, A. W., Gorman, J. M., Hofmann, S. G., . . . Woods, S. W. (1998). Pretreatment patient factors predicting attrition from a multicenter randomized controlled treatment study for panic disorder. *Comprehensive Psychiatry*, *39*(6), 323–332.

Gunzburger, D. W., Henggeler, S. W., and Watson, S. M. (1985). Factors related to premature termination of counseling relationships. *Journal of College Student Personnel*, *26*(5), 456–460.

Hansen, A. M., Hoogduin, C. A., Schaap, C., and de Haan, E. (1992). Do drop-outs differ from successfully treated obsessive-compulsives? *Behaviour Research and Therapy*, *30*(5), 547–550.

Hayes, S. A., Hope, D. A., VanDyke, M. M., and Heimberg, R. G. (2007). Working alliance for clients with social anxiety disorder: Relationship with session helpfulness and within-session habituation. *Cognitive Behaviour Therapy*, *36*(1), 34–42.

Hollon, S. D., DeRubeis, R. J., Fawcett, J., Amsterdam, J. D., Shelton, R. C., Zajecka, J., . . . Gallop, R. (2014). Effect of Cognitive Therapy With Antidepressant Medications vs. Antidepressants Alone on the Rate of Recovery in Major Depressive Disorder: A Randomized Clinical Trial. *JAMA Psychiatry*, *71*(10), 1157–1164. doi: 10.1001/jamapsychiatry.2014.1054.

Hunot, V. M., Horne, R., Leese, M. N., and Churchill, R. C. (2007). A cohort study of adherence to antidepressants in primary care: the influence of antidepressant concerns and treatment preferences. *Primary Care Companion to the Journal of Clinical Psychiatry*, *9*(2), 91–99.

Huppert, J. D., Roth Ledley, D., and Foa, E. B. (2006). The use of homework in behavior therapy for anxiety disorders. *Journal of Psychotherapy Integration*, *16*(2), 128–139. doi: 10.1037/1053-0479.16.2.128.

Husain-Gambles, M., Neal, R. D., Dempsey, O., Lawlor, D. A., and Hodgson, J. (2004). Missed appointments in primary care: questionnaire and focus group study of health professionals. *British Journal of General Practice*, *54*(499), 108–113.

Interian, A., Lewis-Fernández, R., Gara, M. A., and Escobar, J. I. (2013). A randomized-controlled trial of an intervention to improve antidepressant adherence among Latinos with depression. *Depression and Anxiety*, *30*(7), 688–696. doi: 10.1002/da.22052

Issakidis, C., and Andrews, G. (2004). Pretreatment attrition and dropout in an outpatient clinic for anxiety disorders. *Acta Psychiatrica Scandinavica, 109*(6), 426–433. doi: 10.1111/j.1600-0047.200 4.00264.x

Julius, R. J., Novitsky, M. A., and Dubin, W. R. (2009). Medication adherence: a review of the literature and implications for clinical practice. *Journal of Psychiatric Practice, 15*(1), 34–44. doi: 10.1097/01. pra.0000344917.43780.77

Kardas, P., Lewek, P., and Matyjaszczyk, M. (2013). Determinants of patient adherence: a review of systematic reviews. *Frontiers in Pharmacology, 4*, 91. doi: 10.3389/fphar.2013.00091.

Keller, S. M., Zoellner, L. A., and Feeny, N. C. (2010). Understanding factors associated with early therapeutic alliance in PTSD treatment: Adherence, childhood sexual abuse history, and social support. *Journal of Consulting and Clinical Psychology, 78*(6), 974–979. doi: 10.1037/a0020758.

Levensky, E. R. (2006). Nonadherence to Treatment. In J.E. Fisher and W. O'Donohue (Eds.). *Practitioner's Guide to Evidence-Based Psychotherapy* (pp. 442–452). Springer.

Loh, A., Simon, D., Wills, C. E., Kriston, L., Niebling, W., and Härter, M. (2007). The effects of a shared decision-making intervention in primary care of depression: a cluster-randomized controlled trial. *Patient Education and Counseling, 67*(3), 324–332. doi: 10.1016/j.pec.2007.03.023

Lucas, G. M., Gratch, J., King, A., and Morency, L.-P. (2014). It's only a computer: Virtual humans increase willingness to disclose. *Computers in Human Behavior, 37*, 94–100. doi: 10.1016/j.chb.2014.04.043.

Maher, M. J., Wang, Y., Zuckoff, A., Wall, M. M., Franklin, M., Foa, E. B., and Simpson, H. B. (2012). Predictors of patient adherence to cognitive-behavioral therapy for obsessive-compulsive disorder. *Psychotherapy and Psychosomatics, 81*(2), 124–126. doi: 10.1159/000330214.

Maltby, N., and Tolin, D. F. (2005). A brief motivational intervention for treatment-refusing OCD patients. *Cognitive Behaviour Therapy, 34*(3), 176–184. doi: 10.1080/16506070510043741

Mancebo, M. C., Pinto, A., Rasmussen, S. A., and Eisen, J. L. (2008). Development of the Treatment Adherence Survey-patient version (TAS-P) for OCD. *Journal of Anxiety Disorders, 22*(1), 32–43. doi: 10.1016/j.janxdis.2007.01.009.

Martin, L. R., Williams, S. L., Haskard, K. B., and Dimatteo, M. R. (2005). The challenge of patient adherence. *Journal of Therapeutics and Clinical Risk Management, 1*(3), 189–199.

Miranda, J., Azocar, F., Organista, K. C., Dwyer, E., and Areane, P. (2003). Treatment of depression among impoverished primary care patients from ethnic minority groups. *Psychiatric Services, 54*(2), 219–225.

Mitchell, A. J., and Selmes, T. (2007). A comparative survey of missed initial and follow-up appointments to psychiatric specialties in the United kingdom. *Psychiatric Services, 58*(6), 868–871. doi: 10.1176/appi.ps.58.6.868

Mobile Technology Fact Sheet. Retrieved September 30, 2014, from http://www.pewinternet.org/fact-sheets/mobile-technology-fact-sheet/

Mukherjee, S., Sullivan, G., Perry, D., Verdugo, B., Means-Christensen, A., Schraufnagel, T., . . . Roy-Byrne, P. P. (2006). Adherence to treatment among economically disadvantaged patients with panic disorder. *Psychiatric Services, 57*(12), 1745–1750.

Newman, M. G., Szkodny, L. E., Llera, S. J., and Przeworski, A. (2011). A review of technology-assisted self-help and minimal contact therapies for anxiety and depression: Is human contact necessary for therapeutic efficacy? *Clinical Psychology Review, 31*(1), 89–103. doi: 10.1016/j.cpr.2010.09.008.

Prins, M. A., Verhaak, P. F., Bensing, J. M., and van der Meer, K. (2008). Health beliefs and perceived need for mental health care of anxiety and depression—the patients' perspective explored. *Clinical Psychology Review, 28*(6), 1038–1058. doi: 10.1016/j.cpr.2008.02.009

Prochaska, J. O., and DiClemente, C. C. (1992). Stages of change in the modification of problem behaviors. *Progress in Behavior Modification, 28*, 183–218.

Rainie, L., and Fox, S. (2012). Just-in-time information through mobile connections. *Pew Research Center's Internet x0026 American Life Project [Internet].*

Reger, G. M., Hoffman, J., Riggs, D., Rothbaum, B. O., Ruzek, J., Holloway, K. M., and Kuhn, E. (2013). The "PE coach" smartphone application: An innovative approach to improving implementation, fidelity, and homework adherence during prolonged exposure. *Psychological Services, 10*(3), 342–349. doi: 10.1037/a0032774.

Rokke, P. D., Tomhave, J. A., and Jocic, Z. (1999). The role of client choice and target selection in self-management therapy for depression in older adults. *Psychology and Aging, 14*(1), 155–169.

Santana, L., and Fontenelle, L. F. (2011). A review of studies concerning treatment adherence of patients with anxiety disorders. *Journal of Patient Preference and Adherence, 5*, 427–439. doi: 10.2147/ppa.s23439

Santana, L., Versiani, M., Mendlowicz, M. V., and Fontenelle, L. F. (2010). Predictors of adherence among patients with obsessive-compulsive disorder undergoing naturalistic pharmacotherapy. *Journal of Clinical Psychopharmacology, 30*(1), 86–88. doi: 10.1097/JCP.0b013e3181c8272a.

Sherman, M. D., Fischer, E., Bowling, U. B., Dixon, L., Ridener, L., and Harrison, D. (2009). A new engagement strategy in a VA-based family psychoeducation program. *Psychiatric Services, 60*(2), 254–257. doi: 10.1176/appi.ps.60.2.254.

Simpson, H. B., Maher, M. J., Wang, Y., Bao, Y., Foa, E. B., and Franklin, M. (2011). Patient adherence predicts outcome from cognitive behavioral therapy in obsessive-compulsive disorder. *Journal of Consulting and Clinical Psychology, 79*(2), 247–252. doi: 10.1037/a0022659

Sirey, J. A., Bruce, M. L., and Kales, H. C. (2010). Improving antidepressant adherence and depression outcomes in primary care: The Treatment Initiation and Participation (TIP) Program. *The American Journal of Geriatric Psychiatry, 18*(6), 554–562. doi: 10.1097/JGP.0b013e3181cdeb7d.

Slagle, D. M., and Gray, M. J. (2007). The utility of motivational interviewing as an adjunct to exposure therapy in the treatment of anxiety disorders. *Professional Psychology: Research and Practice, 38*(4), 329–337. doi: 10.1037/0735-7028.38.4.329.

Social Networking Fact Sheet. Retrieved September 30, 2014, from http://www.pewinternet.org/fact-sheets/social-networking-fact-sheet/

Soroudi, N., Perez, G. K., Gonzalez, J. S., Greer, J. A., Pollack, M. H., Otto, M. W., and Safren, S. A. (2008). CBT for medication adherence and depression (CBT-AD) in HIV-infected patients receiving methadone maintenance therapy. *Cognitive and Behavioral Practice, 15*(1), 93–106. doi: 10.1016/j.cbpra.2006.11.004.

Stein, M. B., Cantrell, C. R., Sokol, M. C., Eaddy, M. T., and Shah, M. B. (2006). Antidepressant adherence and medical resource use among managed care patients with anxiety disorders. *Psychiatric Services, 57*(5), 673–680. doi: 10.1176/appi.ps.57.5.673

Taylor, S., Abramowitz, J. S., and McKay, D. (2012). Non-adherence and non-response in the treatment of anxiety disorders. *Journal of Anxiety Disorders, 26*(5), 583–589. doi: 10.1016/j.janxdis.2012.02.010.

van Servellen, G., Heise, B. A., and Ellis, R. (2011). Factors associated with antidepressant medication adherence and adherence-enhancement programmes: a systematic literature review. *Mental Health in Family Medicine, 8*(4), 255–271.

Vergouwen, A. C., Bakker, A., Katon, W. J., Verheij, T. J., and Koerselman, F. (2003). Improving adherence to antidepressants: a systematic review of interventions. *Journal of Clinical Psychiatry, 64*(12), 1415–1420.

Vigne, P., de Menezes, G. B., Harrison, B. J., and Fontenelle, L. F. (2014). A study of poor insight in social anxiety disorder. *Psychiatry Research, 219*(3), 556–561. doi: 10.1016/j.psychres.2014.05.033.

Wagner, A. W., Bystritsky, A., Russo, J. E., Craske, M. G., Sherbourne, C. D., Stein, M. B., and Roy-Byrne, P. P. (2005). Beliefs about psychotropic medication and psychotherapy among primary care patients with anxiety disorders. *Depression and Anxiety, 21*(3), 99–105. doi: 10.1002/da.20067

Walitzer, K. S., Dermen, K. H., and Connors, G. J. (1999). Strategies for preparing clients for treatment. A review. *Behavior Modification, 23*(1), 129–151.

Westra, H. A., and Dozois, D. J. A. (2006). Preparing clients for cognitive behavioral therapy: A randomized pilot study of motivational interviewing for anxiety. *Cognitive Therapy and Research, 30*(4), 481–498. doi: 10.1007/s10608-006-9016-y.

White, K. S., Allen, L. B., Barlow, D. H., Gorman, J. M., Shear, M. K., and Woods, S. W. (2010). Attrition in a multicenter clinical trial for panic disorder. *Journal of Nervous and Mental Disease, 198*(9), 665–671. doi: 10.1097/NMD.0b013e3181ef3627.

Williams, M. V., Parker, R. M., Baker, D. W., Parikh, N. S., Pitkin, K., Coates, W. C., and Nurss, J. R. (1995). Inadequate functional health literacy among patients at two public hospitals. *JAMA*, 274(21), 1677–1682. doi:10.1001/jama.1995.03530210031026.

World Health Organization. (2003). Adherence to long-term therapies: evidence for action. Switzerland: World Health Organization.

Zayfert, C., and Black, C. (2000). Implementation of empirically supported treatment for PTSD: Obstacles and innovations. *The Behavior Therapist*, 23(8), 161–168.

Zullig, L. L., Peterson, E. D., and Bosworth, H. B. (2013). Ingredients of successful interventions to improve medication adherence. *JAMA*, 310(24), 2611–2612. doi:10.1001/jama.2013.282818.

31

COMPUTER TOOLS AS NOVEL
TREATMENT FOR DEPRESSION
AND ANXIETY

ANETT GYURAK AND AMIT ETKIN

INTRODUCTION

The past two decades generated important insights into the neurobiological and information processing deficits of depression and anxiety. However, this work has so far failed to
generate a broad staple of novel, widely applicable therapies. Recent work on the malle-
ability of these processes and the plasticity of the brain network that underlie these processing deficits shows promise for developing therapeutic interventions that are rooted in
our neurobiological understanding of mood and anxiety disorders.

Patients with depression or anxiety manifest deficits in executive functions such
as task switching, working memory, and sustained attention (Castaneda, Tuulio-
Henriksson, Marttunen, Suvisaari, and Lönnqvist, 2008; Etkin, Gyurak, and O'Hara,
2013; Snyder, 2013). Similarly, biased processing also manifests in attention to and
memory for emotional stimuli (MacLeod, Mathews, and Tata, 1986; Mathews and
MacLeod, 2005). These perturbations reflect dysfunction in distributed brain regions
that function as part of networks encompassing prefrontal, parietal, and medial temporal regions (Figure 31.1). Brain imaging research quantifies the relationships among
these networks. For example, activation in the default mode network (dark grey in
Figure 31.1) is reduced to support executive functions changes activation in the fronto-
parietal executive control networks (light grey in Figure 31.1) to allow successful executive function (Dosenbach et al., 2007). Particularly important interactions occur in
networks supporting executive control and processing of emotional stimuli, including
the dorsal anterior cingulate cortex (dACC) and bilateral insulae (Browning, Holmes,
Murphy, Goodwin, and Harmer, 2010 medium grey in Figure 31.1). Recent meta-analyses
establish the way in which functioning in these networks relates to depression (Graham
et al., 2013; Hamilton et al., 2012) and anxiety (Sylvester et al., 2012). Deficiencies in
networks supporting attention appear particularly well replicated (Bijsterbosch, Smith,
Forster, John, and Bishop, 2013; Etkin, Prater, Schatzberg, Menon, and Greicius, 2009;
Seeley et al., 2007; Sylvester et al., 2012).

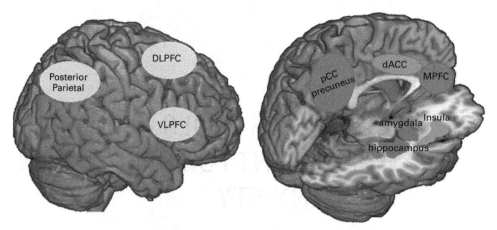

FIGURE 31.1 Neural networks with documented deficits in depression and anxiety. *Light grey:* fronto-parietal executive control network. DLPF = dorsolateral prefrontol cortex, VLPC = ventrolateral prefrontal cortex; *Medium grey:* limbic salience network. dACC = dorsal anterior cingulate cortex; *Dark grey:* default mode network. pCC = posterior cingulate cortex, MPFC = medial prefrontal cortex.

This work suggests that interactions between cognitive and affect-related brain networks support shared features of anxiety and depression (Etkin et al., 2013; Menon, 2011). Current, widely available interventions do not systematically target these networks (Insel, 2014), despite the recognized importance of doing so (National Institutes of Health Blueprint for Neuroscience Research focused on neuroplasticity in 2009; the National Institute of Mental Health sponsored Cognitive Training in Mental Disorders: Advancing the Science workshop in 2012). The current chapter reviews how computerized training might target cognitive and affect dysfunction in anxiety and depression with a focus on challenges and research gaps to be addressed in future work.

BASIC NEUROSCIENCE FOUNDATION OF NEUROPLASTICITY

Plasticity at the broadest level can range from molecular to cellular to brain circuits to behavior (Buonomano and Merzenich, 1998). Plasticity occurs in many contexts, including during normal development (Neville and Bavelier, 2002), in response to environmental changes, during learning, and in response to disease. It also can be harnessed in therapeutic interventions. Interventions targeting brain plasticity have a long history in medicine. This includes interventions deployed following neurological disorders such as stroke and traumatic brain injury as well as in the retraining language and motor functions (Nudo, 2006). This work shows that behavioral training impacts adaptive plasticity after brain injury (Cramer et al., 2011).

Plasticity is not just relevant to injured brains. Recent research examines plasticity after targeted training at the neural networks level in neurologically and physically intact brains as well. To foster neuroplasticity and facilitate transfer to untrained general domains, recent work suggests that training tasks need to meet three critical features (Anguera et al., 2013; Klingberg, 2010; Vinogradov, Fisher, and de Villers-Sidani, 2012): (1) extensive: training needs to focus on general functional abilities as opposed to simple, narrow skills; (2) targeted: training tasks have to engage the target function; and (3) adaptive: training tasks need to adjust continuously forward or backward for participants' performance to keep the participants engaged at their optimal level of difficulty in order to maximize the potential for new learning. Studies using these principles document volumetric changes in the cortex after learning new skills such as juggling (Draganski et al., 2004) or memorizing detailed spatial maps in taxi drivers (Maguire et al., 2000 and see Zatorre, Fields, and Johansen-Berg, 2012 for a review).

Beyond changing brain volume, research shows that training can induce functional level reorganization in brain networks in healthy participants. Most such work targets cognitive executive control functions that allow humans to keep information in mind and that can influence emotions (Gyurak et al., 2009). Some research suggests that computerized training enhances multitasking abilities in older adults (Anguera et al., 2013). These changes were associated with changes in frontal cortex activation as measured by electroencephalography and perfusion (Buschkuehl, Jaeggi, and Jonides, 2012). Other research suggests that such training might improve executive attention and associated brain functions in children (Rueda, Rothbart, McCandliss, Saccomanno, and Posner, 2005). A third set of studies suggest that working memory changes following targeted training relate to changes in fronto-parietal executive control network (Buschkuehl, Jaeggi, and Jonides, 2012; Olesen, Westerberg, and Klingberg, 2004; Westerberg and Klingberg, 2007).

More recently, studies have begun to investigate the effects of computerized training in affective domains among healthy individuals. A series of studies suggest that such training influences attention to emotionally salient information. Specifically, Dandeneau and Baldwin (2009) found that training attention away from threat using a visual search task attenuated feelings of rejection elicited in a social interaction. This training required participants to look for positive faces in a matrix of negative/frowning faces. Another study using the same paradigm among telemarketers (Dandeneau, Baldwin, Baccus, Sakellaropoulo, and Pruessner, 2007) found increased self-esteem and reduced perceived stress along with lower cortisol release and cortisol reactivity in a simulated social interaction designed to induce negative affect. A third study found the training to reduce anxiety in children (Waters et al., 2013).

Considerable research in this area focuses on the training of attention. Much of this work relies on the dot probe task, which requires the subject to repeatedly identify a small probe that appears in the same spatial location as an emotionally laden or neutral stimulus. The most consistent finding with this paradigm demonstrates successful training of affective bias away from threat to neutral stimuli. Browning and colleagues found that such training altered functioning in fronto-parietal executive control networks in healthy individuals (Browning, Holmes, Murphy, et al., 2010). Other work trains attention in the context of working memory tasks. For example, following the training of working memory, Schweizer and colleagues (Schweizer, Grahn, Hampshire, Mobbs, and Dalgleish, 2013) found improvements in behavioral markers of affect regulatory ability and frontal networks previously implicated in emotion regulation. Taken together, this relatively broad series of studies shows that training induces plasticity, reflected in behavioral and neural-level changes in healthy individuals.

BEHAVIORAL TRAINING IN PATIENT POPULATIONS

Research during the past ten years has begun to extend this work to patients with mental illnesses (Vinogradov et al., 2012). These approaches applied finely targeted methods and matched training to documented deficits of the disorders.

For example, in children with attention deficit disorder, Klingberg and colleagues found that intensive computerized working memory training improved executive functions and parent-rated symptoms (Klingberg et al., 2005). Nevertheless, these findings have not consistently emerged in subsequent research (Sonuga-Barke, Brandeis, Holtmann, and Cortese, 2014). Applying a similar approach in schizophrenia, Vinogradov and colleagues demonstrated that computerized sensory discrimination training improved verbal memory and brain responses in auditory and prefrontal cortex. Most importantly, these gains were positively associated with quality of life six months later (Dale et al., 2010; Fisher, Holland, Merzenich, and Vinogradov, 2009). Bell, Bryson, Greig, Corcoran, and Wexler (2001) showed that the training results in improved functional outcomes in this population with serious mental disorders. Another study found that a similar training regimen produced improvements in behavioral performance of reality monitoring and related neural functions (Subramaniam et al., 2012) and working memory performance with corresponding functional changes six-months after the intervention (Subramaniam et al., 2014).

BEHAVIORAL TRAINING IN ANXIETY AND DEPRESSION

Collectively, these findings provide a foundation for other computerized training approaches, targeting an array of psychiatric disorders. Such training might have clinical utility by changing symptoms. Moreover, these clinically relevant changes also might be linked to changes in brain networks, providing insights on the mechanisms that producing clinically meaningful changes.

In the area of anxiety and depression, work finds relationships among computerized training, changes in symptoms, and changes in brain networks. For example, training affective functions, through interventions that target attention bias using a dot-probe paradigm, may change attention, symptoms, and brain function (for a review see Browning, Holmes, and Harmer, 2010). These interventions were developed following consistent observations linking attention biases to individual differences in anxiety, which raised questions about the causal nature of associations between attention biases and anxiety (Mathews and MacLeod, 2005). Over one hundred studies have been conducted on this topic (for reviews see: Browning, Holmes, and Harmer, 2010; Hallion and Ruscio, 2011; Colin MacLeod and Mathews, 2012). Notably, one study found reduced remission rates among previously depressed adults (Browning, Holmes, Charles, Cowen, and Harmer, 2012) and another documented improved social anxiety symptoms during emotional challenge among those with social anxiety (Amir, Weber, Beard, Bomyea, and Taylor, 2008). Similar approaches have been used in children with pediatric anxiety disorders. Some studies find no differences in anxiety symptoms among children randomized to active as opposed to controlled computer-training regimens (Britton et al., 2013), whereas other studies have found greater improvements in the active training condition (Eldar et al., 2011). Overall, these interventions show promise (Browning, Holmes, and Harmer, 2010), although one meta-analytic study indicated that anxiety might be more effectively targeted by these interventions than depression (Hallion and Ruscio, 2011). There is a trend that newer studies are showing smaller effects than earlier studies, consistent with the wider adoption of these techniques.

As opposed to training targeting attention, treatments that target other information-processing functions have a less substantial research foundation, despite widespread documented deficits in cognitive executive functions in both anxiety and depression. To our knowledge, there is one study, to date, that documented improvements in neural markers of affective reactivity and depression symptoms after using a combination of an auditory discrimination task aimed at training sustained attention and a serial arithmetic training task aimed at reducing frustration tolerance as adjuncts to treatment as usual in depressed patients (Siegle, Ghinassi, and Thase, 2007).

TOWARD A CIRCUIT-BASED COGNITIVE-AFFECTIVE REMEDIATION TRAINING IN ANXIETY AND DEPRESSION

Brain imaging research demonstrates perturbations in networks that link cognitive and affective functions. As such, promising approaches might involve computerized tasks that combine cognitive and affective components. As in research on attention, such cognitive-affective remediation training research also could occur in tandem with brain imaging research. This research could assess functioning in three brain networks that support specific cognitive-affective operations: the fronto-parietal executive, the default mode, and the salience networks (see Figure 31.1). In order to facilitate plasticity, such computerized training tasks might incorporate the three critical features of other successful training approaches. Specifically, training tasks should be: (1) extensive: train multiple cognitive and affective functions, (2) targeted: they will need to be derived based on the understanding of the disorders and aimed to engage deficient cognitive and affective functions and the supporting circuitry, and (3) adaptive: they need to adjust to the participants' performance level. Based on existing literature in anxiety and depression, it would be necessary to train domains of executive cognitive functions through several exercises such as working memory, set-shifting and focused sustained attention. The affective functions trained would need to include emotion bias training, preferably across multiple visual and verbal domains. Outcomes of this training would be behavioral markers of cognitive (e.g., inhibition, task-shifting and working memory tasks) and affective functions (e.g., emotion labeling, emotion bias tasks), neural markers of cognitive executive and affective network functions (resting state connectivity and functional tasks) in addition to symptoms and well-being. Target engagement during the training (e.g., learning during the intervention) could be related to these outcomes to validate the effects of the intervention. Development and validation of such a protocol is the necessary next step in developing a viable circuit-based intervention for anxiety and depression.

SUMMARY: WHAT CAN COMPUTERIZED COGNITIVE-AFFECTIVE REMEDIATION TRAINING ACCOMPLISH?

Despite the high prevalence of depressive disorders, most affected individuals do not seek treatment (Kendler, 1995). Even for those who do get treatment, existing interventions provide lasting remission in a minority of patients (Nelson, 2006), particularly in the presence of comorbid anxiety (Fava et al., 2008). This demonstrates the need for scalable, effective treatments. Overcoming both the treatment effectiveness and the treatment access/acceptance and barriers require an intervention that can effectively engage a wide spectrum of individuals without invoking stigma. Behavioral trainings may offer such methods, but these efforts are in their infancy, and much more work is needed. Such work might be encouraged, given the potential to answer several key questions, both at the basic science level and for clinical care.

1. Behavioral training protocols leverage neuroscience understanding to target dysfunctional neural circuitry in anxiety and depression. The extent to which the training *causally* changes these functions will shape our understanding of these

disorders, allowing interventions to serve as experiments evaluating theory as they provide tests of efficacy. As a causal intervention, this provides a powerful, controlled way of linking changes in the functioning of brain networks to symptoms. For example, if results show that behavioral readouts during training causally influence brain function and symptoms following training, then the findings would confirm neuroscientific views of disorders (Etkin et al., 2013).

2. Behavioral training evaluates relations between cognition and affect, a long-standing topic in psychology and neuroscience (e.g., Blair et al., 2007; Chiew and Braver, 2011; Egner et al., 2008). Clearly, cognitive and affective processes frequently interact in both health and psychopathology. Behavioral remediation training offers a controlled way of addressing how changes in cognition drive changes in affect and vice versa.

3. Behavioral training sheds light on plasticity. Adjunct therapies, such as pharmacological agents and exogenous electrical stimulation such as transcranial magnetic stimulation, may provide a more receptive environment through which the efficacy of behavioral training would improve. In addition, recent research on new language acquisition shows that fully developed cognitive control in adults might hinder acquisition of more implicit aspects of language learning (Finn, Lee, Kraus, and Hudson Kam, 2014). To alter behaviorally more implicit forms of affective and social skill learning thus might require specific approaches that engage relevant circuits and bypass cognitive effort. Finally, different developmental trajectories of different brain networks (Gogtay et al., 2004) might keep windows of opportunities open for cognitive and affective networks. First episode of depression is usually reported in late adolescents and early adulthood when the development of frontal lobes that govern executive control are still underway (Beesdo, Knappe, and Pine, 2009). This opportunity of plasticity on top of developmental plasticity might require adjusting current interventions and could offer a great interventional opportunity for preventing the development of anxiety disorders and depression.

4. Behavioral training affords a scalable, easily accessible method of treatment. With the advances in Internet delivery and technological innovations in web application framework programming, it is now possible to deliver highly engaging graphical interfaces that can achieve millisecond precision reaction time recordings allowing for adaptive exercises to be delivered online to anyone with a computer and broadband Internet connection. Further research is needed to understand the baseline moderators of treatment response (e.g., baseline cognitive executive functioning, baseline affective biases). With knowledge of these moderators, tasks can be further personalized and targeted based on patients' needs. Our current treatment modalities afford this level of personalization only in intensive in-person settings at the clinic.

CLOSING COMMENTS

The brain is not a passive organism, rather it actively reorganizes and adjusts based on incoming input and anticipated outcomes. Viewed this way, many of the current methods used in clinical practice engage processes of plasticity. Early childhood behavioral interventions promoting cognitive control and self-regulatory skills have proven to be remarkably effective in improving school grades, affect regulation, and intelligence (Bryck and Fisher, 2011; Diamond, Barnett, Thomas, and Munro, 2007). Cognitive behavioral therapy (Goldin et al., 2013) and mindfulness-based interventions (Allen et al., 2012), two evidence-based therapeutic modalities, both alter cognitive and affective circuitry. As such, psychiatry research has been engaging in behavioral interventions that foster neural-circuit plasticity for a long time. However, recent advances in understanding psychiatric disorders as disorders of brain network opened up a new frontier in creating more precisely targeted behavioral interventions. In addition, advances in computerized technology and Internet delivery methods now offer a way of creating a defined and constrained learning environment to engage the brain in a targeted way. We are at a point where we can engineer highly targeted training programs that drive precise functional and symptom level changes in psychiatric disorders, specifically tailored to the deficient functions. The work is just emerging and its future success will depend on advancing the basic science understanding of these therapeutic approaches to improve their efficacy.

ACKNOWLEDGMENTS

Writing of this manuscript was supported by the Office of Academic Affiliations, Advanced Fellowship Program in Mental Illness Research and Treatment, Department of Veterans Affairs for AG and by NIH F32 MH 86261 awarded to AG and R21 MH097984 to AE. The ideas and the research discussed here greatly benefited from productive scholarly discussions with Drs. James Gross, Ozlem Ayduk, Ruth O'Hara, and Leanne Williams, for which we are grateful.

REFERENCES

Allen, M., Dietz, M., Blair, K. S., van Beek, M., Rees, G., Vestergaard-Poulsen, P., . . . Roepstorff, A. (2012). Cognitive-affective neural plasticity following active-controlled mindfulness intervention. *The Journal of Neuroscience: The Official Journal of the Society for Neuroscience, 32*(44), 15601–15610. doi:10.1523/JNEUROSCI.2957-12.2012

Amir, N., Weber, G., Beard, C., Bomyea, J., and Taylor, C. T. (2008). The effect of a single-session attention modification program on response to a public-speaking challenge in socially anxious individuals. *Journal of Abnormal Psychology, 117*(4), 860–868. doi:10.1037/a0013445.

Anguera, J. A., Boccanfuso, J., Rintoul, J. L., Al-Hashimi, O., Faraji, F., Janowich, J., . . . Gazzaley, A. (2013). Video game training enhances cognitive control in older adults. *Nature, 501*(7465), 97–101. doi:10.1038/nature12486

Beesdo, K., Knappe, S., and Pine, D. S. (2009). Anxiety and anxiety disorders in children and adolescents: Developmental issues and implications for DSM-V. *The Psychiatric Clinics of North America, 32*(3), 483–524. doi:10.1016/j.psc.2009.06.002

Bell, M., Bryson, G., Greig, T., Corcoran, C., and Wexler, B. E. (2001). Neurocognitive enhancement therapy with work therapy: Effects on neuropsychological test performance. *Archives of General Psychiatry, 58*(8), 763–768.

Bijsterbosch, J., Smith, S., Forster, S., John, O. P., and Bishop, S. J. (2013). Resting state correlates of subdimensions of anxious affect. *Journal of Cognitive Neuroscience*, 1–13. doi:10.1162/jocn_a_00512

Blair, K. S., Smith, B. W., Mitchell, D. G. V., Morton, J., Vythilingam, M., Pessoa, L., . . . Blair, R. J. R. (2007). Modulation of emotion by cognition and cognition by emotion. *NeuroImage, 35*(1), 430–440. doi:10.1016/j.neuroimage.2006.11.048

Britton, J. C., Bar-Haim, Y., Clementi, M. A., Sankin, L. S., Chen, G., Shechner, T., . . . Pine, D. S. (2013). Training-associated changes and stability of attention bias in youth: Implications for attention bias modification treatment for pediatric anxiety. *Developmental Cognitive Neuroscience, 4*, 52–64. doi:10.1016/j.dcn.2012.11.001

Browning, M., Holmes, E. A., and Harmer, C. J. (2010). The modification of attentional bias to emotional information: A review of the techniques, mechanisms, and relevance to emotional disorders. *Cognitive, Affective & Behavioral Neuroscience, 10*(1), 8–20. doi:10.3758/CABN.10.1.8

Browning, M., Holmes, E. A., Charles, M., Cowen, P. J., and Harmer, C. J. (2012). Using attentional bias modification as a cognitive vaccine against depression. *Biological Psychiatry, 72*(7), 572–579. doi:10.1016/j.biopsych.2012.04.014

Browning, M., Holmes, E. A., Murphy, S. E., Goodwin, G. M., and Harmer, C. J. (2010). Lateral prefrontal cortex mediates the cognitive modification of attentional bias. *Biological Psychiatry, 67*(10), 919–925. doi:10.1016/j.biopsych.2009.10.031

Bryck, R. L., and Fisher, P. A. (2011). Training the brain: Practical applications of neural plasticity from the intersection of cognitive neuroscience, developmental psychology, and prevention science. *The American Psychologist, 67*(2), 87–100. doi:10.1037/a0024657

Buonomano, D. V., and Merzenich, M. M. (1998). Cortical plasticity: from synapses to maps. *Annual Review of Neuroscience, 21*, 149–186. doi:10.1146/annurev.neuro.21.1.149

Buschkuehl, M., Jaeggi, S. M., and Jonides, J. (2012). Neuronal effects following working memory training. *Developmental Cognitive Neuroscience, 2 Suppl 1*, S167–179. doi:10.1016/j.dcn.2011.10.001

Castaneda, A. E., Tuulio-Henriksson, A., Marttunen, M., Suvisaari, J., and Lönnqvist, J. (2008). A review on cognitive impairments in depressive and anxiety disorders with a focus on young adults. *Journal of Affective Disorders, 106*(1–2), 1–27. doi:10.1016/j.jad.2007.06.006

Chiew, K. S., and Braver, T. S. (2011). Positive affect versus reward: emotional and motivational influences on cognitive control. *Frontiers in Psychology, 2*, 279. doi:10.3389/fpsyg.2011.00279

Cramer, S. C., Sur, M., Dobkin, B. H., O'Brien, C., Sanger, T. D., Trojanowski, J. Q., . . . Vinogradov, S. (2011). Harnessing neuroplasticity for clinical applications. *Brain, 134*, 1591–1609.

Dale, C. L., Findlay, A. M., Adcock, R. A., Vertinski, M., Fisher, M., Genevsky, A., . . . Vinogradov, S. (2010). Timing is everything: neural response dynamics during syllable processing and its relation to higher-order cognition in schizophrenia and healthy comparison subjects. *International Journal of Psychophysiology: Official Journal of the International Organization of Psychophysiology, 75*(2), 183–193. doi:10.1016/j.ijpsycho.2009.10.009

Dandeneau, S. D., and Baldwin, M. W. (2009). The buffering effects of rejection-inhibiting attentional training on social and performance threat among adult students. *Contemporary Educational Psychology, 34*(1), 42–50. doi:10.1016/j.cedpsych.2008.05.004.

Dandeneau, S. D., Baldwin, M. W., Baccus, J. R., Sakellaropoulo, M., and Pruessner, J. C. (2007). Cutting stress off at the pass: reducing vigilance and responsiveness to social threat by manipulating attention. *Journal of Personality and Social Psychology, 93*(4), 651–666. doi:10.1037/0022-3514.93.4.651

Diamond, A., Barnett, W. S., Thomas, J., and Munro, S. (2007). Preschool Program Improves Cognitive Control. *Science, 318*(5855), 1387–1388. doi:10.1126/science.1151148

Dosenbach, N. U. F., Fair, D. A., Miezin, F. M., Cohen, A. L., Wenger, K. K., Dosenbach, R. A. T., . . . Petersen, S. E. (2007). Distinct brain networks for adaptive and stable task control in humans. *Proceedings of the National Academy of Sciences of the United States of America, 104*(26), 11073–11078. doi:10.1073/pnas.0704320104

Draganski, B., Gaser, C., Busch, V., Schuierer, G., Bogdahn, U., and May, A. (2004). Neuroplasticity: Changes in grey matter induced by training. *Nature, 427*(6972), 311–312. doi:10.1038/427311a

Egner, T., Etkin, A., Gale, S., and Hirsch, J. (2008). Dissociable neural systems resolve conflict from emotional versus nonemotional distracters. *Cerebral Cortex (New York, N.Y.: 1991), 18*(6), 1475–1484. doi:10.1093/cercor/bhm179

Eldar, S., Apter, A., Lotan, D., Edgar, K. P., Naim, R., Fox, N. A., . . . Bar-Haim, Y. (2011). Attention bias modification treatment for pediatric anxiety disorders: A randomized controlled trial. Retrieved from http://www.ncbi.nlm.nih.gov/pubmed/22193536

Etkin, A., Gyurak, A., and O'Hara, R. (2013). A neurobiological approach to the cognitive deficits of psychiatric disorders. *Dialogues in Clinical Neuroscience, 15*(4), 419–429.

Etkin, A., Prater, K. E., Schatzberg, A. F., Menon, V., and Greicius, M. D. (2009). Disrupted amygdalar sub-region functional connectivity and evidence of a compensatory network in generalized anxiety disorder. *Archives of General Psychiatry*, 66(12), 1361–1372. doi:10.1001/archgenpsychiatry.2009.104

Fava, M., Rush, A. J., Alpert, J. E., Balasubramani, G. K., Wisniewski, S. R., Carmin, C. N., . . . Trivedi, M. H. (2008). Difference in treatment outcome in outpatients with anxious versus nonanxious depression: a STAR*D report. *The American Journal of Psychiatry*, 165(3), 342–351. doi:10.1176/appi.ajp.2007.06111868

Finn, A. S., Lee, T., Kraus, A., and Hudson Kam, C. L. (2014). When it hurts (and helps) to try: The role of effort in language learning. *PLoS ONE*, 9(7), e101806. doi:10.1371/journal.pone.0101806

Fisher, M., Holland, C., Merzenich, M. M., and Vinogradov, S. (2009). Using neuroplasticity-based auditory training to improve verbal memory in schizophrenia. *The American Journal of Psychiatry*, 166(7), 805–811. doi:10.1176/appi.ajp.2009.08050757

Gogtay, N., Giedd, J. N., Lusk, L., Hayashi, K. M., Greenstein, D., Vaituzis, A. C., . . . Thompson, P. M. (2004). Dynamic mapping of human cortical development during childhood through early adulthood. *Proceedings of the National Academy of Sciences of the United States of America*, 101(21), 8174–8179. doi:10.1073/pnas.0402680101

Goldin, P. R., Ziv, M., Jazaieri, H., Hahn, K., Heimberg, R., and Gross, J. J. (2013). Impact of cognitive behavioral therapy for social anxiety disorder on the neural dynamics of cognitive reappraisal of negative self-beliefs: Randomized clinical trial. *JAMA Psychiatry*, 70(10), 1048–1056. doi:10.1001/jamapsychiatry.2013.234

Graham, J., Salimi-Khorshidi, G., Hagan, C., Walsh, N., Goodyer, I., Lennox, B., and Suckling, J. (2013). Meta-analytic evidence for neuroimaging models of depression: state or trait? *Journal of Affective Disorders*, 151(2), 423–431. doi:10.1016/j.jad.2013.07.002

Gyurak, A., Goodkind, M. S., Madan, A., Kramer, J. H., Miller, B. L., and Levenson, R. W. (2009). Do tests of executive functioning predict ability to downregulate emotions spontaneously and when instructed to suppress? *Cognitive, Affective and Behavioral Neuroscience*, 144–152.

Hallion, L. S., and Ruscio, A. M. (2011). A meta-analysis of the effect of cognitive bias modification on anxiety and depression. *Psychological Bulletin*, 137(6), 940–958. doi:10.1037/a0024355

Hamilton, J. P., Etkin, A., Furman, D. J., Lemus, M. G., Johnson, R. F., and Gotlib, I. H. (2012). Functional neuroimaging of major depressive disorder: A meta-analysis and new integration of base line activation and neural response data. *The American Journal of Psychiatry*, 169(7), 693–703. doi:10.1176/appi.ajp.2012.11071105

Insel, T. R. (2014). The NIMH Research Domain Criteria (RDoC) Project: Precision Medicine for Psychiatry. *American Journal of Psychiatry*, 171(4), 395–397. doi:10.1176/appi.ajp.2014.14020138

Kendler, K. S. (1995). Is seeking treatment for depression predicted by a history of depression in relatives? Implications for family studies of affective disorder. *Psychological Medicine*, 25(4), 807–814.

Klingberg, T. (2010). Training and plasticity of working memory. *Trends in Cognitive Sciences*, 14(7), 317–324. doi:10.1016/j.tics.2010.05.002

Klingberg, T., Fernell, E., Olesen, P. J., Johnson, M., Gustafsson, P., Dahlström, K., . . . Westerberg, H. (2005). Computerized Training of Working Memory in Children With ADHD-A Randomized, Controlled Trial. *Journal of the American Academy of Child and Adolescent Psychiatry*, 44(2), 177–186. doi:10.1097/00004583-200502000-00010

MacLeod, C., and Mathews, A. (2012). Cognitive bias modification approaches to anxiety. *Annual Review of Clinical Psychology*, 8, 189–217. doi:10.1146/annurev-clinpsy-032511-143052

Maguire, E. A., Gadian, D. G., Johnsrude, I. S., Good, C. D., Ashburner, J., Frackowiak, R. S., and Frith, C. D. (2000). Navigation-related structural change in the hippocampi of taxi drivers. *Proceedings of the National Academy of Sciences of the United States of America*, 97(8), 4398–4403. doi:10.1073/pnas.070039597

Mathews, A., and MacLeod, C. (2005). Cognitive vulnerability to emotional disorders. *Annual Review of Clinical Psychology*, 1, 167–195. doi:10.1146/annurev.clinpsy.1.102803.143916

Menon, V. (2011). Large-scale brain networks and psychopathology: a unifying triple network model. *Trends in Cognitive Sciences, 15*(10), 483–506. doi:10.1016/j.tics.2011.08.003

Nelson, J. C. (2006). The STAR*D Study: A Four-Course Meal That Leaves Us Wanting More. *Am J Psychiatry, 163*(11), 1864–1866. doi:10.1176/appi.ajp.163.11.1864

Neville, H., and Bavelier, D. (2002). Human brain plasticity: Evidence from sensory deprivation and altered language experience. *Progress in Brain Research, 138,* 177–188. doi:10.1016/S0079-6123(02)38078-6

Nudo, R. J. (2006). Plasticity. *NeuroRX, 3*(4), 420–427. doi:10.1016/j.nurx.2006.07.006

Olesen, P. J., Westerberg, H., and Klingberg, T. (2004). Increased prefrontal and parietal activity after training of working memory. *Nature Neuroscience, 7*(1), 75–79. doi:10.1038/nn1165

Rueda, M. R., Rothbart, M. K., McCandliss, B. D., Saccomanno, L., and Posner, M. I. (2005). Training, maturation, and genetic influences on the development of executive attention. *Proceedings of the National Academy of Sciences of the United States of America, 102*(41), 14931–14936. doi:10.1073/pnas.0506897102

Schweizer, S., Grahn, J., Hampshire, A., Mobbs, D., and Dalgleish, T. (2013). Training the emotional brain: improving affective control through emotional working memory training. *The Journal of Neuroscience: The Official Journal of the Society for Neuroscience, 33*(12), 5301–5311. doi:10.1523/JNEUROSCI.2593-12.2013

Seeley, W. W., Menon, V., Schatzberg, A. F., Keller, J., Glover, G. H., Kenna, H.,. . . Greicius, M. D. (2007). Dissociable intrinsic connectivity networks for salience processing and executive control. *The Journal of Neuroscience: The Official Journal of the Society for Neuroscience, 27*(9), 2349–2356. doi:10.1523/JNEUROSCI.5587-06.2007

Siegle, G. J., Ghinassi, F., and Thase, M. E. (2007). Neurobehavioral therapies in the 21st century: Summary of an emerging field and an extended example of cognitive control training for depression. *Cognitive Therapy and Research, 31*(2), 235–262. doi:10.1007/s10608-006-9118-6.

Snyder, H. R. (2013). Major depressive disorder is associated with broad impairments on neuropsychological measures of executive function: a meta-analysis and review. *Psychological Bulletin, 139*(1), 81–132. doi:10.1037/a0028727

Sonuga-Barke, E., Brandeis, D., Holtmann, M., and Cortese, S. (2014). Computer-based cognitive training for ADHD: A review of current evidence. *Child and Adolescent Psychiatric Clinics of North America, 23*(4), 807–824. doi:10.1016/j.chc.2014.05.009

Subramaniam, K., Luks, T. L., Fisher, M., Simpson, G. V., Nagarajan, S., and Vinogradov, S. (2012). Computerized cognitive training restores neural activity within the reality monitoring network in schizophrenia. *Neuron, 73*(4), 842–853. doi:10.1016/j.neuron.2011.12.024

Subramaniam, K., Luks, T. L., Garrett, C., Chung, C., Fisher, M., Nagarajan, S., and Vinogradov, S. (2014). Intensive cognitive training in schizophrenia enhances working memory and associated prefrontal cortical efficiency in a manner that drives long-term functional gains. *NeuroImage.* doi:10.1016/j.neuroimage.2014.05.057

Sylvester, C. M., Corbetta, M., Raichle, M. E., Rodebaugh, T. L., Schlaggar, B. L., Sheline, Y. I., . . . Lenze, E. J. (2012). Functional network dysfunction in anxiety and anxiety disorders. *Trends in Neurosciences, 35*(9), 527–535. doi:10.1016/j.tins.2012.04.012

Vinogradov, S., Fisher, M., and de Villers-Sidani, E. (2012). Cognitive training for impaired neural systems in neuropsychiatric illness. *Neuropsychopharmacology: Official Publication of the American College of Neuropsychopharmacology, 37*(1), 43–76. doi:10.1038/npp.2011.251

Waters, A. M., Pittaway, M., Mogg, K., Bradley, B. P., and Pine, D. S. (2013). Attention training towards positive stimuli in clinically anxious children. *Developmental Cognitive Neuroscience, 4,* 77–84. doi:10.1016/j.dcn.2012.09.004

Westerberg, H., and Klingberg, T. (2007). Changes in cortical activity after training of working memory—a single-subject analysis. *Physiology & Behavior, 92*(1–2), 186–192. doi:10.1016/j.physbeh.2007.05.041

32

INTERNET-BASED TREATMENT FOR ANXIETY AND OBSESSIVE-COMPULSIVE AND RELATED DISORDERS

CHRISTIAN RÜCK, ERIK ANDERSSON, AND ERIK HEDMAN

INTRODUCTION

Cognitive behavior therapy (CBT) for anxiety and obsessive-compulsive and related disorders has shown large effects in numerous clinical trials, and it is often recommended as first line treatment for several disorders. However, despite strong evidence in terms of efficacy, most patients do not receive the treatment they need. Some possible barriers for this include too few trained CBT therapists (Mataix-Cols and Marks, 2006); financial, practical, and logistic problems related to treatment-seeking; and embarrassment due to symptoms (B. M. Wootton, Titov, Dear, Spence, and Kemp, 2011). These barriers have prompted the development of multiple strategies to increase access to CBT, including bibliotherapy self-help, telephone-based interventions, and various computer-aided interventions. This chapter focuses on Internet-based cognitive behavior therapy (ICBT).

WHAT IS INTERNET-BASED COGNITIVE BEHAVIOR THERAPY?

ICBT is a self-help treatment that adopts the same treatment components as in regular CBT, which are accessed through the Internet. Structurally, most of these treatments are made up of modules or lessons, which are chapters that are designed to provide the patient with the same knowledge and tools as in conventional face-to-face CBT. Throughout the treatment, the patient has access to a named therapist whose main task is to provide written feedback (emaillike) on homework exercises and provide treatment guidance. The role of the therapist is also to grant access to the next module after the patient is done with the homework exercises. Integrated in the Internet-based platform is a self-report assessment system and online worksheets, so the therapist easily can follow the patient's work progress

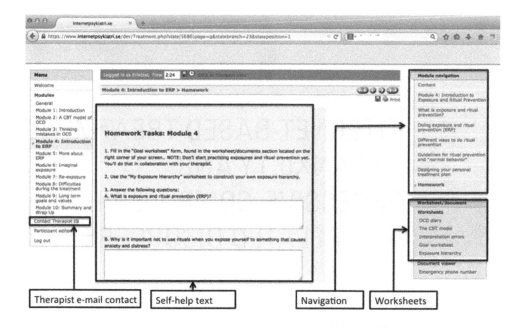

FIGURE 32.1 A screenshot of the Swedish OCD ICBT treatment (Andersson et al.) with high-lighted components.

through the treatment but also monitor symptom change during therapy. The different types of ICBT are similar but vary in some aspects, perhaps mainly regarding technical features. In general, the Swedish type of ICBT is relatively simple from a technical point of view; it could be described as therapist-guided online bibliotherapy, as it relies heavily on text material (Figure 32.1). Other types use some slightly more advanced features, such as video films and interactive scripts (Berger, Hohl, and Caspar, 2009; Botella et al., 2010; Stott et al., 2013). Although these technical features are certainly useful, it is worth emphasizing that technical complexity has not been found to relate to overall outcome in ICBT.

SOCIAL ANXIETY DISORDER

According to DSM-5, social anxiety disorder (SAD) is characterized by a marked and persistent fear about one or more social situations in which the person is exposed to possible scrutiny by others (American Psychiatric Association, 2013).

Internet-Based Treatment for Social Anxiety Disorder

ICBT for SAD is heavily based on the empirically supported psychological treatments designed for a conventional face-to-face format, mainly developed by Heimberg and co-workers (Heimberg and Becker, 2002), and individual cognitive therapy (ICT) developed by Clark and coworkers (Clark et al., 2003). These treatments have a duration of about 12 to 16 weeks and are aimed at breaking the vicious cycle among anxiety symptoms, catastrophic interpretations, attention to internal and external threat, safety behaviors, and avoidance behaviors. Both treatments put a strong emphasis on weekly

TABLE 32.1 Example of Module Content in ICBT for SAD.

MODULE	MAIN THEME	NUMBER OF PAGES
1	Introduction, information on CBT and SAD	19
2	A CBT-model for SAD	20
3	Cognitive restructuring, part I	30
4	Cognitive restructuring, part II	4
5	Behavioural experiments	24
6	Exposure, part I	24
7	Exposure, part I continued	2
8	Exposure, part I continued	2
9	Safety behaviour manipulation, part I	19
10	Safety behaviour manipulation, part II	2
11	Exposure, part II	17
12	Exposure, part II continued	2
13	Psychoeducation on assertiveness	19
14	Summary and relapse prevention	16
15	Relapse prevention	6
	Total number of pages	**246**

Abbreviations: CBT, cognitive behavior therapy; SAD, social anxiety disorder.

homework assignments and include exercises in which exposure to social stimuli and cognitive restructuring are integrated. Table 32.1 presents the principal content of the ICBT for SAD that our research group has used.

Efficacy of Internet-Based Treatment for Social Anxiety Disorder

In a recent systematic review, ICBT for SAD was judged to be a well-established treatment based on the classification criteria of the American Psychological Association (Hedman, Ljótsson, and Lindefors, 2012). At least 16 randomized controlled trials (RCTs) have been conducted and three RCTs have shown that ICBT is as effective as CBT delivered face-to-face (G. Andersson, Cuijpers, Carlbring, Riper, and Hedman, 2014). The treatment has been shown to be effective in a university setting as well in a psychiatric setting, and about two out of three patients make clinically meaningful improvements (Hedman, Andersson, Ljótsson, et al., 2011). The effects of ICBT for SAD endure for long periods, over at least five years, and health economic analyses have shown that the treatment is highly cost-effective compared to face-to-face CBT (Hedman, Andersson, Ljotsson, et al., 2011).

PANIC DISORDER

Panic disorder (PD) is characterized by two main features: recurrent, unexpected panic attacks and persistent worry about additional panic attacks or a significant maladaptive behavior change related to the attacks. PD is often accompanied by agoraphobic avoidance, that is, avoidance of situations that could trigger a panic attack or where escape would be difficult if early signs of panic would occur, such as crowded places or driving on the freeway (American Psychiatric Association, 2013).

Internet-Based Treatment for Panic Disorder

Three independent research groups, based in Sweden and Australia, have developed ICBT programs for PD. The structure of these treatments is the same as in ICBT for SAD outlined above, and the main components of the treatments are best practice interventions such as interoceptive exposure, agoraphobic exposure and cognitive restructuring. The treatments are relatively brief, with about 10 weeks of duration. Our clinical experience is that the straight-forward nature of the treatment model makes it easy and highly suitable to adapt to an Internet format.

Efficacy of Internet-Based Treatment for Panic Disorder

At least nine RCTs have been conducted in which ICBT for PD has been evaluated (Hedman, Ljótsson, et al., 2012). The average effect size (pre–post) of these studies is 1.42 d on measures of panic-related symptoms, indicating that the treatment leads to large improvement (Hedman, Ljótsson, et al., 2012). Three RCTs have compared ICBT for PD with face-to-face CBT and, just as in the case of SAD, the findings indicate that ICBT is equally effective as CBT delivered in a conventional face-to-face format (Bergstrom et al., 2010; Carlbring et al., 2005; Kiropoulos et al., 2008). In a recently conducted effectiveness study using a sample of 570 patients who received ICBT for panic disorder, it was found that the treatment is effective also when given in a psychiatric outpatient setting (Hedman et al., 2013). One study investigated the long-term effects of the treatment and found that improvements were maintained for at least 3 years (Ruwaard, Broeksteeg, Schrieken, Emmelkamp, and Lange, 2010). To conclude, the empirical support for ICBT for PD is substantial, and it can be considered an evidence-based treatment.

GENERALIZED ANXIETY DISORDER

Generalized anxiety disorder (GAD) is marked by excessive worry about a number of events or activities (e.g., job demands, finances, or the safety of one's children) and is also accompanied by symptoms of stress, muscle tension, or sleep disturbance (American Psychiatric Association, 2013).

Internet-Based Treatment for Generalized Anxiety Disorder

At least two independent research groups, based in Australia and Sweden, have developed ICBT programs for GAD that have been tested in RCTs (Paxling et al., 2011; Robinson et al., 2010). These treatments both use psychoeducation, cognitive restructuring, and exposure to worry as central components. The main differences between the treatments are that the Swedish program developed by Paxling and co-workers (Paxling et al., 2011) entails modules focusing on how to solve interpersonal problems and interventions aimed at improving sleep and applied relaxation, whereas the Australian ICBT developed by Titov and coworkers (Titov et al., 2009) entails interventions aimed at challenging core beliefs. There is also another study out that has tested an Internet-based psychodynamic treatment, based on a self-help book called *Make the Leap* (G. Andersson et al., 2012).

Efficacy of Internet-Based Treatment for Generalized Anxiety Disorder

We have found four RCTs that investigate the effect of ICBT for GAD. In a recent systematic review and meta-analysis, the average controlled effect size of those trials was $d = 0.84$ (95% $CI = 0.34–1.23$), indicating a large overall effect, although there was considerable between-group variation in effect sizes (Titov et al., 2009). One long-term follow-up study has shown that the improvements seem to be stable for at least 3 years (Paxling et al., 2011). Another study investigating psychodynamic Internet-based therapy compared ICBT and wait-list control (G. Andersson et al., 2012). In that study, effect sizes were nonsignificant for both Internet-based psychodynamic treatment and ICBT in comparison to wait-list control. In summary, ICBT for GAD is a promising treatment, but too few studies have been conducted, and the empirical support needs to be strengthened before it can be regarded as an evidence-based treatment.

POSTTRAUMATIC STRESS DISORDER

Posttraumatic stress disorder (PTSD) is triggered by exposure to a terrifying stressor, followed for at least one month by intrusive symptoms, avoidance, mood and cognitive alterations, and symptoms of arousal and reactivity (American Psychiatric Association, 2013).

Internet-Based Treatment for Posttraumatic Stress Disorder

Although several treatments have shown promising efficacy in subclinical samples, we focus in the following section only on diagnosed PTSD.

Litz et al. published a small RCT in 2003 where ICBT ("DE-STRESS") was compared to an 8-week Internet-based supportive counseling in PTSD in service members. ICBT did not demonstrate superiority over supportive therapy at 3 months follow-up (Litz, Engel, Bryant, and Papa, 2007). Klein et al. (2010) reported that almost 70% no longer met PTSD criteria after participating in a small open trial of "PTSD Online," a 10-week ICBT program based on standard CBT content. In another study from Australia, Spence et al. randomized 44 PTSD patients to either ICBT for 8 weeks or wait-list control. The ICBT included 7 lessons on psychoeducation, basic cognitive strategies, graded and imaginary exposure as well as relapse prevention. Homework assignments were given each week, participants used an online forum, received automated notifications and reminders, and were also contacted each week by a therapist via email or phone. The ICBT had a superior outcome, with a post-treatment between group effect size of 0.47 (Spence et al., 2011). In conclusion, the evidence for ICBT is still limited for PTSD. Existing randomized studies are very few and small and do not include comparison with gold standard treatment. Clearly, more research is needed.

SPECIFIC PHOBIA

Specific phobia is defined as the persistent fear or anxiety about a specific object or situation. It may concern animals (i.e., spiders, snakes), situations (i.e. airplanes, elevators), injection, natural environments (i.e., heights), and many other stimuli (American Psychiatric Association, 2013).

Internet-Based Cognitive Behavior Therapy for Specific Phobia

There are two small multisession ICBT treatments for snake (G. Andersson et al., 2013) and spider (G. Andersson et al., 2009) phobias that have been tested against the gold standard treatment, that is, a 3-hour single-session exposure. Results showed that ICBT had long-term results equal to the live treatment. In the UK, an ICBT program called "FearFighter," originally developed by Professor Isaac Marks as a stand-alone computerized treatment, has been tested in regular health care settings with some promising findings (Hayward, MacGregor, Peck, and Wilkes, 2007). In conclusion, there is currently limited evidence for ICBT in specific phobias.

OBSESSIVE-COMPULSIVE AND RELATED DISORDERS

In the revision from DSM-IV to DSM-5, obsessive-compulsive disorder (OCD) was moved from the anxiety disorders to a new chapter called "obsessive-compulsive and related disorders," together with body dysmorphic disorder (BDD), trichotillomania, skin picking disorder (SPD), and hoarding disorder (HD; American Psychiatric Association, 2013). These disorders are together highly prevalent and only a fraction of these patients receive evidence-based treatment.

Internet-Based Treatments for Obsessive-Compulsive Disorder

Two ICBT programs have been published, the Swedish and the Australian ICBT programs. The Swedish ICBT program was developed by Andersson, Rück, and colleagues at Karolinska Institutet. This treatment is similar to that previously described for PD and SAD, and the main treatment component is exposure with response prevention (ERP). As therapist support has been shown to be an important factor for both treatment efficacy and compliance in the treatment of OCD (Rosa-Alcazar, Sanchez-Meca, Gomez-Conesa, and Marin-Martinez, 2008), this treatment is supported by high-frequency proactive therapist support, that is, the therapist sends an email in the treatment platform if the patient has not logged in for 3 days and responds to the patient within 24 hours on weekdays. A text message is also sent to the patient's cell phone for every new message. Despite the high frequency duration of communication, the duration of each message is short (total time spent for each patient averages 6–13 minutes per week; E. Andersson et al., 2012).

The Australian ICBT program was developed by Wootton and colleagues, at the eCentreClinic at Macquarie University. This treatment is very similar to the Swedish ICBT program; that is, the treatment is based on ERP, and it is text-based and provided on an encrypted website with consecutive access. The therapist enables further access after the patients have completed their homework assignments. The Australian ICBT treatment also incorporates additional treatment modules to address comorbid mood and anxiety problems. Another difference compared to the Swedish treatment is that the communication between therapist and patients takes place via the telephone (two scheduled phone calls per week).

Efficacy of Internet-Based Treatment for Obsessive-Compulsive Disorders

The Swedish and Australian ICBT treatments have been tested in two pilot trials and two randomized controlled trials, all showing large within- and between-group effect sizes, with 41–61% responders. Results were also sustained up to two years after receiving treatment. The average time spent on each patient was about 7–13 minutes per week (E. Andersson et al., 2012, 2011, 2014; Wootton, Dear, Johnston, Terides, and Titov, 2013; Wootton, Titov, Dear, Spence, Andrews, et al., 2011).

Case Vignette

Mr. J. was a 45-year old man with severe OCD (32/40 on the Yale-Brown Obssesive-Compulsive Scale) who presented with obsessions about contaminating others. He washed his hands up to 100 times per day and was on a disability pension due to OCD, depression, and severe alcohol abuse. However, at the time he commenced treatment he did not meet criteria for depression. Mr. J. had presented with a history of severe alcohol abuse but had been sober during the past two years. Mr. J. was currently living in a group home with daily support from personnel, and he applied to our study after seeing a newspaper advertisement. When considering the history of alcohol abuse and depression and his social situation in general, we first hesitated to include him in the ICBT study. However, he did not fulfill any exclusion criteria and was thus included in the study. Mr. J. had no difficulties reading and writing, and he often used the Internet. Modules 1–4 were completed within two weeks, and Mr. J. worked decisively with response prevention during this time. He had daily email correspondence with his therapist during this time, and sent about t three to four emails per week. At mid-treatment, Mr. J. felt he had made some substantial progress, and the rest of the treatment focused on higher-level exposure tasks such as dating and meeting with friends, which he had previously avoided because of contamination concerns and low mood. Mr. J. had a Y-BOCS score of 3 at post-treatment, 1 at the 3-month follow-up, and 0 at the 12-month follow-up. Although Mr. J. may not have been a typical patient in ICBT, this vignette demonstrates that anyone can potentially benefit from ICBT, even those patients who, at first sight, may not seem appropriate for remote treatment.

Internet-Based Treatment for Youths with Obsessive-Compulsive Disorder

BIP OCD is an ICBT program for adolescents with OCD that has been developed at Karolinska Institutet. In this treatment, youths and their parents work through treatment using a self-help manual provided through a secure Internet platform. The platform is especially designed with age-appropriate appearance, animations, and interactive scripts. Parents and adolescents have separate login accounts and the treatment is supported by a therapist through e-mails, phone calls, and standardized forms within the program. To date, the BIP OCD program has been tested in an open trial, ($n = 21$) showing large within-group effect sizes ($d = 2.29$) with 76% in remission (Child Y-BOCS score <12) at a 6-month follow-up. Average clinician support time was less than 20 minutes per patient per week. A wait-list controlled trial of BIP OCD is currently under way (Lenhard et al., 2014).

INTERNET-BASED TREATMENTS FOR OCD-RELATED DISORDERS

Although several studies have shown that ICBT is effective in the treatment of OCD, the development of such clinician extenders for other OCD-related conditions lags considerably behind. Below follows the few treatments that have been empirically tested.

Body Dysmorphic Disorder

BDD-NET is an ICBT treatment specifically developed for body dysmorphic disorder (BDD). This treatment was developed by the same research group at Karolinska Institutet that developed the OCD treatment and, although the content is BDD-specific, the main features are about the same (web-based design, therapist contact, etc.). The BDD-NET has been tested in an open pilot study, where 23 patients receive a 12-week treatment. Results showed large improvements (d = 2.01, 82% responders) and sustained effects at 3-months. A randomized controlled trial of BDD-NET is currently under way (Enander et al., 2014).

Hoarding

DITCH is a private Yahoo group for people with hoarding difficulties. Patients have access to psycho-education material and are encouraged to email regarding their progress once per month, and they receive feedback from other hoarding sufferers (Muroff, Steketee, Himle, and Frost, 2010). The DITCH study analyzed self-rated outcomes from 105 active users compared to 155 users on a wait-list. Results showed that all members experienced significant reductions in clutter and hoarding symptoms over 15 months (Muroff et al., 2010).

Trichotillomania

StopPulling.com is an Internet-based self-help program for trichotillomania, where the patient has access to self-help material based on habit-reversal therapy. This program is unguided (i.e., not supported by any therapist) and costs about $30 per month. One study analyzed data from 265 users during the first year it was available online. Results indicated significant symptom reductions, with about 32% being classified as responders on the self-rated outcome. A subsequent randomized trial tested StopPulling.com as a free adjunct treatment in a stepped-care program (Rogers et al., 2014), showing small effects compared to wait-list (Mouton-Odum, Keuthen, Wagener, and Stanley, 2006).

Skinpicking

StopPicking.com is similar to StopPulling.com but, content wise, it is tailored for patients suffering from skin picking disorder (Flessner, Mouton-Odum, Stocker, and Keuthen, 2007). This program costs about $30 per month, and data from 372 users showed significant improvements with higher responder rates than StopPulling.com (63%). No controlled studies have been published to date.

CONCLUSIONS

Access to evidence-based treatment such as CBT is a rate-limiting step in mental health care, and the development of ICBT is one way to combat that. A recent review identified more than 100 ICBT RCTs conducted over the last decade (Hedman, Ljotsson, and Lindefors, 2012). There are large differences in the evidence base for ICBT across disorders. Although there are many large RCTs in social phobia, including gold-standard live CBT as control groups and collection of long-term data, there are other disorders, such as PTSD and the obsessive-compulsive and related disorders, for which the evidence is still weak. As ICBT has been shown to be effective in so many different disorders, this probably reflects differences in the pace of development of ICBT for different disorders, rather than the alternative possibility that ICBT may be ineffective for certain disorders where live CBT has demonstrated efficacy. ICBT clearly has great potential to dramatically increase access to evidence-based treatment, but more definitive trials by independent groups, using non-inferiority and other designs, are warranted.

ICBT can help both clinicians and patients in a number of different ways. First, these interventions are much more accessible for patients and can help overcome logistic barriers, such as geographical distances and travel expenses. Patients can conveniently access their treatment materials around the clock without needing to set up appointments to see their therapists, thus making these treatments potentially accessible for patients who would not have sought care. Second, the ICBT programs reviewed in this chapter require considerably less therapist time compared to face-to-face CBT. Third, ICBT is also a highly structured treatment in terms of content and context of delivery, and this can minimize the risk of therapist drift (i.e., the therapist and the patient start to talk about things that are irrelevant to the specific treatment).

Another promising feature with ICBT is that it can serve as a platform for training therapists. For example, in the Andersson et al. (2012) trial, the therapists were psychology students in their final year of training. Our experience from this trial was that ICBT could provide a good basis for junior therapists to learn the basics of CBT for OCD. It is also easy for the supervisor to monitor the therapist feedback.

Does the therapist matter in ICBT for OCD? The answer is yes. When comparing treatments that use therapist support compared to unguided treatments, it seems that ICBT needs therapist support in order to provide clinically useful effects. However, this is probably not a linear relationship in the sense that more therapist support is always better. The exact amount of therapist support needed to achieve optimal cost-effectiveness will be an important research question for the future.

For whom is ICBT suitable? The answer is that we still do not know. Although there has been some research on predictors and moderators of ICBT (e.g., Hedman, Andersson et al., 2012), it is still too soon to give any definite answers. Our experience, from having treated many patients with ICBT, is that it is important that the patients are motivated and have good insight into their difficulties. It is important to note that most of the trials conducted to date have recruited patients via advertisement; it is plausible that patients seeking ICBT are somewhat different compared to the patients that clinicians meet at a regular psychiatric clinic. Clearly, ICBT should not replace standard care for OCD and related disorders, and it will not be indicated for all patients. Furthermore, specialist input will continue to be required for complex patients with very severe symptoms, complex comorbidities, absent insight, or high suicide risk.

We conclude that ICBT has several advantages compared to face-to-face CBT. It is an effective treatment for social anxiety disorder and panic disorder and is a promising treatment for OCD. However, more research is needed for OCD-related conditions, specific phobias, and PTSD. Furthermore, more research is needed that targets youth populations.

DISCLOSURE STATEMENT

The authors have nothing to disclose.

REFERENCES

American Psychiatric Association. (2013). *Diagnostic and statistical manual of mental disorders (5th ed.)*. Arlington, VA: American Psychiatric Publishing.

Andersson, E., Enander, J., Andren, P., Hedman, E., Ljótsson, B., Hursti, T., . . . Rück, C. (2012a). Internet-based cognitive behaviour therapy for obsessive-compulsive disorder: A randomized controlled trial. *Psychological Medicine, 42*(10), 2193–2203. doi: 10.1017/s0033291712000244

Andersson, E., Ljótsson, B., Hedman, E., Kaldo, V., Paxling, B., Andersson, G., . . . Rück, C. (2011). Internet-based cognitive behavior therapy for obsessive compulsive disorder: a pilot study. [Clinical Trial Research Support, Non-U.S. Gov't]. *BioMed Central Psychiatry, 11,* 125. doi: 10.1186/1471-244X-11-125

Andersson, E., Steneby, S., Karlsson, K., Ljótsson, B., Hedman, E., Enander, J., . . . Rück, C. (2014). Long-term efficacy of Internet-based cognitive behavior therapy for obsessive-compulsive disorder with or without booster: a randomized controlled trial. *Psychol Med,* 1–11. doi: 10.1017/S0033291714000543

Andersson, G., Cuijpers, P., Carlbring, P., Riper, H., and Hedman, E. (2014). Internet-based vs. face-to-face cognitive behaviour therapy for psychiatric and somatic disorders: a systematic review and meta-analysis. *World Psychiatry, 3,* 288–295.

Andersson, G., Paxling, B., Roch-Norlund, P., Ostman, G., Norgren, A., Almlöv, J., . . . Silverberg, F. (2012). Internet-based psychodynamic versus cognitive behavioral guided self-help for generalized anxiety disorder: A randomized controlled trial. *Psychotherapy and Psychosomatics, 81*(6), 344–355. doi: 10.1159/000339371

Andersson, G., Waara, J., Jonsson, U., Malmaeus, F., Carlbring, P., and Öst, L. G. (2009). Internet-based self-help versus one-session exposure in the treatment of spider phobia: A randomized controlled trial. *Cogn Behav Ther, 38*(2), 114–120. doi: 912392743 [pii]10.1080/16506070902931326

Andersson, G., Waara, J., Jonsson, U., Malmaeus, F., Carlbring, P., and Öst, L. G. (2013). Internet-based exposure treatment versus one-session exposure treatment of snake phobia: A randomized controlled trial. *Cogn Behav Ther, 42*(4), 284–291. doi: 10.1080/16506073.2013.844202

Berger, T., Hohl, E., and Caspar, F. (2009). Internet-based treatment for social phobia: A randomized controlled trial. *Journal of Clinical Psychology, 65*(10), 1021–1035. doi: 10.1002/jclp.20603 [doi]

Bergström, J., Andersson, G., Ljótsson, B., Rück, C., Andreewitch, S., Karlsson, A., . . . Lindefors, N. (2010). Internet-versus group-administered cognitive behaviour therapy for panic disorder in a psychiatric setting: a randomised trial. *BMC Psychiatry, 10,* 54. doi: 10.1186/1471-244x-10-54

Botella, C., Gallego, M. J., Garcia-Palacios, A., Guillen, V., Banos, R. M., Quero, S., and Alcaniz, M. (2010). An internet-based self-help treatment for fear of public speaking: a controlled trial. *Cyberpsychol Behav Soc Netw, 13*(4), 407–421. doi: 10.1089/cyber.2009.0224 [doi]

Carlbring, P., Nilsson-Ihrfelt, E., Waara, J., Kollenstam, C., Buhrman, M., Kaldo, V., . . . Andersson, G. (2005). Treatment of panic disorder: Live therapy vs. self-help via the internet. *Behav Res Ther, 43*(10), 1321–1333. doi: S0005-7967(04)00237-2 [pii] 10.1016/j.brat.2004.10.002

Clark, D. M., Ehlers, A., McManus, F., Hackmann, A., Fennell, M., Campbell, H., . . . Louis, B. (2003). Cognitive therapy versus fluoxetine in generalized social phobia: a randomized placebo-controlled trial. *Journal of Consulting and Clinical Psychology, 71*(6), 1058–1067. doi: 10.1037/0022-006X.71.6. 1058 [doi] 2003-09784-011 [pii]

Enander, J., Ivanov, Z. V., Andersson, E., Mataix-Cols, D., Ljótsson, B., and Rück, C. (2014) Therapist-guided Internet-based Cognitive Behavioral Therapy for Body Dysmorphic Disorder (BDD-NET): A Feasibility Study. *BMJ Open, 4,* e005923. doi: 10.1136/bmjopen-2014-005923

Flessner, C. A., Mouton-Odum, S., Stocker, A. J., and Keuthen, N. J. (2007). StopPicking. com: Internet-based treatment for self-injurious skin picking. *Dermatology Online Journal, 13*(4).

Hayward, L., MacGregor, A. D., Peck, D. F., and Wilkes, P. (2007). The Feasibility and effectiveness of computer-guided CBT (FearFighter) in a rural area. *Behavioural and Cognitive Psychotherapy, 35*(04), 409–419. doi: 10.1017/S1352465807003670

Hedman, E., Andersson, E., Ljótsson, B., Andersson, G., Andersson, E., Schalling, M., . . . Rück, C. (2012). Clinical and genetic outcome determinants of internet- and group-based cognitive behavior therapy for social anxiety disorder. *Acta Psychiatrica Scandinavica, 126*(2), 126–136. doi: 10.1111/j. 1600-0447.2012.01834.x

Hedman, E., Andersson, E., Ljótsson, B., Andersson, G., Rück, C., and Lindefors, N. (2011). Cost-effectiveness of Internet-based cognitive behavior therapy vs. cognitive behavioral group therapy for social anxiety disorder: results from a randomized controlled trial. *Behaviour Research and Therapy*, *49*(11), 729–736. doi: 10.1016/j.brat.2011.07.009

Hedman, E., Andersson, G., Ljótsson, B., Andersson, E., Rück, C., Mortberg, E., and Lindefors, N. (2011). Internet-based cognitive behavior therapy vs. cognitive behavioral group therapy for social anxiety disorder: a randomized controlled non-inferiority trial. *PLoS ONE, 6*(3), e18001. doi: 10.1371/journal.pone.0018001

Hedman, E., Ljotsson, B., and Lindefors, N. (2012). Cognitive behavior therapy via the Internet: a systematic review of applications, clinical efficacy and cost-effectiveness. *Expert Rev Pharmacoecon Outcomes Res, 12*(6), 745–764. doi: 10.1586/erp.12.67

Hedman, E., Ljótsson, B., and Lindefors, N. (2012). Cognitive behavior therapy via the internet: A systematic review of applications, clinical efficacy and cost-effectiveness. *Expert Review of Pharmacoeconomics and Outcomes Research, 12*(6), 745–764. doi: 10.1586/erp.12.67

Hedman, E., Ljotsson, B., Rück, C., Bergström, J., Andersson, G., Kaldo, V., . . . Lindefors, N. (2013). Effectiveness of Internet-based cognitive behaviour therapy for panic disorder in routine psychiatric care. *Acta Psychiatrica Scandinavica, 128*(6), 457–467. doi: 10.1111/acps.12079

Heimberg, R. G., and Becker, R. E. (2002). *Cognitive-behavioral group therapy for social phobia. Basic mechanisms and clinical strategies*: New York: Guilford Press.

Kiropoulos, L. A., Klein, B., Austin, D. W., Gilson, K., Pier, C., Mitchell, J., and Ciechomski, L. (2008). Is internet-based CBT for panic disorder and agoraphobia as effective as face-to-face CBT? *Journal of Anxiety Disorders, 22*(8), 1273–1284. doi: 10.1016/j.janxdis.2008.01.008

Klein, B., Mitchell, J., Abbott, J., Shandley, K., Austin, D., Gilson, K., . . . Redman, T. (2010). A therapist-assisted cognitive behavior therapy internet intervention for posttraumatic stress disorder: pre-, post- and 3-month follow-up results from an open trial. *J Anxiety Disord, 24*(6), 635–644. doi: 10.1016/j.janxdis.2010.04.005

Lenhard, F., Vigerland, S., Andersson, E., Rück, C., Mataix-Cols, D., Thulin, U., . . . Serlachius, E. (2014). Internet-delivered cognitive behavior therapy for adolescents with obsessive-compulsive disorder: an open trial. *PLoS One, 9*(6), e100773. doi: 10.1371/journal.pone.0100773

Litz, B. T., Engel, C. C., Bryant, R. A., and Papa, A. (2007). A randomized, controlled proof-of-concept trial of an Internet-based, therapist-assisted self-management treatment for posttraumatic stress disorder. *Am J Psychiatry, 164*(11), 1676–1683. doi: 10.1176/appi.ajp.2007.06122057

Mataix-Cols, D., and Marks, I. M. (2006). Self-help with minimal therapist contact for obsessive-compulsive disorder: a review. *Eur Psychiatry, 21*(2), 75–80. doi: 10.1016/j.eurpsy.2005.07.003

Mouton-Odum, S., Keuthen, N. J., Wagener, P. D., and Stanley, M. A. (2006). StopPulling.com: An Interactive, Self-Help Program for Trichotillomania. *Cognitive and Behavioral Practice, 13*(3), 215–226. doi: http://dx.doi.org/10.1016/j.cbpra.2005.05.004

Muroff, J., Steketee, G., Himle, J., and Frost, R. (2010). Delivery of internet treatment for compulsive hoarding (D.I.T.C.H.). *Behav Res Ther, 48*(1), 79–85. doi: 10.1016/j.brat.2009.09.006

Paxling, B., Almlov, J., Dahlin, M., Carlbring, P., Breitholtz, E., Eriksson, T., and Andersson, G. (2011). Guided internet-delivered cognitive behavior therapy for generalized anxiety disorder: A randomized controlled trial. *Cognitive Behaviour Therapy, 40*(3), 159–173. doi: 10.1080/16506073.2011.576699

Robinson, E., Titov, N., Andrews, G., McIntyre, K., Schwencke, G., and Solley, K. (2010). Internet treatment for generalized anxiety disorder: A randomized controlled trial comparing clinician vs. technician assistance. *PLoS ONE, 5*(6), e10942. doi: 10.1371/journal.pone.0010942

Rogers, K., Banis, M., Falkenstein, M. J., Malloy, E. J., McDonough, L., Nelson, S. O., . . . Haaga, D. A. (2014). Stepped care in the treatment of trichotillomania. *J Consult Clin Psychol, 82*(2), 361–367. doi: 10.1037/a0035744

Rosa-Alcazar, A. I., Sanchez-Meca, J., Gomez-Conesa, A., and Marin-Martinez, F. (2008). Psychological treatment of obsessive-compulsive disorder: A meta-analysis. *Clin Psychol Rev, 28*(8), 1310–1325. doi: 10.1016/j.cpr.2008.07.001

Ruwaard, J., Broeksteeg, J., Schrieken, B., Emmelkamp, P., and Lange, A. (2010). Web-based therapist-assisted cognitive behavioral treatment of panic symptoms: A randomized controlled trial with a three-year follow-up. *Journal of Anxiety Disorders, 24*(4), 387–396. doi: 10.1016/j.janxdis.2010.01.010

Spence, J., Titov, N., Dear, B. F., Johnston, L., Solley, K., Lorian, C., . . . Schwenke, G. (2011). Randomized controlled trial of Internet-delivered cognitive behavioral therapy for posttraumatic stress disorder. *Depress Anxiety, 28*(7), 541–550. doi: 10.1002/da.20835

Stott, R., Wild, J., Grey, N., Liness, S., Warnock-Parkes, E., Commins, S., . . . Clark, D. M. (2013). Internet-delivered cognitive therapy for social anxiety disorder: A development pilot series. *Behavioural and Cognitive Psychotherapy, 41*(4), 383–397. doi: 10.1017/s1352465813000404

Titov, N., Andrews, G., Robinson, E., Schwencke, G., Johnston, L., Solley, K., and Choi, I. (2009). Clinician-assisted internet-based treatment is effective for generalized anxiety disorder: Randomized controlled trial. *Australian and New Zealand Journal of Psychiatry, 43*(10), 905–912. doi: 10.1080/00048670903179269

Wootton, B. M., Dear, B. F., Johnston, L., Terides, M. D., and Titov, N. (2013). Remote treatment of obsessive-compulsive disorder: A randomized controlled trial. *Journal of Obsessive-Compulsive and Related Disorders, 2*(4), 375–384. doi: http://dx.doi.org/10.1016/j.jocrd.2013.07.002

Wootton, B. M., Titov, N., Dear, B. F., Spence, J., Andrews, G., Johnston, L., and Solley, K. (2011). An Internet administered treatment program for obsessive-compulsive disorder: A feasibility study. *J Anxiety Disord, 25*(8), 1102–1107. doi: 10.1016/j.janxdis.2011.07.009

Wootton, B. M., Titov, N., Dear, B. F., Spence, J., and Kemp, A. (2011). The acceptability of Internet-based treatment and characteristics of an adult sample with obsessive compulsive disorder: an Internet survey. *PLoS ONE, 6*(6), e20548. doi: 10.1371/journal.pone.0020548

INDEX